Contents

Dedication

Levine's Pharmacology: Drug Actions and Reactions is dedicated to Ruth R. Levine, PhD, who first authored this text in the early 1970s and enriched it through six editions. This seventh edition, now named in her honor, continues her visionary goal of elucidating the basic principles of pharmacology in a style accessible to the nonspecialist reader. Dr Levine was a remarkable pharmacologist and educator. She earned her undergraduate degree in chemistry and education from Hunter College, a master's degree in organic chemistry from Columbia University, and her doctoral degree in pharmacology from Tufts University. In 1958 she joined the faculty of Boston University, where she continued until her death in February 2003. As Professor of Pharmacology

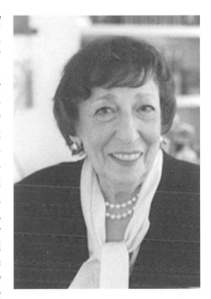

and Experimental Therapeutics, Dr Levine conducted investigations in the field of pharmacokinetics, especially in the area of drug absorption, with support from NIH, the Department of Defense, and a number of pharmaceutical companies. She was promoted to Chairman, and later Associate Dean, of the Division of Graduate Medical and Dental Sciences and in that capacity developed the MA and PhD degree programs offered at Boston University School of Medicine. In the early 1970s, convinced that the important concepts of pharmacology should be understood widely, not just by the pharmacologist or physician, she created a new course in pharmacology for undergraduates. This novel undertaking, as well as her many contributions throughout the university, led to her prestigious appointment as University Professor of Boston University. Dr Levine extended her influence to the national and international arena. The first woman elected to serve as Secretary-Treasurer of the American Society of Pharmacology and

Experimental Therapeutics, she also served on scientific advisory boards and committees of the EPA and NIH. During the 1980s and 1990s she organized seven international symposia on 'Subtypes of Muscarinic Receptors' and edited the proceedings. Throughout her long and productive career Dr Levine cared deeply for her students and her worldwide cadre of colleagues in pharmacology. She took extraordinary pride in her textbook and its successful dissemination of pharmacologic principles. We dedicate this seventh edition to her, with appreciation of her exceptional accomplishments and with gratitude and love for her as our devoted mentor.

Preface to the
Seventh Edition

The philosophy guiding the writing of this textbook, as stated in the preface to the first edition, was to present a comprehensive and coherent explanation of the science of pharmacology in terms of its basic concepts and general principles. The book's continued wide acceptance by undergraduate and graduate students majoring in diverse fields of both science and humanities, as well as by students in medicine, nursing, and veterinary medicine affirms that this was a logical approach to use. More than 20 years after publication of the first edition by Dr Ruth R. Levine, she initiated a collaborative effort with us, Dr Carol T. Walsh and Dr Rochelle Schwartz-Bloom, to reaffirm and strengthen the original conceptual approach. The fifth edition incorporated our knowledge and experience, as we had been using this text in teaching pharmacology at several different levels at Boston University and Duke University, respectively. This partnership has, indeed, proved successful, and although we mourn the passing of our mentor, Dr Levine, we have continued as collaborators in the preparation of this textbook, now in its seventh edition.

We have worked carefully to preserve the focus and the flavor of Dr Levine's original text. Indeed, the basic concepts and general principles presented in the original text remain in the seventh edition. However, the entire text and references have been updated to reflect current understanding of biological processes and their modification by drugs and other exogenous chemicals. The drugs chosen to exemplify pharmacologic principles are of current therapeutic importance, although references to some older and less frequently used agents of historical or developmental significance have been retained. We have also made major revisions and added new sections in several chapters. Chapter 3 now incorporates a summary of receptor families that are targets of drug action. Chapter 8 now includes a discussion of the fundamental properties of the cytochrome P450 family of enzymes, important in drug biotransformation. A new section has been added to Chapter 14 that describes the action of drugs on the autonomic nervous system. To illustrate the principles of such drug action, we have included a section highlighting how drugs affect cardiovascular function. Chapter 15 has been rewritten extensively to reflect the current pharmacologic and neurobiologic knowledge in the field of substance abuse.

The appendixes have also been revised considerably and updated. We have added Appendix 4 to supplement the new overview in Chapter 14 on drugs that affect cardiovascular function. In this new appendix we address the pharmacology of the classes of drugs used in the treatment of hypertension. We have removed the former appendix on weights and measures, because of its lesser importance to the mission of this text. The appendixes have proved useful to students to supplement their knowledge of basic principles with more specific information about some of the therapeutic agents currently in widespread use. The material is presented in an introductory style to be consistent with the purpose of this text. Comprehensive sources, including online resources, are provided in Chapter 2 for more detailed information about the drugs and drug classes that are discussed in this book.

Finally, many of the graphics and figures have been redrawn and updated with the help of Dr Mark Williams, of Pyramis Studios, Inc. An accomplished neurobiologist, Dr Williams has created high quality informative graphics that add a pleasing feature to the seventh edition of this book.

We are very grateful to Parthenon Publishing, now a division of Taylor and Francis Publishing, and especially to Mr Nick Dunton and Ms Dinah Alam for their work in the publishing of the seventh edition of this textbook. Mr Nat Russo, who played a critical role in the publishing of the sixth edition, was instrumental in the planning for a seventh edition under our authorship. In addition to acknowledging our debt to all those who helped launch the first edition of this book, our thanks are due to the many students, teachers, and readers whose steadfast reception of the previous editions encouraged and promoted the preparation of this seventh edition. Finally, we thank Dr Ruth R. Levine for her guidance, for the relentless energy that she put into this book, and for her thoughtfulness in handing us the opportunity to continue her dream.

C.T.W. and R.D.S.

Boston, MA and Durham, NC

Preface to the
First Edition

Pharmacology is the unified study of the properties of chemical agents (drugs) and living organisms and all aspects of their interactions. So defined, it is an expansive science encompassing areas of interest germane to many other disciplines. The specific pharmacologic knowledge needed by the physician, who uses chemicals as therapeutic agents, differs from that of the biochemist or physiologist, who uses chemicals as tools in research. Likewise, this knowledge is different for the ecologist or legislator, who is sensitive to the consequences or responsibilities inherent in the widespread use of chemical agents. There is, however, a body of information dealing with the basic concepts and principles that is fundamental to understanding the actions of drugs in every aspect of this science, theoretical or applied, and at any level of complexity.

The purpose of this book is to provide a concise source of that core of pharmacologic knowledge that can be shared by all wishing to acquire an understanding of how chemical agents affect living processes. The emphasis is placed, therefore, on fundamental concepts as they apply to the actions of most drugs. In order to illustrate the underlying principles, some agents that are in general use or are subjects of public concern are singled out for fuller discussion. Certain therapeutic conditions are also discussed in order to provide an understanding of the basis of drug therapy. The nontherapeutic or toxicologic aspects of drug action are given special attention since the widespread exposure of living organisms to a multitude of chemicals is of grave public significance.

This book is written for individuals of diverse backgrounds who have in common a working knowledge of general chemistry and biology. The biochemical and physiologic principles needed to understand pharmacologic principles form an integral part of the text. In order to provide more coherence and greater ease in reading, individual statements have not been scientifically documented with the references to the pertinent literature. At the end of each chapter, however, some specific as well as some general references are listed for those who desire more extensive information. And in the body of the text certain words or phrases are printed in boldface type to indicate that a fuller explanation of the term is contained in the Glossary. The Glossary of nearly two hundred entries also provides a handy reference for most terms defined throughout the text.

I have tried to prepare a text that alone will provide the nonprofessional with a basic understanding of pharmacology but that may also serve as an introduction for those who will be professionally concerned with the interactions of drugs and living organisms. I hope, too, that this book will serve the further purpose of implementing the presentation of pharmacology in nonprofessional schools so that students in biology, chemistry, psychology, physical education, and premedical programs as well as those in other fields will have the opportunity to acquire some training in one of the youngest of the experimental medical sciences – pharmacology.

R.R.L.

Boston

1   The Heritage of Pharmacology

An acquaintance with the history of a subject frequently reveals the true nature of the subject. Tracing the growth of pharmacology, then, from its earliest beginnings will give us a sharper perspective of the scope of the field and a clearer understanding of what distinguishes pharmacology today as an orderly science in its own right. In the words of the Nobel laureate Albert Szent-Györgyi, 'If we want to see ahead we must look back.'

THE BEGINNINGS

The use of medicinals by humans is as old as the human race itself, since the need to find measures to combat sickness was as important to survival as the need for food and shelter. Early efforts in dealing with disease, colored as they were by superstitious concepts of the causes of illness, led to the search for animate and inanimate objects in the environment with which to drive away the evil spirits. But the successes of science frequently have their roots in the absurdities of magic, and some of our important drugs were discovered through primitives' experiments with the plants that grew around them. The use of alcohol and opium to ease pain, of cinchona bark (the source of quinine) to treat malaria and of ipecac for amebic dysentery can be cited as examples of early therapeutic success despite ignorance of the causes of these ailments. Some of the failures can also be called valuable discoveries, since drugs like curare, known only as fatal poisons by primitive cultures in various regions of the world, became valuable therapeutic agents when used in proper amounts. Thus the accumulation of this primitive medical lore and its dissemination and use by midwives, priests, witch doctors and other practitioners were the beginnings of **materia medica**[1], medicine and toxicology.

---

[1] Terms appearing in **boldface type** are defined in the Glossary.

Egypt and Babylonia

The Egyptians are to be credited with handing down to us the oldest known records of medicine, even though the medical systems of Sumaria, Babylonia and India are probably of equal antiquity. The most ancient of the records devoted entirely to medicine is the Papyrus of Smith (ca. 1600 BCE[2]). It clearly indicates that the Egyptians had developed a codified and conventionalized form of therapy for a great variety of diseases and had differentiated between those clinical conditions that could be treated successfully and those that could not. The Ebers Papyrus (1550 BCE), the largest of the Egyptian medical papyri, lists more than seven hundred remedies and describes in detail the procedures for their preparation and administration for specific ailments. Many of the ancient prescriptions plainly show their magical origins in the inclusion of incantations together with ingredients such as lizard's blood, an old book boiled in oil, the thigh bone of a hanged man and excreta or organs of various domestic animals. But there is also reference to liver as a remedy for anemia and to modern drugs, such as castor oil and opium. This close alliance of medicine and religious beliefs was to continue for many, many centuries and even today has not been completely broken.

As Egyptian medicine developed, it gave rise to great physicians and surgeons whose knowledge was unsurpassed even by the famous Greek physicians who came later. The Egyptians not only advocated professional standards of conduct that were to influence the Hippocratic code of medical ethics but also developed medical specialization. For example, some physicians limited their practice to obstetrics, gynecology, or gastric disorders. For the first time the patient was given the choice of witch doctor or which doctor. The Egyptians can also take credit for some of the earliest concerns about public health in their promotion of public sanitation through a system of copper pipes for the collection of rainwater and the disposal of sewage.

The known contributions of the Babylonians to medicine appear to be fewer and of lesser consequence than those of the Egyptians. This may be related to the differences in their religious philosophies. The Egyptians had a comforting mythology that made them feel secure in their world; they believed that the supernatural powers were concerned with promoting their welfare. The Babylonians, on the other hand, lived in a hostile world in which demons were everywhere and were always ready to descend upon a victim in the form of sickness. Although the code of Hammurabi (2123–2081 BCE) established the profession of physician as separate from that of clergy, with doctors' fees set by law, the highly superstitious populace demanded the irrational treatment purveyed by the sorcerers. Yet despite this contrast in medical culture between the Egyptians and the Babylonians, it was the latter who transmitted the foundations of medicine to India and Greece and even supplied the names of many drugs used in Greek medical practice.

---

[2] BCE: before the common (Christian) era; CE: common era.

Greece and India

In both the Greek and Indian cultures, the earliest records disclose that secular medicine was practiced but still had to compete with that of the priesthood. For even though disease was treated by both medicinals and charms, the most common place for treatment was the temple. In Greece, with its luxuriant mythology and its plethora of deities, separate temples were built to Asclepios, the God of Healing, and these became virtually sanatoria or hospitals for the sick. The greatest of these temples was built atop a high mountain peak at Epidaurus, to which people flocked from all parts of the Mediterranean area. Near the present-day ruins of this temple-sanatorium is an almost perfectly preserved theater built in the fourth century BCE and paid for by the fees and largess of the temple's patients.

Secular medicine was fostered by and developed around the celebrated centers of learning. In India, the universities at Taxila (present-day Pakistan) and Benares, famous for their medical schools, and in Greece the four prestigious schools at Kos and Cnidus (in Asia Minor), Crotone (in Italy) and Acragas (in Sicily) produced some of the most illustrious men associated with the medical sciences of antiquity.

Sushruta (ca. 500 BCE), one of the renowned names of Hindu science, was professor of medicine at the University of Benares. He described and laid down elaborate rules for many surgical procedures and was also probably the first to graft skin from one portion of the body to another and to attempt aseptic surgery by sterilization of wounds. Sushruta also recommended diagnosis by inspection, palpation and auscultation for the detection of the 1120 diseases he described.

In the sixth century BCE, vaccination for smallpox was known and probably practiced in India. Evidence for this appears in writings attributed to one of the earliest Hindu physicians, Dhanwantari (500 BCE): 'Take the fluid of a pock on the udder of the cow . . . upon the point of a lancet, and lance with it the arms between the shoulders and the elbows until the blood appears; then, mixing the fluid with the blood, the fever of the small-pox will be produced.' Yet vaccination for smallpox and the aseptic surgery practiced by Sushruta were unknown in Europe for another two thousand years. It may well be that there were still other advances that the Hindus could have contributed to Europeans, if the latter had had wider acquaintance with the culture of India and if there had been better transmission and acceptance of Indian knowledge.

The impact of the Indians on the advancement of medicine depends on whether one speaks about their contributions to European medicine or about the practice of medicine in India itself. In contrast, the preeminent Greek physicians of this period had a far-reaching effect on medicine and pharmacy; their influence was to pervade the ensuing years.

Development of Medical Ethics

It was the great teacher Hippocrates (460–377 BCE) and his successors who strove to free medicine from mysticism and philosophy and made it reliant upon rational therapy. Hippocrates taught the doctrine that disease stems from natural causes and that knowledge is gained only through study of the natural laws; he sought to explain Nature in Nature's terms. Since Hippocrates believed that the body has ample natural resources for recuperation and that the role of the physician was to remove or reduce the impediments to this natural defense, he made little use of drugs. He relied mainly upon fresh air, good food, purgatives and enemas, blood-letting, massage and hydrotherapy, and used sparingly only a few of the four hundred drugs mentioned in his writings. However, Hippocrates is known as the Father of Medicine not just for his rational doctrine but mainly for his emphasis on medical ethics. The famous oath attributed to him did much to ennoble the medical profession by setting a standard of professional conduct to which subsequent generations of physicians have sworn fealty.

The emancipation from religious beliefs and the setting of high standards of ethics were the two most important contributions that the Greeks made directly to medicine; the art itself was not advanced to any degree beyond that achieved by the Egyptians of a millennium earlier. The Age of Greece did contribute to some important progress, however, in pharmacy, anatomy, and physiology.

Development of Pharmacy

Theophrastus (372–287 BCE), in his classic treatise *The History of Plants*, provided a summary of all that was known about the medicinal properties of plants. This work was later used by Dioscorides (57 CE), Nero's surgeon, in the preparation of a materia medica which scientifically described six hundred plants, classified for the first time by substance rather than by disease. It remained the chief source of pharmaceutical knowledge until the sixteenth century, and Dioscorides is honored as the Father of Materia Medica.

Development of Anatomy and Physiology

Herophilus, perhaps the greatest anatomist of antiquity, and Erasistratus, probably the most outstanding physiologist of ancient times, were contemporaries of Theophrastus. They developed their respective disciplines to heights which would be attained only once again before the Renaissance. Herophilus carried out remarkable dissections, named various parts of the human body and even understood the role of nerves, differentiating for the first time between **sensory** and **motor nerves**. He understood so completely the function of the artery that he might well be credited with the discovery of the circulation of blood nineteen centuries before Harvey.

Erasistratus also made noteworthy advances in dissection and in understanding the function of arteries, veins, and nerves as well as some of their interrelationships. Although Hippocratic medicine developed the rational approach to therapy, it was Erasistratus who rejected the final ties of medicine to mystical entities. Hippocratic medicine was bound to the doctrine of so-called humors, the composition of the body being blood, phlegm, yellow bile and black bile, and illness or pain being brought about by a change in the proportion of these humors. Erasistratus abandoned this humoral theory and tried to account for all physiological phenomena on the basis of natural causes. Unfortunately, it was the Hippocratic theory which became the heritage of medicine, being ultimately discarded only in the nineteenth century.

The Roman Era

After the conquest of Greece, the heritage of Greek medicine migrated to Rome. With their great sense of order, the Romans organized medicine, trained physicians in state schools, built military and private hospitals and provided for public sanitation. But their most useful contribution was the compilation of encyclopedic summaries of knowledge which prepared the way for future advances. In medicine, the foremost was that of Aurelius Celsus (first century BCE); when rediscovered in the fifteenth century, his *De Medicina* played a major role in fostering the reconstruction of medicine.

Although the Romans formulated and applied their borrowed medicine in able fashion, they contributed little of real significance to the development of Western medical science. Even the one outstanding original scientist of this period – Galen (131–201 CE) – was a Greek physician.

Galen was one of the first true experimental physiologists. For example, in neurology he performed experiments by which, in serial sectioning of the spinal cord, he was able to distinguish the sensory and motor functions of each segment of the cord. Galen also made many contributions to the field of pharmacy; most noteworthy are his extensions of the work of Dioscorides, introduction of a complicated polypharmacy and origination of the use of **tincture** of opium and preparations of vegetable drugs, still known as '**galenicals**'.

Galen missed anticipating the science of pharmacology, however, since he did not carry over the experimental approach to the study of the drugs he used. He further tarnished his record as an experimentalist by ignoring the work of Erasistratus and adopting and enlarging the Hippocratic doctrine of the origin of human illness. Galen added the four elements – earth, air, fire and water – to the four humors – blood, phlegm, yellow bile and black bile – and ascribed the cause of all diseases to derangement of these elements and humors. In Galen's voluminous writings (of the 500 books imputed to him, 118 have survived), he set forth his ideas and his system of medicine and pharmacy with such authority and conviction in his own invincibility that he profoundly affected medicine for fifteen hundred years. Unfortunately, to the detriment of medieval medicine, it was the serious errors embodied in Galen's system of the cause of disease which went uncriticized; these far outweighed in influence his valuable contributions as an accurate observer and experimentalist.

The Middle Ages

In the long span of years between the distinguished Greek physicians and Paracelsus (1493–1541), there were no significant new advances in medical science. This is not to say, however, that progress was not made during the Dark Ages. While the medical sciences were marking time in Europe, the wealth of knowledge that had been accumulated and preserved in the Roman manuscripts passed to the East. Sustained and enriched in turn by the Arab and Jewish physicians, this medical knowledge came back to Europe with the Western movement of the Arabs and the travels of the Crusaders. The diligence of the Christian religious orders in copying manuscripts and in making their monasteries the repositories of all the learning of the past also helped in preserving this knowledge. Notable among those responsible for maintaining the continuum of medicine during the Dark Ages were the Muslim physicians Abu Bekr Muhammad Al-Razi (844–926), famous in Europe as Rhazes, and Abu Ali al-Husein ibn Sina (980–1037), known as Avicenna, and the Jewish physicians Isaac Israeli (ca. 855–ca. 955) and Moses Maimonides (1135–1204). The medical writings of these men left their mark on European medicine for hundreds of years, being used as authoritative texts as late as the seventeenth century. In addition, Avicenna and his successors preserved the pharmaceutical art of the sixth to sixteenth centuries by compiling and condensing the detailed directions for concocting hundreds of drugs.

The Arab Influence

Although the synthesis of accumulated knowledge, rather than original findings of scientific research, was characteristic of all medieval science, the Arabs between the seventh and eleventh centuries made certain contributions that would prove to be of great consequence to the future development of pharmacology. In chemistry and alchemy, the Saracens, by introducing precision in observation, control in experimentation and meticulous record keeping, developed the experimental method that was to stimulate the growth of European chemistry five hundred years later. Second, the Muslims, by establishing the first apothecary shops and dispensaries and by founding the first medieval school of pharmacy, dissociated the practice of pharmacy from the profession of medicine. Third, the Arabs, by subjecting pharmacists to state regulations and inspections and by producing the first pharmaceutical formulary, developed standards for preparing and storing drugs. Since druggists who violated these standards by selling deceptive or deteriorated drugs were subject to punishment by law, the medieval Muslims can also be credited with one of the earliest efforts at consumer protection.

Pharmacies as separate establishments for the compounding and dispensing of medicinals began to appear and spread throughout Europe only after the thirteenth century. An illustration contained in a book published shortly after the invention of printing permits us to visualize one of these medieval apothe-

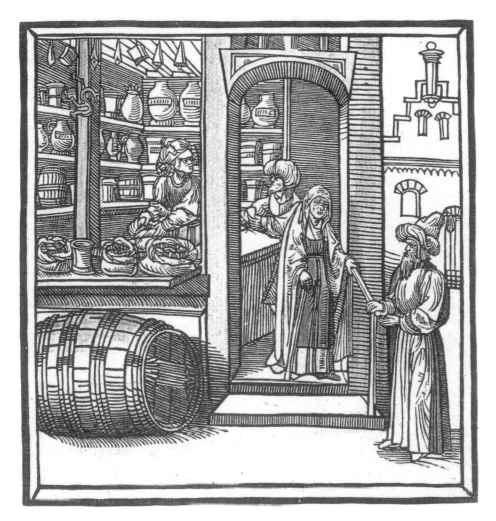

Figure 1-1. *A medieval apothecary shop. (From Quiricus de Augustis,* Dlicht d'Apotekers, *Brussels, 1515, National Library of Medicine, Bethesda.)*

cary shops (Fig. 1-1). What this early drawing does not show, however, is the close resemblance between the fifteenth-century drugstore and that of the present day. Even in medieval times, the druggist sold stationery, confections, jewelry and miscellany, along with drug preparations, in order to augment his income. But the kind of pharmacy practiced in Europe at the end of the Middle Ages was really an art that required special training. This is perhaps best exemplified by the most popular of all drugs, triaca or theriaca, a mixture which in the lifetime of Dioscorides had 57 components and by the fifteenth century had grown to 110 constituents.

As the alchemy of the Arabs swept over Europe in the fifteenth century, it brought, together with its search for the elixir of life and the philosopher's stone, new chemical methods and simpler, relatively pure substances (sulfur, iron and arsenic) which were diverted to medical use. In this period, too, the awakening of medicine and its reliance on ancient therapy, the introduction of new drugs from the East and the proliferation of formularies for the preparation of a vast arsenal of medicinals all pointed toward the necessity of having official regulations and standards. The city of Florence, Italy, is credited with issuing the first European book endowed with legal sanction for standardization and uniformity in drug preparation. This *Nuovo Receptario*, published in 1498, was distinguished not only as the first official European pharmacopeia, but also as the first *printed* compilation of medicinal preparations. The sixteenth century saw pharmacy come into its own in the Western world, and it will not serve our purpose here to trace further the varied endeavors to standardize drugs which have culminated in national and international pharmacopeias, formularies and other publications in current use.

The Influence of Paracelsus

Aureolus Paracelsus (1493–1541), whose real name was Philippus Theophrastus Bombastus von Hohenheim, has been called the Grandfather of Pharmacology. As such he deserves special attention.

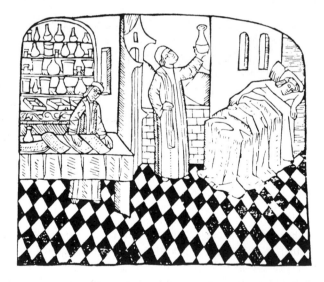

Figure 1-2. *A pharmacist at work, while a physician examines a urine sample from the patient. It may be the earliest depiction of the concept of the 'triad of medical care' to appear in an English book. (The illustration introduces Book 7 of the encyclopedia* On the Properties of Things *by Bartholomew [13th century], Westminster, 1495.) (From G. Sonnedecker [ed.].* History of Pharmacy, *by Kremers and Urdang [4th ed.]. Philadelphia: Lippincott, 1976. p. 34.)*

Paracelsus was one of the angry young men of his day. He possessed a brilliant mind, but his restlessness, arrogance and defiance – his bombast – frequently brought him into conflict with the law as well as with the medical profession. He studied medicine but never obtained a degree, giving it up to experiment with chemistry and alchemy. Even though he never completely separated science from magic, he nevertheless revolutionized therapy by boldly advancing the application of chemistry to medicine. Paracelsus believed that man's body is composed of chemicals; he discarded Galen's theory of humors and advocated the theory that illness is a disturbance of the chemical constituents of the body. He popularized the use of chemical tinctures and extracts and compounded laudanum, the tincture of opium which remains in use today. He spoke out against the indiscriminate use of drug mixtures derived from the plant and animal world, recognizing that any useful substance which they contained was probably diluted to ineffective concentrations by their inert ingredients. He stressed the curative powers of single agents, particularly inorganic materials, such as the use of mercury to treat syphilis. He recognized the relationship between the amount of a drug administered and the beneficial or harmful effects produced, for he wrote: 'All things are poisons, for there is nothing without poisonous qualities. It is only the dose which makes a thing a poison.'

THE RISE OF PHARMACOLOGY

The advances made by a few men like Paracelsus frequently are too far ahead of most people, and contemporary society as a whole remains almost completely indifferent to their value. Perhaps a maverick like Paracelsus is too hostile, intolerant and impatient to be able to infuse his influence into his own time. The experimental methods and work of Paracelsus certainly forecast the modern approach to pharmacology, but a century was to elapse before another significant milestone appeared along the road of progress. This noteworthy event followed close on the heels of William Harvey's (1578–1657) explanation of the circulation of the blood.

The Forecasters of Experimental Pharmacology

The publication of Harvey's *Exercitatio anatomica de motu cordis et sanguinis in animalibus* in 1628 not only was the most momentous event in medicine to occur in the fifteen centuries since Galen, but also signaled the beginning of the scientific study of drug action. It opened the way for administering drugs in a new manner – by the intravenous route – and thus made it possible to demonstrate temporal connections between the administration of a drug and biologic effects produced. It is interesting to note that it was not a physiologist but a great chemist and physicist, Robert Boyle, who apparently was among the first to use this new route to investigate drug action in animals. About the year 1660, Boyle and an associate, Timothy Clarke, showed by well-controlled pharmacologic experiments that drugs are active when administered by vein. They also indirectly proved that these drugs, when taken by mouth, could produce the same effects only after being absorbed into the circulation.

There are only a few other events in the science of the seventeenth and eighteenth centuries that can be singled out as meaningful to the development of pharmacology. Those that are notable herald the great advances of the nineteenth century. The work of the Swiss physician John Jacob Wepfer (1620–1695) was the first critical publication of careful and large-scale pharmacologic experiments designed and carried out to determine the toxicity of drugs and poisons in animals. Felix Fontana (1720–1805), following the example set by Wepfer, also performed thousands of experiments on the toxicity of various crude drugs. His results suggested to him that a crude drug contains an *active principle* which preferentially acts upon one or more discrete parts of the organism to produce a characteristic effect. Thus Fontana's premise was preamble to the pioneering demonstrations of François Magendie (1783–1855) and Claude Bernard (1813–1878) that the site of action of a drug could be located in specific structures of the body.

The work of a young pharmacist's apprentice, Peter John Andrew Daries, in the late eighteenth century, was of equal or perhaps greater importance to pharmacology than that of Fontana. The results of Daries' carefully controlled studies were published as his doctoral dissertation in 1776. Through his astute deductions, he anticipated by many years the establishment of one of the fundamental pharmacologic principles, namely, that there is a relationship between the amount of a drug administered and the magnitude of the biologic response evoked.

The Influence of Advances in Physiology and Chemistry

The aforementioned pharmacologists of the seventeenth and eighteenth centuries recognized the need and value of animals as experimental tools and used them in their studies. They were hampered in their investigations, however, by a lack of refined physiologic techniques and methods with which to pinpoint where and how drugs interact with living tissue. In the early nineteenth century this impediment to the development of pharmacology as a science was removed by the achievements of illustrious French physiologists. To pioneers like Magendie and Bernard, modern pharmacology owes a debt equal to that owed by modern physiology. The methods of physiologic experimentation which they established and employed were as fundamental and essential to understanding normal physiologic processes as they were to understanding the dynamic actions of chemicals on biologic processes and materials. They provided the means for discovering what drugs do in the living organism.

The revolutionizing changes that occurred in chemistry almost simultaneously with those in physiology were of equal import to the subsequent rapid rise of pharmacology. Until this time, most of the drugs in medical or experimental use were impure, crude preparations or extracts of plants; the chemical methods needed to separate active ingredients were unknown. The German apothecary Frederick W.A. Sertürner (1783–1841) altered all this in 1806 when he isolated a white crystalline substance, morphine, from opium. This *first isolation* of an active principle of a medicinal plant stimulated so much enthusiastic research on other botanical drugs that Magendie was able to publish a medical formulary in 1821 which contained only single chemical entities.

After the momentous discovery of Sertürner, pharmaceutical chemistry rapidly took its place as an important branch of chemistry. With new isolation procedures, many natural drugs became available for investigation and use, and with the invention of chemical syntheses, many derivatives of natural products were made. The advances in organic chemistry also resulted in the production of totally synthetic drugs, many of which had chemical structures entirely different from compounds of plant origin.

Pharmacology as a Separate Discipline

Once chemistry had provided the pure chemicals, and physiology the experimental methods with which to determine their biologic activity, pharmacologists had the implements they needed to advance their science to a discipline in its own right. From this time on, new developments in all aspects of pharmacology followed one another in quick succession.

Localization of Site of Drug Action

The investigations of the pioneering physiologist Magendie ushered in this new era in pharmacology. He not only studied the action of a number of the newly purified drugs, but, more importantly, by using his new methods of experimentation, he was able to show that their effects were the results of actions within specific organs of the body. Thus, 50 years after Fontana had made the suggestion that each active component of a crude drug exerts its own characteristic effect at one or more specific sites in the body, Magendie concluded the experiments which established this as fact.

Magendie's work was continued and extended by his brilliant pupil Claude Bernard, one of the most outstanding physiologists of all time. Among the many valuable contributions Bernard made to our understanding of the sites and modes of action of various drugs, his studies of the arrow poison curare are perhaps the most remarkable. In a series of ingenious experiments culminating around 1856, he clearly demonstrated that curare exerts its paralyzing effect by acting at the junction between skeletal muscle and the nerve stimulating the muscle. He further showed that the drug does not affect the nerve or the muscle itself. Therefore, by pharmacologic means, Bernard proved that there is a specialized area between the nerve and the muscle which is directly concerned with muscular activity. From this time on, the determination of the locus of action of a drug became an essential part of the study of the drug.

Cellular Mechanisms of Drug Action

Claude Bernard stated that drugs are the means of 'dealing with the elementary parts of organisms where the elementary properties of vital phenomena have their seat.' He therefore inferred that to understand the action of a given drug, it is essential both to know which tissues are primarily involved and to explain how the drug interacts with the biologic system to produce its effect. Rudolf Buchheim (1820–1879), in his masterly experiments with various drugs, advanced the thesis that drug activity could be explained on the basis of physicochemical reactions between cell constituents and the particular drug. The work of Buchheim foreshadowed the great conceptual contributions made at the turn of the twentieth century by J.N. Langley (1852–1926) and Paul Ehrlich (1854–1915) concerning the nature of the cellular combining sites for drugs – **receptors** – and by A.J. Clark (1885–1941) on the quantitative aspects of this interaction between drug and cell. The work of these men is discussed in more detail in later chapters.

Chemical Structure and Biologic Activity

In 1841 James Blake (1815–1893), a British physician who emigrated to the United States in 1847, employed a novel methodologic approach that was to be profitably exploited by the future developers of synthetic drugs. By using a systematic series of chemically related inorganic salts, Blake established the principle that *the chemical structure of drugs determines their effect on the body*. The first steps toward disclosing the relationship between the chemical structure of organic compounds and their pharmacologic activity were made by the British physician T.R. Fraser (1841–1920) in collaboration with the chemist A. Crum Brown (1838–1923). Paul Ehrlich's work in the preparation of hundreds of arsenical compounds in the course of his search for a drug effective in the treatment of syphilis is a classic example of the structure-activity approach to the development of new and effective agents. The use of structure-activity relationships was also to become a powerful tool in the twentieth century in helping to bring to light the ultimate mechanisms by which drugs interact with biologic materials to produce their characteristic effects.

Fate of Drugs in the Body

James Blake, in the studies already referred to, also established the fact that drugs are effective only if, after administration, they are able to reach a responsive tissue. Oswald Schmiedeberg (1838–1921), a pupil of Buchheim, enlarged upon this and added the concept that drug activity is the consequence of a dynamic equilibrium, i.e. that the activity of a given drug is related to its ability to reach its site of action and to be removed from it. The means by which the body is able to eliminate drugs and terminate their action therefore became an important concern.

That the body eliminates many chemical substances, particularly in the urine, had been known for centuries. But clear-cut proof that the living organism can also turn off the activity of a drug by carrying out chemical reactions which change the drug was obtained for the first time in 1842 by W. Keller. Schmiedeberg and his co-workers discovered a number of additional chemical reactions carried out by the body on various groups of drugs and strengthened the concept that drug activity can be terminated by chemical conversion within the body.

Pharmacology as a Profession

Buchheim and Schmiedeberg are important figures in pharmacology not only for their contributions to its substantive content but also for the stature to which they raised the discipline. Buchheim was the first professor of pharmacology as well as the founder of the first laboratory devoted exclusively to experimental pharmacology as an independent part of physiology. The excellent textbook of pharmacology that he authored grouped drugs according to their chemical and pharmacologic actions rather than by their therapeutic effects.

Oswald Schmiedeberg, as professor of pharmacology at Strasburg, Germany, continued this transformation of the traditional materia medica into the modern science of pharmacology. He defined the purpose of pharmacology – to study the reactions brought about in living organisms by chemically acting substances (except foods) whether used for therapeutic purposes or not. Schmiedeberg, with Naunyn and Klebs, also founded *Archiv für Experimentelle Pathologie und Pharmakologie*, the first modern journal devoted to reports of pharmacologic experimentation. But it was Schmiedeberg's renown as a teacher that drew students to him from all over the world. Through these students, many of whom attained eminence in their own right, he influenced the worldwide development of professional pharmacology. Noteworthy among Schmiedeberg's pupils were John Jacob Abel (1857–1938) and Arthur Robertson Cushney (1866–1926).

Abel officially founded pharmacology in the United States and became the Father of American Pharmacology. He occupied the first full-time professorship of pharmacology at the University of Michigan in 1891 and started the American Society for Pharmacology and Experimental Therapeutics (ASPET) in 1908 and its journal, *Journal of Pharmacology and Experimental Therapeutics* (*JPET*), thereafter. When Abel left Ann Arbor in 1893 to chair the Department of Pharmacology at the Johns Hopkins University, Cushney took Abel's place at the University of Michigan and established an outstanding laboratory of pharmacologic research.

The Modern Era

Together with the tremendous achievements in the advancement of pharmacology to the status of a science, the nineteenth and early part of the twentieth centuries witnessed dramatic discoveries of new pharmacologic agents. The

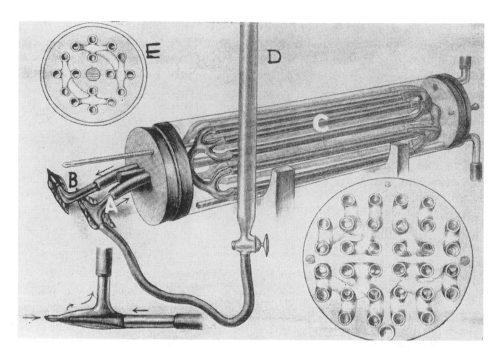

Figure 1-3. *'Artificial kidney' as envisioned by John Jacob Abel years before one was finally developed that would work on human patients. The view, reproduced from an old drawing, shows the artificial kidney used by Dr Abel on animals in 1913. A cannula (tube) was inserted in the animal's artery* (A) *to lead blood into the device's apparatus* (C), *a series of collodion tubes through which the blood flowed and from which substances in the blood were diffused into a fluid introduced from outside. A cross-section of these tubes is shown in the circle at the upper left* (E). *Anticoagulant was introduced through the burette in the center of the drawing* (D). *Blood was returned to the animal's vein through the upper cannula at left* (B). *(From J.J. Abel, L.G. Rowntree and B.B. Turner,* Trans. Assoc. Am. Physicians, *p. 28, 1913.)*

character of surgery and obstetrics was changed by W. Morton (1819–1868) with the introduction of ether and by J. Lister (1827–1912) and I. Semmelweis (1818–1865) with the use of antiseptics to prevent infection. Ehrlich's work showing that drugs can be developed which are capable of destroying invading organisms without disabling the host ushered in the era of chemotherapy. The discovery of insulin by Banting and Best in 1921 led to dramatic success in the treatment of diabetes; it also focused attention on the therapeutic use of normally occurring substances as replacement for what the body is unable to provide in adequate quantities to maintain health. All these events and more formed the basis for the rational therapy of disease. And the growth of the pharmaceutical industry, with its extensive programs of research and development, ensured the availability of an ever-increasing number of new drugs for the treatment and prevention of more and more diseases.

We end our narration of the history of pharmacology at this point, for as Albert Szent-Györgyi has stated: 'The future is the continuum of the past, the present being the dividing line between the two.' The progress made in the recent past, greater than in all the years before, becomes our present and forms the subject matter of this book.

SYNOPSIS

Primitive peoples used drugs with about as much logic as they used magic, charms and incantations to drive away the evil spirits that they thought responsible for their illness. The rational use of drugs began only in the more recent past with the understanding of the true causes of disease. The emergence of pharmacology from a purely empiric part of medicine to a science in its own right was dependent on the development of sound medical therapy. But the real impetus for the growth of pharmacology was supplied by advances in chemistry and physiology. Chemistry provided pure compounds, and physiology provided the experimental techniques and knowledge essential in evaluating the biologic effects of pure chemicals. Many able scientists contributed significantly to the rise of pharmacology, but certain ones may be singled out as the innovators and pathfinders. Among these are:

Paracelsus (Philippus Theophrastus Bombastus von Hohenheim) (1493–1541), who united chemistry with medicine; he discarded the ancient theories of the causes of disease and advocated the belief that illness is a derangement of body chemistry to be treated by simple chemical therapeutic agents.

William Harvey (1578–1657), who explained the circulation of the blood; this momentous discovery signaled the beginning of the scientific study of the medical sciences.

François Magendie (1783–1855), who pioneered the experimental approach to the study of pharmacology as well as physiology.

Frederick W.A. Sertürner (1783–1841), who isolated morphine from opium in 1806, the first isolation of an active ingredient from a botanical drug source.

Claude Bernard (1813–1878), the first to demonstrate and explain how a drug produces its action in the body.

James Blake (1815–1893), who first set forth the principles that drugs are effective only after reaching a responsive tissue and that there is a relationship between the structure of drugs and the effects that they produce.

Rudolf Buchheim (1820–1879), the first professor of pharmacology as well as founder of the first laboratory devoted exclusively to experimental pharmacology; he raised pharmacology to a position of equal importance with other branches of medicine.

Oswald Schmiedeberg (1838–1921), the first great teacher of pharmacology; his textbook, techniques and students set the pattern for the worldwide development of pharmacology.

Paul Ehrlich (1854–1915), who ushered in the era of chemotherapy by showing that chemicals can be made which are capable of destroying particular invading organisms; he also formulated the concept of receptors, i.e. that part of a chemical component of living tissue with which a drug combines to produce its biologic effect.

John Jacob Abel (1857–1938), the Father of American Pharmacology, who occupied the first full-time professorship of pharmacology in the United States and founded the American Society for Pharmacology and Experimental Therapeutics and its journal.

GUIDES FOR STUDY AND REVIEW

Which great physiologist was the first to demonstrate and explain how a drug produces its action in the body?

Who ushered in the era of chemotherapy and formulated the concept of receptors?

Who is known as the Father of American Pharmacology? What were some of his major contributions to pharmacology as a profession?

SUGGESTED READING

Annual Review of Pharmacology and Toxicology. Palo Alto: Annual Reviews, Inc., Chapter 1, 1960–present, autobiographies of eminent pharmacologists.

Black, W.G. *Folk-Medicine: A Chapter in the History of Culture.* London: Eliot Stock, 1883.

Bryan, C.P. *The Ebers' Papyrus.* London: Geoffrey Bales, 1930.

Castiglioni, A. *A History of Medicine.* (Translated and edited by E.B. Krumbhaar.) New York: Knopf, 1947.

Chatard, J.A. Avicenna and Arabian medicine. *Johns Hopkins Hosp. Bull.* 19:157, 1908.

Estes, J.W. *The Medical Skills of Ancient Egypt.* Canton: Science History Pub., 1993.

Fisher, J.W. Origins of American Pharmacology. *Trends Pharmacol. Sci.* 7:41, 1986.

Garrison, F. *History of Medicine* (4th ed.). Philadelphia: Saunders, 1929.

Homstedt, B. and Liljestrand, G. (eds). *Readings in Pharmacology.* Oxford, UK: Pergamon, 1963.

Jarvis, D.C. *Folk Medicine.* New York: Holt, 1958.

Krantz, J.C., Jr. *Historical Medical Classics Involving New Drugs.* Baltimore: Williams & Wilkins, 1974.

La Wall, C.H. *Four Thousand Years of Pharmacy.* Philadelphia: Lippincott, 1927.

Leake, C.D. *A Historical Account of Pharmacology to the 20th Century.* Springfield, IL: Charles C. Thomas, 1975.

Maehle, A.-H. *Drugs on Trial. Experimental Pharmacology and Therapeutic Innovation in the Eighteenth-Century.* Amsterlands, Clio Medica/The Wellcome Institute Series in the History of Medicine 53, Rodopi Bv Editions, 1999.

Meek, W.J. *Medico-Historical Papers: The Gentle Art of Poisoning.* Madison: University of Wisconsin Press, 1954.

Paracelsus. *Four Treatises of Theophrastus von Hohenheim Called Paracelsus* (Edited by H.E. Sigerist). Baltimore: Johns Hopkins University Press, 1941.

Parascandola, J. *The Development of American Pharmacology: John J. Abel and the Shaping of a Discipline.* Baltimore: Johns Hopkins University Press, 1992.

Schwartz, R.S. Paul Ehrlich's magic bullets. *N. Engl. J. Med.* 350:1079–1080, 2004.

Shuster, L. (ed.). *Readings in Pharmacology.* Boston: Little, Brown, 1962.

Withering, W. An account of the foxglove, and some of its medical uses; with practical remarks on dropsy, and other diseases. *Med. Classics* 2:305, 1937.

2   The Scope of Pharmacology

The word *pharmacology* is derived from the Greek *pharmakon*, equivalent to 'drug', 'medicine' or 'poison', and *logia*, meaning 'study'. But the question 'What is pharmacology?' is only partially answered by the derivation of the term. We have seen that it is a branch of biology, because it is concerned with living organisms, and as such it borrows heavily from kindred subjects like physiology and biochemistry for much of its substantive matter and experimental techniques. Pharmacology is equally related to chemistry, because it deals with chemical agents and is dependent upon knowledge of their sources and properties. Also, pharmacology is an essential part of medicine. For although a *drug*, in broad terms, is any chemical agent other than food that affects living organisms, in its medicinal sense a drug is any chemical agent used in the treatment, cure, prevention or diagnosis of disease. Pharmacology makes use of mathematics to express its principles in quantitative terms and of behavioral sciences, such as psychology, to understand the actions of drugs that lead to changes in mood or emotion. Thus *pharmacology is the unified study of the properties of chemicals and living organisms and all aspects of their interactions*; it is an *integrative* rather than an autonomous science, drawing on the techniques and knowledge of many allied scientific disciplines.

The broad science of pharmacology may be divided into four main categories: pharmacodynamics, toxicology, pharmacotherapeutics and pharmacy. In each of these subdivisions the emphasis is on those aspects of pharmacology that meet the specific requirements and objectives of the professional engaged in the particular field of specialized study.

Pharmacodynamics may be defined as *the study of the actions and effects of chemicals at all levels of organization of living material and of the handling of chemicals by the organism.* The similarity of the definition of pharmacodynamics to that of pharmacology itself is indicative of the fundamental nature of this aspect of pharmacology and of its place as the foundation on which the study of all other facets of pharmacology must be based. Indeed, pharmacodynamics is frequently referred to simply as pharmacology. Pharmacodynamics may also be used in a narrower sense to mean the science and study of how chemicals produce their biologic effects; this definition distinguishes pharmacodynamics from **pharmacokinetics**, *the science and study of the factors that determine the amount of drug at sites of biologic effect at various times after application of an agent to a biologic system.* The professional pharmacologist, whether physician or nonphysician, depends on his knowledge of pharmacodynamics for a productive career.

Pharmacodynamics includes the study of (1) the biologic effects produced by chemicals; (2) the site(s) at which and mechanism(s) by which the biologic effects are produced; (3) the fate of a chemical agent in the body: its absorption, distribution and elimination; and (4) the factors which influence the safety and effectiveness of an agent, i.e. the factors attributable to the physicochemical properties of the agent and those attributable to the biologic system.

General pharmacodynamics includes the fundamental principles or properties involved in the actions of all drugs and *special pharmacodynamics* the additional factors necessary to understand the action of individual drugs or drugs of similar action. In this book we are concerned primarily with the study of general pharmacodynamics. We shall deal with certain aspects of the specific pharmacology of some common drugs only to help in elucidating the general principles applicable to most drugs. We shall use the term *drug* in its broad sense to apply to *any chemical agent that affects living organisms.*

Toxicology is *the study of the toxic or harmful effects of chemicals as well as of the mechanisms and conditions of occurrence of these harmful effects.* It is also concerned with the symptoms and treatment of poisoning as well as the identification of the poison.

As Paracelsus pointed out, all drugs are toxic in overdosage. But what may constitute an overdose of insecticide for a particular insect may be entirely harmless to animals and human beings. Thus toxicity, while always indicating a harmful effect on some biologic system, is a relative term and requires definition of the system on which the toxic effect is produced. Although the toxic effects of therapeutic agents are part of their pharmacodynamics, the study of toxicology has developed into a separate discipline because large masses of people are exposed to a great variety of other potentially toxic substances. The toxicologist, in addition to training in pharmacodynamics, requires special training in drug identification and poison control.

The field of toxicology has developed into three principal subdivisions:

1. *Environmental toxicology* is concerned with the toxic effects of chemicals that become incidental or occupational hazards as contaminants of the atmosphere, water or food.
2. *Economic toxicology* deals with the toxic effects of those chemicals that are intentionally administered to a living organism in order to achieve a specific purpose. Thus economic toxicology deals with (a) all the therapeutic agents for human and veterinary use; (b) the chemicals used as food additives and cosmetics; and (c) the chemical agents used by humans to eliminate selec-

tively another species. In the last case, the human is considered the economic species, and the undesirable species, e.g. an insect, is considered the uneconomic species.

3. *Forensic toxicology* refers to the medical aspects of the diagnosis and treatment of poisoning and the legal aspects of the relationships between exposure to and harmful effects of the chemical. It involves both intentional and accidental exposure to chemicals.

Pharmacotherapeutics is *the application of drugs in the prevention, treatment or diagnosis of disease and their use in purposeful alteration of normal functions,* such as in the prevention of pregnancy or in the use of anesthetics for surgical procedures. Pharmacotherapeutics is of primary concern to those individuals engaged in the healing professions. It is that division of pharmacology which correlates pharmacodynamics with the pathologic physiology or microbiologic or biochemical aspects of disease.

Pharmacy is concerned with *the preparing, compounding and dispensing of chemical agents for therapeutic use.* It includes (1) *pharmacognosy*, the identification of the botanical source of drugs; (2) *pharmaceutical chemistry*, the synthesis of new drugs either as modifications of older or natural drugs or as entirely new chemical entities; and (3) *biopharmaceutics*, the science and study of the ways in which the pharmaceutical formulation of administered agents can influence their pharmacodynamic and pharmacokinetic behavior.

We have seen that pharmacy was the first branch of pharmacology to achieve professional status in its own right. But pharmacists today bear little resemblance to their predecessors. They are no longer called upon to prepare or package drugs, which is now done by the pharmaceutical manufacturing companies. The role they now play, and which will become progressively more important as the complexity of therapeutics increases, is that of essential assistants to the physician, since pharmacists have specific knowledge of the properties of drugs and drug preparations.

DRUG NOMENCLATURE

Drugs used as therapeutic agents may be conveniently divided into two main groups: (1) nonprescription drugs, which may be sold 'over the counter' (OTC) since they are judged safe for use without medical supervision; and (2) prescription drugs, which are considered to be unsafe for use except under supervision and which are, therefore, dispensed only by the order of practitioners licensed by law to administer them, e.g. physicians, dentists and veterinarians. In the United States, the OTC drug evaluation division of the Food and Drug Administration (FDA) is empowered to make decisions on which drugs require prescription and which may be sold OTC.

Drugs may also be classified *generically* to designate a chemical or pharmacologic relationship among a group of drugs, such as sulfonamides, local anesthetics, sedatives and so forth. This is a particularly useful categorization, because it focuses attention on the pharmacologic similarities among the members of a class as a whole. Usually, attention is directed within the group to one or two drugs chosen as representatives, or prototypes, of the entire class. Procaine, for example, is commonly used as the prototype of the drugs classified as local anesthetics. The use of prototypes also permits easy recognition of the member of a group that displays different or unique properties. In this text, we shall use this prototype device to characterize a generic class of drugs.

The problems in drug nomenclature arise in naming individual therapeutic agents. Not only are an overwhelming number of agents available for use, but each of these agents has at least three names. Every drug has a *chemical* name, a *nonproprietary* name and a *proprietary*, or *trade*, name. Many of the older drugs, in addition, have an *official* name, whereas the official name of newer drugs is usually synonymous with their nonproprietary name. The non-proprietary name is frequently referred to as the *generic* name of the drug. The latter by strict definition is inappropriate, however, and should be reserved to designate a family relationship among drugs, as already indicated.

The chemical name of a drug – its first name – is a precise description of its chemical constitution and indicates the arrangement of atoms or atomic groups. For example, the chemical name of a drug prototypic of a class of drugs used to treat anxiety is 7-chloro-2-methylamino-5-phenyl-3H-1,4-benzodiazepine-4-oxide. Although meaningful to a chemist, this name obviously is too complex and unwieldy for most persons to use. Consequently, chemical names are rarely employed to designate drugs except for the simplest compounds, such as sodium bicarbonate.

The nonproprietary name of a drug is the name assigned to it when it is found to be of demonstrated or potential therapeutic usefulness. New drugs are now given nonproprietary names by the United States Adopted Name (USAN) Council, an enterprise jointly sponsored by the United States Pharmacopeial (USP) Convention, Inc., the American Pharmaceutical Association and the American Medical Association (AMA), and with representation from the FDA. The USAN Council replaced the older AMA–USP Nomenclature Committee. The nonproprietary name usually becomes the *official* name of the drug as well when the drug is finally admitted to official compendia, *The United States Pharmacopeia* or *The National Formulary* (see p. 26). The names selected by the USAN Council for newer drugs may also be adopted for use on a worldwide basis through the mediation of the World Health Organization (WHO). Such uniformity of nomenclature is very desirable in view of the rapid proliferation of new agents and the frequency with which people travel from one country to another.

The nonproprietary names selected for many drugs, however, have frequently defeated the purpose for which they were originally established. These assigned names are, for the most part, too long, too difficult to pronounce or spell and, consequently, too hard to remember. For example, chlordiazepoxide is the nonproprietary name given to the previously mentioned agent widely used for the treatment of anxiety. The *trade* name selected by the pharmaceutical company for the same drug is LIBRIUM. And it is the rule rather than the exception that the proprietary name is shorter, more euphonious and easier to recall than the nonproprietary name. As a result, it is the trade name that is most frequently remembered and used. The USAN Council is now trying to correct this situation for newly introduced drugs by selecting nonproprietary names that are easier to pronounce and remember, and that also suggest the nature of the drug.

Confusion about proprietary names arises from the fact that a single drug may have many different trade names. Unlike the nonproprietary or official name, which is public property, the trade name is registered and its use restricted to the owner of the copyright. Even when a drug is new and is protected by a patent, it may be licensed for use by a number of companies, and it then appears under a variety of trade names. The patent which covers the drug as a chemical entity, or protects its method of manufacture or use, expires at the end of either 17 years after its issue date for patents filed before June 8, 1995 or 20 years from filing, whichever is greater. After June 8, 1995, the term of a patent was set to end 20 years from the date on which the application was filed. After that time, a single agent may be marketed under 10 or 20 different trade names. For example, the names by which a local anesthetic – known in the United States by the nonproprietary name procaine – has been designated in various parts of the world include the following:

NOVOCAINE	ATOXICOCAINE	AMINOCAINE
ETHOCAINE	BERNACAINE	EUGERASE
NEOCAINE	CHLOROCAINE	SEVICAINE
SYNCAINE	IROCAINE	TOPOKAIN
SCUROCAINE	JUVOCAINE	WESTOCAINE
ALLOCAINE	KEROCAINE	ISOCAINE-ASID
ANESTHESOL	PARACAIN	NAUCAINE
CETAIN	PLANOCAINE	ALOCAINE

The nonproprietary name should be used, however, to designate a particular therapeutic agent in order to minimize confusion and ensure accurate recognition. This is the nomenclature that we shall use throughout this book. When widely known or popular proprietary names are used, they will be designated by SMALL CAPITALS as above.

SOURCES OF INFORMATION ABOUT DRUGS

In this text we will focus on the principles and mechanisms that are fundamental to understanding all aspects of pharmacology and discuss specific drugs only to illustrate and exemplify. In the standard textbooks, the emphasis is on drugs and their application to therapeutics, with only a relatively small section being devoted to basic principles. For those who desire supplemental information about drugs per se, these systematic textbooks provide a concise catalog and detailed descriptions of prototypes that serve as standards of reference for the various classes of therapeutically useful agents. Certain periodically published monographs and journals which feature comprehensive reviews of selected subjects or fields are also excellent sources of pharmacologic information. The data which eventually find their way into review articles and textbooks are collected and synthesized from papers in the numerous journals of pharmacology and related medical sciences. These journals publish the wealth of experiments and rechecked observations on which our present generalizations are founded.

Although textbooks and reviews provide information about established drugs and furnish the bases for understanding new ones, they obviously cannot include details on many older agents or keep abreast of those most recently introduced. This type of encyclopedic information is the province of the numerous compendia, only two of which, *The United States Pharmacopeia* and *The National Formulary*, are recognized as official in the United States.

A number of the compendia are revised annually with several supplements per year as well. But even this frequency is often insufficient and too slow to keep up with the constant advances in the field of pharmacology. So to meet the need for current and critical sources of information, there are also several publications which furnish prompt and pointed assessment of new drugs and of recent developments in drug therapy and toxicity. Many of these compendia, texts, and journals are available in electronic format and online versions. An example of a frequently updated online resource is the website of the Food and Drug Administration (www.fda.gov), which contains documents about decisions on drug approvals, withdrawals, and changes in labeling.

Some of these sources of general and current drug information are listed below. Although the sources are representative of those considered pertinent, the list is by no means complete.

Current Textbooks

Goodman and Gilman's *The Pharmacological Basis of Therapeutics* (J.G. Hardman and L.E. Limbard, eds.-in-chief) (10th ed.). New York: McGraw-Hill, 2001. A multi-authored textbook of pharmacology, toxicology and therapeutics that has become a classic since the first edition was published in 1941.

Katzung, B.G. (ed.) *Basic & Clinical Pharmacology* (9th ed.). New York: McGraw-Hill, 2004. A comprehensive text on principles of pharmacology, therapeutic classes of drugs, and topics of relevance to their use in therapeutics.

Pratt, W.B. and Taylor, P. *Principles of Drug Action: The Basis of Pharmacology.* New York: Churchill Livingstone, 1990. An excellent advanced text on molecular mechanisms of receptors, drug metabolism and distribution, pharmacogenetics, chemical mutagenesis, carcinogenesis and teratogenesis, drug tolerance and resistance.

Rang, H.P., Dale, M.M., Ritter, J.M. and Gardner, P. *Pharmacology* (4th ed.). New York: Churchill Livingstone, 2001. A well-written text, with clear descriptions of mechanisms of drug action, effective figures and helpful summaries of clinical use.

Reviews

Pharmacological Reviews. Baltimore: Williams & Wilkins. Quarterly (The American Society for Pharmacology and Experimental Therapeutics).

Molecular Interventions: Pharmacological Perspectives from Biology, Chemistry, and Genomics. (The American Society for Pharmacology and Experimental Therapeutics.)

Annual Review of Pharmacology and Toxicology. Palo Alto: Annual Reviews, Inc. Annual.

Journals of Pharmacology and Therapeutics

Some of the journals containing original articles dealing with the effects of drugs in animals and humans also regularly feature reviews on selected topics. These journals are identified by an asterisk.

Publications of the American Society for Pharmacology and Experimental Therapeutics:

Journal of Pharmacology and Experimental Therapeutics
Molecular Pharmacology
Drug Metabolism and Disposition
Molecular Interventions

Other journals:

Annals of Internal Medicine
Biochemical Pharmacology
British Journal of Pharmacology (British Pharmacological Society)
British Medical Journal
Canadian Journal of Physiology and Pharmacology
Clinical Pharmacology and Therapeutics
Clinical Pharmacokinetics
Drugs
European Journal of Pharmacology
* JAMA (Journal of the American Medical Association)*
Journal of Pharmacy and Pharmacology (Canadian Society for Pharmaceutical Sciences)
Journal of Pharmaceutical Sciences (American Association of Pharmaceutical Scientists)
Lancet
Nature Review. Drug Discovery
New England Journal of Medicine
Toxicology and Applied Pharmacology
Toxicological Sciences (Society of Toxicology)
Trends in Pharmacological Sciences

Compendia

Official Compendia

The Pharmacopeia of the United States of America (USP) (27th revision). Rockville, MD: United States Pharmacopeial Convention, Inc., 2004.

The first pharmacopeia was published in the United States in 1820, but was only given official status in 1906 by the Federal Food, Drug and Cosmetic Act. It is now revised regularly by expert pharmacologists, physicians and pharmacists who donate their services to the USP Convention, held every 5 years.

The drugs included in the *USP* are selected on the basis of their proven therapeutic value and low toxicity. Included are prescription and nonprescription drugs and botanical and nonbotanical dietary supplements. Trademarked or patented drugs of therapeutic usefulness may be included as long as their content and method of preparation are not secret; they are listed under their official names. Drugs may be deleted from the *USP* when they have been supplanted by newer or better drugs or when there is a high incidence of toxic reactions after extensive use.

The official drugs in the *USP* are defined according to source; physical and chemical properties; standards for identity, quality, strength and purity; method of storage; and dosage range for therapeutic use. However, the *USP* does not provide information about the pharmacologic actions or therapeutic uses of the drugs.

The National Formulary (NF) (22nd ed.) Rockville, MD: United States Pharmacopeial Convention, Inc., 2004.

The *NF* was also given status in 1906 and was similar in purpose, format and content to the *USP*. When it was originally published in 1888 under the name *National Formulary of Unofficial Preparations*, it contained only formulas for drug mixtures. This changed slowly over the years to include single drugs, but the *NF*, unlike the *USP*, still listed drug mixtures along with a variety of materials of plant origin. In 1980 the scope of the *USP* and *NF* was changed, the *Pharmacopeia* being limited to drug substances and dosage forms and the *National Formulary* to pharmaceutical ingredients such as excipients. The *NF* is now published annually together with the *USP* in a single volume, the USP-NF, available in print and online. Both continue as distinct official compendia.

The *British Pharmacopoeia (BP)*, published by the British Pharmacopoeia Commission under the direction of the General Medical Council, and the *British Pharmaceutical Codex (BPC)*, published by the Pharmaceutical Society of Great Britain, are counterparts of the *USP* and *NF*, respectively. Other countries also have their official compendia. A committee of the World Health Organization publishes *The Pharmacopoeia Internationalis (PhI)* (3rd ed., 2003). This compendium is not intended to convey official status, but to encourage the development of international standards and unification of national pharmacopeias.

Unofficial Compendia

USP DI: Vol. 1. *Drug Information for the Health Care Professional*. Rockville, MD: US Pharmacopeial Convention, Inc., Thomson MICROMEDEX, Greenwood Village, CO. Annual.

Medically accepted uses of more than 10,000 nonproprietary (generic) and trade name drug products including indications, pharmacokinetics, side-effects and dosage forms.

American Drug Index. Facts and Comparisons Staff (ed.). Philadelphia, PA: Lippincott, Williams & Wilkins. Annual.

Essentially a dictionary providing a useful cross-indexed source of drug products and dosage forms, listed by both nonproprietary and trade names.

The Merck Index (13th ed.). Whitehouse Station, NJ: Merck, 2001.

Contains the structural formulas and chemical and physical properties of more than 10,000 chemical compounds, including many therapeutic agents. The *Index* is also an excellent source for the many synonyms by which an individual drug is known. Available in print and electronic editions that facilitate searches by chemical structure.

Physicians' Desk Reference. Montvale, NJ: Medical Economics. Annual with two supplements per year.

The *PDR,* as it is best known, lists the products of all the major drug manufacturers and is supported by them. Although a convenient source of information about available products, dosage forms, composition and untoward reactions of the listed preparations, it is not useful as a critical guide to the pharmacologic actions or uses of drugs. The information provided is almost the same as that contained in the drug package insert (the FDA-approved 'label') but includes no comparative data on efficacy and safety.

The Medical Letter on Drugs and Therapeutics, New Rochelle: Drug and Therapeutic Information, Inc. Biweekly.

Contains concise, informative and critical comments on newly promoted drugs and those being currently evaluated. The comments are written by a board of distinguished physicians affiliated with teaching hospitals and medical schools. The *Medical Letter* compares new drugs with older agents, critically analyzes the claims made for new drugs and also alerts physicians to reports of adverse drug reactions.

USP Dictionary of USAN and International Drug Names. Rockville, MD: United States Pharmacopeial Convention, Inc., 2003.

A compilation of United States Adopted Names (USANs), International Nonproprietary Names (INNs), British Approved Names (BANs), Japanese Approved Names (JANs), and other names for drugs both current and retrospective. Includes chemical formulas. Available online and in print.

GUIDES FOR STUDY AND REVIEW

What distinguishes 'pharmacodynamics' from 'pharmacokinetics'? How are toxicology, pharmacotherapeutics and pharmacy related to pharmacology?

What do we mean by the chemical name of a drug? the nonproprietary name? the proprietary name? the official name? Why is 'generic name' an inappropriate synonym for 'nonproprietary name'?

What are the names of the compendia that have official status in the United States? How are drugs selected for inclusion in these official compendia? What are some of the other compendia that furnish encyclopedic information about established and new drugs?

3   How Drugs Act on the Living Organism

The eminent Canadian physician Sir William Osler made the witty comment, 'The desire to take medicine is perhaps the greatest feature which distinguishes man from the animals.' Whatever truth there be to this quip, it is certainly true that from the dawn of history people have exercised a desire to assuage suffering and combat illness by concocting thousands of medicinals and avidly partaking of them. But of this legion, only a handful continually enjoyed popularity through the ages and made their way to our own time. Why did the juice of the poppy seed, the beverages made from fermented fruits and vegetables, the infusion of the autumn crocus, the extract of willow bark or the seeds of the castor oil plant survive as useful remedies? These and similar nostrums (Fig. 3-1) survived not because they actually contain *effective* drugs, but because to both physician and patient the *effects they produced were immediately evident and unmistakable*. Opium and alcohol quickly relieved the patient's pain and suffering; within a few hours colchicine terminated the agony of an acute attack of gout; salicin (an ancestor of our aspirin) rapidly reduced fever; and castor oil was equally conspicuous in its activity. The effects of these agents were easily recognizable and readily measured as significant changes in the recipient's physiologic state. Physician and patient alike could answer the question 'What does the drug do?'.

The effect produced by a drug can be recognized only as an alteration in a function or process that maintains the existence of the living organism, since all drugs act by producing changes in some known physiologic function or process. Drugs may increase or decrease the normal function of tissues or organs, but they do not confer any *new* functions on them; effects of drugs are quantitative, never qualitative. As in the examples previously cited, the effects produced by a drug can be identified as an *increase* in the normal rate of evacuation of the bowels, a *reduction* in an elevated body temperature or the *lessening* of pain and return to the normal painless state. Thus the particular effect of a drug is always expressed in relative terms – relative to the physiologic condition that exists at the time of drug administration. The primary factor in the facility with which the

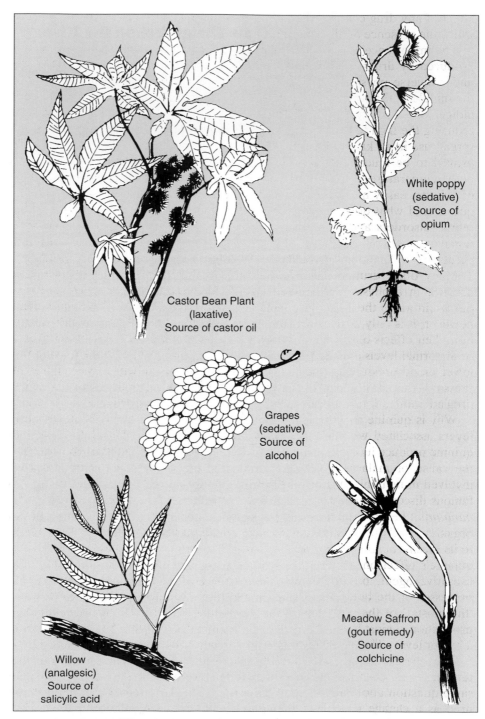

Figure 3-1. *Sources of ancient remedies and modern drugs.*

effect of any drug can be evaluated is that there are yardsticks or standards by which the presence or absence of an effect can be measured.

The importance of having an appropriate yardstick to measure the changes produced by drugs is well illustrated by an analysis of quinine's effectiveness under diverse physiologic conditions. Quinine was introduced into Europe in the middle of the seventeenth century as the powdered bark of cinchona, a tree indigenous to South America. The powder was found to have a striking effect in reducing the high fever of patients with malaria. This discovery led to its widespread use in all kinds of febrile illnesses. However, the cinchona preparations proved to be much less effective in fevers of nonmalarial origin. On normal body temperature, the effect of cinchona was found to be negligible. The effect of quinine, easily measured as a change in body temperature, answers only the question of what quinine does. Evaluating quinine's effect in malaria, in other febrile disorders and in healthy individuals provides the answer to the additional question 'When does the drug act?' It also tells us that normal body temperature is an inappropriate standard to choose for measuring quinine's effect.

Many other drugs resemble quinine in this respect; i.e. the changes they produce in a physiologic process can be detected only in the presence of a disease in which the process is functioning at an abnormal level. For most drugs, however, it is only necessary to know the conditions at the time of administration; their effects on a physiologic process can be measured using either normal or abnormal levels as the appropriate standard. For example, certain drugs that lower blood pressure produce this effect in patients with high, low or normal pressure; the yardstick in each condition is the blood pressure present before drug administration, and the lowering is measured relative to the initial state.

Why is quinine so much more effective in the treatment of malaria than in fevers associated with other disorders? Now we are really asking, 'How does quinine produce its effect?'. The answer to this had to await the identification of the cause of malaria as well as the disclosure of the physiologic processes involved in maintaining normal body temperature. Following C.L.A. Laveran's famous discovery in 1880 that malaria is caused by the infecting parasite *Plasmodium*, it became relatively simple to show that quinine kills and destroys this organism. Quinine's significant effect on malarial fevers can now be attributed to its *specific action* on the agent responsible for the disease. On the other hand, quinine's effect on nonmalarial fevers can be explained not as an action on a causative agent, but in terms of what we now know about the regulatory processes of the body (Fig. 3-2). Certain distinct areas in the brain act as the 'thermostat' of the body and maintain normal temperature by balancing heat production against loss of body heat. Fever results when the thermostat is 'set at a higher level'. The action of quinine is to readjust the controls to normal levels.

The answers to the question of how does quinine produce its effect on body temperature incorporate several points that are fundamental in answering this same question about any drug. First, they tell us that a particular effect measured as a change in a definite physiologic process may be brought about in several ways. The action of the drug may be *specific*, i.e. aimed directly at the

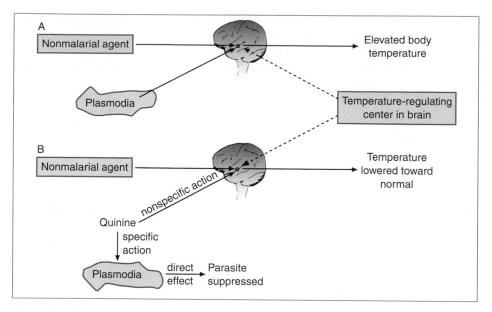

Figure 3-2. *Site of action of quinine in fevers of malarial and nonmalarial origin. (A) Both the nonmalarial vector and the plasmodia act directly or indirectly on the temperature-regulating center in the brain to produce an elevation in body temperature. (B) In fevers of nonmalarial origin, quinine produces a lowering of body temperature by acting on the temperature-regulating center to alter its response to the nonmalarial vector. In malaria, quinine acts directly on the plasmodia, thereby eliminating the cause of the elevation in body temperature.*

agent responsible for the disease, or *nonspecific*, i.e. ameliorating a symptom of the disease, such as fever, without getting to the basis of the disorder. Clearly, the distinction between what is produced by an agent – its *effect* – and where and how the effect is produced – its *action* – becomes of consequence in determining the use to which the drug may be put. But the most salient point is that, while the effects of many drugs are amenable to measurement, their actions can be identified and characterized only in terms of what we know about physiologic functions and processes. New actions of drugs can be found only after a new physiologic or biochemical process is uncovered on which the drugs may act. And what effect or action a drug has in a particular disease depends on a basic knowledge of the disease – its cause and the changes in normal body function brought about by the illness. For example, not until the thyroid gland was revealed to be an organ with a definite physiologic role was it possible to relate certain clinical symptoms to disturbances in the functioning of this gland. Only then was it feasible to develop, test and find agents capable of counteracting these disorders.

In arriving at an understanding of how drugs interact with a living organism, we must address ourselves to some specific questions: 'What is the action of the drug?,' which includes 'Where does it act?,' 'By what means does it act?,' 'When does it act?,' 'What does the drug do?' and 'What are its effects?.' In discussing general pharmacodynamics we will be concerned only with answers common to most or all drugs. In this chapter we will consider the general answer to 'What is the action of the drug?' by considering, first, where it acts and then the means by which it acts.

SITE OF ACTION

The part of the body – organ, tissue or cell – where a drug acts to initiate the chain of events leading to an effect is known as *the site of action of the drug*. For quinine, the site of action in malaria is the plasmodium, the cell invading the host; in nonmalarial fever it is the discrete areas of the brain involved in the regulation of body temperature.

It should be obvious that different experimental approaches were required in order to arrive at these two conclusions about quinine's sites of action. For malaria, once the cause of the disease had been discovered and the fever shown to be one of its accompanying symptoms, it was only necessary to determine the effect of quinine on isolated plasmodia. For other fevers, various surgical procedures had to be carried out in febrile experimental animals in order to demonstrate that quinine could lower temperature only when the areas within the brain involved in temperature regulation were left intact. Although the two experimental approaches were markedly different, the 'system' used in each case was identical. Each system included both the effector tissue, organ or cell – that entity in which the change in function could be observed or measured as an effect – and the site of action of the drug – that entity in which the drug acted to produce the response.

We saw earlier that an appropriate physiologic state had to be chosen as a standard in order to measure the effect of quinine on body temperature. In an entirely analogous fashion, it is essential to choose a suitable 'intact living system,' not only to disclose the site of action of the drug but also to determine its effect. The site of action and the effect of a drug are mutually dependent – one cannot be demonstrated in the absence of the other.

Let us consider the effects of drugs on the pupil of the eye as another example of the need for relevance in choosing the system on which these effects are to be measured. The muscles of the iris control the size of the pupillary opening in response to light; in bright light the opening is made smaller, in dim light, larger. Some drugs, like atropine, when applied to the *external* surface of the eyeball cause the pupil to become larger than it would be normally under the same light conditions (Fig. 3-3). The ophthalmologist frequently uses atropine or similar agents in just this way to dilate the pupil for eye examinations. Other drugs analogous to the organic phosphorus insecticides, when applied externally, cause the pupil to constrict. Application of drug solutions to the external surface of the eye can be used in these cases as a simple test system, since the system includes both the site of action – the muscles of the iris – and

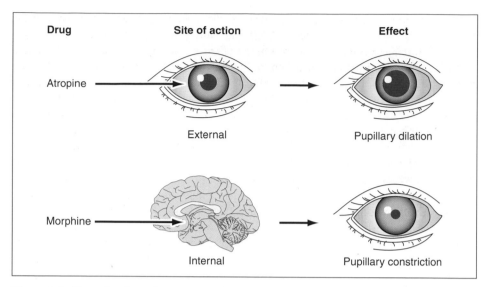

Figure 3-3. *Sites of action of atropine and morphine in producing effects on pupillary diameter.*

the target – the pupil, where the effect may be perceived as a change in diameter.

In contrast, if solutions of morphine are applied externally to the eyeball, no change in the size of the pupil is observed. Yet when morphine is administered internally it produces marked pupillary constriction, and this effect is so characteristic that the presence of 'pinpoint pupils' always leads to the presumption that an individual has taken morphine. These observations lead us to conclude that morphine cannot act directly on the muscles of the iris to produce its effect. Since the simple test system includes only part of what is essential – it does not include the site where morphine acts – no effect can be produced or seen. The site of action of morphine is within the brain, on the oculomotor nerve that influences the response of the pupil to light (Fig. 3-3). Thus, when morphine is taken internally, it has an opportunity to reach this site of action within the central nervous system (the brain and the spinal cord).

From the examples cited, we can see that a particular effect may be produced by a drug acting at a site close to the structure that ultimately responds or by a drug acting at a site distant from the target organ. The more complex the physiologic process, the more sites at which drugs may act to produce the same alteration in function. For instance, blood pressure is regulated in the normal individual by the diameter of blood vessels, the rate at which the heart beats and the amount of blood forced out of the chambers of the heart at each beat, as well as by influences coming to the heart or blood vessels from several areas of the brain. A substance may lower blood pressure by acting at any one of these sites involved in its regulation: directly on the muscle of the blood vessel walls; indirectly through action on the heart muscle; or within the brain. Knowing only the effect of the drug tells us little about its site of action.

All that is necessary to determine the effect of a drug is to choose an appropriate standard and method of measurement and a relevant system that includes the effector organ and the site of action. Although determination of the effect of a drug is not always straightforward, determining the site at which a drug acts to produce a specific effect necessarily requires more experimental finesse. For example, it took little work to show that the iris of the eye was not the site at which morphine acts to constrict the pupil. But to delineate the site at which morphine does act required extensive investigation to obtain knowledge of the manner in which individual areas of the brain influence physiologic function.

Even when we can localize the site of action of a drug to a certain tissue or organ, this knowledge in itself may be insufficient, since different drugs producing the same or different effects may have different sites of action within the same tissue or organ. For example, caffeine, histamine and nitrates, such as nitroglycerin, all act on the muscle of blood vessels to increase their diameter, whereas cocaine acts to produce constriction. It is then necessary to consider the separate components of the tissue or organ and to determine which of them is the specialized, functional element on which the drug acts. Ultimately it may be possible to show that the site of action is a particular kind of cell within an organ and that the drug acts either at the surface of this cell or within the cell itself. Alternatively, the site of action may be identified as extracellular, i.e. the site of action may be a component not contained within a cell. One of the fundamental objectives of pharmacodynamics is to be able to identify the site of action of each drug with this kind of precision. Although there are many drugs for which this has been possible, for many other important drugs we still do not have sufficient information to achieve this objective.

MECHANISM OF ACTION

When the site of action of a drug has been identified to be either at the surface of the cell, intracellular or extracellular, we are still at least one step away from understanding *how* the drug acts. We know where the drug acts. Now knowledge is needed of the *mechanism of action* – the means by which the presence of the drug produces an alteration in function at the site and initiates the series of events that we measure or observe as the effect (Fig. 3-4). The mechanism of action of some agents, particularly those that act extracellularly, is relatively uncomplicated and easy to understand. Other mechanisms, especially those of drugs that act intracellularly, are complex, and our understanding of them is frequently not explicit. For still other agents we have only a superficial explanation of how they act, since too little is known of the cellular, biochemical, or physiologic functions involved in the effects they produce.

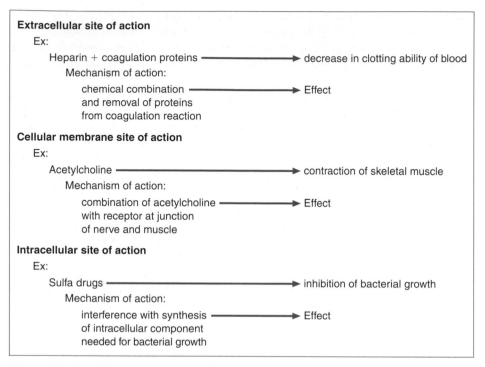

Figure 3-4. *The different sites at which drugs may produce their effects.*

Actions at Extracellular Sites

Let us consider first some of the drug reactions that occur extracellularly and that are aimed at noncellular constituents of the body. One of the simplest examples is that of the neutralization of gastric acid by antacid drugs. In this reaction a base, such as sodium bicarbonate, reacts chemically with the hydrochloric acid of the stomach and removes the acid by formation of new products, salt, water and carbon dioxide:

$$NaHCO_3 + HCl \rightarrow NaCl + H_2O + CO_2$$

Another type of extracellular mechanism is illustrated by the action of heparin in preventing the coagulation of blood. Heparin is a high-molecular-weight **polymer** in which the repeating units contain sulfuric acid. Such a structure makes heparin a highly acidic organic substance with a negative charge. The strong electronegativity allows heparin to react with substances of opposite charge. **Proteins**, also macromolecular substances, contain a number of groups in their structure that are positively charged. The electronegative heparin combines with the electropositive groups of a variety of proteins to form new compounds. The anticoagulant effect of heparin is the consequence of its combination with a protein in the blood, which is essential for coagulation. The new compound formed by this combination, although containing heparin and the essential protein, no longer has the properties of the uncombined protein and, thus, cannot enter into the reactions involved in coagulation. The result is that clotting is inhibited.

The specific **antidote**, calcium disodium edetate, used to treat lead poisoning provides another example of the type of reaction that can take place extracellularly. The drug removes lead that is free in blood and tissue fluids by a reaction in which the calcium of the drug is displaced by the lead. The attractive force between the drug and lead – its affinity for lead – is many orders of magnitude greater than that between the drug and calcium. Thus the antidote renders the lead inert by complexing it so tightly that the lead can be excreted from the body as the soluble lead-edetate complex.

In each of these examples, the action of the drug was the result of a chemical reaction. And this chemical reaction was easily definable since, in addition to the drugs involved, the other reactants could also be specifically identified. Thus, whenever a drug can be shown to interact with a distinct biologic entity and when the identified material is also a functionally important molecule in a living system, the mechanism of action of the drug can be readily explained.

Actions at Cellular Sites

Most functions of the living organism, however, do not take place extracellularly but are cellular in origin. Therefore, the vast majority of drugs produce their effects by interactions with cells, either with components of the interior of the cell or with those on the surface of the cell comprising the cellular membrane. Many of the constituents of the cell interior have been obtained as separate entities by complicated methods of isolation following careful disruption of the intact cell; using sophisticated techniques and instrumentation, it has also been possible to chemically identify or characterize many of these cellular substances and to determine their function. These efforts have been particularly fruitful in identification of the various molecules functioning to maintain the life of the *individual cell* – those involved in the processes of cellular respiration, energy production and reproduction.

When a drug is shown to act intracellularly, it may be possible to determine whether it affects one of these vital processes, since its effects can be measured in terms of the change in the function, e.g. a change in the utilization of oxygen or of a sugar. Just as with heparin, it then becomes feasible to determine the mechanism of drug action, since most of the reactants as well as the chemical reactions of a particular process have been identified. The mechanisms of action of many drugs used to treat infectious diseases have been elucidated, since they produce their effects on single-celled organisms. However, with a tissue like muscle or an organ like the heart, the specialized function of the tissue or organ is not dependent solely on the vital processes going on in the individual cells; it is also determined by the way in which the cells are integrated to form the organized structure. Breaking the heart up into its chemical components and showing that one or more of them can react chemically with a particular drug will not necessarily tell us how the drug acts to produce a slowing of the rate of the beating, intact heart. But even when our understanding of the mechanism of action is incomplete, the general concepts of the ways in which drugs act are valuable in analyzing specific drug effects. These concepts are based on the propositions that a drug can produce an effect on a living organism only through *interaction* with a *functionally important molecule*, whether that molecule exists as a free entity or as part of an organized structure, and that this interaction triggers events that lead to the physiologic response.

The Concept of Receptors

The overwhelming majority of drugs show a remarkable amount of **selectivity** and **specificity** in their actions. That is to say, they act at some sites to produce their characteristic biologic effects, whereas their presence at other cells, tissues or organs leads to no measurable biologic response. This suggests that (1) there is something exceptional in the physicochemical properties of the biologic molecule at the sites where the responses are produced by drug interaction and (2) this uniqueness is absent at other sites. There is also a definite relationship between the chemical structure of a drug and the biologic effect it produces at a particular site. Sometimes a very slight modification in the chemical structure of the drug molecule yields a compound that no longer produces the same effect at the site as did the parent compound. In other instances a variety of substitutions or additions can be made in some parts of the molecule without producing a qualitative change in the characteristic pharmacologic effects, provided that certain fundamental structural features are not altered. In still other cases, changes in the effect produced at a site can be shown to occur when there are no changes in the chemical formula of the agent, but only changes in the way a few atoms are arranged in the three dimensions of space – when the compounds are **stereoisomers**.

Even from these few brief statements about the relationship of the chemical structure of drugs to their activity at a particular site, it is possible to infer (1) that there is something unique in the physicochemical properties of the tissue constituent at the site of action and (2) that the three-dimensional aspect of the site – its shape or configuration – also plays a role in determining whether an interaction with a drug will lead to a biologic effect. The macromolecules of tissue – substances such as proteins or nucleic acids – have physicochemical and spatial characteristics well suited to permit certain drugs, but not others, to interact with them. When this interaction initiates the events that lead to a biologic effect, these macromolecules are considered to be the functionally important tissue components at a site of drug action. These substances with which drugs interact to produce their characteristic biologic effects are called *receptors*.

The concept of receptors originated with the work of Paul Ehrlich (1845–1915) and J.N. Langley (1852–1926). Ehrlich coined the word receptor to help explain the high degree of specificity which he first noted in his early work on the interaction between **antibodies** and the **antigens** that stimulated their production, and later in his pioneering investigations on the reactions between synthetic organic materials and microorganisms. He postulated that all cells have 'side-chains' and that side-chains of different cells have different chemical compositions as well as a definite three-dimensional arrangement of their chemically reactive groups. He believed that drugs can be active only when bound to these side-chains, or receptors as he called them, and that chemicals can be attached only when they fit the receptors, as a key fits the lock.

Langley coined the term *receptive substance* to describe the specialized material in muscle on which drugs act. Much earlier, Claude Bernard had established that the site of action of curare, when it prevents the contraction of a muscle in response to stimulation of its motor nerve, is at the junction between the end of the nerve and the muscle. Langley showed that nicotine acts at this same site to elicit a muscular contraction and that curare can prevent this contractile response to nicotine. He then postulated that both nicotine and curare could bind to the same receptive substance, which was neither muscle nor nerve, but that only the combination of nicotine with the receptive substance triggers the contraction of the muscle. When curare combines with the receptive substance, no muscle action is elicited and, furthermore, the presence of curare prevents the binding of nicotine. Thus Langley used the concept of receptors to explain how drugs act to initiate a biologic effect as well as to inhibit one. The term receptor as used currently is defined as a specialized macromolecule that is able to recognize drugs with exquisite selectivity and, as a consequence of this recognition, sets in motion events that ultimately result in biologic response.

Binding Forces in the Drug-Receptor Interaction – Types of Bonds

According to the receptor theory of drug action, the drug must interact by *combining or binding* with the macromolecular tissue element at the site of action in order to initiate the series of events that produce its characteristic biologic effect. Therefore, there must be some forces that not only attract the drug to its receptor, but also hold it in combination with the receptor long enough to initiate the chain of events leading to the effect. These forces are the chemical bonds that hold two atoms, groups of atoms or molecules together with sufficient stability that the combination may be considered an independent molecular species. Since these forces underlie all interactions between drugs and the tissue elements of a living system, we shall briefly consider each of the four types of bonds that may be formed.

Let us first recall some features of the structure of the atom. The internal structure of the atom consists of a nucleus that has a positive electric charge and accounts for most of the mass of the atom. The nucleus is surrounded by electrons in sufficient number that their total negative charge is equal to the positive charge of the nucleus. This makes the atom electrically neutral. The simplest atom is hydrogen, which contains a single positively charged proton in its nucleus and a single negatively charged electron moving about the nucleus. Atoms larger than hydrogen also contain neutrons in their nucleus, and these, as the name implies, carry no charge. For example, carbon has six protons and six neutrons in its nucleus and six surrounding electrons; oxygen has eight protons and eight neutrons with eight surrounding electrons. The extranuclear electrons are the seat of chemical reactivity, and this reactivity is dependent on the configuration of the external electrons.

The external electrons move about the nucleus in groups and subgroups, referred to respectively as shells and subshells, each shell and subshell having a definite number of electrons that may be situated in it. The number of shells and subshells is determined by the total number of external electrons of the atom. The simplest atoms, hydrogen and helium, have only one external shell; two is the maximum number of electrons that can be accommodated in this shell. Successive shells may contain eight or more electrons, but there can be no more than eight electrons in the outermost shell of an atom *before* the next shell is started. In other words, in shells that can contain more than eight electrons, only eight enter initially, then a new shell is started and the incomplete shell is left to be filled in later. This electronic configuration of eight electrons in the outermost shell (two in the case of helium) corresponds to the structure of the inert, noble or rare gases. The chemical inactivity of these gases indicates that their configuration must be a highly stable arrangement of electrons.

All atoms try to reach chemical stability and to attain the configuration of a rare gas. They do this by giving up or taking on electrons. For example, the sodium atom, with eleven external electrons, has two closed shells, the first with two electrons corresponding to helium, the second with eight electrons corresponding to neon and the remaining electron in the third outermost shell. When the sodium atom gives up this electron to reach the configuration of neon, the resulting particle is positively charged because it now has one more proton in its nucleus than it has electrons in its surrounding shells. Chlorine, with seventeen electrons, has seven of these in its outermost shell. When chlorine accepts an electron to attain the configuration of the inert gas argon, it also loses its neutrality and becomes negatively charged. Charged particles are called *ions*. Thus, chemical reactivity is associated primarily with the electrons in the outermost shell.

THE IONIC BOND. The atoms of metallic elements, such as sodium, tend to give up their electrons easily, whereas the nonmetallic atoms, such as chlorine, tend to add electrons. These natural tendencies come into play when a metallic atom and a nonmetallic atom approach one another to form a stable molecule or crystal. In the electronic formulation of the interaction, the symbol of the element, i.e. Na for sodium, Cl for chlorine, represents the kernel of the atom, standing for the nucleus and the closed shells of electrons. The electrons of the outermost shell, the **valence** shell, are shown by dots, thus:

$$Na\cdot\ +:\ddot{\underset{..}{C}}l\cdot \longrightarrow Na^+\ +[:\ddot{\underset{..}{C}}l:]^-$$

An electron is transferred from the Na to the Cl to yield a positively charged sodium *cation* and a negatively charged chloride *anion*, each with the configuration of a rare gas. These ions are stable and retain their electronic configuration essentially independently of each other in solution and even in the solid, crystalline form. However, they are held together to form a molecule by the electrostatic attraction between them. The bond formed between atoms involving the *outright transfer* of one or more electrons from one atom to the other is called the *ionic bond*. The ionic bond is defined, then, as the electrostatic attraction between oppositely charged ions. The strength of this bond depends on the distance between the two ions and diminishes as the square of the distance between them.

THE COVALENT BOND. Whereas electrostatic attraction can explain the binding found in a simple salt like sodium chloride, or in a more complicated molecule such as that formed by heparin with a protein of the coagulation process, this type of binding can hardly account for the formation of molecules such as the gases hydrogen, H_2, or methane, CH_4, in which no ions can be detected. To explain this latter type of binding, G.N. Lewis proposed in 1916 that not only can a bond between atoms arise from outright transfer of electrons, but a rare gas configuration can also be attained from the *sharing* of a pair of electrons by the two bonded atoms. Thus we can write electronic structures such as

$$\text{H}\cdot + \text{H}\cdot \longrightarrow \text{H:H} \quad \text{or} \quad \cdot\overset{\cdot}{\text{C}}\cdot + 4\text{H}\cdot \longrightarrow \text{H:}\overset{\overset{\text{H}}{\cdot\cdot}}{\underset{\text{H}}{\text{C}}}\text{:H}$$

in which a pair of electrons held jointly by two atoms is doing double duty and is effective in completing a stable electronic configuration for each atom. Each hydrogen can claim the shared pair and thereby attain the structure of helium. And the carbon, by being able to share in its own as well as in the four acquired electrons of hydrogen, has the configuration of the rare gas neon. The bond formed when two atoms share a pair of electrons is known as a covalent bond. It is about twenty times stronger than the ionic bond and is responsible for the chemical stability of organic molecules.

Covalent bonding resulting from electron sharing also accounts for the formation of double and triple bonds in molecules. Moreover, a covalent bond can result from the sharing of electrons supplied by one atom only, the resulting bond being called a *coordinate covalent bond*. The atom contributing the electron pair is called the donor atom and in biologic systems is usually nitrogen, oxygen or sulfur. Consider the formation of ammonium ion (NH_4^+) from ammonia (NH_3) and hydrogen ion:

$$\text{H:}\overset{\overset{\text{H}}{\cdot\cdot}}{\underset{\text{H}}{\text{N}}}\text{:} + \text{H}^+ \longrightarrow \left[\text{H:}\overset{\overset{\text{H}}{\cdot\cdot}}{\underset{\text{H}}{\text{N}}}\text{:H}\right]^+$$

The ammonia molecule has four electron pairs, of which only three are shared; thus each hydrogen has attained a stable helium configuration, and the nitrogen atom with five electrons in its outermost shell has attained its complete octet. When a hydrogen ion approaches the ammonia, the nitrogen allows the hydrogen proton to share with it the free pair of electrons. But the positive charge associated with the hydrogen ion is retained by the ammonium ion complex, since there has been no net gain or loss of electrons. We shall see that this coordinate covalent bond formation is important in the ionization of drugs and in certain interactions with receptors.

THE HYDROGEN BOND. The hydrogen atom, with only a single electron, can form only one covalent or one ionic bond with another atom. The hydrogen nucleus, however, being a bare proton, is strongly electropositive. When hydrogen is bound by an ionic or covalent bond to a strongly electronegative atom, the hydrogen may further coordinate two more electrons donated by another strongly electronegative atom, such as oxygen (O), nitrogen (N) or fluorine (F). This second bond of hydrogen is referred to as the *hydrogen bond,* and it forms a bridge between two strongly electronegative groups. Hydrogen bonding may form this bridge between different molecules or may lead to the association between like molecules, as in acetic acid:

$$
\begin{array}{ccc}
& H & & & & H \\
& | & & O \cdots H-O & & | \\
H-C-C & & & & C-C-H \\
& | & & O-H \cdots O & & | \\
& H & & & & H
\end{array}
$$

The dotted lines represent hydrogen bonds; the solid lines are covalent bonds.

Although the hydrogen bond is ionic in character, its strength is less than that of a true ionic bond. A single hydrogen bond confers little stability on the association of two molecules, but *several* such hydrogen bonds can stabilize an interaction significantly. For example, in a compound like water, which can form hydrogen bonds readily, the hydrogen bonding does not stop at two molecules but may extend throughout the entire mass:

$$
\begin{array}{c}
H \quad H \\
O \\
\end{array}
$$

This association between molecules of water in the liquid state makes it more resistant to disruption by heat. This is why water has a higher boiling point than organic solvents such as chloroform, $CHCl_3$, which do not exist as associated liquids. Chloroform cannot form hydrogen bonds, since the hydrogen is attached by a covalent bond to carbon, which is not a strongly electronegative atom.

VAN DER WAALS FORCES. These are very weak attractive forces between any two neutral atoms or atomic groupings; they operate only at close range. Since the force of attraction is inversely proportional to the seventh power of the distance between the atoms, these forces decrease rapidly with a slight increase in interatomic distance.

Drug Binding at Receptors

We have stated that a drug can produce an effect on a living organism only through interaction with a functionally important molecule of that organism, and that for most drugs this means combining with a macromolecular tissue element, the receptor. We have also said that most drugs are selective in their action, combining only with certain receptors and not with others, and that receptors also show specificity by binding with some agents and not with others. Still another important characteristic of the drug-receptor interaction is that it is of sufficient stability to permit the initiation of the action-effect sequence. However, what is equally true is that for most drugs the binding to receptors is not so stable that it cannot be readily broken. In other words, the binding of most drugs to receptors is a reversible reaction. It is obvious that this selectivity, specificity and reversibility of drug-receptor interaction cannot be brought about by a single force but requires the synchronous operation of numerous bonds of the several types mentioned to achieve all these conditions.

Factors and processes involved in getting a drug to its site of action are discussed in the next two chapters. Let us consider now only what may happen once the drug is present in the immediate vicinity of its receptor. As the drug molecule approaches, the first force to be exerted must be one that can overcome the random thermal agitation of the drug molecule and draw it to its receptor. What is needed, then, is a bond that can form rapidly, is of sufficient strength to hold the molecule to the receptor and, most importantly, can exert its influence when the drug molecule is still distant from its receptor. The ionic bond formed by electrostatic attraction is best suited to this purpose. The ionic bond acts at high velocity and is stronger than the hydrogen bond and the bond formed by Van der Waals forces. Also, whereas the force of the latter diminishes as the seventh power of the interatomic distance, the force of the ionic bond diminishes only as the square of the distance. The strength of the covalent bond is many times that of the ionic bond; so strong, in fact, that unlike the other three bonds, it is essentially irreversible at ordinary body temperature. Since the drug-receptor combination of most drugs can dissociate at body temperature, covalent bond formation in their interaction is rather improbable; covalent binding to receptors is characteristic of long-lasting drug actions.

Of course, what is needed for ionic bond formation is the presence of oppositely charged groups on a drug and on its receptor. This condition is readily satisfied for most drugs: the macromolecules of the receptors contain charged groups that are available for interaction, and most drugs have one or more groups that can act as either negatively or positively charged centers of attraction. Thus, even though only one or two ionic bonds may be formed, it is probably this electrostatic attraction that first ties a drug to its receptor.

Whereas the formation of one or two ionic bonds may be sufficient to initiate drug-receptor combinations, the strength of these bonds by themselves would be insufficient to hold the drug molecule in combination long enough to promote the action-effect sequence. The ionic bond must be reinforced by other bond formation in order to overcome the energy of thermal agitation, which is great enough at 37°C to break a single ionic bond. Thus the additional attractions of hydrogen bonds and Van der Waals forces must be called upon to give the drug-receptor combination the stability essential for drug action.

The formation of one or even two ionic bonds would also be insufficient to confer much specificity or selectivity on the drug-receptor interaction. The inference was made earlier, from brief statements about the relationship between the structure of a drug molecule and its activity, that the receptor requires not only unique physicochemical properties, such as charge, but also a definite shape in order to account for specificity. To use Ehrlich's analogy, a drug can produce an effect only when it fits its receptor as a special key fits a well-designed lock. The ionic bonds can be visualized, then, as the first major notches made in the blank key which permit it to approach the lock, to penetrate, as it were, the exterior of the lock – the keyhole. The electrostatic attraction of hydrogen bonds, weaker than that of ionic bonds but still felt at a distance from the receptor, may be analogous to smaller notches in the key which bring it in still closer contact with the lock mechanism by allowing it to turn part way in the keyhole. The Van der Waals attraction, the weakest of all the binding forces, nevertheless is the force most critically dependent on the

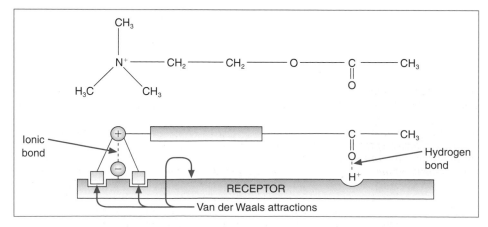

Figure 3-5. *A model for the combination of acetylcholine with a receptor (see text for explanation).*

interatomic distance between reacting molecules. The Van der Waals forces may be considered, then, as special small notches in the key whose spatial arrangement is such as to fit the lock perfectly and permit it to turn the mechanism once the key is in position to do so. The Van der Waals forces may well be the major contributing forces in determining the specificity of drug-receptor interactions. A slight misfit, one tiny notch out of place, may hinder the perfect association of the drug molecule with the complementary aspects of the receptor and, despite the other bond formations, may prevent the drug action, i.e. the turning of the lock. Thus the concerted operation of ionic bonds, hydrogen bonds, Van der Waals forces and, in some cases, covalent bonds is needed to initiate the action of most drugs and to confer specificity on this action.

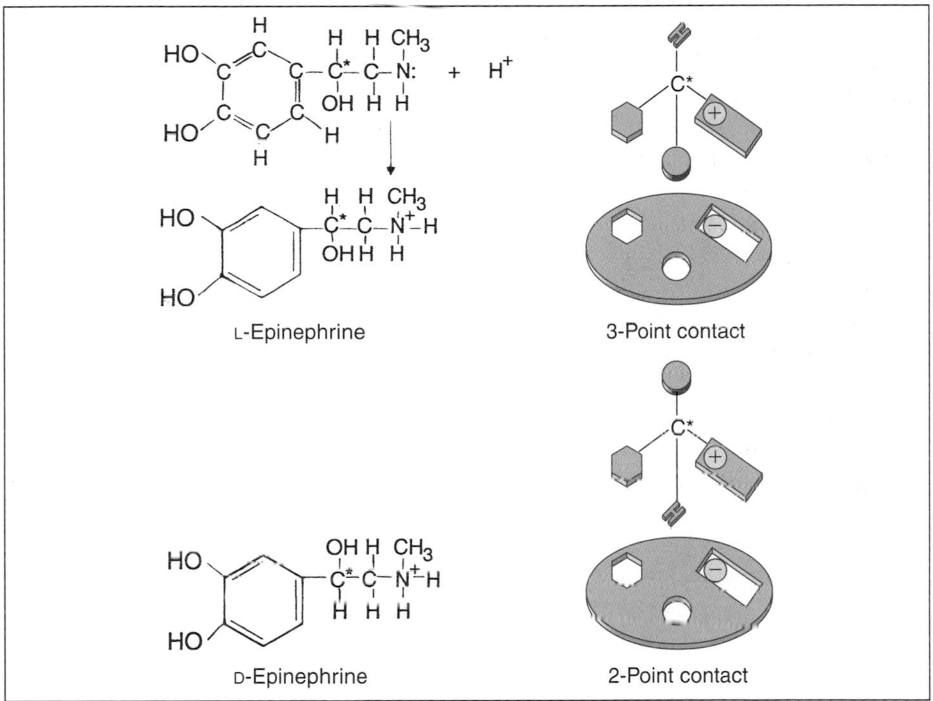

Figure 3-6. *Combination of epinephrine with its schematic receptor, illustrating the influence of the three-dimensional structure of the receptor surface. The positively charged nitrogen forms an ionic bond with an anionic portion of the receptor site; the hydrogen of the hydroxyl group attached to the asymmetric carbon engages in hydrogen bonding with an atom of the receptor site which can donate a pair of electrons; Van der Waals forces probably account for the binding of the ring to the receptor. In L-epinephrine, the spatial arrangements of the hydrogen atom and the three radicals bound to the asymmetric (*) carbon atom permit a three-point attachment to the complementary receptor. This perfect fit cannot be achieved with the D isomer. The symbol ◯ , written with or without double bonds, is the diagrammatic representation of benzene and indicates a ring structure of six carbons, each with one hydrogen atom, and alternating double and single bonds between the carbon atoms of the ring. (Modified from T.Z. Csaky,* Introduction to General Pharmacology. *New York: Appleton-Century-Crofts, 1969. p. 29.)*

Figures 3-5 and 3-6 are schematic representations of the ways in which drugs are postulated to interact with receptors. A model for the combination of naturally occurring acetylcholine with a receptor is shown in Figure 3-5. In acetylcholine, the nitrogen group has a strong positive charge which it acquired by donating its unshared pair of electrons to carbon to form a coordinate covalent bond. This is like the situation previously described for the formation of the ammonium ion, NH_4^+, in which the nitrogen atom of ammonia donated its unshared pair of electrons to the hydrogen proton. When a nitrogen atom donates this unshared pair to an atom other than hydrogen, the resulting compound is called a *quaternary ammonium compound*. The positively charged quaternized nitrogen in acetylcholine forms an ionic bond with a negatively charged group of the receptor. This electrostatic attraction may be sufficient to draw acetylcholine close to the receptor. But the stability of the bond is increased by Van der Waals forces, produced by the close fit of two of the CH_3, or methyl, groups into the cavity in which the charged site of the receptor is embedded. Van der Waals attractions may contribute additional stability to the overall binding, since the chain of carbons between the nitrogen and oxygen is pictured as lying close to and fitting a flat part of the surface of the receptor. Finally, the formation of a hydrogen bond with oxygen may draw the other end of the molecule close to the receptor and thus further increase the stability as well as specificity of the entire acetylcholine-receptor combination.

The inferences concerning individual points of binding of acetylcholine to its receptor are based on the results of studies of structure-activity relationships. That is, the structure of acetylcholine was systematically altered, for example, by changing the groups attached to the nitrogen or by changing the length of the middle chain of carbons. The ability of the new compound to produce a specific biologic effect of acetylcholine, such as contraction of muscle, was then determined. A model of the receptor for acetylcholine was subsequently formed, which was consistent with all the data obtained.

The three-dimensional aspects of the drug-receptor combination may be seen more clearly, perhaps, by the interaction diagrammed in Figure 3-6. L-Epinephrine and D-epinephrine are identical molecules with respect to the number and kinds of atoms and the distances between atoms in their structures. They differ only in the arrangement in space of the groups attached to one carbon atom. The two structures cannot be superimposed but are mirror images of each other and are, therefore, optical stereoisomers or **enantiomers**. Since the biologic effects of these two isomers differ, the inference may be drawn that the receptor surface can distinguish between these two enantiomers. Both L-epinephrine and D-epinephrine could be bound to the receptor by hydrogen bonding of the two hydroxyl (OH) groups at one end of the molecule and by ionic bond formation at the other end, where nitrogen has become positively charged by coordinate covalent bonding with a hydrogen ion. But only the entire spatial arrangement of all the atoms in L-epinephrine, the naturally occurring isomer, permits a three-point attachment to the receptor, a condition which appears to be consistent with maximum biologic effect. A molecule that has at least one pair of enantiomers is a **chiral compound** and chiral molecules frequently differ in **potency** (cf. pp. 194–196), pharmacologic action and pharmacokinetics.

That receptors do exist and are not merely conceptual constructs is now incontrovertible in light of the notable progress in the isolation, purification and determination of the molecular structures of a variety of different receptors. For example, using highly specialized and sophisticated techniques, membrane-bound receptors for acetylcholine have been isolated from various sources and shown to be high-molecular-weight **proteolipids**. Then studies utilizing radioactive chemicals as **ligands** with high affinity and specificity for the individual receptor isolated from each source yielded evidence that the putative receptor displayed binding patterns and functional properties consistent with the known pharmacologic activities of acetylcholine at the site under study. Successes have also been obtained in the isolation and identification of receptors for epinephrine as well as the insulin receptor and in the detection of highly specific binding sites for a variety of chemicals that occur naturally in the body and for drugs such as morphine or the anti-anxiety benzodiazepines (cf. Chapter 15). We can anticipate that the recent explosion in genomic information and in biotechnology will lead to the discovery of more and more important new proteins and other macromolecules as well as to knowledge of their function.

Advances in establishing the complete three-dimensional structures for nucleic acids and many proteins, including receptors, also indicate the feasibility and potential validity of many inferences made concerning the binding of drugs to receptors that may not yet have been isolated. These recent advances also provide some insight into how this binding may lead to drug action. For example, the elucidation of the three-dimensional configuration of the red blood cell protein, hemoglobin, has shown us how and where the reversible attachment of oxygen occurs in the structure. Moreover, the discovery that the *shape* of hemoglobin changes when oxygen combines with it suggests that perhaps a drug can also change the spatial configuration of a receptor upon combining with it. This drug-induced change in the shape of the macromolecular receptor may be the trigger for the biologic effect seen, for example, as muscular contraction or increased secretion.

Types of Receptors

Over the past several decades, techniques have become available to identify how the structure of a receptor is coupled to its function. Receptor binding assays have been used to identify the existence of specific receptors on membranes of various cell types that are bound by endogenous ligands (e.g. neurotransmitters, hormones) as well as drugs. Antibodies that recognize certain domains on receptor proteins have been used in immunoblotting assays to identify expression levels of receptor protein and in immunohistochemistry assays to identify specific cell types that express the receptor. The protein structure of many kinds of receptors has been elucidated with the help of x-ray crystallography and cloning using cDNA probes. In general, receptors comprise four categories, including: ion channels, G-protein-coupled receptor proteins, hormone receptors, and tyrosine kinase or growth factor receptors (see Fig. 3-7 and Table 3-1). Consider ion channels, or *ionotropic* receptors first. Ligand-gated ion channels open and close in response to the binding of a neurotransmitter or a drug to a critical binding site within the protein structure. The response, an influx or efflux of Na^+, K^+, Ca^{2+} or Cl^-, is fast – within milliseconds upon binding of a ligand. The movement of ions changes the membrane potential of excitable cells (e.g. neurons, muscle cells) to increase or decrease the rate at which the cell fires an electrical impulse. The family of ion channel receptors

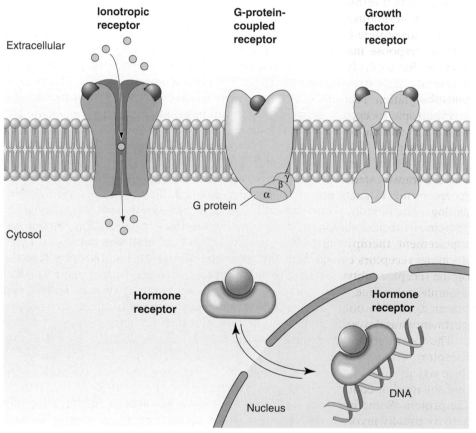

Figure 3-7. *Different types of receptors that are targets for drugs. Four major types of receptors, localized within the plasma membrane, the cytosol, or the nucleus, are targets of drugs. The ionotropic receptor contains an ion channel, which is opened or closed in response to membrane voltage or ligand binding; the metabotropic G-protein-coupled receptor regulates many intracellular signals, including enzymes and membrane permeability for ions; growth factor receptors, such as that for insulin, contain an enzymatic portion that phosphorylates other proteins; and hormone receptors, located in the cytosol or the nucleus, bind to specific sites on DNA to alter transcriptional activity, and thus, protein synthesis.*

generally have five subunits, with a central pore that is gated to allow or restrict the passage of ions. Each subunit typically has four membrane-spanning regions of the protein, with an extracellular portion and an intracellular tail. Examples of receptors that are ligand-gated ion channels are listed in Table 3-1. Drugs that act at ligand-gated ion channels include nicotine, diazepam (VALIUM), alcohol, and phencyclidine (PCP or angel dust).

Probably the most ubiquitous types of receptors are the G-protein-coupled receptors. These *metabotropic* receptors belong to a family of proteins that contain a single subunit of seven hydrophobic membrane-spanning regions. The membrane-spanning regions form extracellular and intracellular loops with extensions that terminate extracellularly (N-terminus) and intracellularly (cytoplasmic C-terminus) ('tails'). The metabotropic receptors are coupled to a guanine nucleotide-binding protein in order to elicit a cellular response. The cellular response may include activation or inhibition of adenylyl cyclase, an enzyme that controls the production of cAMP. This nucleotide derivative plays a role in signal transduction by affecting the activity of enzymes involved in phosphorylation reactions (kinases). Many clinically effective drugs act at metabotropic receptors, including compounds such as beta-blockers for hypertension, dopamine receptor antagonists for the treatment of schizophrenia, and opioids for pain.

Receptors for hormones, such as glucocorticoids, reside within the cytoplasm and are translocated into the nucleus on binding to the steroid hormone. These receptors are bifunctional, binding both to the endogenous hormone or drug analog and then to a responsive element on DNA to produce a change in protein synthesis. Often, the hormones themselves are used as drugs for replacement therapy, such as estrogen or thyroid hormone. In some cases hormone receptors can mediate opposing effects in different tissues depending on the receptor subtype or the accessory proteins to which they are coupled. For example, raloxifene (EVISTA) is an estrogen antagonist in the breast and uterus, but an agonist in bone, making it a useful drug for preventing osteoporosis in postmenopausal women.

The fourth group of receptors includes the tyrosine kinase or growth factor receptors. These receptors are typically membrane-spanning proteins that transduce signals through enzyme activation. Some receptors of this type, such as the one for insulin, contain the enzymatic function on the intracellular portion of the protein. Sometimes a separate cytosolic enzyme is involved. This enzyme activity usually involves a phosphorylation reaction such as addition of a phosphate group to a tyrosine moiety in another protein.

Other proteins act like receptors, although they are not usually classified as receptors *per se*. However, they do deserve some mention here. Transporters and enzymes are common targets of drugs (Table 3-2). The binding of a drug to these proteins follows the same laws as the binding of a drug to a receptor. Transporters belong to a family of proteins that can contain up to 12 membrane-spanning regions. They transport endogenous compounds such as neurotransmitters (e.g. monoamines, GABA, glutamate) and ions (e.g. Na^+, K^+, Cl^-)

Table 3-1. *Categorization of types of receptors that are drug targets*

Ionotropic	Metabotropic	Hormone	Tyrosine kinase/growth factor
Nicotinic acetylcholine	Muscarinic acetylcholine	Thyroid	Insulin
Glutamate (NMDA)	Glutamate (AMPA)	Estrogen	VEGF
$GABA_A$	$GABA_B$	Testosterone	Her2
Glycine	α, β-adrenergic	Gluococorticoid	BCR-ABL
$5\text{-}HT_3$	$5\text{-}HT_1$, $5\text{-}HT_2$	Mineralocorticoid	
	Dopamine		
	Opioid		
	Prostaglandins		

Abbreviations: NMDA, *N*-methyl-D-aspartate; AMPA, α-amino-3-hydroxy-5-methylisoxazole-4-propionic acid; GABA, γ-aminobutyric acid; 5-HT, serotonin; VEGF, vascular endothelial growth factor; Her2, expressed in breast cancer; BCR-ABL, expressed in chronic myeloid leukemia.

Table 3-2. *Categorization of other proteins that are drug targets*

Transporters	Enzymes
Dopamine	Cyclooxygenase
Norepinephrine	Monoamine oxidase
Serotonin	Acetaldehyde dehydrogenase
GABA	Na^+-K^+ ATPase
Glutamate	Protein kinases
NKCC	
Glucose	

Abbreviations: NKCC, Na^+-K^+-Cl^- cotransporter

across cell membranes. Most drugs that bind to transporters inhibit rather than stimulate their function. Some of the most well-known transporter inhibitors include selective serotonin reuptake inhibitors (SSRIs) for the treatment of depression; the dopamine reuptake inhibitor, cocaine; and the sodium/chloride cotransporter inhibitor, chlorothiazide (DIURIL), a diuretic used commonly for the treatment of hypertension.

Enzymes often contain a catalytic subunit. These proteins may be membrane bound, cytoplasmic, or extracellular. In general, drugs that interact with enzymes inhibit their function. Drugs that are enzyme inhibitors include non-steroidal anti-inflammatory compounds (e.g. aspirin, ibuprofen), which inhibit cyclooxygenase; the anti-arrhythmic digoxin, which inhibits the Na^+-K^+ ATPase; and selegilene (ELDEPRYL), a monoamine oxidase inhibitor for the treatment of Parkinson's disease.

Actions Not Involving Receptors

We have already noted that certain drugs act extracellularly to produce their characteristic effects without combining directly with a receptor. The neutralization of gastric acid by antacid drugs and the interaction of a small molecule like lead with an antidotal drug are true chemical reactions that produce biologic effects. However, they are not considered *receptor* interactions by the definition of a receptor, since no macromolecular tissue elements are involved. Still other mechanisms of drug action are not mediated directly by receptors. These actions may occur at cellular sites and may involve macromolecular tissue components, but the biologic effects produced are nonspecific consequences of the physical or chemical properties of the drugs.

Drugs that are used primarily to destroy living tissue, such as germicides to kill bacteria, are obvious examples of agents with a nonspecific, and thus nonreceptor, mechanism of action. Detergents, alcohol, oxidizing agents such as hydrogen peroxide and phenol derivatives like lysol all act by irreversibly destroying the functional integrity of the living cell through disruption of cellular membranes or cellular constituents, such as nucleic acids or proteins.

Another group of agents whose mechanism of action has not been shown as yet to involve direct combination with specific receptors, as they are defined, are the volatile general **anesthetics**. Their action on the living organism, however, is entirely different from that of the antiseptic agents, in that the action of the former is completely reversible and appears to involve no readily discernible chemical reactions. The inert gas xenon, the inorganic gas nitrous oxide and organic gases used in general anesthesia, along with volatile substances like ether and ethanol, all produce similar effects on the brain. Such a diversity of chemical structure, indeed the remarkable lack of any obvious common molecular feature, made it untenable that these agents produce a common pharmacologic effect by acting at a receptor with structural specificity. These agents do have some physicochemical properties – such as their solubilities in various solvents – which may be partially correlated with their pharmacologic activity. Older theories on their mechanism of action have been built around these correlations, suggesting that general anesthetic agents act by perturbing the lipid structure of cell membranes. However, newer evidence suggests that the sites of action for volatile anesthetic agents are protein in nature, indeed possibly receptors in the central nervous system, and that interaction with these sites modulates neuronal excitability. And so, until more definitive evidence is available, we can conclude that the action of general anesthetic agents involves a complex interaction with membrane lipids, proteins, and water.

On the other hand, the mechanism of action of certain other types of drugs can be adequately explained on the basis of their physicochemical properties. Certain water-soluble cathartics, such as magnesium sulfate (Epsom salt), are almost completely retained within the alimentary canal after oral administration, since both the magnesium and the sulfate of the salt are only slightly absorbed. This excess of a salt within the intestinal lumen creates a solution that is much more concentrated than normal body fluids. The body tends to compensate for this high concentration by adding water, from the blood carried in vessels within the wall of the bowel, to the intestinal contents to bring them back to a normal level, i.e. to **isotonicity**. Thus magnesium sulfate acts as a cathartic by exerting an **osmotic effect** within the lumen of the intestine to bring fluid into the intestine, to retain fluid therein and to increase the total fluid bulk of the feces. The macromolecular blood plasma substitutes used in acute blood loss act by the same principle. These substances are administered directly into blood vessels and remain within them. By exerting an osmotic effect, they help to restore and maintain an adequate volume of blood.

SYNOPSIS

The action of a drug is the process by which the drug brings about a change in some preexisting physiologic function or biochemical process of the living organism. The effects produced by a drug can be measured and expressed only in terms of an alteration of some known function or process that maintains the existence of the organism. The alteration brought about by the action of a drug may be one that either returns a function or process to normal operating levels or changes a function or process in a direction away from normal levels. Drugs may also act to prevent changes by other factors, such as disease or other drugs. Although drugs do not confer any new function on the living cell or organism, they may be precise tools to disclose and analyze, as Claude Bernard said, 'the most delicate phenomena of the living machine.'

The part of the body in which the drug acts to initiate the chain of events leading to the response – the effect – is the site of action. It may be close to the effector organ or distant from the tissue or organ that ultimately responds. It may be at the surface of the cell, inside the cell or extracellular.

The means by which a drug in the immediate vicinity of its site of action initiates the series of events measured or observed as an effect is known as its mechanism of action. The mechanism of action of most drugs is believed to involve a chemical interaction between the drug and a functionally important component of the living system. When this component is identifiable as a distinct entity, the mechanism of action can be readily explained. This is frequently the case for drugs that act at extracellular sites. However, the majority of drugs do not act extracellularly, and to help understand their mechanisms of action, the concept of receptors was formulated.

The receptor is regarded as a macromolecular tissue constituent of functional significance at the site of drug action. Drugs combine reversibly with receptors by means of ionic bonds, hydrogen bonds and Van der Waals forces. The concomitant formation of a number of these different types of bonds gives the drug-receptor complex sufficient stability to initiate the events that ultimately lead to the pharmacologic effect. For the most part, these interactions are readily reversible. The specificity and selectivity of drug-receptor interactions arise not just from the number and types of bonds formed, but also from the spatial configuration of the sites for bond formation at the surface of the receptor.

Whereas the majority of drugs produce effects by mechanisms involving a drug-receptor interaction, certain drugs produce their characteristic effects without combining directly with a functionally important macromolecule or with a receptor. The most notable among those drugs whose actions may not involve combination with receptors are the general anesthetic agents.

GUIDES FOR STUDY AND REVIEW

How do you distinguish between the effect of a drug and the action of a drug?

What are the only terms in which the effects of any drug can be expressed or measured? Do drugs produce quantitative or qualitative changes in bodily functions?

What is the site of action of a drug? What parts of the body can serve as sites of drug action? What is the relationship between the site of action of a drug and the tissue or organ of the body that ultimately responds to the drug?

The mechanism of action of most drugs involves what type of interaction? For most drugs, where does this interaction take place with respect to the cell?

What is a drug receptor? How do drugs interact with receptors? What are the forces responsible for this interaction? What force is best suited to initiate a drug-receptor interaction? What forces largely determine the specificity of drug-receptor interactions? How can the receptor concept explain the difference in the pharmacologic effect of two isomers?

What are the different classes of receptors? How does their general structure impact on their function?

May some drugs produce effects by chemical interactions other than drug-receptor interactions? Are these actions relatively specific or nonspecific? What are some examples of such interactions?

Does the mechanism of action of drugs such as the general anesthetics involve discernible chemical reactions? How have the pharmacologic effects of such agents been explained? Are there classes of drugs other than the general anesthetics whose mechanism of action may not involve a chemical reaction?

SUGGESTED READING

Campagna, J.A., Miller, K.W. and Forman, S.A. Drug therapy: mechanisms of action of inhaled anesthetics. *N. Engl. J. Med.* 348:2110–2124, 2003.

Clark, A.J. *The Mode of Action of Drugs on Cells.* London: Arnold, 1933.

Cooper, J.R., Bloom, F.E. and Roth, R.H. *The Biochemical Basis of Neuropharmacology.* New York: Oxford University Press, 2003.

Ehrlich, P. *Collected Papers* (Edited by F. Himmelweit). London: Pergamon, 1957.

Foreman, J.C. and Johansen, T. (ed.) *Textbook of Receptor Pharmacology* (2nd ed.). Boca Raton: CRC Press, 2002.

Furchgott, R.F. Receptor mechanisms. *Annu. Rev. Pharmacol.* 4:21, 1964.

Kenakin, T.P., Bond, R.A. and Bonner, T.I. Definition of pharmacological receptors. *Pharmacol. Rev.* 44:351, 1992.

Pierce, K.L.., Premont, R.T. and Lefkowitz, R.J. Seven transmembrane receptors. *Nat. Rev. Mol. Cell Biol.* 3:639, 2002.

Pauling, L. *The Nature of the Chemical Bond* (3rd ed.). Ithaca, NY: Cornell University Press, 1960.

Van Rossum, J.M. The relation between chemical structure and biologic activity. *J. Pharm. Pharmacol.* 15:285, 1963.

Zwick, E., Bange J. and Ullrich A. Receptor tyrosine kinases as targets for anticancer drugs. *Trends Mol. Med.* 8:17, 2002.

4   How Drugs Reach Their Site of Action

I. General Principles of Passage of
Drugs Across Biologic Barriers

We have seen that a drug can produce an effect only when it is in the immediate vicinity of its site of action. With the obvious exceptions of chemicals that act like the cathartic magnesium sulfate or the plasma substitutes, drugs do not make their initial contact with the body at, or even near, their locus of action. In almost all cases, drugs must move from where they are administered to the tissues or cells where they will act. For example, when aspirin is swallowed for the relief of a headache or a **hypnotic** is taken to produce sleep, these agents must go from the gastrointestinal tract to their respective sites of action in the brain to exert their characteristic effects. (One would hardly consider rubbing an aspirin on the forehead to relieve the headache!) To do this, they must pass through various cells and tissues which act as barriers to their movement. Just as receptors show specificity with regard to the drugs with which they combine, so too do barriers show a certain degree of selectivity in the ease with which they permit drugs to pass through them. Thus the anatomic structures which act as barriers to the migration of materials are called *semi-permeable*, allowing certain chemicals to pass freely, others to pass with difficulty and still others to be almost entirely excluded from passage. We have seen that the specificity of a drug-receptor combination is the consequence of the physicochemical properties and structural configuration of the receptor at the site of action as well as of the physicochemical properties and structure of the drug molecule. In an analogous way, the selectivity of migration through the anatomic barrier is the consequence of the physicochemical properties and structural configuration of the barrier as well as of the migrating molecule. We have also noted that the forces responsible for a particular drug-receptor combination are not unique to that combination but underlie all the reactions between drugs and tissue elements of a living system. In a parallel fashion, the mechanisms that serve to move a drug across a particular barrier are those which move any substance across any biologic barrier. This movement is called *biotransport*, and the mechanisms underlying the transfer of chemicals across biologic barriers are called *transport processes* or *transport mechanisms*.

Biotransport is a specific case of the general phenomenon of transport, and *transport* is defined as the translocation of a *solute* from one *phase* to another, the solute appearing in the same form in both phases. A *phase* is a homogeneous, physically distinct part of a system which is separated from other parts of the system by definite bounding surfaces. In the physicochemical sense, the boundary may be any surface we choose to designate as separating two phases, but in the biologic sense we usually mean an anatomic structure which may be the membrane separating the outside from the interior of a cell, or may even be the whole structure, such as the epidermal layer of the skin. In the biologic sense, then, the phases are the environmental conditions on either side of the anatomic barrier. The material that is transferred from one phase to another is a solute, and implicit in any discussion of biologic transport is the fact that we are talking about *chemicals in solution in biologic media*. The explicit statement that the transferred solute must be in the same form in both phases also helps to distinguish biologic transport processes from other biologic processes. For example, when the sugar sucrose is ingested, it quickly disappears from the intestine. However, its disappearance cannot be considered transport across the intestinal wall, since the substances crossing the wall are glucose and fructose, the end products of a digestive process, and not the original sucrose (Fig. 4-1). Thus *biotransport* may be defined as *the translocation of a solute from one side of a biologic barrier to the other, the transferred solute appearing in the same form on both sides of the biologic barrier.*

The principal transport mechanisms underlying movement across biologic barriers are *passive diffusion*, *facilitated diffusion*, *active transport* and *endocytosis*. Each of these will be discussed in terms of the forces responsible for the movement of solute and of the requirements of the process for energy derived from the cells or tissues of the biologic barrier.

PASSIVE DIFFUSION

Definitions

The term *diffusion* denotes the natural phenomenon by which molecules or other particles intermingle as a result of their ceaseless, chaotic motion – their inherent kinetic energy – during which they collide with each other and with the surface of any enclosure. The progression of the diffusion process can be readily observed with the naked eye if distilled water is carefully layered onto the surface of a water solution of a dye. Both water and dye molecules wander across the boundary, so that in the course of time the whole body of liquid attains nearly uniform color, i.e. uniform concentration (Fig. 4-2). If a barrier or membrane permeable to the dye molecule is placed between the two layers, the same phenomenon occurs. When the dye molecules collide with the surface of the membrane, some may pass through it from one side to the other. Obviously, the greater the number of molecules, the greater the number of collisions with the membrane and the greater the probability of transfer through the membrane.

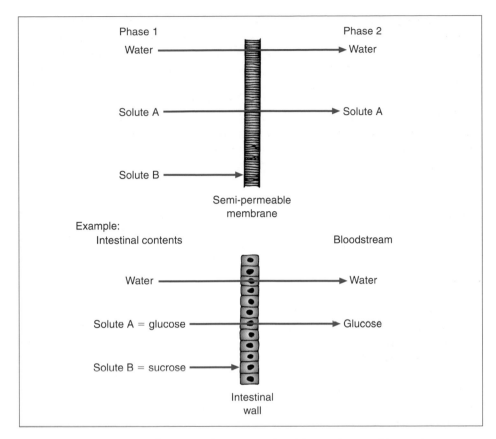

Figure 4-1. *Translocation from one phase to another. The semipermeable membrane permits the passage of water and solute A (glucose), but not solute B (sucrose) from phase 1, the side of higher concentration, to phase 2, the side of lower concentration. Sucrose may disappear from phase 1 since it is digested by intestinal enzymes and converted to glucose and fructose, which are absorbed.*

The diffusion of dye molecules through the membrane will continue from the side where there are more dye molecules – the side of higher concentration – to the side where there are fewer molecules – the side of lower concentration – until there are equal numbers on both sides, i.e. equal concentrations. When equal numbers of molecules are present on both sides of the membrane, there will still be an exchange of dye molecules between the two sides, but there will be no *net* change in numbers. Thus the transfer of solutes across a membrane by the process of diffusion, analogous to the movement of water 'downhill' from a higher to a lower level, is the consequence of the *tendency of all naturally occurring processes to change spontaneously in a direction which will lead to equilibrium.*

The force which determines the movement of solute is the difference

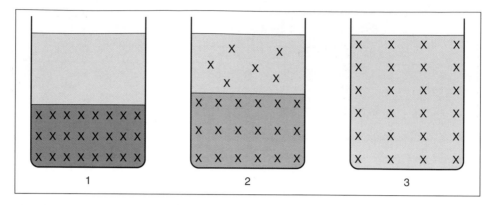

Figure 4-2. *Diffusion. In the first beaker, distilled water is carefully layered over an aqueous solution of dye. Due to thermal agitation (Brownian movement) of both water and dye molecules, the dye molecules (X) migrate into the distilled water layer and water migrates into the solution of dye (beaker 2). Equilibrium is reached with time, and the dye molecules are equally distributed throughout the entire system (beaker 3).*

between concentrations of the solute on the two sides of the membrane – the *gradient* between the two phases. No energy has to be supplied to the system since no work is done to make the molecules move from a higher to a lower concentration. Thus the process is said to be a *passive* process. We may define *passive diffusion*, then, *as the directed movement of a solute through a biologic barrier from the phase of higher concentration to the phase of lower concentration, the process requiring no direct expenditure of energy by the biologic system.*

In diffusion, any increase in concentration leads to a proportional increase in the amount of solute transferred in a unit of time. Thus the rate of migration or diffusion of the solute is proportional to the gradient between the two phases. This is illustrated in Figure 4-3 for the transfer of ethyl alcohol from the lumen of the intestine to the blood. As the ethanol crosses the intestinal wall and diffuses into the blood vessels in the tissue, it is rapidly carried away from the intestine by the circulation. Therefore the concentration of the alcohol on the nonluminal side of the intestinal barrier tends to be negligible compared with that on the luminal side. As a result, the amount of alcohol that leaves the intestine in one hour is directly proportional to the concentration of alcohol in the intestine.

Although a concentration gradient is indispensable for the passive diffusion of a solute, it does not follow that a solute will be able to diffuse across a biologic barrier just because it is in higher concentration on one side of the barrier. The concentration gradient is merely the force responsible for movement. The facility with which a solute diffuses depends on the nature of the biologic barrier itself – on those factors determining the barrier's selective permeability: the physicochemical properties of its individual constituents and the way in which

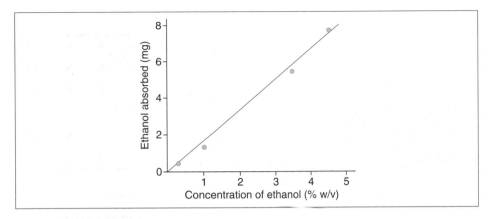

Figure 4-3. *Relationship between the amount of ethanol absorbed from the small intestine of the rat in 1 hour and the concentration of ethanol in the intestine (concentration of ethanol expressed as per cent, weight/volume × 100). (After T.Z. Csaky, First International Pharmacological Meeting Symposia, 1963. Vol. 3, p. 230.)*

these constituents are organized within the barrier structure. One would anticipate, then, that the rate of diffusion of a particular solute across the wall of the intestine might be different from that across the wall of a blood capillary even if the concentration were the same at both barriers. This is indeed true. But even though the *absolute* rates of diffusion of given solutes vary according to the characteristics of the particular barrier, the *relative* rates of diffusion of given solutes appear to be much the same regardless of the barrier involved. In other words, if we rank a group of compounds according to the rate at which they diffuse across the intestinal wall, we find that they arrange themselves in much the same order with regard to rate of diffusion across most other biologic barriers. This implies that the diverse anatomic structures that serve as barriers to the free migration of solutes must have certain similarities in their properties and organization which are noteworthy with respect to the diffusion of solutes. Knowing the characteristics which biologic barriers have in common, we should be able to formulate some general principles of passive diffusion that would be applicable to all barriers.

Membrane Structure

Regardless of whether we designate the biologic barrier as a complete tissue or organ, e.g. the wall of a capillary or of the intestine, or as particular cells which make up the tissue or organ, the organizational architecture of the tissue is such that in most cases the migration of solutes occurs through cells and not between them. In order for a solute to pass through a cell, it must, of course, first penetrate the enclosure of the cell, the *cell membrane*. The membrane, then, becomes the ultimate barrier to the migration of solutes through any biologic structure. Moreover, studies have shown that the membranes of all types of cells are remarkably alike in their overall chemical composition and in the spatial arrangement of their chemical components. Therefore the characteristics which biologic barriers share in common and which make for similarities in solute diffusion at diverse sites reduce to *the characteristics common to cell membranes*. What is this generalized view of the cell membrane and how do its structure and properties regulate the diffusibility of chemicals?

Chemical analyses of various cell membranes show that, despite differences in specific details, all cell membranes are composed chiefly of lipids and proteins. The lipids of the membrane consist mainly of cholesterol and **phospholipids**. These compounds, like proteins, have groups that can form ionic or hydrogen bonds with other appropriate groups. We have seen that water can form hydrogen bonds within itself or with other molecules having suitable atomic groupings. Compounds with groups like —OH or —NH acquire solubility in water through this tendency toward hydrogen bond formation. Accordingly, the groups which can readily form hydrogen bonds are called *hydrophilic groups*, from the Greek *hydro*, for 'water,' and *philos*, meaning 'loving' or 'a tendency toward.' The membrane lipids also have numerous groups which cannot form hydrogen bonds, such as the —CH_2— groups of the long hydrocarbon chains of the fatty acid esters in the phospholipids. They are called *hydrophobic groups*, from the Greek *phobos*, meaning 'to fear.' The hydrophobic groups of molecules tend to make the compounds insoluble in water but soluble in organic solvents. Since lipids are characterized by relative insolubility in water and by solubility in organic solvents (or fat solvents), substances which acquire fat-like solubility through their hydrophobic groups are said to be *lipid-soluble* compounds.

It is this dual nature of the membrane lipids, possessing both hydrophilic and hydrophobic groups, that causes them to orient themselves into an orderly configuration within the membrane core. The tendency of the hydrophobic portions of the molecule is to withdraw from the aqueous phase, whereas the tendency of the hydrophilic portions is to be surrounded by water. Both these tendencies must be satisfied simultaneously. This can be achieved most economically when the lipid organizes itself into two layers in which all the hydrophobic chains face each other and are surrounded by other hydrophobic chains, and all hydrophilic portions are oriented toward the water phase – toward the outer and inner membrane surfaces. In early studies of the membrane, it was thought that this bimolecular lipid layer was covered on both sides by sheets of protein. Evidence now establishes that proteins as globular molecules are dispersed throughout the lipid and, in many instances, extend from one side of the membrane to the other (Fig. 4-4). The hydrophilic groups of the protein protrude from the membrane surface and are in contact with an aqueous phase; the hydrophobic residues are buried in the interior of the membrane sequestered from contact with water. The surfaces of the membrane have the appearance of tightly packed hydrophilic groups of phospholipids interspersed with globular proteins.

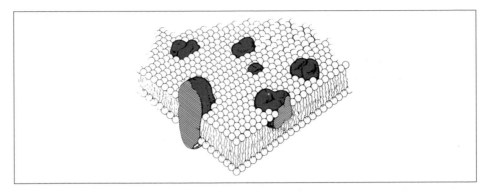

Figure 4-4. *The lipid-globular protein mosaic model of the cell membrane with a lipid matrix. Schematic three-dimensional and cross-sectional views. The circles represent hydrophilic groups of the phospholipid molecules; wavy lines represent the hydrophobic fatty acid chains; solid bodies represent the globular integral proteins.*

The interior of the membrane is more loosely ordered, since the embedded proteins produce discontinuities in the lipid bilayer that forms the matrix of the mosaic. Thus the characteristic feature of the cell membrane is a bimolecular lipid layer, oriented perpendicular to the plane of the membrane, and forming the matrix of a mosaic in which globular proteins are embedded.

Diffusion Across Membranes

The barrier action of the membrane, its ability to restrict and sometimes prevent the passive penetration of many solutes, is believed to arise from the compact arrangement of the hydrocarbon chains of the lipids within it. Historically, the concept that the cell is surrounded by a lipid membrane which acts as a barrier to free diffusion arose indirectly from studies of the actual rates of penetration of various substances into cells; it did not come from morphologic evidence obtained by microscopic examination. We have stated earlier, in the discussion of the actions of drugs which do not involve a receptor-drug interaction, that there is great diversity of chemical structure among compounds which produce the common pharmacologic effect of general anesthesia. Ernest Overton and Hans H. Meyer, at the turn of the twentieth century, carried out independent investigations intended to explain the action of general anesthetics. In doing so, they found a systematic relationship between the solubility properties of the chemicals they studied and the rates at which the chemicals entered cells.

These investigators used intact plants and animals to study the permeability characteristics of living cells. For example, Overton placed tadpoles in solutions of different alcohols and used disappearance of movement of the tadpoles as an indication of penetration of the agents into cells. He noted both the concentration at

Table 4-1. *Effect of alcohols on the movement of tadpoles in aqueous medium*

Alcohol	Formula	Concentration to produce equivalent cessation of movement (moles/liter[1])	Partition coefficient (oil/water)
Methyl	CH_3OH	0.57	0.001
Ethyl	C_2H_5OH	0.29	0.036
Propyl	C_3H_7OH	0.11	0.156
Isobutyl	C_4H_9OH	0.045	0.588

Notes

[1]See Glossary for definition of **molarity**.

Data from E. Overton, *Studien über die Narkose zugleich ein Beitrag zur allgemeinen Pharmakologie.* Jena, Germany: Gustav Fischer, 1901, p. 101; and from K.H. Meyer and H. Hemmi, Beiträge zur Theorie der Narkose: III. *Biochem. Z.* 277:39, 1935, p. 45.

which the various alcohols produced this cessation of movement and the time required for the alcohols to act. Results typical of those obtained are shown in Table 4-1. The relative rates of penetration of these four alcohols are expressed in terms of the concentration of each agent that produced equivalent effects on tadpoles. The alcohols differ from each other by the length of their hydrocarbon chains. A series of compounds whose successive members possess, in addition to structural similarity, a regular difference in formula (in this case a —CH₂— group) is known as a *homologous* series. It can be seen that the concentration required to produce an equivalent disappearance of movement of the tadpoles becomes lower and lower as the length of the hydrocarbon chain of the alcohols increases. Thus the rate of penetration increases within the homologous series, since it takes less and less of a concentration gradient to move successive members of the series to the site of action.

As might be anticipated, the addition of a hydrophobic —CH₂— group makes successive compounds less water-soluble and more lipid-soluble – it makes them less **polar** and more **nonpolar**. These changes in solubility cannot be measured, however, in terms of *absolute* solubility, i.e. how much of an agent will dissolve in water or in a lipid solvent. If absolute solubility alone were measured, we would see no differences among methyl, ethyl and propyl alcohols, since they are all infinitely soluble in water and in a fat solvent such as ether. Only isobutyl alcohol would appear to be different, since it has limited solubility in water. Differences in solubility characteristics can be demonstrated when *relative* solubilities are determined, i.e. when the tendency of an agent to *distribute* between water and lipid is measured in the presence of both an aqueous and a lipid phase. The tendency of an agent to distribute between these two phases can be expressed as the *ratio* of its concentration in the lipid phase to its concentration in the aqueous phase after the agent has come to equilibrium in the two-phase system. This ratio is known as the *lipid/water partition* *coefficient.* The lipid phase may be any fat solvent, such as ether, chloroform or a vegetable oil. Overton chose cottonseed oil as the lipid phase for his determination of the lipid/water partition coefficients of the alcohols in Table 4-1. He found that in this homologous series, the partition coefficient between the two solvents water and oil changed in favor of the latter as the chain length increased. It follows that the rate of cellular permeability of the alcohols also increased as the oil/water partition coefficient increased. Thus the lipid/water partition coefficient can be an external measure of the relative tendency of agents to leave the aqueous medium outside a cell and enter the lipid within the membrane.

Overton and Meyer summarized the results of their studies by suggesting that (1) the cell membrane is lipoid in nature; (2) the facility of substances to diffuse across the membrane is determined by their ability to dissolve in the membrane; and (3) this ability is proportional to their lipid/water partition coefficients. This view was later supported by the classic experiment of Collander and Bärlund. These investigators found a high correlation between olive oil/water partition coefficients of an extensive series of organic substances and their rates of penetration into plant cells (Fig. 4-5). Many other studies since then, using various two-phase solvent systems to determine lipid/water partition coefficients, have shown that these early findings are generally applicable to the permeability of many other types of cells. Thus one of the general principles governing the passive diffusion of substances across membranes may now be stated: *the rate of passive diffusion is dependent on the degree of lipid solubility, and compounds that are highly soluble in lipids diffuse rapidly, whereas those that are relatively lipid-insoluble diffuse more slowly.*

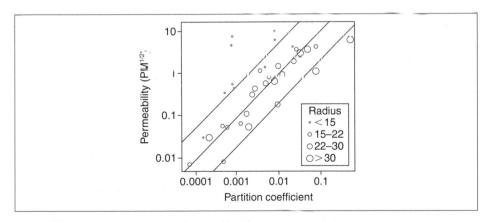

Figure 4-5. *Permeability of cells of* Chara certatophylla *to organic nonelectrolytes of different lipid solubility and different molecular size. Abscissa: olive oil/water partition coefficient. Ordinate: permeability* ($PM^{1/2}$)*; P is the permeability constant in centimeters per hour, and M is the molecular weight of the penetrating substance. Each circle represents a single compound; the radius of each circle symbolizes the molecular radius in angstroms, as indicated. (Modified from A. Collander,* Physiol. Plant. *2:300, 1949.)*

As we have said, these first deductions about the lipoid nature of the cell membrane were based on its functional properties. Only much later, after the tools of electron microscopy, polarized light microscopy and x-ray diffraction analysis became available, was it possible to obtain evidence of structure directly from observations of the cell membrane. The structure of the cell membrane that has emerged from these studies incorporates the earlier deductions concerning the bimolecular arrangement of its phospholipids. The latest findings present a different conceptual organization and role, however, for the membrane proteins.

Although Collander and Bärlund found good correlation between rates of penetration and lipid/water partition coefficients for the majority of the compounds they examined, they noticed that certain very small molecules penetrate more rapidly, and some very large molecules somewhat more slowly, than would be predicted on the basis of their partition coefficients. In Figure 4-5 the size of the symbol used for each compound indicates its relative molecular size, or molecular radius. It can be seen that many of the compounds of radius below 15 angstroms[1] are high above the line and some of those of larger size fall well below the line, indicating a deviation from the relatively good proportionality shown by the other compounds. The small molecules that diffused faster than predicted were water-soluble compounds like urea (NH_2CONH_2) and thiourea, and water itself was found to penetrate with extreme rapidity. These findings led Collander and Bärlund to propose that the surface of the cell membrane is not a continuum of lipid, but is interspersed with tiny holes through which certain molecules can leak in spite of their relative lipid insolubility.

As this 'pore theory' developed, the assumption was made that water-filled channels extend through the membrane from one side to the other and that small molecules diffuse through these hydrophilic passageways. In the fluid-mosaic model of the structure of the cell membrane, these aqueous channels are formed by the proteins that protrude from the outer surface of the membrane and traverse its entire breadth. Such passageways can open and close as the proteins are induced to undergo conformational changes; thus the membrane is not a static system but a dynamic one in constant change. In addition, the geometry and charge distribution of the proteins make the channels selective for certain ions or water molecules. On the basis of their selective permeability, these *channels* can be classified as *sodium, potassium, calcium, chloride, or water* channels. The driving force for transport of ions and other molecules is the concentration gradient between the outside and inside of the membrane. The rates at which these water-soluble entities passively diffuse are related inversely to their molecular size (the smaller the molecule, the faster it penetrates).

The slower-than-predicted rate of diffusion for relatively large organic molecules has another explanation. When a substance traverses a membrane, not only does it have to diffuse through the interior lipid of the membrane but, in

---

[1] An angstrom is a unit of length equal to one ten-thousandth of a micron or one hundred-millionth of a centimeter.

order to reach or to leave the lipid core, it has to diffuse through water-lipid interfaces on both sides of the membrane. Large organic molecules with a great number of hydrophobic groups are so water-insoluble that they may encounter difficulty in passing through the water-lipid interface, and therefore their rate of passage across the cell membrane is slowed despite the high degree of lipid solubility. Thus some water solubility conferred on a molecule by the presence of hydrophilic groups is also essential for rapid diffusion across cell membranes. We can now modify our statement of the principles governing passive diffusion to include this factor of molecule size and say that *the rate of diffusion of a solute across a biologic barrier is dependent on its lipid solubility and on its molecular size.*

Weak Electrolytes

The early investigators, in arriving at the theory concerning the relationship of the rate of passive diffusion to lipid solubility, used organic compounds which do not form ions when dissolved in water, in other words, nonelectrolytes. But the majority of the agents of pharmacologic interest are organic compounds which do form ions in aqueous solutions and which are electrolytes. Their ability to ionize, however, is different from that of inorganic compounds like sodium chloride or hydrochloric acid. Whereas inorganic electrolytes exist in water almost completely as their respective ions, only a fraction of the molecules of most organic electrolytes dissociate into ions in aqueous solution. Thus most organic electrolytes may be present in aqueous solution as both undissociated and dissociated entities. Since the conductance of electricity in solution is dependent on the number of ions present, substances like the inorganic salts are known as *strong electrolytes*, and the organic compounds, which ionize only partially, as *weak electrolytes*. The way in which these weak electrolytes diffuse across the cell membrane needs some additional clarification.

Some weak electrolytes form ions by giving up, or donating, a proton (hydrogen ion) and are called *weak acids*. Thus, for the weak electrolyte acetic acid:

$$CH_3COOH \rightleftharpoons CH_3COO^- + H^+$$

or for aspirin:

Other weak electrolytes are *bases*, which ionize by accepting a proton. In the discussion of bond formation we pointed out that certain atoms like oxygen, sulfur and nitrogen can donate an electron pair to the naked proton of the hydrogen ion to form a coordinate covalent bond and retain the positive charge associated with the hydrogen ion. Since so many drugs are organic compounds containing nitrogen, this type of coordinate covalent bond formation plays an

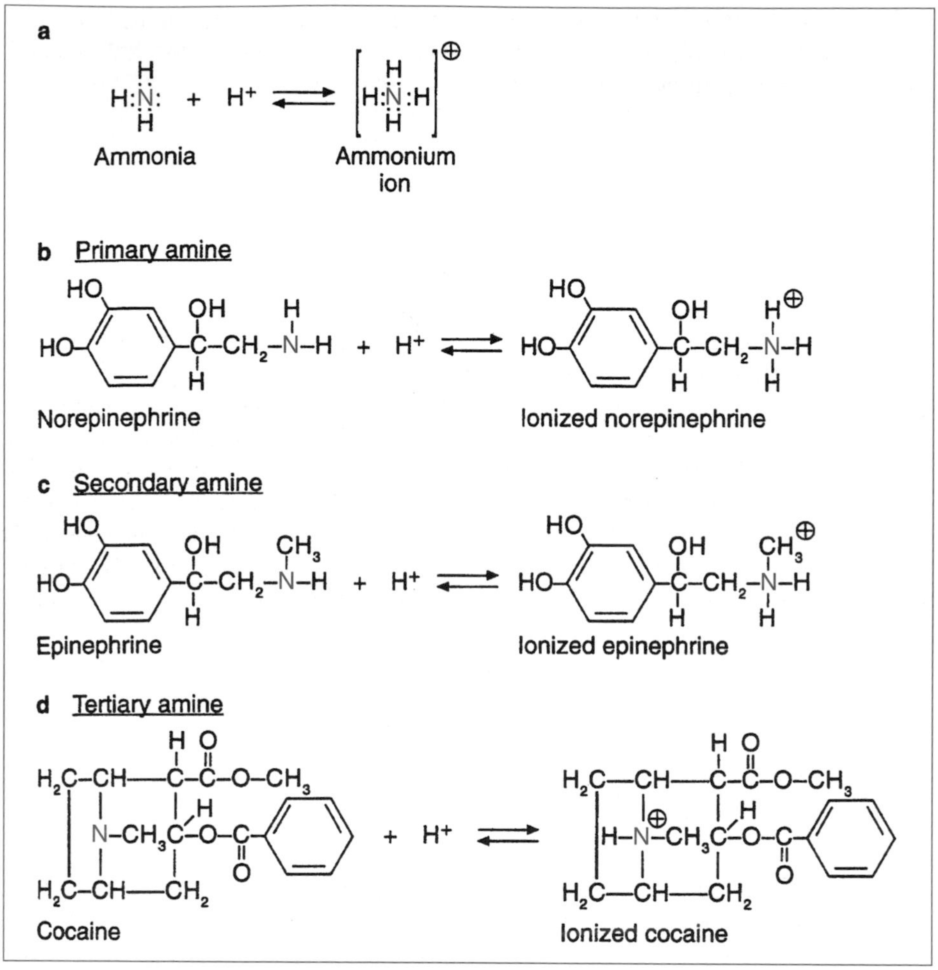

Figure 4-6. *Ionization of amines by coordinate covalent bond formation.*

important role in the ionization of drugs. Figure 4-6 shows this ionization for three different drugs. Norepinephrine, which has a nitrogen attached to only one carbon, is an example of a *primary amine*; epinephrine, with its nitrogen attached to two carbon atoms, is an example of a *secondary amine*; and cocaine, with three carbons attached to the nitrogen, is an example of a *tertiary amine*. All drugs which have one of these structures are *weak bases* and have the potential of becoming positively charged ions (cations) by the mechanism illustrated earlier for ammonia (see p. 41).

The degree to which a weak electrolyte will ionize is an inherent property of the molecule and is determined by the electron-attracting and electron-repelling properties of its constituent atoms. This tendency to ionize is a constant for a given weak electrolyte when measured in pure water at a given temperature and is expressed as the *ionization constant*. Moreover, the fraction that is ionized is always in equilibrium with the fraction that is unionized. Thus:

$$HA \rightleftharpoons H^+ + A^-$$

and

$$B + H^+ \rightleftharpoons BH^+$$

where HA symbolizes the undissociated acid and B, the unionized base.

Since such equilibria exist for the ionization of weak electrolytes, the law of mass action is applicable to them, and it is possible to change the fraction of ionized or unionized material present in solution by changing the hydrogen ion concentration. You will recall that the law of mass action states: when a chemical reaction reaches equilibrium at a constant temperature, *the product of the active masses on one side of a chemical equation, when divided by the product of the active masses on the other side of the equation, is a constant regardless of the amount of each substance present at the beginning of the action*. Thus, for an acid:

$$\frac{[H^+] \times [A^-]}{[HA]} = \text{a constant}$$

where [ ] stands for concentration. For a base:

$$\frac{[BH^+]}{[B] \times [H^+]} = \text{a constant}$$

If we add hydrogen ions to a solution of a weak acid, the concentration of the ionized portion, $[A^-]$, in the numerator must decrease and the concentration of the undissociated acid, $[HA]$, in the denominator must increase in order to keep the relationship constant. The converse would be true for the addition of hydrogen ions to a solution of a weak base. In both cases, an excess of hydrogen ions drives the ionization reaction of the weak electrolytes to the *side of the equation which does not have free hydrogen ions*. Therefore, an excess of hydrogen ions in a solution of a weak acid tends to decrease the extent of ionization of the weak acid, and an excess of hydrogen ions in a solution of a weak base tends to increase the extent of ionization of the weak base.

It is much simpler to use the convention **pH** to express the hydrogen ion concentration of a solution. The term pH refers to the negative logarithm of the hydrogen ion concentration in molar units; i.e. the logarithm of the *reciprocal* of the hydrogen ion concentration. Therefore, the higher the pH of a solution, the lower the hydrogen ion concentration, and vice versa. From the relationships between the ionization of weak electrolytes and pH, we can now draw the following generalizations: (1) the degree of ionization of a weak electrolyte is dependent on its ionization constant and on the pH of the aqueous medium in which it is dissolved; (2) the degree of ionization of a weak acid tends to be greater at higher pHs and lower at lower pHs; and (3) the degree of ionization of a weak base tends to be greater at lower pHs and lower at higher pHs.

The degree of ionization of weak acids and bases has a great deal of significance when we consider their diffusion across biologic barriers. At the pHs of biologic fluids, weak electrolytes are present partly in the ionized form and partly in the unionized form. The ionized groups of the weak electrolytes interact strongly with water, which makes them more water soluble and less fat soluble than the unionized molecule. If we consider diffusion only in terms of a solute's ability to dissolve in the membrane lipid, then the ionized form of a weak electrolyte would diffuse across the membrane much more slowly than the more lipid-soluble, unionized form. However, in the case of ions, an additional barrier to passage through the membrane may arise from their interaction with negatively or positively charged groups at the protein surfaces. These two factors – the greater electrical resistance to passage and the much lower lipid solubility – combine to make the rate of penetration of the ionized form so slow that, for all practical purposes, the rate of diffusion of a weak acid or base may be entirely attributed to the concentration gradient of the unionized fraction itself. For weak electrolytes, then, we must now add another factor to the general principles governing their passive diffusion across cell membranes: *The rate of passive diffusion of weak electrolytes is dependent on their degree of ionization: the greater the fraction that is nonionized, the greater the rate of diffusion, since the rate of diffusion is mainly determined by that of the* nonionized *portion*.

The stability of the pH of most fluids within the body is vigorously maintained at levels near neutrality by the body's regulatory mechanisms. But the fluids within the stomach are characteristically at a low pH, whereas those within the intestines vary from a relatively acid pH near the stomach to more neutral values farther from it. The pH of the urine as it is formed in the kidney can be either lower or higher than 7 under various normal conditions. In certain abnormal states, even the pH of plasma or other body fluids may be above or below their normal range.

It can be readily appreciated, then, that the degree of ionization of a given compound may vary considerably at different biologic barriers or at a particular barrier under different conditions of pH. It follows from the relationship between rate of diffusion and degree of ionization that the rate of penetration of a weak electrolyte across a particular barrier also depends on the pH of its solution at the barrier site. This is well illustrated by the results obtained in studies of the effect of pH on the absorption of the weak base strychnine from the stomach of animals (Table 4-2). At pH 8, more than half of strychnine exists in solution in the more lipid-soluble, unionized form. Consequently, when strychnine was administered in alkaline medium, it rapidly crossed the stomach wall as measured by the fact that the animals died within a relatively short time. In contrast, when an equivalent amount of strychnine was administered in solution at pH 3, the concentration gradient of the unionized form was markedly

Table 4-2. *Effect of pH on rate of absorption of strychnine from the stomach*[1]

pH of solution in stomach	% Undissociated strychnine	Interval to death following injection (min)
8	54.0	24
6	1.2	83
5	0.1	150
3	0.001	Survived

[1]Strychnine (5 mg) was injected into the ligated stomach of anesthetized animals.
Source: Modified from J. Travell, *J. Pharmacol. Exp. Ther.* 69:21, 1940.

reduced. As a result, the rate of absorption of the poison from the ligated stomach was insufficient to produce any deleterious effects.

In summary, then, passive diffusion may be defined as a transport process in which the driving force for movement across the cell membrane is the concentration gradient of the solute, the rate of diffusion being proportional to this gradient and dependent on the lipid solubility, degree of ionization and molecular size of the solute. For drugs that are weak electrolytes, the rate of passive diffusion will depend on the pH of the fluid on both sides of the membrane. In contrast, for drugs that have fixed negative or positive charges regardless of pH, the rate of passive diffusion through cell membranes does not depend on pH and is likely to be relatively slow.

SPECIALIZED TRANSPORT PROCESSES

If cell membranes were simple lipid barriers interspersed with aqueous channels, cells would have little discriminatory power to move material into or out of its environment, except by virtue of size, solubility and charge of the solutes. Cells must have greater latitude than this for acquiring substances needed as energy sources or building materials and for getting rid of waste products. Indeed, cell membranes are able to distinguish between optical isomers of sugars and amino acids as well as among a variety of other substances, irrespective of their lipid solubility, molecular size and charge. Also, many substances of physiologic importance, such as glucose, penetrate membranes at rates much faster than would be predicted merely on the basis of passive diffusion and the properties of an inert barrier. Specialized transport processes in which the barrier plays an active role can account for these and many other experimental observations. These specialized transport processes give the cell membrane the flexibility and selectivity it requires to control the movement of specific substances into and out of the cell.

Facilitated Diffusion

Many molecules, especially those which are primarily hydrophilic, show peculi-
arities in their diffusion through membranes even though their movement is
with the concentration gradient and ceases when the gradient disappears. First,
as already mentioned, the rate of penetration for many substances is greater
than would be expected on the basis of either their lack of lipid solubility, as in
the case of glucose, or the presence of a charge, as in the case of many ions such
as the sodium ion. Furthermore, optical isomers with the same lipid solubility
and the same charge may have very different rates of penetration. What is also
observed is that the rate of penetration is initially proportional to the concentration gradient, but as the gradient increases, the rate no longer increases and,
instead, reaches a limiting or maximal value (Fig. 4-7). This phenomenon differs
from what happens in passive diffusion, in which the rate of diffusion always
increases with a rise in the concentration gradient, provided that the cell membrane is not structurally damaged by high concentrations of solute. One may
also frequently observe that the rate of diffusion of a particular compound is
markedly reduced by the presence of another compound of similar chemical
structure.

   The transport processes with these characteristics are obviously diffusion
processes since, by definition, the driving force is a concentration gradient. But
how can we account for the other characteristics which are so different from
those of simple passive diffusion? To explain the specificity and selectivity of
drug action, the concept of receptor was developed. And to account for the
analogous properties of specialized transport processes, a similar concept was

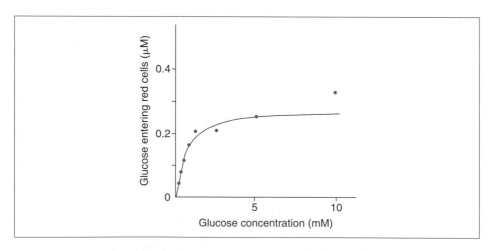

Figure 4-7. *Facilitated diffusion of glucose into human red blood cells. Abscissa: glucose
concentration (mM) in the bathing medium. Ordinate: μM glucose entering intracellular
water (1 ml) of red blood cells during 15-second incubation at 5°C. (Modified from W.D.
Stein,* The Movement of Molecules Across Cell Membranes. *New York: Academic, 1967.
p. 134.)*

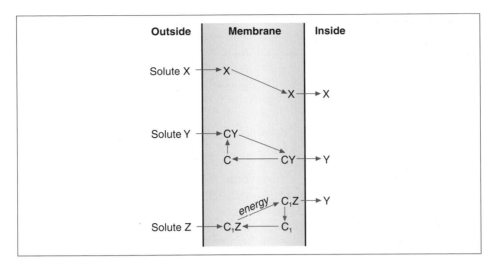

Figure 4-8. *Passive diffusion, facilitated diffusion and active transport.* X *is a lipid-soluble drug, freely diffusible in the membrane.* Y *is a lipid-insoluble drug which combines with carrier,* C, *at the outside surface of the membrane to form a complex,* CY, *which moves across the lipid membrane. At the inner surface of the membrane,* CY *dissociates to release* Y *into the intracellular space. Both* X *and* Y *are transferred with the concentration gradient.* Z *is a drug, insoluble in the membrane, which combines with carrier* C_1. Z *is actively transported against a concentration gradient.*

formulated. The specificity and selectivity of solute transport was postulated as arising from temporary binding of solute to some site or component of the membrane. This postulated binding site was given the name *carrier*, and since binding of carrier and solute facilitates the transmembrane movement of solute, the process has been termed *facilitated diffusion* (Fig. 4-8). Carriers are now also referred to as *transporters*.

Transporters, as in the case of receptors, have special groups or structural configurations that lead to their binding only with solutes that are complementary. Also, the interaction between the transferred molecules and the transfer system is reversible and does not modify the solute or the carrier. This implies that the temporary binding involves the same kind of bond formation that can occur between a drug and its receptor – hydrogen bonding, ionic bonding and Van der Waals attractive forces. Proteins have the properties necessary to impart the specificity characteristic of carrier transport systems. And the molecular structures of many membrane transport proteins now have been determined.

The binding of a solute to a membrane transporter and the subsequent process of movement through the membrane may markedly increase the rate at which the solute can diffuse into or out of a cell. However, the availability of binding sites on the carrier protein is necessarily limited; the rate of diffusion will be proportional to the concentration gradient only as long as there is sufficient carrier to accommodate all the solute. A limit to the rate of diffusion is reached at higher concentration gradients, when the carrier ability is saturated.

Facilitated diffusion may be defined, then, as a transport process in which the driving force for movement across the cell is the concentration gradient of the solute, the rate of diffusion being dependent on the binding capacity of the solute and its carrier and being limited by the availability of carrier. As in passive diffusion, no cellular energy is required beyond that needed to maintain the integrity of the cell and cell membrane. But in facilitated diffusion, the membrane can no longer be considered an inert barrier, as it is in passive diffusion, since it participates by making carrier available for the transfer of solute.

A number of physiologically important facilitated diffusion systems have been adequately characterized. Their presence at most cell membranes favors the cell's acquisition of essential substances, such as sugars, amino acids and various ions. For drugs, there is evidence to conclude that facilitated diffusion processes exist for the transport of some water-soluble agents.

Active Transport

In some cases of carrier-mediated transport, the solute continues to move across the membrane even though there no longer is a concentration gradient in the direction of movement. Obviously, the driving force cannot be the concentration gradient, since the migration proceeds beyond the concentration equilibrium and, in fact, against a higher concentration. This movement across the membrane from the side of lower concentration to that of higher concentration is analogous to water being raised from a lower to a higher level. In both instances work has to be done, and this requires energy. The energy needed to transport a solute 'uphill' must be supplied by the cell. Generally, this energy is derived from adenosine triphosphate (ATP), which releases energy upon removal of a phosphate group. Thus the cell is now actively involved in the transport process, and these processes are accordingly termed *active transport* (Fig. 4-8). With the exception of this requirement for expenditure of energy by the cell, the characteristics of active transport are the same as those for facilitated diffusion. Thus, *active transport* is defined as a transport process requiring energy of cellular origin to move solute across a biologic barrier from a lower to a higher concentration, the rate of transport being dependent on the binding capacity of the solute and its carrier and being limited by the availability of carrier.

The physiologic need for transport systems that will allow a cell to accumulate substances essential for growth and maintenance and to eliminate waste products against concentration gradients is obvious. It is not surprising that active transport processes have been shown to exist for ions, sugars, amino acids, some vitamins and various other substances vital to the cell. The active transport of drugs includes, but is not limited to, those agents that bear structural similarities to normal body constituents and to water-soluble compounds that share processes used for elimination of waste products. The active transport of drugs has been demonstrated in many sites in the body, including the kidneys, the liver, the intestinal tract, and the vasculature of the central nervous system. Determination of the molecular compositions of membrane transporter proteins has revealed common structural features, including binding sites for ATP and weaving of the protein strand in and out of the cell membrane with twelve 'membrane-spanning' regions. Transporters are expressed not only in normal mammalian cells, but also in cancer cells and in microorganisms such as bacteria and malaria-causing protozoa. Changes in the amount and function of these transporters can modify the effect of drug substrates and represent one mechanism of drug resistance to chemotherapeutic agents (see Chapter 12).

Endocytosis

Endocytosis involves the infolding of a microscopic part of the cell membrane, local invagination, and the subsequent budding off within the cell interior of this small sac, or vesicle (Fig. 4-9). Substances outside the cell engulfed by the invagination enter the cell without crossing the cell membrane. Endocytotic transport includes pinocytosis, phagocytosis, and receptor-mediated endocytosis. The transfer process of pinocytosis almost defines itself in its derivation from the Greek *pino*, meaning 'I drink', *kytos*, meaning 'hollow vessel' (denoting a cell), and *osis*, 'a process'. Pinocytosis is just that: the engulfing of fluid by a cell. In some cases, particulate matter can also be transferred by local invagination of the cell membrane; but then the process is more properly termed *phagocytosis*, from the Greek *phagein*, 'to eat'. Endocytosis may also result from the interaction of a solute with a membrane protein. The interaction triggers the invagination process, a phenomenon called receptor-mediated endocytosis. This form of endocytosis only occurs at sites where the receptor is present in the membrane and is only elicited by substances that bind the receptor. The process of engulfing particles or dissolved materials by vesiculation is the most primitive mechanism for the ingestion of food. In the course of evolution the process was lost, but not completely, since the intestinal cells of newborn mammals still possess the ability to absorb certain substances by pinocytosis. In the newborn calf, for example, the capacity for absorbing soluble protein by pinocytosis is present at birth but disappears shortly thereafter. Poisoning by botulinus toxin and allergic reactions resulting from the ingestion of offending proteins (cf. **antigens** in the Glossary) are well-known phenomena in humans and certainly leave no doubt that the adult mammal can absorb intact macromolecules. The amount absorbed appears to be extremely small, however, and mechanisms other than pinocytosis may be responsible. Pinocytotic activity is rather marked at other biologic barriers, such as the alveoli of the lungs and the walls of blood vessels. Whether the numerous vesicles that are seen at these barriers account for the transfer of solute has not always been related as cause and effect. Certainly this process cannot represent the transfer mechanism for large quantities of materials, since the number of vesicles that would have to be formed would be beyond possibility.

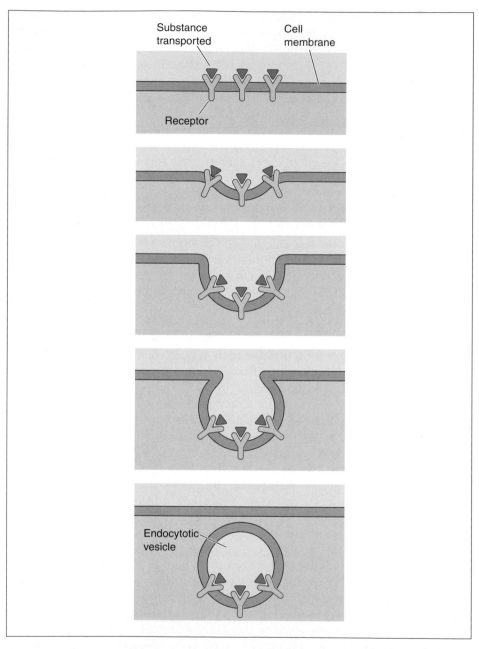

Figure 4-9. *Stages of endocytosis. Macromolecular solutes in contact with the membrane are trapped in microscopic cavities or cups – invaginations – formed on the surface of the membrane. The membrane fuses around and completely encloses the fluid to form a vesicle. The vesicle is pinched off, passing some fluid and solutes across the membrane into the interior of the cell. Some solutes may bind a membrane receptor which triggers the endocytotic process.*

Receptor-mediated endocytosis is an important transport mechanism for targeting drugs to certain cells. That strategy has been used successfully by designing drugs to mimic an endogenous protein, transported by receptor-mediated endocytosis. The protein analog can be synthesized using new techniques of biotechnology so that it binds to specific membrane receptors and therefore gains access by endocytosis only to those cells that have the receptor.

FILTRATION

Filtration is the process in which the solids and liquid of a system are separated by means of a porous membrane that allows passage of fluid, solutes and some particulate materials, while retaining particles too large to pass through the pores. It is a purely physical process in which the driving force for movement is a *pressure gradient*, the rate of filtration being dependent on this gradient and on the size of the particle to be filtered in relation to the size of the pore. Thus filtration is markedly different from the transfer processes already described.

We know that intact proteins can pass through various biologic barriers such as the capillary wall, and at the capillary level at least, their rate of movement is strongly dependent upon a pressure gradient. So when we consider filtration in terms of a biologic barrier, the process generally does not occur *across cell membranes* but *through spaces between cells*. Filtration can be important for the movement of large macromolecules and is an especially important process in the formation of urine and the ultimate elimination of substances from the body.

SYNOPSIS

Drugs or chemicals foreign to the body move across biologic barriers using the preexisting processes that serve to transport substances required for the maintenance and growth of living organisms. This movement of solutes across complex barriers is determined by the general principles governing transport across the membranes of cells which constitute the barrier. The membranes of all cells have functional similarity derived from their similar structural organization and chemical composition. The cell membrane is a structure containing a bimolecular layer of lipids with the hydrophobic groups of the lipid oriented toward each other and the hydrophilic groups aligned at both surfaces. This lipid bilayer forms the matrix of a mosaic in which proteins are embedded; the highly polar and ionic groups of the proteins protrude into the aqueous phase, and the nonpolar residues are largely buried in the interior of the membrane. These membrane proteins perform many important functions, including (1) contributing to the strength of the membrane; (2) acting as enzymes (cf. p. 154) to catalyze chemical reactions; (3) acting as carriers for transport of substances through the membrane; (4) providing discontinuities in the lipid bilayer which then serve as 'pores' for passage of water-soluble materials through the membrane, and (5) acting as receptors.

The mechanism underlying biotransport can best be defined in terms of the forces responsible for movement of the solute and of the requirements of the process for cellular energy. Basic to all the mechanisms is the cellular energy needed to maintain the integrity and organization of the cell and its membrane. *Passive*, or *simple, diffusion* requires no additional expenditure of cellular energy, and movement occurs in the direction of the concentration gradient and in proportion to the physical force provided by the gradient. The rate of passive diffusion is also determined by the lipid solubility, the degree of ionization and the molecular size of the solute. *Facilitated diffusion*, like passive diffusion, requires no further expenditure of cellular energy, and movement occurs only with the concentration gradient. It differs from passive diffusion in that the physicochemical properties of the constituents of the membrane and those of the solute are insufficient to account for the rate of movement of the solutes. Therefore, the concept of temporary combination of solute with a particular chemical structure or site – *carrier* – of the membrane must be invoked to explain the total phenomenon. *Active transport* also requires the concept of carrier-mediated passage across the membrane, but it is clearly distinguished from facilitated diffusion by the movement of the solute in a direction opposite to that of the concentration gradient. Thus active transport requires an energy source for the work to be done in moving the solute 'uphill.' *Endocytosis* is a transport mechanism also requiring an expenditure of cellular energy. It entails the local invagination of the cell membrane and subsequent budding off of a vesicle containing fluid, particulate, or solute bound to a membrane protein.

Nonelectrolytes, with the exception of very small or very large molecules, can diffuse passively across biologic barriers at rates proportional to their lipid/water partition coefficients. Very small molecules appear to move faster, and very large ones slower, than would be predicted on the basis of their lipid/water partition coefficients. Weak electrolytes, among them the majority of compounds of pharmacologic interest, diffuse passively across cell membranes at rates which are relatively proportional to their degree of ionization and to the lipid/water partition coefficient of their unionized form. These general principles apply equally to substances of physiologic and pharmacologic importance. Many of the former are nonelectrolytes such as glucose, weak electrolytes such as amino acids or strong electrolytes such as inorganic ions. For these poorly lipid-soluble substances, the specialized transport processes of facilitated diffusion and active transport are available to assist their rapid ingress into or egress from cells. Agents of pharmacologic interest may also use the specialized transport processes that entail reversible interactions with a membrane transporter protein.

Relatively small water-soluble molecules and charged ions may diffuse across cell membranes at rates inconsistent with their nonlipophilic structures. This biotransport may result from direct passage of water through channels within large protein molecules that are embedded in the lipid bilayer and traverse the entire thickness of the membrane. At some biologic barriers the spaces *between* cells provide a means of more ready passage for some substances. At these barriers, the process of filtration, proportional to a *pressure* gradient and related to the size of the transferred molecules, can account for the movement of these solutes.

GUIDES FOR STUDY AND REVIEW

What common characteristics do diverse biologic barriers have that account for similarities in solute movement at different sites? What is the general view of the cell membrane and how do its structure and properties regulate solute transport?

What are the mechanisms that account for the transfer of drugs (or other solutes) across biologic barriers? How do these mechanisms differ from one another?

In passive diffusion, what is the force responsible for solute movement and what are the requirements of the process for cellular energy? How do lipid solubility, degree of ionization and molecular size influence the rate of passive diffusion? How does an alteration in pH affect the diffusion of a weak acid? a weak base? Does a change in pH affect the diffusion of a strong acid? a strong base?

In facilitated diffusion, what is the force responsible for solute movement, and what are the requirements of the process for cellular energy? How does facilitated diffusion differ from passive diffusion? What factor determines and what factor limits the rate of facilitated diffusion?

What factor clearly distinguishes the process of active transport from the processes of passive and facilitated diffusion? Why is active transport essential for the life of the cell?

What is endocytosis? What role may this process play in the movement of drugs across biologic barriers?

How does the process of filtration differ from other transport processes with respect to the pathway of solute movement across a cellular barrier? How does the process of filtration differ from other transport processes with respect to the force responsible for transfer across a barrier? How does molecular size influence filtration? At what biologic barrier is filtration an important transport process?

SUGGESTED READING

Ambudkar, S.V., Dey, S., Hrycyna, C.A., Ramachandra, M., Pastan, I. and Gottesman, M.M. Biochemical, cellular, and pharmacological aspects of the multidrug transporter. *Annu. Rev. Pharmacol. Toxicol.* 39:361–398, 1999.

Ayrton, A. and Morgan, P. Role of transport proteins in drug absorption, distribution and excretion. *Xenobiotica* 31:469–497, 2001.

Berne, R.N. and Levy, M.N. (eds) *Principles of Physiology* (3rd ed.). St Louis: Mosby, 1999.

Clark, D.E. and Grootenhuis, P.D. Predicting passive transport in silico – history, hype, hope. *Current Topics in Medicinal Chemistry* 3:1193–1203, 2003.

Cohn, V.H. Transmembrane movement of drug molecules. In: B.N. La Du, H.G. Mandel and E.L. Way (eds), *Fundamentals of Drug Metabolism and Drug Disposition*. Melbourne: Krieger Publishing Co., 1979.

Conner, S.D. and Schmid, S.L. Regulated portals of entry into the cell. *Nature* 422:37–44, 2003.

Davson, H. and Danielli, J.F. *Permeability of Natural Membranes*. New York: Cambridge University Press, 1952.

Lodish, H.F. and James, E. The assembly of cell membranes. *Sci. Am.* 240:48, 1979.

5   How Drugs Reach Their Site of Action

II. Absorption

In order for a drug to exert its characteristic effects, it must reach its site of action. This usually entails movement, since most drugs make initial contact with the body some distance away from where they act. Although the transport processes described in Chapter 4 can account adequately for passage of drugs across any biologic membranes that impede their progress, they can hardly explain movement over a great distance. The forces that drive passive or facilitated diffusion, or active transport and endocytosis, are sufficient only to move solutes across the very short span of cellular membranes themselves. How, then, is the movement of drugs over greater distances accomplished? Just as oxygen from the lungs or food substances from the intestine gain access to every cell of the organism by way of the bloodstream, so too does the circulatory system serve as the *common pathway* for carrying drugs from the *inner side* of a biologic barrier to any tissue or organ. Hence, unless a drug is administered purposely to produce its effect locally or is injected directly into the bloodstream, access to its site of action involves two separate processes. The first of these is *absorption*, the movement of the solute into the bloodstream from the site of administration. The second process is *distribution*, the movement of solute from the blood into the tissue (Fig. 5 1).

The rate at which a drug reaches its site of action depends on both its rate of absorption and its rate of distribution. These rates, in turn, are determined by the rates of translocation across the specific barriers interposed between the sites of absorption and action. We have already seen that there are notable similarities in the movement of materials across any biologic barrier. No matter how grossly different the barriers, the mechanisms responsible for solute movement are those that serve to transfer material across any cell membrane. In addition, the principles governing these transport mechanisms apply equally at all barriers. However, barriers may differ with respect to the contribution of filtration, carrier-mediated, and endocytotic transport to the overall translocation process. In addition, the overall movement of materials across different biologic barriers depends upon the anatomic arrangement of the barriers themselves within their contiguous environment.

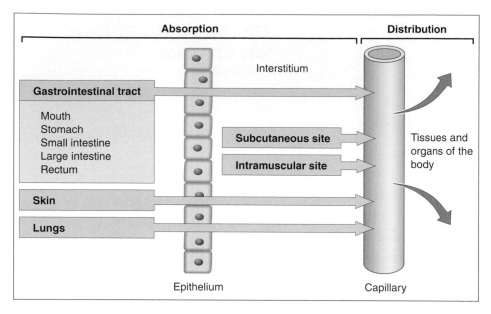

Figure 5-1. *Absorption and distribution. Drugs entering the body by way of the gastrointestinal tract, skin or lungs must first traverse an epithelial barrier before entering the interstitium. Drugs given subcutaneously or intramuscularly bypass the epithelial barrier. Drugs given by any of the routes shown must traverse the capillary wall in order to enter the circulation.*

From the physiologic viewpoint, the differences in the structure of biologic barriers subserve their particular function in relation to their normal external environment. For example, an alcohol sponge bath can be used to cool the body of a fevered child without the danger of producing any of the symptoms that would follow if the same quantity of alcohol were ingested by the child. The normal function of the skin is to protect the individual from material of the external environment, whereas that of the alimentary canal is to afford a more or less open gateway into the body for materials of exogenous origin. And the structure of each of these barriers is such that its main function can be realized.

Let us now examine some of these biologic barriers more closely to see how each structure with its normal physiologic function and its normal environmental conditions influences the absorption of drugs. In Chapter 6 we shall consider these same variables with respect to the distribution of drugs.

ROUTES OF ADMINISTRATION

We defined absorption as the movement of solute from the site of administration across a biologic barrier into the bloodstream. To be more explicit, this definition should also embrace the movement of solute into the *lymphatic system* – the tubular system that supplements the blood circulation. This second vascular

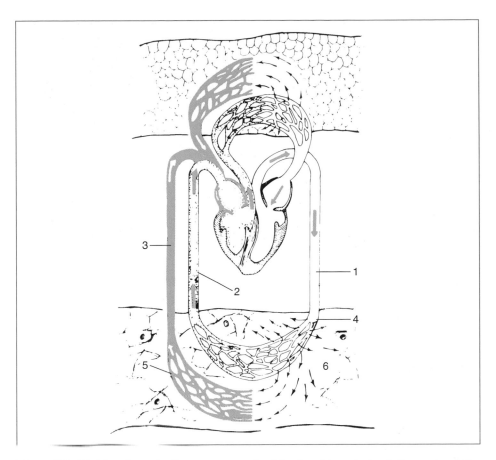

Figure 5-2. *Highly schematic diagram comparing blood and lymph circulation: artery (1); vein (2); lymphatic vessel (3); blood capillary (4); lymph capillary system (5); and interstitial space (6).*

system is like the blood vasculature, in that the smaller lymphatic tubules resemble capillaries and the large vessels, called lymphatic ducts, are comparable to veins. But the lymphatic system has no vessels corresponding to arteries; its fluid, lymph, does not flow in a circuit and is not self-contained. Lymph flow begins in the lymphatic capillaries, which collect fluid from the tissue spaces, and ends at the level of the neck where the chief vessels, the thoracic duct and the right lymphatic duct, empty into the large veins (Fig. 5-2). Thus the lymph functions only to deliver or carry back to the bloodstream substances, particularly water and macromolecules, that have entered the extracellular fluid from the cells or the blood capillaries. Indeed, in the intestinal tissue, the lymphatics serve as the chief route by which nutrients like fat and proteins make their way to the blood after leaving the intestine. Since the lymphatics can act as potentially important channels for absorption of materials that have gained access to interstitial fluid, we should amplify our statement of absorption: *only after a substance has entered the blood or lymph capillaries can it be said to be truly absorbed.*

It follows from the definition of absorption that an important factor in determining the rate of entry of a solute into the circulation after its passage through the barrier is the vascularity at the site of absorption. The greater the vascularity, the greater the flow of blood and lymph within the tissue, and the greater the opportunity for removal of a drug from tissue into the circulation. Since the rate of blood flow is many hundred times that of lymph flow, the *amount of blood flowing* through the tissues on the inner side of the biologic barrier is really the determinant of the rate of absorption for most substances. Consequently, one of the environmental variables we shall have to consider with respect to the overall absorption at each site of administration is blood flow. This factor is equally important, as we shall see, in determining the rate of distribution of drugs to various organs and tissues.

In humans and other terrestrial mammals, the lungs, the alimentary canal and the skin represent the most important sites of absorption of material from the external environment. When a drug or chemical is a *therapeutic agent* used in the treatment, prevention, cure or diagnosis of disease, the gastrointestinal tract is the most commonly used route of administration. Placement of a drug directly into any part of the gastrointestinal tract is called *enteral* (Gk. *enteron*, 'an intestine') administration. This includes the usual mode of administration, i.e. swallowing the drug (oral, per os, p.o.), as well as placing the drug under the tongue (sublingual) and administration into the rectum. Other routes are called *parenteral* (Gk. *para*, 'aside from'), since they bypass the gastrointestinal tract. Thus the administration of drugs by injection, by topical application to the skin, or by inhalation through the lungs are all parenteral. The most common routes of injection are subcutaneous (s.c.), intramuscular (i.m.) and intravenous (i.v.).

From the standpoint of absorption, the various routes of administration can be more conveniently classified into those used primarily for *local effects* and those used for *systemic effects* (Table 5-1). The former do not require the intervention of the vascular system to get the drug to its site of action; agents may be regarded as acting locally when the manner of their placement ensures effects without the necessity of being distributed by the blood. As examples we can cite the application of hydrocortisone cream to the skin for treatment of poison ivy, the use of nose drops to ease nasal congestion, and the intradermal injection (placement into the upper layers of the skin) of local anesthetics for minor surgical procedures on the skin itself. The routes used for systemic effects require both absorption of the agents into the circulation and their distribution by the blood to the cells and tissues capable of responding to them. Only after intravascular administration is absorption completely bypassed; drugs are ready for immediate distribution to the various tissues of the body. We shall discuss only those routes that involve the more important sites from which chemicals or therapeutic agents enter the body.

Table 5-1. *Administration of drugs*

For local effect	For systemic effect
Application to skin	Application to skin (transdermal delivery device)
Application to mucous membranes	Sublingual administration
Nose	Oral administration
Throat	Rectal administration
Mouth	Inhalation
Eye	Subcutaneous administration
Genitourinary tract	Intramuscular administration
Oral administration (limited) – only for	Intravenous administration
cathartics, antacids, or drugs used to treat	Intrathecal (injection into spinal
parasitic or bacterial infections of	subarachnoid space)
gastrointestinal tract	
Various techniques for administering local	
anesthetics or agents useful in pulmonary diseases	

ABSORPTION FROM THE GASTROINTESTINAL TRACT

The tissue covering the surface of the skin and lining every canal, tract, and cavity that communicates with the external air is *epithelial* tissue. This tissue is made up of closely associated cells with intercellular junctions that preclude passage of material between cells. Thus, the barriers to absorption common to all parts of the alimentary canal as well as to the respiratory tract and skin are the epithelial cells themselves. After a substance passes through the epithelial barrier and reaches the inner side – the interstitial tissue containing vascular vessels – it comes in contact with internal environmental conditions that are nearly identical for each site, regardless of whether it is part of the gastrointestinal, respiratory, or integumental epithelium. The fluids on the interior of these barriers are maintained at relatively constant composition, pH, and temperature. On the inside of each of these barriers the resistance to movement of solutes into the blood or lymphatics is also nearly the same. However, the organization of the epithelium and the environmental conditions on its *external* surface are different for each site. Even in the alimentary canal, the epithelial lining, and intraluminal environment vary from one part to another in accordance with the function of the particular segment. And it is these factors that account for differences in absorption in different parts of the gastrointestinal tract and at the different sites of entry into the body.

The Oral Cavity

The oral cavity is lined with a smooth-surfaced epithelium made up of several layers of cells. Its normal function is to secrete saliva into the mouth in order to moisten dry foodstuffs and start digestion. As a result of these secretions, the normal external environment of the epithelial cells has a slightly acidic pH and is composed mainly of water.

The thin epithelium and the rich vascularity of the oral mucosa are highly conducive to rapid absorption. At least theoretically, the unionized form of lipophilic drugs with low molecular weights can be expected to undergo rapid absorption from solutions in the oral cavity. But not much absorption occurs in the mouth, mainly because it is so difficult to keep solutions in contact with the oral mucosa for any length of time.

Placement of solid drugs under the tongue – sublingual administration – so that they may be retained for longer periods can prove a very effective method of administration if the drugs meet certain requirements. It was stated earlier that transport across biologic barriers is almost exclusively the prerogative of *solutes*. Hence, drugs given as solids by the sublingual route must be able to dissolve rapidly in the salivary secretions before they are ready for absorption. From the standpoint of patient comfort, the drug also must be able to produce its desired effects when given in small amounts. These two restrictions, combined with the need for the patient's cooperation in keeping the drug under the tongue until it has dissolved and is absorbed, limit the potential usefulness of this route of administration. Similar absorption issues are associated with the use of chewing tobacco or snuff, which is placed between the cheek and the teeth. Nicotine within the tobacco must first be released from the plant before it passes through the epithelial cells lining the cheeks.

When the sublingual route *can* be used, it has certain advantages over the other enteral routes. Following absorption within the oral cavity, the drug gains access to the general circulation without first traversing the liver. All the blood leaving the stomach or small intestine passes first through the liver before entering the general circulation to be distributed to other tissues and organs. In the large intestine, only the blood coming from the lower part of the rectum circumvents the liver on its way to the heart. The liver is the principal organ for the chemical reactions (to be discussed in Chapter 8) that, for the most part, inactivate a drug or transform it into a less effective substance. In some cases chemical reactions within the liver are needed to activate a drug. For almost any drug *on which the body acts*, more drug will be available to *act on the body* when it is administered in a region served by veins that bypass the liver and go directly to the heart. Removal of drug by the liver during absorption is referred to as the *first-pass effect*.

The effectiveness of sublingual administration is well demonstrated by the rapidity with which nitroglycerin relieves the pain of *angina pectoris*[1]. A nitroglycerin tablet placed under the patient's tongue usually acts within two minutes to terminate the attack. The same quantity of nitroglycerin is totally ineffective if swallowed, since it must pass through the liver before reaching its site of action and is subject to an extensive first-pass effect.

---

[1] Angina pectoris, a transient interference with the flow of blood, oxygen and nutrients to heart muscle, is associated with severe pain.

The Stomach

Beyond the oral cavity the alimentary canal becomes a hollow tube extending from the larynx to the anal sphincter. Throughout its length the tube is surrounded by four concentric layers of tissue: *mucosa, submucosa, muscularis* and *serosa*. The mucosa is made up of three components: a superficial epithelium composed of a single layer of cells; an underlying layer, the *lamina propria*, containing connective tissue, blood vessels and lymphatics; and, innermost, a relatively thin layer of muscle fibers.

The superficial epithelium of the gastric mucosa, in contrast to that of the oral cavity, is not a smooth surface but contains many folds. These folds increase the number of epithelial cells and, thereby, the total area available for absorption over that afforded by a flat, smooth lining.

The normal function of the stomach is to act as a storage depot for food and to assist in its digestion. It accomplishes the latter by secreting hydrochloric acid and the enzyme pepsin, the catalytic protein that accelerates the initial digestion of food proteins. The secretions are usually sufficient to make the gastric contents very acidic (in healthy humans about pH 2).

Although the stomach does not function primarily as an organ for absorption, its considerable blood supply combined with the potential for prolonged contact of an agent with a relatively large epithelial surface is conducive to the absorption of various drugs. However, the length of time a substance remains in the stomach is the greatest variable determining the extent of gastric absorption. The rate at which the stomach empties its contents into the small intestine is influenced by the volume, viscosity, and constituents of its contents; by physical activity; by the position of the body; by drugs themselves; and by many other factors. For example, lying on the left side decreases the rate of stomach emptying compared with lying on the right side; the presence of fat in the gastric contents also leads to a decreased rate of emptying compared with the effect of carbohydrate foods. The sum total of so many influences makes any prediction concerning the length of sojourn of an agent in the stomach highly unreliable. Only when a drug is taken with water on a relatively empty stomach is it possible to say that it will reach the small intestine fairly rapidly.

From our considerations of the principles governing transport across cell membranes, it follows that water, small molecules, lipid-soluble nonelectrolytes, and weakly acidic drugs can pass through the gastric epithelium by passive diffusion. The low pH of the stomach contents decreases ionization of weak acids while promoting that of weak bases. Consequently, a larger fraction of weak acids than of weak bases is present in the unionized form, and the former are more rapidly absorbed than the latter. For example, studies on drug absorption have shown that at normal gastric pH, weak acids such as aspirin and phenobarbital are absorbed from the stomach, whereas weak bases such as morphine and nicotine are not absorbed to any significant degree. We have already seen that the base strychnine was negligibly absorbed when the gastric pH was 3, but when the pH was made increasingly alkaline, increasingly greater amounts of

Table 5-2. *Influence of lipid solubility on rate of absorption*

Drug	Relative partition coefficient[1]	% Absorbed from stomach in 1 hour
Barbital	1	4
Secobarbital	52	30
Thiopental	580	46

[1]Concentration in organic solvent, methylene chloride, divided by concentration in water. Partition coefficient data from M.T. Bush, Sedatives and hypnotics: 1 Absorption, fate, and excretion. In: Root, W.S. and Hofman F.G. (eds). *Physiological Pharmacology*. New York: Academic, 1963. Vol. I, pp.185–218. Absorption data from Schanker, L.S., Shore, P.A., Brodie, B.B. and Hogben, C.A.M., *J. Pharmacol. Exp. Ther.* 120:528, 1957.

strychnine reached the general circulation (cf. Table 4-2). The absorption of alcohol from the stomach is also in conformity with the concept that lipid-soluble, small nonelectrolytes diffuse relatively readily across biologic barriers. However, the influence of lipid solubility on transport is more strikingly illustrated by the observed rates of gastric absorption of three derivatives of barbituric acid (Table 5-2). Barbital, secobarbital, and thiopental are each present in excess of 99.99% as nonionized molecules when placed in the stomach at normal gastric pH. There is, however, considerable dissimilarity in lipid solubility among the undissociated forms of the three drugs (as indicated by the large differences in their partition coefficients), and this condition leads to marked differences in their rates of absorption.

Absorption of various drugs can and does occur in the stomach. Nevertheless, under the normal conditions of oral administration, the contribution of gastric absorption to total absorption is not only variable but, at best, exceedingly small compared with that of the small intestine.

The Small Intestine

The epithelial lining of the mucosal layer of the small intestine, like that of the stomach, is composed of a single layer of cells. But the unique arrangement of this lining makes the intestine exquisitely suited to its prime function of absorbing the end products of digestion for utilization by the organism. These exceptional features provide the small intestine with the means for increasing the surface area of its absorbing epithelium out of all proportion to that of the area of its flat serosal surface. In humans, the mucosal surface is heaped up into folds, known as the folds of Kerckring. These folds are more numerous and deeper than the folds of the gastric epithelium; they alone increase the intestinal epithelial surface about three times relative to that of the serosal surface (Fig. 5-3). Using the light microscope, one sees that these folds give rise to slender, delicately ruffled projections called *villi*. These projections make an additional tenfold relative increase in the luminal surface area. Individual villi are lined with the primary absorbing units – epithelial cells – and with goblet cells, the

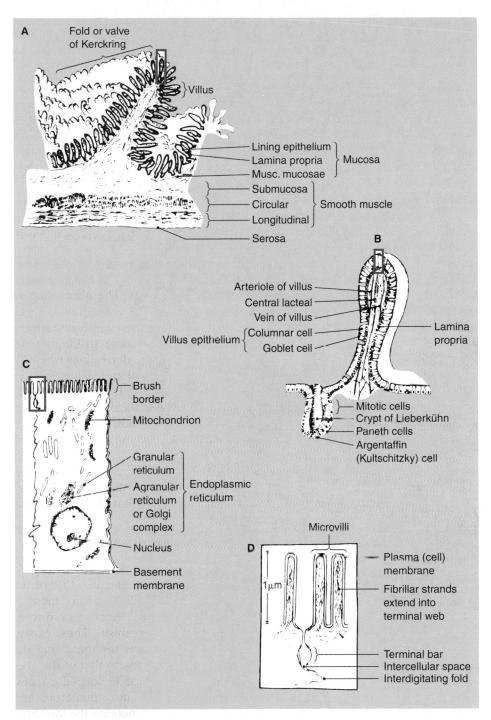

Figure 5-3. *The small intestine. The boxed-in area of figure portions A to C is shown in greater magnification in the succeeding figure portion. (A) The several layers forming the wall of the small intestine; (B) the villus and the crypts of Lieberkühn; (C) highly schematic interpretation of the electron microscopic appearance of the columnar absorbing cell; (D) details of the brush border and the intercellular space. (Modified from L. Laster and F.J. Ingelfinger.* N. Engl. J. Med. *264:1138, 1961.)*

mucus-secreting cells. The central portion of each villus contains the blood and lymph capillaries. Visualized with the electron microscope, the free surface of the epithelial cell at the luminal (or brush) border is seen to bear an array of finger-like structures called *microvilli*. It has been estimated that there are about 600 microvilli per cell, which produce another 20-fold increase in relative epithelial surface area. As Figure 5-4 illustrates, the human small intestine, approximately 280 cm long and 4 cm in diameter, would have about 200 m^2 of available absorbing surface area!

The environmental conditions within the intestinal lumen change somewhat along its length. In the duodenum – the segment of the intestine closest to the stomach – the pH remains acidic, about 4–5, due to the gastric contents that have been emptied into it. However, the somewhat alkaline secretions of the pancreas and the secretions of bile and of the intestine itself quickly neutralize this acid. From about the first quarter of the small intestine to the end of the large intestine, the intraluminal pH changes only from slightly acidic to barely alkaline. Obviously, the ingestion of food and liquids markedly affects

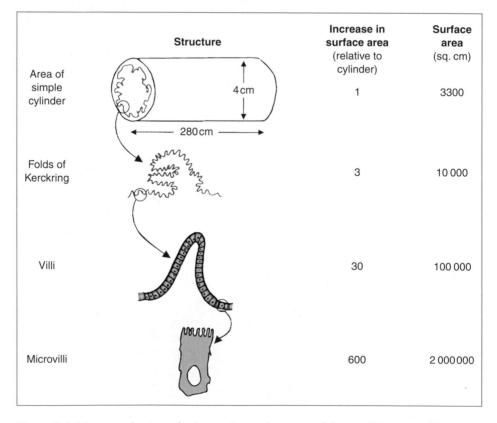

Figure 5-4. *Three mechanisms for increasing surface area of the small intestine. (From T.H. Wilson.* Intestinal Absorption. *Philadelphia: Saunders, 1962. p. 2.)*

the composition of the contents of the entire alimentary canal and also stimulates gastrointestinal secretions.

For *any* substance that can penetrate the gastrointestinal epithelium in measurable amounts, *the small intestine represents the area with the greatest capacity for absorption*. This is true whether the molecule is relatively lipid-soluble and nonionizable, like alcohol, or is a weak electrolyte, either base or acid. For example, in animal studies, when the rates of absorption were determined for various agents placed directly into the intestine or into the stomach and prevented by a ligature from emptying into the intestine, the following results were obtained (Table 5-3): alcohol was found to be at least *six times*, and weak acids such as phenobarbital *twelve times* more rapidly absorbed from the small intestine than from the stomach. A weakly basic antihistamine drug, promethazine, was insignificantly absorbed from the stomach but was absorbed relatively quickly from the intestine. These data may at first glance appear to be a partial contradiction of the stated general principles of biotransport. For although one would predict that a weak base would be more completely absorbed under the pH conditions of the intestine, one would hardly anticipate faster absorption from the intestine than from the stomach for drugs like alcohol, whose absorption is independent of pH, or for weak acids, which are more ionized at the higher intestinal pH. These are not, however, deviations from the general rules governing transport across biologic barriers. They are simply manifestations of the *qualitative difference* in the primary function of the stomach and intestine and of the enormous *quantitative difference* in the *area available for absorption* in these two regions of the gastrointestinal tract.

The large epithelial area of the intestine provided by the villi and microvilli presents many more surfaces than the gastric mucosa for the absorption of neutral, lipid-soluble substances and more than compensates for the decrease in the relative proportion of the nonionized molecules of weak acids. It follows from this that the rate at which the stomach empties its contents into the intestine can markedly affect the overall rate at which drugs reach the general circulation after oral administration. The absorption of weak bases, which constitute the majority of commonly used drugs, would be particularly dependent on the speed with which they arrive in the intestine. But for all drugs, it is

Table 5-3. *Comparison of absorptive capacity of rat stomach and small intestine*[1]

Drug	% Absorbed from stomach in 1 hour[2]	% Absorbed from small intestine in 10 minutes[3]
Phenobarbital	17.1 ± 4.7	52.4 ± 2.3
Pentobarbital	23.7 ± 3.8	54.6 ± 4.6
Promethazine	-0.2 ± 3.2	38.2 ± 6.1
Ethanol	37.7 ± 8.6	64.1 ± 7.5

[1]All values are means ± standard deviation of 6–22 determinations.
[2]Drugs dissolved in 0.01 N HCl.
[3]Drugs dissolved in solution, pH 6, containing NaCl, KCl and $CaCl_2$.
Data from Magnussen, M.P. *Acta Pharmacol. Toxicol. (Kbh.)* 26:130, 1968.

essentially valid to predict that slowing the rate at which the stomach empties will decrease the overall rate of gastrointestinal absorption, and vice versa. That is why so many agents are administered on an empty stomach with sufficient water to ensure their rapid passage into the intestine.

Under normal conditions, substances usually take several hours to pass from one end of the small intestine to the other. In contrast to the stomach, this slow transit through the intestine enhances absorption, since absorption can take place along the entire length. Only when intestinal motility is abnormally increased, as in marked diarrhea, is the residence time in the small intestine too short to ensure maximal absorption.

Passive diffusion and the laws governing it appear to be sufficient to account for the intestinal absorption of the majority of drugs that are either lipid-soluble or weak electrolytes. Usually these drugs are completely absorbed. In contrast, lipid-insoluble drugs and agents that are completely ionized at all physiologic pH levels, such as the quaternary ammonium compounds referred to earlier (cf. p. 46), undergo limited absorption from the small intestine. This poor yet partial absorption was a demonstrated fact long ago. Although primitive hunters did not know that the active ingredient in their arrow poison, curare, was a quaternary ammonium compound, they were well aware that they could eat with impunity the flesh of animals killed with it. The hunter absorbed too little tubocurarine, the active ingredient of the curare present in the meat, to produce deleterious effects. On the other hand, the ingestion of certain species of mushroom has long been known to produce poisonous effects. It was not until Schmiedeberg isolated muscarine from *Amanita muscaria* that it was shown to be the culprit and subsequently identified chemically as a quaternary ammonium compound. The mushroom contains sufficient muscarine so that poisoning results even from partial absorption. Even large macromolecules like proteins, although they undergo substantial degradation in the gastrointestinal lumen, may be absorbed, as such, to a very small degree. An excellent example of this is the poisoning by botulinus toxin, which occurs after eating canned foods contaminated with the causative microorganism. Mechanisms such as carrier-mediated transport and endocytosis may contribute to the absorption of quaternary ammonium compounds and proteins, respectively. Active transport has been shown to account for the absorption of those drugs that closely resemble the normal nutrients known to be actively absorbed. An example is the drug levodopa, an amino acid of importance in the treatment of Parkinson's disease.

More recently, it has been discovered that carrier proteins in the luminal membrane of intestinal epithelial cells, such as the p-glycoprotein (MDR1) transporter, actively pump drugs from the cell back into the lumen. This process reduces the absorption of drugs that bind to these transporters. In addition, the gastrointestinal epithelium contains enzymes like those in the liver. An especially important one in the intestinal mucosa is the oxidative enzyme of the cytochrome P450 family, CYP3A4, which will be described in more detail in Chapter 8. Although generally not as quantitatively significant as those in the liver, these intestinal enzymes can contribute to the first-pass effect that reduces the absorption into the systemic circulation of some drugs taken orally. A classic example of this is the enzyme that converts alcohol into actetaldehyde. Alcohol dehydrogenase is present in the mucosa of males, and to a lesser degree in females. The gastrointestinal metabolism of alcohol can account for up to 30% of its first-pass effect.

The Large Intestine

The structure of the epithelial lining of the large intestine reflects the change in primary function of this part of the gastrointestinal tract compared with the small intestine. The epithelial cells of the colon do not possess microvilli, and their function is primarily that of secreting mucus rather than of absorption. However, the large intestine retains the ability to transport sodium ions actively and to reabsorb water.

Even though the function of the colon is not fundamentally that of absorption, drugs that escape absorption in the small intestine may continue to be absorbed during their passage out of the body. Moreover, the terminal segment of the large intestine – the rectum – can serve as a useful site for drug administration, particularly when the oral route is unsuitable. Rectal administration, commonly referred to as a suppository, is advantageous in the unconscious patient, in patients unable to retain material given by mouth, and for drugs with objectional taste or odor, or those destroyed by digestive enzymes. This route protects susceptible drugs not only from alteration by the digestive processes of the mouth, stomach, and small intestine, but also from the chemical reactions occurring in the liver. It should be recalled that the blood supply leaving the lower part of the rectum bypasses the liver on its way to the heart.

Absorption of Drugs Administered as Solids

Under normal conditions, ingested material is transferred across the gastrointestinal epithelium as a *solute* in the fluid at the site of absorption. While there may be a few exceptions to this rule in the case of nutrients absorbed by pinocytosis, no such exceptions have been demonstrated for therapeutic agents. However, for convenience and for practical reasons of solubility, stability, and consumer acceptance, most drugs are administered orally in some form of solid dosage. Therefore, drugs administered as solids must first go into solution in the fluids of the gastrointestinal lumen. And the rate at which dissolution takes place determines how much of the drug is made available for absorption and how quickly:

$$\text{Solid drug} \xrightarrow[\substack{\text{gastrointestinal} \\ \text{contents}}]{\overset{1}{\text{Dissolution in}}} \text{Dissolved drug} \xrightarrow{\overset{2}{\text{Absorption}}} \text{Drug in circulation}$$

In this two-step process, if the rate of dissolution is slower than the rate of absorption, then the second step becomes initially dependent on the physico-chemical principles that apply to the dissolution of substances in aqueous media. Only after dissolution would the rate of absorption be governed by the principles established for the passage of solutes across biologic barriers. If the rate of dissolution is faster than the rate of absorption, however, then the first step is no longer rate limiting, and the rate of absorption will be governed entirely by the principles of biotransport.

Of course, the greater the inherent aqueous solubility of a drug, the greater its rate of dissolution from the solid dosage form. The salts of acidic or basic drugs are usually more soluble in water than the parent compounds, which is why many acidic drugs are prepared as salts of sodium or other cations (e.g. sodium salicylate or potassium penicillin G), and basic drugs as salts of hydrochloric or other acids (e.g. epinephrine hydrochloride). But formation of salts is only one of many ways in which the pharmaceutical chemist has successfully manipulated the form or formulation of an agent to change its dissolution rate.

The size of the drug particle presented to the dissolving medium is one of the more important factors determining rate of dissolution. The smaller the particle size, the greater the rate of solution, since the proportion of surface area exposed to the solvent compared to the volume of the particles increases with decreasing particle diameter. For example, in human subjects, the administration of sulfadiazine as microcrystalline particles results in a more rapid and complete absorption than when the same drug is given in 'ordinary' particle size with a surface area approximately one-seventh that of the micronized substance. However, reduction in particle size, while almost always increasing rate of solution, is potentially beneficial to absorption only for substances with dissolution rates slower than their rates of absorption. Equal amounts of the antibiotic tetracycline hydrochloride, for instance, administered to humans either as capsules containing small particles or as compressed pellets, were equally well absorbed despite the 30-fold difference in surface area between the two dosage preparations. Tetracycline hydrochloride dissolves rapidly in the acidic gastric environment but is only poorly absorbed from the stomach, and even from the intestine its absorption is slow and incomplete.

Almost all solid dosage forms of drugs contain other ingredients besides the active agent. The **excipients** are considered pharmacologically inert but are included in the pharmaceutical preparation for a variety of reasons, e.g. to mask an unpleasant taste, to increase solubility or stability or to add bulk to active agents used in small quantities. But the inclusion of these inert constituents adds another dimension to be considered in the availability of a drug for absorption – the disintegration of the dosage form itself and the dispersion of the active ingredients within the gastrointestinal tract. Thus:

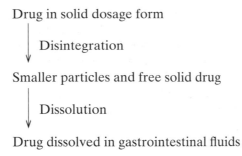

Drug in solid dosage form

    Disintegration

Smaller particles and free solid drug

    Dissolution

Drug dissolved in gastrointestinal fluids

Hence, in the majority of instances of drug administration by the oral route, drug absorption is not only dependent on the rate of dissolution of the *therapeutic agent*, but also influenced by rates of disintegration of the solid dosage form.

These points were well illustrated by the results of studies carried out with twelve brands of tablets of a single agent, phenylbutazone (Table 5-4). A 15-fold variation was found among the different brands with respect to the time required for tablet disintegration. The time necessary for 50% of the phenylbutazone to dissolve showed a more than 70-fold difference among the tablets

Table 5-4. *Disintegration and dissolution data for 12 brands of the anti-inflammatory agent phenylbutazone*

Brand	Disintegration time[1] (min)		Dissolution data[2] (mg in solution)			
	Mean	Range	2h	4h	6h	$t_{1/2}$[3] *(min)*
A	17	11–22	80	94	99	54
B	12	8–16	60	83	93	86
Cq	4	3–4	99	99	99	9
D	20	19–21	78	98	104	57
E	41	18–83	21	56	76	210
G	43	30–45	98	100	100	31
H	35	20–48	75	96	99	80
L	41	28–52	80	94	99	54
Pq	42	28–55	86	87	88	36
Q	44	39–53	39	59	70	174
W	61	46–120	29	64	88	188
X	51	23–62	0	7	48	369
Pure drug	...	...	99	100	100	5

[1]Mean of six tablets from each brand.
[2]Average of two tablets from each brand, subjected separately to the dissolution test.
[3]$t_{1/2}$ is the time required for 50% of the quantity of drug to be dissolved.
Data from Searl, R.O. and Pernarowski, M. *Can. Med. Assoc. J.* 96:1513, 1967.

tested. Additionally, there was no significant correlation between disintegration and dissolution times. From the clinical viewpoint, however, the most important finding was the wide variation in the rate and extent of absorption among the four brands chosen for study in human subjects, despite the fact that equal amounts of drug were administered (Fig. 5-5). That different brands of the same drug could produce quantitatively different therapeutic responses and that equality of the analytic content of a given agent in a particular preparation was no guarantee that there would be equality of availability for absorption or for therapeutic effectiveness were important findings.

A comparison of the absorption rates of three different commercial aspirin tablets also documented the dependence of absorption on the pharmaceutical formulation (Fig. 5-6). This particular example also demonstrates the effect of another variable in oral administration – the quantity of water ingested along with the solid dosage form. The amount of each preparation absorbed by the subjects in group B, who ingested a large quantity of water with the aspirin tablets, was greater than in group A, even though the same relationship between absorption and dissolution rate was maintained.

Recognition of the fact that different formulations of the identical quantity of the same drug might not result in equal therapeutic response led the Food and Drug Administration (FDA) to set standards for biologic availability or **bioavailability**. The term bioavailability as defined by the FDA refers to the rate and extent to which a drug is absorbed from its formulation and is available to

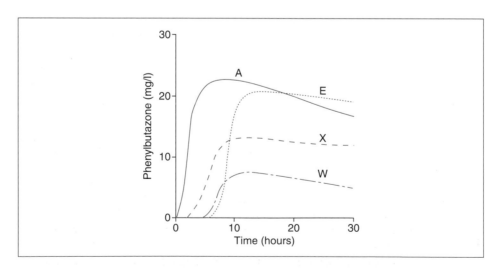

Figure 5-5. *Concentration of phenylbutazone in serum of patients after the oral administration of four different products (A, E, X and W). Each product contained the same amount of phenylbutazone. Curves are composite curves of results obtained in three subjects per product, but the individual data points were sufficiently close to permit the construction of reasonably accurate composite curves. (Modified from R.O. Searl and M. Pernarowski. Can. Med. Assoc. J. 96:1513, 1967.)*

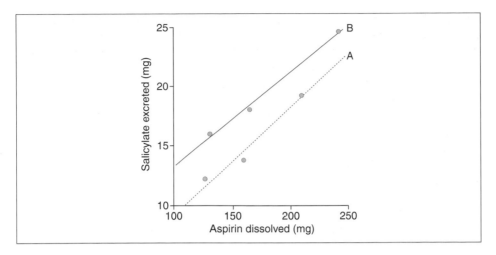

Figure 5-6. *Mean amount of apparent salicylate excreted in one hour after administration of three different commercial aspirin tablets (two tablets of 0.3 g each) as a function of in* vitro *dissolution rate (mean amount of aspirin dissolved in 10 minutes from one tablet). Lower line, group A: 14 subjects ingested aspirin with exactly 100 ml water. Upper line, group B: 10 subjects ingested aspirin with exactly 200 ml water. (Adapted from G. Levy.* J. Pharm. Sci. 50:388, 1961. *Reproduced with permission of the copyright owner.)*

its site of action. The Federal Food, Drug and Cosmetic Act as amended in 1977 requires sponsors of drugs to provide data of **bioequivalence** whenever there is evidence that drug products containing the same active drug are intended for the same therapeutic effect (cf. Chapter 16). As we shall see (Chapter 10), data to establish bioequivalence include the plasma concentrations of the drug at various times after administration, in order to assess the rate and extent of drug absorption.

For some drugs it is desirable to use pharmaceutical methods to decrease the rate of disintegration and dissolution from solid formulations. Tablets or capsules can be externally coated to prevent their disintegration within the stomach. When such *enteric* coatings are used, the drug is not presented to an absorbing surface until it reaches the small intestine, where the environment is conducive to destruction of the coating and release of the drug. This is a particularly useful procedure to protect drugs that are prone to alteration by the acidity of the gastric medium.

Other types of oral preparations contain drugs coated in various ways so as to release only a limited amount of active agent at any one time and thus provide for sustained therapy by making additional small quantities of drug available for absorption over a relatively long period. However, if the *sustained-release medication* leaves the intestine before all of the drug has been delivered for absorption, an unused portion will be excreted in the feces. Still other disadvantages, of a more serious nature, may be associated with the use of sustained-release preparations. Since the liberation of the drug depends upon certain reactions taking place in appropriate segments of the gastrointestinal tract, there may be greater variability in the rate of release among individuals, and even in the same individual at different times. A single sustained-release tablet or capsule contains a larger amount of drug than does a conventional form. If release is more rapid than expected, too much drug may be absorbed too quickly and thus lead to adverse effects. Conversely, if the rate of discharge is slower than expected, amounts of drug may be provided that are inadequate to produce the desired therapeutic effect. Sustained-release preparations are justified only when a drug is so rapidly absorbed – and, following absorption, so quickly eliminated – that a sufficient amount reaches the site of action for only a short period following administration. If continued action of such a drug is needed, it would require taking the drug more than three or four times a day. In such cases, sustained-release preparations provide the means to avoid fluctuations in the amount of drug delivered and to obviate the necessity of repeated ingestion of the more usual oral preparations.

A different form of oral dosage for controlled drug release may overcome some of the problems previously associated with such preparations, since the rate of release of drug is made independent of changing conditions within the gut. These dosage forms, the size and shape of ordinary tablets, comprise a core of solid drug surrounded by a layer of osmotically active material and an outer polymeric membrane that is permeable to water (Fig. 5-7). Water entering from the gastrointestinal lumen gradually dissolves the osmotically active material. The resulting pressure within the core forces the drug into the gut lumen through a single, small orifice. The rate at which these osmotic pumps release drug can be controlled and made constant for up to 24 hours, thereby minimiz-

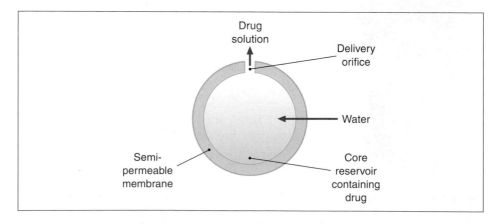

Figure 5-7. *Schematic diagram of an oral controlled-release dosage form. Drug delivery depends upon the development of osmotic pressure within the drug-containing core and is independent of pH and motility variations in the gut.*

ing the fluctuations in plasma concentrations observed with tablets or capsules. Nifedipine, a drug used to treat hypertension, is available in this type of dosage form.

ABSORPTION THROUGH THE SKIN

The epidermis, the outer layer of the skin, is composed of epithelial cells. From a functional point of view, it is a two-ply structure consisting of the dead *stratum corneum*, or the *cornified or horny layer*, and an underlying layer of living cells, the *stratum germinativum* (Fig. 5-8). The stratum corneum is normally made up of many tiers of cells bound tightly together into a dense, coherent membrane whose intercellular spaces are submicroscopic. The function of the skin as a barrier to the movement of solutes resides almost entirely in its dead product. 'The raison d'être of the viable layer is to make the horny layer; this is its

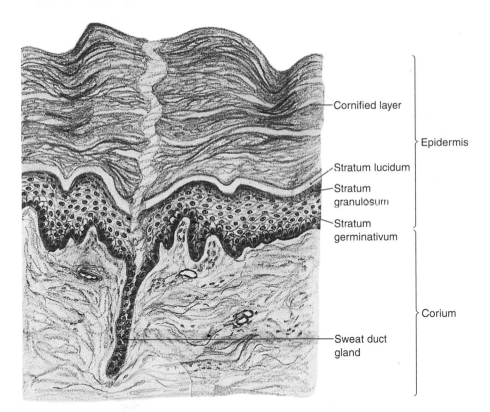

Figure 5-8. *Structure and layers of the skin. A thick, cornified layer is characteristic of areas such as the fingertip. The cornified layer is made up of flat, dead, dry, keratinized cells. Cell division in the epidermis takes place in the stratum germinativum. The corium, or dermis, is a compact layer of connective tissue containing sweat glands and numerous collagenous and elastic fibers. (Modified from G. Bevelander.* Outline of Histology *[6th ed.]. St Louis: Mosby, 1967.)*

specific biologic mission. Its aim in life is to die usefully so that its horny shroud forms a continually renewable wrapping around the body.'[2]

The integumental epithelium differs in still other ways from the rest of the epithelial barriers. With the possible exception of a portion of the mucous lining of the nose, the skin is the only tissue whose free surface is usually exposed to relatively dry air. This dry outer environment leads to a comparatively low water content of the several cell layers on the outside of the skin and, generally speaking, of the entire stratum corneum. In no other normal epithelium is there dry tissue on the environmental side. The cells of the horny layer also contain less phospholipid and lipid than those of other epithelia and are unique in being densely packed with the complex protein keratin. Thus this horny layer may derive its true barrier function from its lack of water and lipid and the presence of keratin, which together account for the density and packing of the cells.

The epidermis affords the body protection; this is really its exclusive function, and it is a two-way process. Its dead product, the horny layer, obstructs the passage of materials both to and from the environment. No multicellular membrane of biologic origin is as 'waterproof' as the skin, and water loss from the body by diffusion and evaporation is equally retarded, except at the sweat glands. It is well to note that there is no evidence that sweat or sebaceous glands act as the entrance pathways for exogenous materials. It is not surprising, then, that absorption through the skin, when it does occur, is ordinarily extremely slow. Once a solute passes this barrier, it encounters no further significant obstacles to absorption. The underlying tissue, the dermis, is well supplied with lymph and blood capillaries.

Passage of chemicals through the skin, as determined by direct measurement, appears to be simply by passive diffusion. Although rates of penetration of various agents are relatively slower than at other biologic barriers, they conform qualitatively to the general principles governing this transport process. In humans, no evidence of active transport processes has been obtained even though various inorganic ions can traverse the skin. This might be anticipated since the horny layer is really dead tissue. But the point that needs emphasis is that, even though the skin is an effective barrier against the transport of almost all substances, letting no molecule through readily, *it is a perfect barrier to very few substances.* Even a heavy metal like mercury can be absorbed to some degree through the skin. Indeed, absorption through the skin represents one of the most common routes by which poisoning in man and animals occurs following accidental exposure to foreign chemicals. For example, many insecticides – particularly those containing parathion, malathion, or nicotine – may cause serious poisoning as a result of percutaneous absorption following inadvertent contamination of the skin or even clothing.

When drugs are purposely applied to the skin, or for that matter to any external mucous membrane (nasal sprays, intravaginal jellies, and the like), they are

---

[2] A.M. Kligman. The biology of the stratum corneum. In: Montagna, W. and Lobitz, W.C. Jr (eds). *The Epidermis.* New York: Academic, 1964.

ordinarily expected to produce their desired effects only in the local area of administration. Little thought is usually given to the fact that the skin is not an *absolute* barrier and that there may be absorption of the drug leading to systemic effects, sometimes of a serious nature. For example, tannic acid, once widely used in the treatment of burns, was abandoned during World War II when it was discovered that it produces toxic effects on the kidney. Some of the preparations presently available for decreasing the pain of sunburn contain local anesthetics. Again, if these preparations are not used as directed and are placed over large areas of the body, the quantity of local anesthetic absorbed through the skin may prove harmful. Of course, any time the skin is broken by cuts or wounds, it no longer retains its barrier function in the injured area, and substances can be readily absorbed through the exposed tissues underlying the epidermis.

Although sustained-release preparations for enteral administration do not appear to be the desired panacea for prolonged, uniform drug absorption, more promising results have been obtained using such preparations for topical application to the intact skin or mucous membranes. Some of these preparations have been designed for placement and prolonged delivery of drug directly at the site where therapy is required. Other preparations placed on the intact skin are designed for systemic therapy and provide relatively long periods of continuous delivery of drug to distant sites of action. For example, a class of dosage forms known formally as transdermal drug delivery devices, or more commonly as the *transdermal patch*, is available for delivery of drugs to the surface of the intact skin for systemic therapy. This method of drug administration is desirable for drugs with an extensive first-pass effect by the oral route or with a short duration of action by enteral and parenteral routes. The device is a multilayer disk comprising a reservoir of drug sandwiched between an impermeable backing membrane and a rate-controlling microporous membrane. On the dermal side of the latter is an adhesive gel which serves to secure the system to intact skin (Fig. 5-9). Drug is delivered to the skin at a rate controlled by the choice of the appropriate polymeric material for the microporous membrane. Hence the rate of drug absorption into the systemic circulation is determined primarily by the drug delivery system, and not by the skin. Drug administration for systemic effect using transdermal therapeutic systems provides continuous, unattended, controlled drug input for long periods while avoiding problems associated with other parenteral or oral administration, e.g. gastrointestinal or hepatic drug inactivation prior to systemic circulation and the inconvenience of injections. Examples of transdermal delivery devices include a 'birth control' patch that delivers estrogen and progesterone over one week, a 3-day continuous-release form of scopolamine for the treatment of motion sickness and preparations that deliver constant amounts of nitroglycerin over a 24-hour period for the treatment and prevention of angina. Now nitroglycerin patches of shorter duration or their removal overnight is recommended for angina patients, since the drug has been shown to lose effectiveness when administered on a round-the-clock basis. The development of **drug tolerance** or **tachyphylaxis** (cf. pp. 300–305) is largely avoided with intermittent therapy.

One of the first of this type of sustained-release preparation was developed for local effects following topical administration. Pilocarpine, a drug useful in the treatment of glaucoma[3], was successfully incorporated into a drug delivery system for placement in the cul-de-sac between the skin and the conjunctival surface of the eye. This therapeutic system is biocompatible during prolonged contact with body tissues and consists of a drug-containing reservoir bounded by membranes that control the rate of drug diffusion (Fig. 5-9). Drug is delivered at a slow but essentially constant rate for the 7-day prescribed lifetime of the system. The rate of pilocarpine release is sufficient to maintain a constant reduction in intraocular pressure, but the amount released is too small to produce significant systemic effects. A single weekly administration of the drug is obviously more convenient than periodic daily application of eye drops. Other methods of sustained drug delivery to mucous membranes include a variety of devices for release of contraceptive agents. The T-shaped intrauterine contraceptive device that provides continuous and precisely controlled release of progesterone within the uterus for more than one year is one such example (Fig. 5-9).

ABSORPTION FROM THE RESPIRATORY TRACT

As air is inhaled, it passes first into the pharynx, a region common to both the respiratory and gastrointestinal tracts. From there it moves into the *trachea*, the principal air tube of the vertebrate respiratory system, and then into the *bronchi*, the major branches connecting the trachea with the lungs. Food and water are normally prevented from entering the air tube by the *epiglottis*, a flap that covers the opening into the trachea upon swallowing. Within the lungs the bronchial tubes subdivide into the finer bronchioles, whose branches communicate with the *alveoli* (Fig. 5-10). It is the anatomic structure and organization within the lung of these minute, sac-like chambers, the alveoli, that enable the lung to carry out its primary function of rapidly supplying oxygen to the body and removing carbon dioxide.

The pulmonary alveolus is lined with a single layer of flat epithelial cells forming an extremely thin barrier between alveolar air and an interstitium richly supplied with capillaries. The alveolar epithelium and capillary wall are so closely associated that the total air-blood barrier is only 0.5–1.0 μm thick (Fig. 5-11). This is quite different from the space separating the epithelial cells of the intestinal villus from their underlying capillaries, or from the space separating the surface of the skin from the dermal layer; these spaces are about 40 and 100 μm,

---

[3] Glaucoma is a disease of the eye marked by increased pressure within the eyeball. Untreated, there may be damage to the optic disk and gradual loss of vision. Drugs useful in the treatment of glaucoma reduce intraocular pressure by providing better drainage of the aqueous humor – the fluid occupying the space between the crystalline lens and the cornea of the eye. Contraction of muscles of the eye by pilocarpine widens the passage through which fluid drains from the aqueous humor back to the blood.

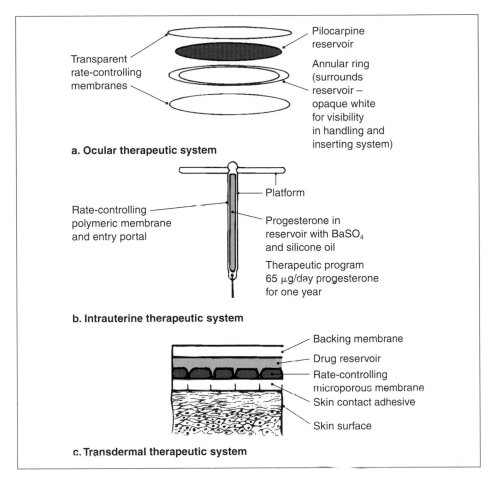

a. Ocular therapeutic system

Pilocarpine reservoir

Transparent rate-controlling membranes

Annular ring (surrounds reservoir – opaque white for visibility in handling and inserting system)

b. Intrauterine therapeutic system

Platform

Rate-controlling polymeric membrane and entry portal

Progesterone in reservoir with $BaSO_4$ and silicone oil

Therapeutic program 65 μg/day progesterone for one year

c. Transdermal therapeutic system

Backing membrane

Drug reservoir

Rate-controlling microporous membrane

Skin contact adhesive

Skin surface

Figure 5-9. *Schematic diagrams of various therapeutic systems for drug delivery. (Modified from J.E. Shaw. Drug delivery systems. Annu Rep, Med. Chem. 15:302, 1980.)*

respectively. The number of alveoli in human lungs is estimated to be from 300 to 400 million, providing a total surface area of about 200 m². Of equal importance to absorption is the fact that the pulmonary vasculature is functionally structured to ensure the rapid removal of material which has crossed this huge surface. First, the pulmonary capillaries have a surface area of about 90 m². Second, all the blood coming from the right side of the heart passes through the lungs, and since the same volume of blood is ejected by both sides of the heart, the lungs receive in one minute an amount of blood equal to that passing through the remainder of the entire body in the same interval. All these factors combine to make the lungs the most effective absorptive area of the body.

As air is inhaled, its water content increases quickly, and it becomes virtually saturated by the time it reaches the alveoli. Thus the normal external environment

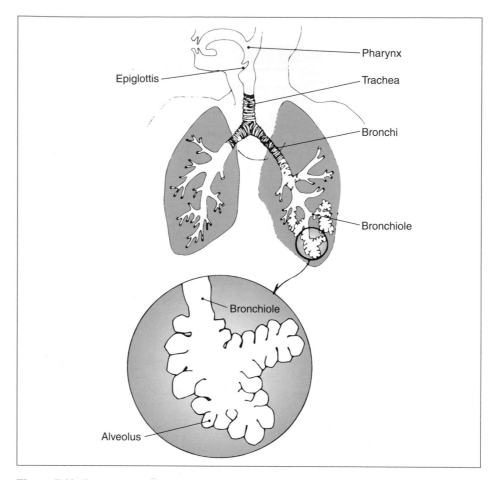

Figure 5-10. *Respiratory apparatus.*

at the primary absorptive surface is really not dry air but moisture-laden air. This is of physiologic importance since it prevents the loss of considerable amounts of water from the body upon expiration. In humans, only about 400 ml of water per day is lost to the environment through the lungs. In animals that have no sweat glands, like the dog, or in humans when body temperature is elevated and respiratory rate is increased, there is a compensatory increase in water loss from the lungs to assist in regulating body temperature.

The cellular membrane in the alveolus or elsewhere is not a barrier to diffusion of gases into or out of a cell, since gases as a rule are small molecules of relatively high lipid solubility. Thus, materials inhaled as gases or as vapors of volatile liquids almost instantaneously cross the alveolar epithelium and enter the blood when they are in higher concentrations in the alveolar air than in the blood. This extremely rapid absorption is a desirable feature for gases like

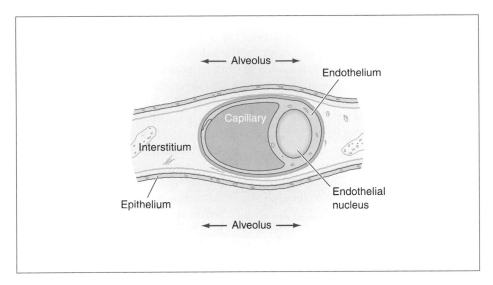

Figure 5-11. *Alveolar capillary membranes. (After F.N. Low.* Anat. Rec. *139:105, 1961.)*

nitrous oxide or volatile liquids when they are used to produce general anesthesia, but it can be disastrous when the inspired air contains poisonous gases or vapors like carbon monoxide or gasoline fumes.

Chemicals can also be inhaled as aerosols, which are liquid droplets or solid particles so small that they remain suspended in air for some time instead of settling out quickly under gravitational pull. Once within the respiratory tract, these suspended particles are deposited along its various segments as the current of air in which they are moving causes them to impact on the tissue. The deposition, or impaction, occurs principally at the points where the pulmonary tree branches and the airstream changes course, since the tendency of a particle is to continue moving in its original direction. Particle size largely determines the site of impaction; the smaller the particle, the deeper into the pulmonary system it is drawn before being deposited. Particles larger than 10 µm in diameter are usually deposited within the nasal passages, and those larger than 2 µm rarely reach the alveolar sac. Pollens, smoke, industrial dusts and fumes, bacteria, viruses and various aerosol preparations used in the treatment of asthma are examples of substances with particle sizes below 10 µm in diameter.

The reactions produced by the deposited particles depend on their solubility and on whether they reach the alveolus. Soluble chemicals can be absorbed anywhere along the respiratory tract in accordance with the principles governing passive diffusion. The smaller the particle size, the greater the rate of solution of the chemical and the greater its rate of absorption. Also, the smaller the particle is in size, the greater the likelihood of its reaching the alveoli, where conditions are most conducive to absorption. Pulmonary drug delivery devices, including nebulizers and metered dose inhalers, are designed to deliver aerosolized particulates into the alveoli of drugs indicated for treatment of lung diseases such as asthma. Delivery by inhalation for a local effect in the lungs greatly improves the safety of these drugs, as compared to their use by the oral route or by injection. Inhalation of particulates of drugs that are proteins, such as insulin, may prove effective for systemic actions and become an alternative to parenteral injection.

The upper respiratory tract is lined as far down as the end of the bronchioles with mucus-secreting epithelial cells bearing many cilia. The constant movement of these hair-like processes propels the mucous secretions and any insoluble particles deposited on them toward the nose and mouth and, in this way, rapidly clears the bronchial epithelium. Insoluble particles reaching the alveolus are in part transported, by some means, to the base of the ciliated epithelium in the bronchioles and are excreted by the ciliary movement. Removal by the phagocytic white blood cells (cf. pp. 73–75, endocytosis) present in the alveoli or other lung tissue is also a mechanism by which the lung rids itself of insoluble material reaching the alveolus. When the airborne concentration of particles is low – less than about ten particles per cubic centimeter of air – the lungs can completely eliminate the insoluble material by these two mechanisms. As a consequence, only a minute quantity of the total particulate material inhaled during a lifetime is retained in the normal, healthy lung. But as the particle concentration in the air increases, the capacity for elimination is overtaxed and some of the particles are retained in the tissue. A small decrease in the lung's capacity to rid itself of solid particles can lead to a great increase in the quantity retained. This may explain the several lung diseases which frequently afflict miners exposed to relatively high concentrations of mineral dust in their work. In this connection it is also interesting to note that cigarette smoke consists primarily of particles measuring less than 1 μm in diameter. Comparison of the number of particles in inhaled and exhaled cigarette smoke has shown that 82% of the particles are retained when the smoke is held for 5 seconds in the lungs. The ability of the lung to rid itself of these particles is then related to whether its capacity is sufficient to keep up with the rate of smoke entry. Some of the vapors contained in cigarette smoke slow down the ciliary action of the bronchial epithelium, and this may work against the lung, decreasing its capacity to rid itself of particulate matter by ciliary excretion.

ABSORPTION FROM SUBCUTANEOUS SITES

Subcutaneous injections of drugs bypass the barrier of the epidermis since they are placed below the dermis directly in contact with channels into the general circulation. Thus, in a sense, we have already discussed some aspects of subcutaneous absorption when we indicated that, once substances pass through the epithelial cells separating the external environment from the internal environment, they enter into the immediate vicinity of blood and lymph capillaries. At subcutaneous sites, just as on the *inside* of the epithelial barrier, the hindrance to entry into the systemic circulation is the wall of the capillary (Fig. 5-12). It is

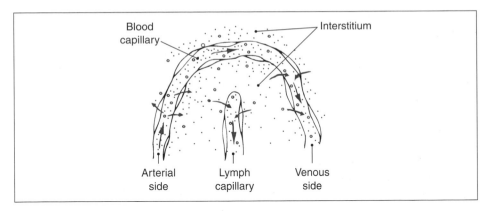

Figure 5-12. *Movement of substances into and out of capillaries (highly idealized). Fluid, solutes and even macromolecules like proteins leave the blood capillary on the arterial side and enter intercellular fluid and tissue cells. At the venous side, fluid, solutes and some proteins enter the blood capillary. Solutes, fluid and particularly proteins are also returned to the circulation by way of the lymph capillary. The proteins and macromolecules are represented as small circles (o) and the fluid and solutes of blood and tissue as dots (·). Arrows show direction of flow. (After A.W. Ham.* Histology. *Philadelphia: Lippincott, 1965.)*

composed of *endothelial* cells, and it is the endothelial tissue which forms the barrier to solute movement into as well as out of the circulation.

The rates at which all substances penetrate endothelial tissue at all sites except the brain are far in excess of those at which these same materials cross epithelial tissue. Even large macromolecules like protein can make their way into and out of capillaries, albeit relatively slowly. The reason for this increased permeability will be discussed more fully in Chapter 6, on distribution. But as a rule, the rates of absorption into capillaries are determined for lipid-soluble substances by their oil/water partition coefficients and for lipid insoluble substances by their molecular size.

The rate of capillary blood flow is the major factor in determining rate of entry into the circulation. The more vascular the subcutaneous area, the greater the rate of absorption. Removal from the site of injection by way of the lymph plays only a minor part in the total absorption of smaller molecules, since the flow of lymph is so slow compared to that of blood. However, lymphatic absorption is significant in the case of larger molecules such as proteins.

This dependence of rate of absorption on rate of blood flow makes it possible to change the rate at which a drug enters the circulation following subcutaneous injection. This can be done by changing either the rate of blood flow through the area of administration or the rate at which the drug is exposed to capillary surfaces. For example, when a local anesthetic is injected subcutaneously around a tooth on which work is to be performed, the dentist wishes to retard absorption and keep the anesthetic in the local area as long as possible.

Therefore, the dentist uses a local anesthetic solution that also contains an agent (e.g. epinephrine) capable of decreasing the diameter of the blood vessels at the site of injection. Under these conditions, the local anesthetic is carried away more slowly since less blood is flowing through the area in a given period compared with the flow when the vessels are not constricted.

It is also sometimes desirable to decrease the rate of absorption from subcutaneous injections, even when the drug is being given to produce its effects systemically. In these instances, special preparations are used which release small amounts of drug continuously over a period of time. Some insulin is prepared in this way so that the diabetic patient need use only a single injection during a day to obtain a long-lasting effect. Certain hormones (e.g. estradiol) are incorporated into a solid pellet form and implanted subcutaneously. These pellets resist rapid disintegration in the fluid at the subcutaneous site, but minute amounts of the hormone go into solution very slowly, and a single administration sometimes lasts as long as 5–6 months (see Fig. 10-6). The effectiveness of both of these preparations is due to the facts that rate of dissolution becomes the rate-limiting factor and that the drug dosage form remains at the site of administration under essentially unchanging environmental conditions – quite different from the conditions imposed on a sustained-release dosage form of a drug given by the oral route. These preparations also differ from the type of sustained-release preparations called therapeutic systems (cf. p. 99), in which the rate-limiting factor is not the rate of drug dissolution but is the rate of drug diffusion through the polymeric membrane.

Increasing the rate of absorption from a subcutaneous site is usually achieved by increasing the total surface area over which absorption can occur. Gentle massage following administration may spread the solution over a wider area so that the drug comes in contact with more capillaries. However, the lateral spread of an injected solution is limited by the connective tissue present in the subcutaneous area, and ordinarily only a small volume of solution, 0.5–2.0 ml, can be comfortably injected. The subcutaneous route is rarely, but can be, used for administration of large fluid volumes, but special means must be used to overcome the resistance of the connective tissue. This is done with an enzyme, hyaluronidase, which breaks down the connective tissue matrix and allows the fluid to spread over larger areas.

Rapid absorption and the relative ease with which subcutaneous injections can be given, compared with intramuscular or intravenous injections, account for the frequent use of the subcutaneous route for drug administration. However, many drugs are too irritating to tissue or produce too much pain to be given in this way, and their injection may even lead to the formation of sterile abscesses (abscesses free of living microorganisms). Infections also occur more readily after subcutaneous than after intravenous injection. Nevertheless, the subcutaneous route offers an advantage over the intravenous one in that the rate of absorption from the subcutaneous site can be retarded when immediate adverse reactions occur in response to the administration of a drug. Once a drug has been given intravenously, it cannot be recalled. But after subcutaneous administration, as well as in some intramuscular administrations, it is possible to place a tourniquet between the site of injection and the heart and thereby block the superficial venous and lymphatic flow from the area. This is also the technique used to slow the rate at which venoms reach the general circulation following bites from poisonous snakes or insects.

ABSORPTION FROM INTRAMUSCULAR SITES

Intramuscular injections are usually made into the muscles of the buttock, the lateral side of the thigh or the upper arm. Thus drugs are introduced into areas that lie below the skin and subcutaneous tissue. The intramuscular route permits the administration of more irritating drugs and of larger volumes of solutions than can be tolerated subcutaneously.

The barrier to absorption from muscles is also the capillary wall. Qualitatively, the permeability of the muscle capillaries is hardly different from that of subcutaneous capillaries. Therefore, all that was said about absorption from subcutaneous sites applies equally to absorption from intramuscular sites. The rates of absorption from both areas also appear to be about the same when the muscles are at rest. But during activity, the blood flow through the muscles may increase markedly as additional vascular channels are opened. During exercise, since the rate of absorption is dependent on rate of blood flow, drugs gain access to the general circulation more rapidly from intramuscular than from subcutaneous sites.

The intramuscular route, like the subcutaneous route, can be used to introduce drugs into the body slowly as well as rapidly. This is accomplished by altering the physical state of the drug so that, after it is deposited in the muscle, it goes into solution gradually, making small fractions of the dose available for absorption over an extended period. For example, special microcrystalline suspensions of penicillin, when injected intramuscularly, dissolve so slowly that a single injection may provide adequate penicillin therapy for a few days. Such preparations, called *depot preparations*, are convenient for patient as well as physician, since they eliminate the necessity and discomfort of frequently repeated injections.

INTRAVENOUS ADMINISTRATION

The injection or infusion of a drug into the bloodstream, usually into a vein of the arm, ensures that the entire quantity of drug administered is available for distribution to its site(s) of action. This procedure obviously has certain advantages over other routes of administration which necessitate absorption before distribution. But at the same time, the immediate availability of a drug given intravascularly entails certain hazards. And the procedure of injection itself, regardless of the nature of the drug, presents certain dangers. Generally, drugs are administered by this route in a sterile aqueous solution. There are examples, however, of drugs administered as a lipid emulsion or in liposomal preparations, which are very small spheres formed by lipid surrounding the drug in an aqueous core.

The intravenous route of drug administration is of greatest value in emergencies when speed is vital. Another advantage is that the amount of drug administered can be controlled with an accuracy not possible by any other procedure. Administration by a route that requires absorption never guarantees that all of the drug given will be absorbed, even though there is the potential for complete absorption from the site. The intravenous route may also be used for drugs that are too irritating to be injected into other tissues without causing undue pain and tissue damage. An example is nitrogen mustard in the treatment of cancer. The irritating drug is quickly diluted by the blood, and the vessel wall is relatively insensitive to damage. Drugs that would be destroyed by chemical reactions before reaching the bloodstream are also given intravenously. Other types of drugs that must be given intravenously are agents with high molecular weights. Examples include the anticoagulant heparin and proteins manufactured using recombinant technology such as the anti-inflammatory monoclonal antibody infliximab. Obviously, blood or plasma substitutes are effective only when given directly into the vascular system. Intravenous administration is also the route of choice when blood circulation is so poor that the rate of absorption from tissue sites would be extremely uncertain.

Once a drug has been injected into the bloodstream there is no retreat, in contrast to the various techniques that can be used to slow absorption from intramuscular or subcutaneous sites or to remove a drug physically from the gastrointestinal tract. From this standpoint, the intravenous route is the least safe method of drug administration. However, if injections are made slowly, danger can be largely averted. It takes about 1 minute for a complete circulation of blood in the normal individual and about 10–15 seconds for material injected in the arm to proceed through the heart to the brain. Thus, if injections are made over a period of at least 1 minute, it may be possible to discontinue further administration in patients in whom adverse reactions, such as loss of consciousness, occur within 15–30 seconds.

Rapid intravenous injections may produce deleterious effects which are unrelated to the effects of the injected drug, since they occur with pharmacologically inert substances as well. These effects usually involve the respiratory and circulatory systems and are seen as shallow and irregular breathing, precipitous fall in blood pressure and stoppage of the heart. They are probably associated with the fact that the material in the rapidly injected solution arrives at the heart as a relatively concentrated solution, since too much is placed in the bloodstream at one time to permit dilution in the circulating blood volume. Still other dangers attend intravenous injections, such as the inadvertent administration of particulate matter or air, which can produce serious complications. This route should be reserved for those instances when it is specifically indicated.

GENERAL CONSIDERATIONS

The oral route is the safest, most convenient and most economic method of administering drugs. However, the daily fluctuations of the gastrointestinal environment produced by food, combined with the dependence of absorption on the rate of gastric emptying, make it the most unpredictable and slowest of the commonly used routes in terms of both amount and rate of drug absorption. Moreover, this route cannot be used for drugs that are susceptible to alteration by the chemical processes involved in digestion. Thus a protein drug like insulin, which is destroyed by the enzymes normally secreted to digest food protein, must be given by a parenteral route despite daily need of long duration. The economy of oral administration also becomes questionable for those drugs that are rapidly destroyed by chemical reactions in the intestinal epithelium and liver. Since all of the drug absorbed from the stomach and small intestine passes through the liver on its way to the general circulation, larger amounts may be required to ensure an adequate biologic effect.

Drugs administered by the other enteral routes, sublingual and rectal, are not changed by the digestive processes and also avoid passage through the liver before reaching the systemic circulation. However, the sublingual route is restricted in usefulness to readily soluble drugs and, like the oral route, it is dependent on the patient's cooperation. Rectal administration can be used in unconscious patients, but it has the disadvantage that retention is frequently unpredictable.

The administration of drugs at other epithelial barriers is usually limited to specific agents or effects. Application to the skin is usually used only when a local drug effect is desired. However, devices for transdermal drug administration provide continuous delivery of drugs to the systemic circulation via the intact skin. Administration by way of the respiratory tract is used for aerosols and other preparations in the therapy of pulmonary diseases such as asthma and for gaseous and volatile agents, including oxygen and substances for general anesthesia.

Subcutaneous and intramuscular administration provides for relatively rapid absorption of drugs since they bypass the epithelial barrier. Absorption from these sites is also more predictable and less variable than from the alimentary canal. The environment at the sites of injection is kept relatively constant, and rates of absorption usually vary only with rates of blood flow through the subcutaneous tissue or muscle. At rest, the rate of absorption following subcutaneous administration is not much slower than that from sites of intramuscular injection, and the latter usually provides more rapid absorption only during muscular activity. Irritating drugs cannot be given by either of these routes, although muscle is less sensitive to damage than is subcutaneous tissue. Both the subcutaneous and intramuscular sites may be used as depots for sustained therapy with formulations of drugs that undergo slow release for solution and absorption. The main disadvantage of both the subcutaneous and intramuscular routes of administration, in common with all routes requiring injection, is the need for special equipment, skill and a suitably prepared form of sterile medication.

The intravascular route completely eliminates the process of absorption and thus represents the most rapid means of introducing drugs into the body. This route has its greatest value in the treatment of emergencies and when absolute control of the amount of drug administered is essential. It is the most hazardous route, since there can be no recall once the drug is given. Intravascular injections require the greatest amount of skill and the most careful attention to the preparation of the injected material. Introduction of particulate matter or air may produce embolism – the obstruction of blood vessels – which may prove fatal. Infections introduced by intravenous injections may also be more widespread than those resulting from injections at other sites. Drugs should never be introduced directly into the bloodstream unless specifically indicated.

GUIDES FOR STUDY AND REVIEW

What distinguishes *enteral* from *parenteral* routes of absorption?

What distinguishes drug administration for local effects from administration for systemic effects? How may drugs be administered for local effects?

From the standpoint of absorption, what distinguishes the subcutaneous, intramuscular, and intravenous routes from the oral route of administration? What are the advantages and disadvantages of each of these routes?

How does the blood flow influence the rate of absorption from different sites of drug administration? What is the role of the lymphatic system in drug absorption?

Which routes of administration avoid exposure of the drug to the liver before its exposure to the general circulation? Why is the initial exposure of a drug to the liver an important factor in the overall pharmacologic effect of some drugs?

What are the factors that modify the gastric absorption of a drug? Why is the rate of gastric emptying a primary determinant of the overall rate of drug absorption following oral administration?

Why is absorption usually greater from the intestine than from the stomach in the case of basic drugs? in the case of acidic and neutral drugs?

When are rates of disintegration and dissolution of solid dosage forms determinants of the rate of drug absorption? of pharmacodynamic effects?

How can the rate of absorption of the drug in solution be altered intentionally for a drug given orally? subcutaneously? intramuscularly?

How are rates of disintegration and dissolution of solid dosage forms modified? Does a change in particle size always affect dissolution rate? absorption rate? How can drugs that are susceptible to chemical alteration in the stomach be protected?

For what types of drugs or clinical situations is the sustained-release preparation a useful dosage form for oral administration? for subcutaneous administration? for intramuscular administration? Why are sustained-release preparations unsatisfactory in some people at certain times?

What are some advantages of transdermal drug delivery devices? For what types of drugs is this a useful system?

What environmental and physiologic factors in addition to pH can modify oral absorption?

When would it be advantageous and feasible to use the sublingual route for drug administration? The rectal route?

How does drug absorption from the skin compare qualitatively and quantitatively with absorption at other epithelial barriers?

Why does drug administration by inhalation closely resemble intravenous drug administration in terms of the rapidity with which the drug enters the general circulation?

How do drug solubility and particle size influence the site and extent of absorption of drugs inhaled as solids?

SUGGESTED READING

Ansel, H.C., Allen, L.V., Popovich, N.G. *Pharmaceutical Dosage Forms and Drug Delivery Systems* (7th ed.). Baltimore: Lippincott Williams & Wilkins, 2004.

Benet, L.Z. Effect of route of administration and distribution on drug action. *J. Pharmacokinet. Biopharm.* 6:559, 1978.

Benet, L.Z. Understanding bioequivalence testing. *Transplant. Proc.* 31:7S–9S, 1999.

Dressman, J.B. and Lennernas, H. (eds) *Oral Drug Absorption: Prediction and Assessment* (Drugs and the Pharmaceutical Sciences, vol. 106). New York: Marcel Dekker, 2000.

Langer, R. Drug delivery and targeting. *Nature* 392 (6679 Suppl):5–10, 1998.

Urquhart, J. Controlled drug delivery: therapeutic and pharmacological aspects. *J. Intern. Med.* 248:357–376, 2000.

Levine, R.R. Intestinal absorption. In Rabinowitz, J.L. and Myerson, R.M. (eds). *Absorption Phenomena.* New York: Wiley, 1972.

Prescott, L.F. and Nimmo, W.S. (eds). *Drug Absorption.* New York: Adis Press, 1981.

Saltzman, W.M. *Drug Delivery: Engineering Principles for Drug Therapy.* New York: Oxford University Press, 2001.

Walters, K.A. (ed.) *Dermatological and Transdermal Formulations* (Drugs and the Pharmaceutical Sciences, vol. 119). New York: Marcel Dekker, 2002.

Zhang, Y. and Benet, L.Z. The gut as a barrier to drug absorption: combined role of cytochrome P450 3A and P-glycoprotein. *Clin. Pharmacokinet.* 40:159–168, 2001.

How Drugs Reach Their Site of Action
III. Distribution

Once a solute has reached the bloodstream, the principal pathway for its distribution, it usually must traverse one or more biologic barriers in order to reach its ultimate site of action. Its accessibility to this site is determined initially by its ability to cross the capillary wall, then by the blood flow through the site and finally, if the drug acts intracellularly, by its rate of passage across cells. Thus the sequence of movement of a solute in the process of its distribution is the *reverse* of that involved in its absorption.

Since the capillary is the initial barrier to distribution, its permeability characteristics will be our first concern. We shall then examine the general factors that influence the amount of drug eventually reaching its site of action. Finally, special attention will be directed to the singular aspects of passage of drugs into the brain and across the placenta into the fetus.

CAPILLARY PERMEABILITY

The tissue covering the surface of internal cavities of the body is *endothelium*. The individual cells comprising the endothelium overlap each other at their margins but are not as closely approximated as are epithelial cells. In the capillaries, this lining is one cell thick and is continuous throughout the closed passages. However, in the liver the smallest channels of its circulation, called *sinusoids*, are even simpler than capillaries. These sinusoids lack a complete endothelial lining, and their walls are, at least in part, nonexistent because there are large gaps in the abutments between the endothelial cells.

We have previously noted that small lipid-soluble molecules like gases pass into, and consequently out of, the capillary so readily that equilibrium on both sides of the vessel wall is reached almost instantaneously. The same holds true for nongaseous lipid-soluble materials, the lipid/water partition coefficient being the most important factor in determining differences in rates among compounds. In fact, the rate at which any molecule diffuses across the capillary endothelium at all sites except the brain is greater than its rate of passage across epithelial tissue. At both types of tissues this diffusion occurs across the *cellular membrane* and not between cells. Thus, whether there is greater separation between endothelial cells than between epithelial cells becomes a moot point with respect to the observed differences in rates of penetration of lipid-soluble substances across these two barriers. Rather, these differences may be attributed to disparities in the rates at which an absorptive surface is made available to a molecule within the capillary compared with that at epithelial tissues. The solutes in the blood are flowing within minute tubes, only 0.005–0.01 mm in diameter, completely surrounded by endothelium with an entire surface that is conducive to diffusion. The flow of blood within these narrow channels affords many more opportunities for molecules of solute to collide with permeable surfaces than are provided for molecules within the intraluminal contents of the intestine, for example. This situation is somewhat analogous to the differences in rates of absorption between the stomach and small intestine: it is the huge difference in the area of available absorptive surface that gives the intestine the much greater capacity for absorption of all materials.

Water-soluble molecules, and water itself, also readily traverse the capillary wall, but at rates slower than compounds with lipid solubility. Molecular size is the major determinant of the rate of transcapillary movement: the smaller the water-soluble molecule, the faster its rate of diffusion. But even relatively large molecules like proteins are able to penetrate the capillary endothelium very slowly. The hypothetical existence of pores penetrating the cell membrane might explain these phenomena. Yet pores are not observed generally in the plasma membrane of normal endothelium, even though the electron microscope can detect pores of the diameter needed to accommodate proteins. Rather, in the case of water-soluble molecules, the gaps that exist *between* endothelial cells have indeed been shown to serve as passageways from the circulation to the extravascular spaces. Furthermore, capillary permeability can be increased by an agent such as histamine, which acts directly on the endothelial cells to enlarge the gaps between them. Thus the difference between the organization of individual cells of the endothelial and epithelial barriers does have some functional significance.

Relatively small water-soluble molecules cross the capillary at rates directly proportional to their concentration gradients, as if they were simply diffusing in water. In contrast, the driving force for movement of the large water-soluble substances appears to be the hydrostatic pressure exerted by the blood. The pressure of the blood on the arterial end of the capillaries is normally higher than that at the venous end (see Fig. 5-12). It is this pressure gradient between the two ends of the capillary bed that largely accounts for the transcapillary movement of high-molecular-weight compounds like protein. Since the pressure gradient normally fluctuates and may also be influenced by various drugs, the permeability of the capillary is characteristically dynamic and continually subject to change. Whereas the rate of movement of macromolecules is strongly dependent on the hydrostatic pressure in the capillary lumen, the actual mechanism of their transfer across the capillary remains in doubt. Pinocytosis has been suggested as a possibility on the basis of microscopy studies that revealed the presence of vesicles at either margin of the endothelial membrane. This mechanism may contribute to the increase in endothelial permeability caused by substances released from tumor cells that stimulate blood vessel growth.

In the liver and kidney the capillaries present less of a barrier to the movement of molecules of all sizes than do capillaries elsewhere. These differences are important since they serve the functions of these organs: the kidney is the organ chiefly responsible for the excretion of water-soluble compounds; the liver not only manufactures many proteins for use by the body, but also receives most substances absorbed from the small intestine before they are distributed. In the kidney the increase in permeability is primarily one of rate rather than kind of material transferred. Two factors contribute to this increase. First, the capillaries associated with the initiation of urine formation in the renal glomeruli contain large pores or *fenestrae* in the endothelial wall at the junctions between cells; these pores are readily visualized by means of the electron microscope. Second, the hydrostatic pressure within these capillaries is very high compared with that of many other capillary beds. This force is responsible for the increased rates of solute movement, since diffusion is supplemented by transcapillary *filtration* through the pores. In the liver the increased permeability relates mainly to the greater rate of translocation of large molecules. Blood from both the heart and the portal vein draining the intestine courses through the hepatic *sinusoids* before being returned to the heart by the hepatic vein. Since these sinusoids have a discontinuous endothelial lining, large molecules, even large proteins, can enter and leave the blood flowing through the liver more readily than the blood flowing through other tissues of the body.

MAGNITUDE OF DISTRIBUTION

It is clear from the foregoing that the blood capillary is a relatively effective barrier only to large molecules. Therefore, when a macromolecular compound is injected intravascularly, it is almost completely retained in the extracellular fluid of the circulation – the plasma – since its size also precludes entry into the blood cells. The action of the heart and the turbulence of the uneven blood flow through various vessels mixes the agent quickly with the circulating plasma. In the average 70-kg man, the volume of plasma is approximately 3 l, a little more than half of the whole blood volume. So within a very few minutes the quantity of drug originally entering the circulation is diluted into this volume of fluid. We can say, then, that a drug which is unable to cross the capillary wall has an **apparent volume of distribution** equal to plasma-water (Fig. 6-1).

In contrast, the volume of distribution of a drug capable of readily traversing the capillary endothelium will be greater than that of plasma-water. Let us, for the moment, specify an ideal situation in which the drug is (1) a free solute, unbound to any tissue components; (2) unchanged by any chemical reactions of the body; and (3) not eliminated during the period of distribution. When such

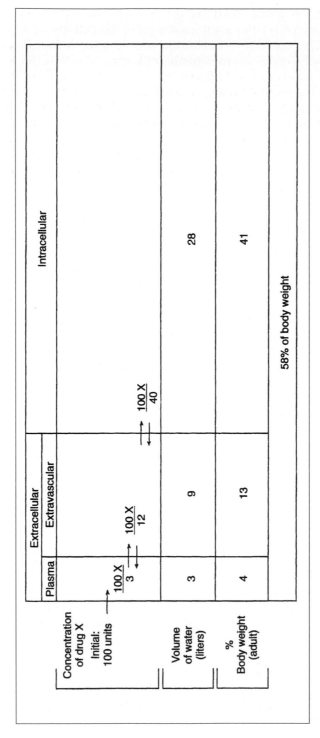

Figure 6-1. *Distribution and concentration of a drug in the various fluid compartments of the body in relation to its permeability characteristics. The values for water content of the plasma and extracellular and intracellular compartments are only approximate. These figures do not include the inaccessible water in bone, or the water in the cavities of the stomach, intestine and tracheobronchial tree, in the cerebrospinal fluid or in the anterior chamber of the eye (total 7–10%).*

an agent enters the circulation, either by direct placement or following absorption, it will be mixed into plasma-water. But as this dilution is taking place, the concentration gradient in the plasma will drive the drug across the capillary wall. It will diffuse at a rate consistent with its molecular size, lipid solubility, and degree of ionization. Let us also assume, for the present, that the permeability characteristics of capillaries are identical all over the body. Then, since all tissues are supplied with capillaries, the drug will be distributed from the plasma to the extracellular fluid of *all* parts of the body. This movement of drug into the interstitial water of the tissues will continue until there is no longer a gradient between the inside and outside of the capillaries supplying the tissues. Obviously, however, the *rate* at which the drug concentration in the extracellular fluid of a particular site reaches this point of equilibrium will depend on the number of capillaries coursing through it. The richer the vascularity, the greater the blood flow and the more rapid the distribution of drug from plasma to the extravascular interstitial fluid. Table 6-1 shows average rates of blood flow through some organs of the body in relation to their mass. These data indicate that a drug will appear in the extracellular fluid of organs like the kidney, heart, brain and liver more rapidly than in that of tissues like muscle or fat.

Yet, eventually, assuming our ideal conditions, the concentration of drug in *all* extracellular water, including plasma-water, will reach the *same* level. When this equilibrium is attained, the quantity of drug that originally entered the bloodstream will be diluted into about 12 l, the sum of extravascular interstitial fluid (about 9 l in the 70-kg adult male) plus the volume of plasma-water. Hence, a drug which can readily leave the capillaries but which cannot enter cells will have an apparent volume of distribution equal to the total extracellular

Table 6-1. *Blood flow in various organs and tissues[1]*

Tissue	Tissue mass (% of total body weight)	Blood flow (l/min)	Blood flow (l/kg of tissue/min)
Rapidly perfused			
Kidneys	0.4	1.27	4.5
Heart (musculature)	0.4	0.21	0.70
Brain	2.0	0.8	0.55
Liver (hepatic artery flow)	2.0	0.27	0.20
Less rapidly perfused			
Skin	7.0	0.27	0.05
Muscle (resting)	45.0	0.8	0.03
Poorly perfused			
Fat tissue	15.0	0.1	0.01
Connective tissue	7.0	0.05	0.01

[1]Values in this table are to be considered as approximations only. Calculations are for a 70-kg man and 5.4 l cardiac output.

fluid. Ions such as iodide or water-soluble molecules the size of sucrose or larger remain, for the most part, distributed within extracellular fluid. And drugs that are so poorly absorbed from the gastrointestinal tract that they must be administered by a route that bypasses epithelial tissues are usually largely confined to this volume of distribution.

If the drug is capable of traversing the cell membrane, it will move from the extracellular space into the fluid within the cell. Assuming no active transport process is involved, the transfer across the cell wall will proceed until the intracellular drug concentration is the same as that outside the cell. Since the permeability characteristics of the cellular membrane are about the same for all cells, it follows that the concentration of the drug will be further diluted by a volume equal to that of the total intracellular water of all cells, approximately 28 l in a 70-kg subject. Consequently, a drug which can readily pass all biologic barriers will have an apparent volume of distribution at least equal to the total water content of the body, about 40 l per 70 kg, or 58% of body weight. All highly lipid-soluble drugs have this type of distribution.

It is both customary and convenient to express the extent of drug distribution, as we have above, in terms of the water content of compartments of the body which are anatomically and functionally distinct, i.e. vascular fluid, extracellular fluid and intracellular fluid (see Fig. 6-1). This convention, however, is based on an idealized situation and, as such, is an oversimplification, ignoring many known variables while incorporating a number of assumptions that may or may not be correct. Nonetheless, this general treatment permits drawing some valid and important conclusions about the distribution of drug from the circulation. First, the quantity of drug reaching an extravascular site of action represents only a *small* fraction of the total amount of drug administered. And the more readily diffusible the drug, the smaller the fraction likely to reach its target, and the greater its distribution to parts of the body not involved with the production of the desired biologic effects. Thus, the very nature of the process for getting most drugs to their various sites of action is responsible for dispersing them throughout the tissues of the body.

BINDING OF DRUGS TO PLASMA PROTEINS AND OTHER TISSUE COMPONENTS AND ACCUMULATION IN FAT

One of the assumptions made in developing the general picture of the distribution of drugs is that the drug remains as a solute in the fluid of various compartments of the body. Obviously, the rate of movement of a drug across biologic barriers is determined by its *own* physicochemical properties only when it exists as an independent entity. This ideal behavior is characteristic of very few drugs. The same kinds of bonds that are formed when a drug interacts with its receptor can be formed between drug molecules and other macromolecular tissue components. The major difference, of course, is that the drug-receptor combination leads directly to a sequence of events measurable as a biologic effect, whereas binding with a nonreceptor substance does not. The binding sites that do not function as true receptors are sometimes referred to as *secondary receptors, silent receptors* or *sites of loss*. The last is the most appropriate designation, since the molecules of a drug that are bound to nonreceptor macromolecules are neither free to move to a site of action nor free to produce a biologic effect. The importance of these interactions with sites of loss will depend on how much drug is bound and on the strength, or reversibility, of the bond formation.

Binding of drugs to tissue constituents can occur at sites of absorption, within the plasma or at extravascular sites following egress from the bloodstream. For example, in the intestine the positively charged quarternary ammonium compounds are strongly bound to highly negatively charged groups of the mucus secreted into the lumen. The large quantities of mucus normally present can act as sites of loss for a considerable quantity of the positively charged molecules and thereby decrease the effective concentration gradient of the drug. This binding has been shown to account in part for the incomplete absorption of quarternary ammonium drugs and for the fact that, to produce equal effects, larger quantities must be administered orally than parenterally. However, the proteins of plasma are the most common and well-characterized site for drug binding, in part because this binding can be so readily detected.

Albumin, the principal protein of plasma, is the protein with which the greatest variety of drugs combine. Antibiotics such as penicillin, tetracycline and sulfa preparations, as well as drugs like aspirin and the anticoagulant warfarin, among many others, exist in plasma to a greater or lesser extent as a reversibly bound albumin complex. But how much and how strongly any drug will be bound to albumin is a property of the drug inherent in its molecular structure; the tendency to bind with protein – its affinity for protein – is a constant for a given drug. Generally, the interaction of drugs with albumin is a reversible reaction. Because of this, the law of mass action is applicable.

$$\text{Free drug + protein} \rightleftharpoons \text{Drug-protein complex}$$

The fraction of drug that is bound will be in equilibrium with the fraction of drug that is free. Ordinarily, the protein concentration of plasma is fixed, and therefore the fraction of drug that is free to leave the plasma is determined only by the concentration of drug and strength of the binding. At low drug concentrations, the stronger the bond between the drug and protein, the smaller the fraction that is free. As drug concentration increases, the concentration of free drug also gradually rises until all the binding capacity of the protein has been saturated. At this point, any additional drug will remain unbound.

How does this binding to plasma protein influence the distribution of a drug to its site of action? Binding to protein, by decreasing the concentration of free drug in the circulation, lowers the concentration gradient driving the drug out of the circulation and slows its rate of transfer across the capillary. The complex of drug bound to plasma protein is generally too large to diffuse out of the capillary even in the relatively porous renal glomerulus. However, as the free drug leaves the circulation, the protein-drug complex begins to dissociate and more free drug is available for diffusion. Thus as long as the binding is reversible, it does not prevent the drug from reaching its site of action but only *retards* the rate at which this occurs. Furthermore, as the drug is eliminated from the body, more can be dissociated from the protein complex to replace what is lost. In this way, plasma-protein binding can act as a reservoir to make a drug available over a longer period. For example, some sulfa drugs are strongly bound to protein and are eliminated slowly in the urine, since only the fraction that is free can diffuse out of the capillaries. Consequently, these compounds remain in the body and are effective for longer periods than those sulfa drugs which have lower affinities for protein. Suramin, a drug used in the treatment of the protozoal infection trypanosomiasis, is an example of an agent still more firmly bound to plasma proteins. It is likewise very slowly eliminated in the urine, but unlike the sulfa drugs, suramin is not appreciably altered by the chemical reactions carried out by the body. These factors combine to yield therapeutically effective levels of suramin for extended periods, sometimes as long as 3 months, following a single intravenous injection.

Other tissues of the body can also act as reservoirs for drugs, but usually the *sites where drugs accumulate are not those where they exert their pharmacologic effect*. For example, tetracycline may be stored in bone, and the cannabinoid THC in fat. These stored drugs are in equilibrium with the drug in plasma and are returned to plasma as the plasma concentration decreases upon elimination of the drug from the body. However, the rate of release from the storage depots in the case of these two agents is ordinarily too slow to provide enough circulating drug to produce biologic effects. Consequently, this type of storage represents a site of loss rather than a depot for continued drug action. A classic example of binding to tissue components is provided by the interaction of the antiparasitic agent chloroquine with nucleic acids of the cell nucleus. The drug may achieve a concentration in the liver 200–700 times the plasma concentration. When chloroquine is used to treat malaria, the liver represents a site of loss which must be saturated before plasma levels adequate for antimalarial therapy can be reached. In contrast, this accumulation of chloroquine in the liver becomes therapeutically useful in amebiasis when the intestinal infestation has spread to the liver.

Fat tissue is an important reservoir site for lipophilic drugs. Due to their solubility characteristics, these drugs accumulate in fat and achieve much higher concentrations in this tissue than in plasma. Because fat tissue contributes a fairly substantial percentage of total body weight, a significant fraction of the amount of drug in the body may be located in this site. The apparent volume of distribution of lipophilic drugs is often considerably higher than total body water, and even body weight, because of the accumulation of drug in fat. This tissue is poorly perfused, however, and so the distribution of drugs into and out of this reservoir site occurs slowly, as compared to other tissues such as the brain. It follows that the binding of a drug to nonreceptor sites or accumulation in some tissues generally means that more drug has to be administered in order to ensure its availability to its site of action. When the phenomenon of

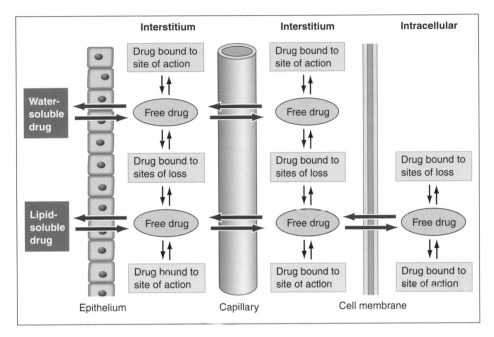

Figure 6-2. *Factors influencing the amount of drug that will reach a site of action following absorption and distribution. In the plasma and interstitium, functionally important small ions or proteins may be sites of action; in the interstitium, the cell membrane may also be a site of action for drugs acting by receptor or nonreceptor mechanisms. Intracellular sites of action may be receptors or identifiable cellular components. The capillary endothelial barrier is not included on the other side of the epithelial barrier for the sake of clarity. Obviously, drugs which are absorbed through an epithelial barrier must also pass through the capillary endothelium before entering the plasma.*

binding and accumulation is added to the generalized dispersal of drug inherent in the process of distribution, it becomes obvious that the amount of drug in the tissue or site where it acts is, indeed, a very small portion of what was originally introduced into the body (Fig. 6-2).

DISTRIBUTION FROM BLOOD TO BRAIN

It has been stated several times that capillaries in the brain do not permit substances to leave the blood as readily as do capillaries elsewhere in the body. Actually, this decreased permeability pertains only to the *diffusion of water-soluble or ionized* molecules. Lipid-soluble substances diffuse across brain capillaries at rates determined by their lipid/water partition coefficients, just as at other capillary barriers. In fact, since the brain receives one-sixth of the total amount of blood leaving the heart, lipid-soluble drugs are distributed to the brain very rapidly compared with a tissue such as muscle (Table 6-1). Water-soluble materials for which active transport processes exist, such as glucose and amino acids, also gain rapid access to brain cells.

A factor that contributes to the slow diffusion of water-soluble materials from capillary to brain tissue is the organization of the endothelium itself. The endothelial cells of brain capillaries are much more firmly joined to one another than is characteristic of other capillary endothelia. Moreover, the increased resistance to the passage of water-soluble and ionized materials is also due to the fact that the brain capillaries do not communicate directly with the interstitium. Interposed between the capillary endothelium and the extracellular space of the brain is another membrane that is very closely attached to the capillary wall. Certain cells within the brain connective tissue, the astrocytes, have long processes that form sheaths around the capillaries. As a result, substances leaving the blood must traverse not only the capillary endothelium, but also the astrocytic sheath in order to reach the interstitial fluid of brain tissue. However, it is the *circumferential tight junctions* of the endothelial cells of the brain capillaries that form the barrier, which is usually referred to as the *blood-brain barrier*. In addition, the endothelial cells in the vasculature of the brain contain transporter proteins that can pump some drugs from the endothelium *back* into the plasma. Inhibition of the function of these transporters can increase drug distribution into brain tissue. So for some drugs, the blood-brain barrier results as well from the role of tranporters.

Passage across the capillary directly into the interstitial fluid represents only one of the ways in which chemicals can reach brain tissue. Materials can also leave the blood and directly enter the *cerebrospinal fluid* (CSF). The CSF system bathes the surfaces of the brain and spinal cord, functioning as a protective layer to cushion the delicate tissue against trauma. The CSF thus represents a third fluid compartment within the brain, the other two being the extravascular extracellular and intracellular fluid compartments. Cerebrospinal fluid is formed in the brain itself, primarily within its cavities, or *ventricles* (Fig. 6-3). From these ventricular sites of formation the CSF circulates to the spaces surrounding the surfaces of the brain and spinal cord, and from these spaces the bulk of the fluid flows directly into the venous drainage system of the brain. Since most of the CSF does not recycle, there is constant need for its regeneration. A specialized vascular organ within each ventricle, the *choroid plexus*, functions in this capacity. It is located between the blood capillary wall and the ventricle and is lined on its ventricular side with epithelial cells. These cells have the same provisions for solute transport as do other epithelial barriers, including active transport processes. Consequently, the transfer of chemical substances from the blood across the choroid plexus into the CSF has the characteristics of passage across epithelium rather than those across simply endothelium. Once in the CSF, material can enter brain tissue at rates typical of passage from interstitial fluid across cell membranes. In this manner the CSF provides a gateway for substances to reach the intracellular spaces of the brain as well as a pathway for solutes to be returned to the venous system (Fig. 6-4). The juxtaposition of epithelial tissue between the blood-CSF barrier and the circumferential tight

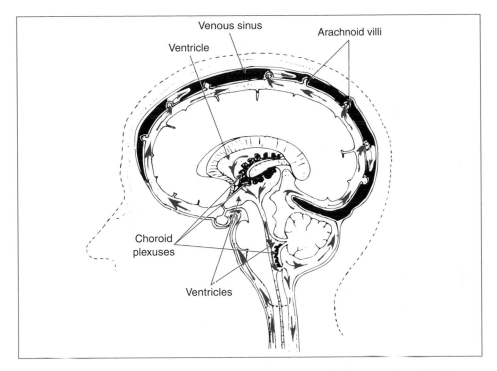

Figure 6-3. *Circulation of cerebrospinal fluid (CSF). Channels through which CSF flows are exaggerated, and structures of the brain are not drawn to scale. The choroid plexuses are tufts of small capillary vessels much like renal glomeruli. The CSF elaborated into the centrally located ventricles (lateral and third) flows downward to the lower ventricle. Fluid is added by the choroid plexus of the lower ventricle (fourth) and then flows either downward to bathe the spinal cord or upward to bathe the convexities of the brain. The fluid finally reaches the arachnoid villi, where it drains into the great venous sinuses. The quantity of CSF in the ventricles and subarachnoid spaces is usually between 125 and 150 ml.*

junctions that characterize the blood capillary – the blood-brain barrier – together account for the slow diffusion of water-soluble materials into brain tissue.

The major portion of the CSF drains directly into venous blood, and drugs may leave the CSF by this bulk flow into the venous sinuses. However, a small portion of the CSF is formed from material returning to the ventricle from the extracellular fluid. This is important from a pharmacologic viewpoint, since some drugs are actively transported by the choroid plexus *out* of the CSF back into the blood. One such drug is penicillin. Because this water-soluble drug also enters the brain and CSF very slowly, as would be expected on the basis of its physicochemical properties, it is not ordinarily as effective an antibiotic in the treatment of infections in this region of the body as it is elsewhere.

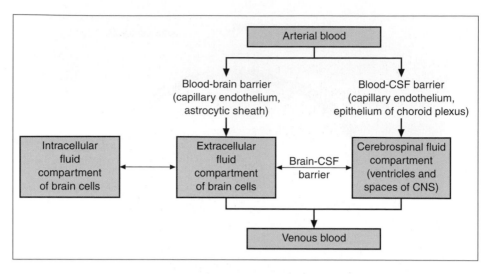

Figure 6-4. *Structural and functional relationships of the blood supply, cerebrospinal fluid and extracellular and intracellular fluid compartments of the brain. A drug may enter the brain by crossing either the blood-brain barrier or the blood-CSF barrier. Material entering by the blood-CSF barrier must cross an additional barrier, the brain-CSF barrier, in order to reach the extracellular fluid compartment of the brain. Material can only enter and leave the intracellular fluid compartment by the extracellular fluid compartment. Materials are returned to the venous blood from either the extracellular fluid compartment or the CSF fluid compartment.*

The slow rate of entry of water-soluble drugs into the brain has still other pharmacologic consequences. As the example of penicillin illustrates, a drug intended for action in the brain must have solubility characteristics that permit its distribution to this site. Conversely, water-soluble drugs may be used purposely when it is desirable to exclude effects on the brain. For example, the antihistamine diphenhydramine (BENADRYL) is often used for relief of allergic symptoms. However, because it has lipid solubility and readily enters brain tissue, it produces sedation, which is usually undesirable. This side effect can be largely avoided by substituting a highly water-soluble agent that has pharmacologic effects outside the brain similar to those of diphenhydramine. The antihistamine fexofenadine (ALLEGRA), which does not produce sedation, adequately fulfills these conditions.

DISTRIBUTION FROM MOTHER TO FETUS

The same pathways that serve to supply the fetus with the substances necessary for development and growth and that act to remove waste material also provide the means by which drugs interchange between the maternal and fetal circulations. This mutual exchange takes place primarily in the placenta, which connects the embryo or fetus with the maternal uterine wall (Fig. 6-5). Within the

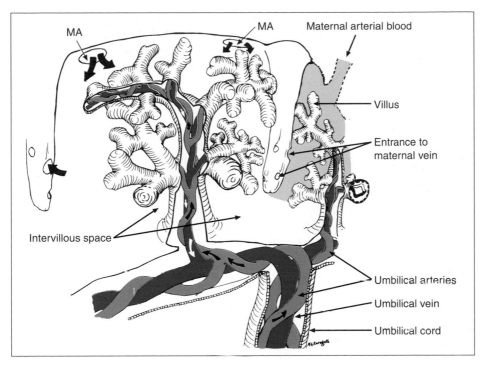

Figure 6-5. *Relationship of maternal and fetal blood vessels. Maternal blood from the uterine arteries (MA) enters a pool (intervillous space) where it is exposed directly to the epithelial membranes of the fetal villus. Materials from the maternal blood cross the villous membrane and enter fetal capillaries, from which they are carried to the fetus by the fetal placental veins which converge into the umbilical vein. Materials to be transferred from the fetal circulation to maternal blood are brought to the fetal side of the placenta by the umbilical arteries. Maternal blood from the intervillous space drains into the maternal uterine veins to be returned to the maternal systemic circulation.*

placenta are relatively large cavities, sinuses, into which the maternal arterial blood empties and from which veins arise to carry blood back to the mother. Fetal capillaries are contained in finger-like processes, villi, protruding into the blood sinuses. Thus, maternal and fetal blood do not mingle, and solute transfer takes place across the epithelial cells of the villi and the endothelium of the fetal capillaries. Material reaching the fetal capillaries is carried to the fetus by the umbilical venous blood, and material to be transferred from fetus to mother returns to the villi by the umbilical arterial blood.

The characteristics of drug diffusion from maternal blood to fetal blood in the capillaries of the villi are very similar to those of passage across any epithelial barrier. Lipid-soluble materials readily move from mother to fetus in accordance with lipid/water partition coefficients and degree of ionization. Water-soluble drugs move much more slowly and in inverse proportion to their molecular size. The rate and direction of this exchange is dependent on the concentration gradients and the rate of delivery to the intervillous spaces and villi.

As indicated above, drug distribution from mother to fetus begins with diffusion of the drug across the villous membrane into the fetal blood capillary. The drug is then carried to the fetus by way of the umbilical vein and finally becomes available for distribution to the various fetal organs and tissues. It is obvious from this pattern of distribution that the cord venous blood will reach equilibrium with maternal blood much more rapidly than will be true for the various tissues of the fetus. It has been estimated that the fastest equilibrium possible between maternal blood and fetal tissues is about 40 minutes, even when the maternal blood has a constant level of a drug over a period of time. The rate of maternal blood flow to the placenta limits the availability of the drug to the fetus. This explains why a wakeful infant can be delivered to an anesthetized mother provided the delivery takes place within about 15–30 minutes after drug administration. If the quantity of drug used to anesthetize the mother is within therapeutic range and the delivery takes place quickly, the fetus is never likely to have blood levels sufficient to produce a state of anesthesia. However, if a drug is administered many hours before delivery, the fetus may, indeed, acquire sufficient drug to produce effects. For example, in the past, some women were deeply anesthetized with a barbiturate 2–3 hours before delivery; their newborn infants remained drowsy for 12–24 hours following delivery. Also, pinpoint pupils have been observed in infants born to mothers who received morphine during labor, well before delivery.

Whereas a single administration of a drug may not necessarily lead to pharmacologic effects in the fetus, frequent administration during gestation may produce adverse effects. Infants born to mothers addicted to drugs like morphine or heroin show all the withdrawal symptoms that addicts show when they, too, are no longer receiving these agents. Newborn infants with a history of intrauterine exposure to cocaine have abnormal electroencephalograms (EEGs) and show other signs of central nervous system dysfunction which can persist for months or longer; some have even suffered heart attacks after delivery. Typical pharmacologic effects are observed in newborn infants, which indicate that other agents also gain ready access to the fetus.

The exposure of the pregnant female to certain agents, particularly during the early stages of fetal development in the first trimester, has been linked to the production of defects of one or more of the infant's organ systems. Agents that increase the risk of fetal malformations are referred to as teratogens. This phenomenon was first recognized in the 1930s when malformed offspring were born to women who had been exposed to X-ray irradiation of the pelvic region during early pregnancy. Another concern is the effect of environmental contaminants such as products of nuclear fission (e.g. radioactive cesium, calcium and strontium) and organic mercury compounds, which readily cross the placental barrier. In 1940 the rubella virus was shown to be capable of producing serious malformations in infants whose mothers had suffered even mild infections of German measles in the first trimester of pregnancy. But it took the thalidomide disaster of 1960–1962 to bring to full awareness the fact that ordinary drugs can be most harmful to the fetus even though they have little potential for adverse effects in the adult female (cf. p. 332). In some cases adverse effects of a drug on the fetus may not become apparent until the offspring have themselves reached adulthood. This has been shown to be the case for diethylstilbestrol (DES), a once widely used estrogen. Large doses of estrogens were used in the past in the unsubstantiated belief that this might prevent threatened miscarriage. Since DES, in contrast to the natural estrogens, was effective orally as well as cheap and plentiful, it was the drug usually administered. In the early 1970s, an increased incidence of vaginal carcinoma was discovered in the female offspring of women who had received DES during the first trimester of pregnancy – a time when the fetal reproductive system is developing. More recently the use of alcohol during pregnancy has been shown to cause fetal growth retardation, a variety of major and minor malformations, and central nervous system dysfunction, referred to as the fetal alcohol syndrome (when only the central nervous system dysfunction is present, the term used is fetal alcohol effects). The uncertainty of the risk to the human embryo that may be associated with the use of any drug certainly dictates that all unnecessary medication be avoided during pregnancy and particularly during the first trimester.

REMARKS

In this chapter we have gained some insight into the ways in which distribution influences the accessibility of a drug to its site of action. The rates at which the processes of both absorption and distribution take place will, of course, determine not only how much drug is made available to a site of action but also how quickly the action will be seen after drug administration – the *onset* of drug action. However, while absorption and distribution are proceeding, other processes are also in operation, namely, those involved in removing the drug from its site of action. In the next two chapters we shall consider how drugs are eliminated, so that we can put all the processes together in proper perspective and determine their combined effects on the entire course of drug action.

GUIDES FOR STUDY AND REVIEW

What distinguishes the process of distribution from that of absorption?

What do we mean by 'apparent volume of distribution'? What is the approximate fluid volume of the major compartments into which the body is conveniently divided?

What factors determine the rate and volume of distribution of different types of drugs? What factors determine the rate of distribution of a particular drug to various organs and tissues?

How do differences in capillary permeability affect drug distribution to various organs and tissues?

How does binding to plasma proteins influence the rate of drug distribution to various tissues and organs? Does binding to plasma proteins alter the actual volume of distribution of the unbound drug? Does binding to plasma proteins alter the rate of drug elimination? If so, how? Does binding to tissue sites or accumulation in fat alter the calculated apparent volume of drug distribution? How?

How are drugs transferred from the blood to the brain? What are the factors that tend to keep many drugs from entering the tissues of the central nervous system (CNS)? What factors tend to make the rate of distribution of some drugs more rapid to the CNS than to tissues like muscle or fat? Which types of drugs gain ready access to the CNS and which do not?

How are drugs transferred between the mother-to-be and the fetus? Why can a wakeful infant be delivered to an anesthetized mother when the delivery takes place within about 15 to 30 minutes of drug administration?

SUGGESTED READING

Begley, D.J. and Brightman, M.W. Structural and functional aspects of the blood-brain barrier. *Prog. Drug Res.* 61:39–78, 2003.

Bertucci, C. and Domenici, E. Reversible and covalent binding of drugs to human serum albumin: methodological approaches and physiological relevance. *Curr. Med. Chem.* 9:1463–1481, 2002.

Briggs, G.G. Drug effects on the fetus and breast-fed infant. *Clin. Obstet. Gyn.* 45:6–21, 2002.

Butler, T. The distribution of drugs. In: La Du, B.N., Mandel, H.G. and Way, E.L. (eds). *Fundamentals of Drug Metabolism and Drug Disposition*. Melbourne: Krieger Publishing Co., 1979.

de Boer, A.G., van der Sandt, I.C. and Gaillard, P.J. The role of drug transporters at the blood-brain barrier. *Annu. Rev. Pharmacol. Toxicol.* 43:629–656, 2003.

Garland, M. Pharmacology of drug transfer across the placenta. *Obstet. Gynecol. Clin. North Am.* 25:21–42, 1998.

Green, T.P., O'Dea, R.F. and Mirkin, B.L. Determination of drug disposition and effect in the fetus. *Annu. Rev. Pharmacol. Toxicol.* 19:285, 1979.

Greenblatt, D.J., Sellers, E.M. and Koch-Weser, J. Importance of protein binding for the interpretation of serum or plasma drug concentrations. *J. Clin. Pharmacol.* 22:259, 1982.

Pardridge, W.M. Drug and gene delivery to the brain: the vascular route. *Neuron* 36:555–558, 2002.

7   How the Actions of Drugs are Terminated

I. Excretion

The processes of absorption and distribution determine not only how but also how quickly a drug will reach its site of action; they determine the *speed of onset* of drug effect. If nothing else happened to a drug after it entered the body, its action would continue indefinitely. Although this would be advantageous in chronic diseases such as epilepsy or diabetes, it would not be so in most other illnesses. But the interactions between a drug and the body are not confined to the changes that the drug brings about in the living organism; the body also acts on the drug. The same processes that the body normally utilizes to eliminate waste products associated with its growth and maintenance, or to stop the actions of chemicals that it has synthesized, e.g. hormones, also put an end to the actions of drugs introduced into the body. The processes of *excretion* and *biotransformation* and, to a lesser extent, *redistribution* terminate the actions of drugs by removing them from their sites of action.

Excretion is the process whereby materials are removed from the body to the external environment. Biotransformation, or metabolism as it is frequently called, is the process by which chemical reactions carried out by the body convert a drug into a compound different from that originally administered. Redistribution, as the term implies, is the removal of a drug from the tissues where it exerts its effect to tissues unconnected with the characteristic pharmacologic response. The combined rates at which these processes occur determine the *duration of action* of a drug.

We shall start our discussion of how the body acts to terminate the action of a drug by considering the process of excretion; this process, by removing the drug from the body, almost always puts an end to the action of a drug. Next, in Chapter 8, on biotransformation, we shall be concerned primarily with the general principles and types of chemical reactions that drugs undergo in the body. We shall see that the process of biotransformation does not necessarily lead to the immediate cessation of drug effect, yet it may yield products that are more readily excreted than are the parent compounds. The topic of the influence of tissue redistribution on the termination of drug effects is deferred to Chapter 10, in which its discussion will be more pertinent.

ROUTES OF EXCRETION

In the process of excretion the direction of movement of a drug is just the opposite of that involved in getting a drug to its site of action – it is the reverse of distribution and absorption. Excretion involves the movement of a drug from the tissues back into the circulation and from the bloodstream back into those tissues or organs separating the internal from the external environment. Thus, we need formulate no new principles to understand the process of excretion; we need only reconsider the principles that generally govern movement of materials across biologic barriers in terms of some additional anatomic structures.

The lung is the major organ of excretion for gaseous substances, and agents remaining as gases in the body are almost completely eliminated by this route. Agents that can be volatilized at body temperature are also excreted in the expired air to a greater or lesser extent, depending on their volatility. Indeed, so much of the foul-smelling liquid drug paraldehyde is eliminated through the lungs that it has found limited use, even though pharmacologically it could be a suitable agent for inducing sleep. Some alcohol is also excreted in expired air; this is the basis for the medicolegal test commonly used to estimate the blood alcohol level in a person who may have ingested alcohol.

Nonvolatile, water-soluble drugs can leave the body by way of any of the media discharged to its external surface. Sweat, tears, saliva, nasal excretion and the milk of the lactating mother are all examples of fluids in which drugs may be excreted. The amount excreted by any of these routes ordinarily represents only a minor fraction of the total amount of drug eliminated from the body. Yet in the case of breast milk, even a small content of drug may be of considerable consequence to the suckling infant, e.g. cocaine intoxication has been reported in breast-fed infants due to maternal use of cocaine. However, the most important vehicle by far for the excretion of nonvolatile, water-soluble drugs is the urine; there are many instances in which a drug or the product of its biotransformation or both are excreted almost entirely by this route.

The alimentary canal is the next most important route of excretion of nonvolatile agents, and not just for drugs incompletely absorbed following oral administration. Drugs may enter the alimentary canal along its entire length from the mouth to the rectum in any of the fluids secreted into it. If the drug entering the gastrointestinal tract is not readily reabsorbed, it leaves the body in the feces. However, the liver, through its secretion of bile into the small intestine, contributes the major portion of material excreted in this manner. We shall confine our detailed discussion to the two major organs of excretion of water-soluble drugs – the kidney and the liver.

Excretion of Drugs by the Kidney

The volume and composition of the body fluids are kept remarkably stable despite the daily fluctuations imposed by the intake of water, food and other materials, and by the many substances produced by the body itself. To maintain these relatively constant conditions – **homeostasis** – the body has to rid itself of

Table 7-1. *Electrolyte composition of normal blood plasma*

Constituent	Concentration in plasma (mEq/l)
Cations	
Sodium (Na^+)	142
Potassium (K^+)	4
Calcium (Ca^{2+})	5
Magnesium (Mg^{2+})	2
Anions	
Chloride (Cl^-)	101
Bicarbonate (HCO_3^-)	27
Phosphate (HPO_4^{2-})	2
Sulfate (SO_4^{2-})	1
Organic acids	6
Protein	16

materials it cannot use or that are present in excess, while conserving substances essential for its very existence and well-being. In this regulation of homeostasis, the kidney plays a very significant and strategic role. As a major organ of the excretory system, it is responsible for eliminating the majority of the non-volatile, water-soluble substances produced or acquired and not needed by the body. But at the same time that the kidney is performing its excretory function, it must also carry out its additional functions: (1) to maintain a constant volume of circulating blood and regulate the fluid content of the body as a whole; (2) to regulate the **osmotic pressure** relationships of the blood and tissues; and (3) to adjust the relative and absolute concentrations of normal constituents of the plasma (Table 7-1). To carry out these functions simultaneously, the kidney cannot be just a waste-disposal unit. It must be, and is, an organ of functional selectivity, capable of handling individually and according to need the many substances brought to it by the blood. Thus the kidneys, as the 'master chemists of the internal environment'[1] are able to regulate and maintain the constancy of the volume and composition of the body's fluids because they are capable of elaborating a urine of variable volume and composition. And nowhere is it more clearly evident than in the kidney that function is related to structure.

Anatomic Considerations

The human kidney is a bean-shaped organ about 6 inches long, composed of a cortex, or outer layer; a medulla, or middle layer; and a central cavity called the pelvis (Fig. 7-1). The funnel-shaped pelvis is continuous with the ureter, the long tube connecting the kidney to the bladder.

---

[1] Attributed to Homer W. Smith (1895–1962), a famous American renal physiologist.

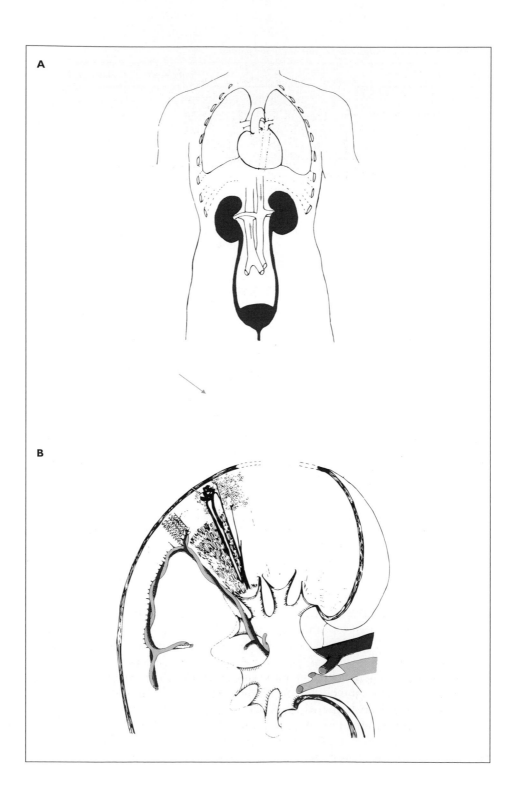

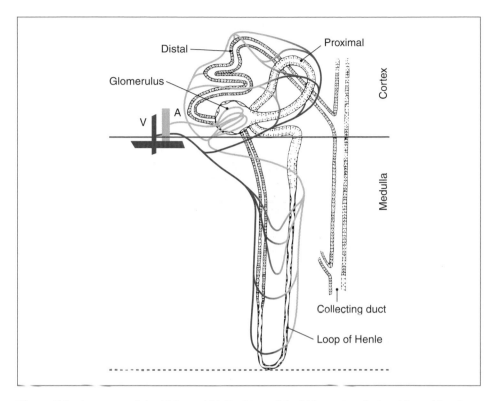

Figure 7-1. *Anatomy of the kidney. (A) Position of the kidneys in relationship to blood vessels and ureters. (B) Gross structure of the kidney, showing relationship of cortex, medulla, pelvis and ureter. The position of a nephron with a long loop of Henle (greatly enlarged) is also indicated. In humans, about 20% of the nephrons extend from the cortex to the papilla. Other nephrons have shorter loops of Henle penetrating to varying depths within the medulla; still other nephrons lie wholly within the cortex. (C) A nephron with a long loop of Henle. The glomerulus and the proximal convoluted, distal convoluted and collecting tubules lie within the cortex. The loop of Henle lies within the medulla, and the collecting duct courses from the cortex through the medulla to the pelvis. The long capillary loop paralleling the loop of Henle is known as the vas recta. V = vein; A = artery.*

The functional unit of the kidney is the nephron. Each nephron consists of a long, unbranched, tortuous tubule originating in the kidney cortex as a closed-ended structure known as *Bowman's capsule*. This capsule envelops a tuft of capillaries called a *glomerulus*. The tubule leading from Bowman's capsule, but continuous with it, is divided into four segments: (1) the proximal segment or proximal convoluted tubule; (2) the loop of Henle; (3) the distal segment or distal convoluted tubule; and (4) the collecting tubule. A single layer of epithelial cells lines the lumen of the nephron throughout its entire length.

Bowman's capsule, created by the invagination of the dilated blind end of the tubule, forms a double-walled enclosure around the glomerular capillaries, the space between the walls of the capsule being continuous with the lumen of the tubule. We may picture the glomerulus then as being surrounded by the capsule in the same way as a fist would be if it were pushed into a large, partially inflated balloon. But the capsule does not represent merely a pouch to receive the capillaries. The inner wall of capsular epithelium has numerous projections that completely cover the fifty or more loops of the glomerular capillaries, much as a finger is covered by a glove. This close contact of capillary and capsule, and the fact that the capsular and capillary lumen are each lined by a single layer of cells, make the biologic barrier between a capillary and the lumen of Bowman's capsule exceedingly thin; normally the total thickness is only about 1 μm.

The proximal segment of the tubule lies within the cortex in the vicinity of the capsule and coils back on itself in a much more complicated fashion than is shown in Figure 7-1. The tubule then proceeds in a straight line for a variable distance into the medulla of the kidney before making a sharp bend and returning to the cortex; this narrow, hairpin-shaped structure is the loop of Henle. The segment distal to the loop of Henle, the distal convoluted tubule, also coils back on itself repeatedly, as its name implies, before emptying into the collecting duct by way of the collecting tubule. The collecting duct then courses straight through the medulla and empties into the renal pelvis. The collecting ducts, the ureter and the urinary bladder are the channels between the nephron and the external environment. They provide a clear path for urine, the fluid formed in the kidney, to pass to the outside of the body. The inside of the tubule itself may be considered a part of the external environment.

It is estimated that there are about one million nephrons per kidney and that the total length of the tubules of both kidneys is in the order of 75 miles (120 km)! This huge surface area and the thinness of the barrier separating the tubular lumen from the internal environment make it obvious that the kidneys are ideally structured to provide maximum contact between the external and internal environments of the body. But in order to serve the body effectively, the kidney must also be able to obtain readily from blood the substances to be eliminated and to return to the blood the essential materials that must be conserved. And the manner in which blood is supplied to the kidney is admirably geared to these functions.

The arteries leading from the heart to the kidney are short and wide, permitting a large supply of blood to reach the kidney at a high hydrostatic pressure. Between one-quarter and one-fifth of the blood pumped out of the heart at every beat is routed through the kidney. This means that a volume of blood equal to the total blood volume of the body is made available to the kidneys about every 4–5 minutes (cf. Table 6-1).

Upon entering the kidney, the renal artery branches into smaller and smaller arteries, and these in turn subdivide into arterioles. Each Bowman's capsule is supplied with one of these arterioles, referred to as the *afferent arteriole.*

The network of capillaries – the glomerulus, formed by the subdivision of the afferent arteriole – has several distinguishing characteristics with respect to structure and location, which are of functional importance. First, as we have seen, the endothelium of the glomerular capillary contains large pores that readily permit passage of all plasma constituents except macromolecules like protein (cf. p. 115). By discriminating against the passage of blood constituents only on the basis of molecular size and charge, the glomerular endothelium resembles an artificial porous structure. And, in common with other porous filters, the force that determines the rate of filtration is pressure; in the case of the glomerulus this pressure is supplied by the work of the heart. The hydrostatic pressure within the glomerulus, the porous nature of the endothelium and the thinness of the total barrier between capillary and capsular lumen provide for rapid movement out of the capillary and into the capsule of water and all dissolved constituents. This filtrate of plasma, lacking only the plasma proteins and blood cells, is termed an *ultrafiltrate*. The formation of this ultrafiltrate is rapid; as blood passes through the glomerulus, one-fifth of its volume is filtered. Nearly all this fluid is recaptured by the bloodstream through a *second set of capillaries*. For another feature of the glomerulus is that it is the first of two capillary beds between the arterial supply and venous drainage of the kidney. The vessel leaving the glomerulus is not a venule but an *efferent arteriole*. It subdivides into another network of capillaries nestling around the tubules of the nephron and forming their blood supply. It is only after passing through this second capillary bed that blood enters the venous side of the circulation to be returned to the heart (see Fig. 7-1).

Thus the unique characteristics of the glomerulus readily provide the means whereby the kidney can easily obtain everything from the blood – the delivery system of the body – that needs to be eliminated. The enormous surface area of the tubules and their intimate contact with blood capillaries throughout their length afford the opportunities necessary to return to the body those substances that need to be conserved. All these factors combine to make the kidney ideally suited for its role as the guardian of the body's economy. Now let us turn our attention to how the dichotomous functions of reabsorption and excretion can be carried out simultaneously by the kidney and, moreover, on a very selective basis. An understanding of these functions is essential for understanding not only how the kidney eliminates drugs from the body, but also how drugs act on the kidney. The renal mechanisms that normally account for the formation and final composition of voided urine are identical with those which account for the rate and extent of the urinary excretion of drugs.

Formation of Urine

In the average, healthy 70-kg adult, about 1200 ml of blood (650 ml plasma) is delivered each minute to the glomeruli of the two kidneys. Of this volume, about one-fifth, or 130 ml/minute, appears in Bowman's capsule as an ultrafiltrate of the plasma. This amounts to about 180 liters of fluid per day being presented to the kidneys for processing. Since all the plasma constituents except proteins and protein-bound compounds pass through the glomerulus, the filtrate contains indispensable substances like water, ions, glucose and other nutrients, in addition to disposable waste materials such as phosphate, sulfate and urea, the end products of protein metabolism. Urine formation begins indiscriminately and lavishly. This is essential, however, if the fluids of the body are to be subjected to a purification process by the kidney. But it would spell rapid and total disaster through exhaustion of body resources were it not for the fact that more than 99% of the original filtrate is reabsorbed and returned to the body (Table 7-2). Under normal conditions, the total quantity of water and solutes lost daily in the urine is equal to that acquired by the body, minus only the amounts excreted through other routes.

It is obvious, however, that the processes responsible for reabsorption from the renal tubules can have little in common with the mechanism involved in the first step of urine formation. Glomerular filtration, the process primarily responsible for excretion, is a physical process dependent for its operation on energy derived from the work of the heart. As such, it is selective only with respect to the molecular size and charge of the substances filtered. On the other hand, the movement of solutes out of the tubular urine, across the tubular epithelial cells and through the interstitium back into the circulation involves physicochemical processes. The driving force for this movement is either a concentration gradient or the energy derived from the work of the renal tubular cells. Thus, passive diffusion and active transport across the tubular epithelium

Table 7-2. *Quantitative aspects of urine formation*[1]

Substance	Per 24 hours				Reabsorbed (%)
	Filtered	*Reabsorbed*	*Secreted*	*Excreted*	
Sodium ion (mEq)[2]	26000	25850		150	99.4
Chloride ion (mEq)	18000	17850		150	99.2
Bicarbonate ion (mEq)	4900	4900		0	100
Urea (mM)[2]	870	460[3]		410	53
Glucose (mM)	800	800		0	100
Water (ml)	180000	179000		1000	99.4
Hydrogen ion			Variable	Variable[4]	
Potassium ion (mEq)	900	900[5]	100	100	100[5]

[1]Quantity of various plasma constituents filtered, reabsorbed and excreted by a normal adult on an average diet.
[2]See Glossary for explanation of **mEq** and **mM**.
[3]Urea diffuses into, as well as out of, some portions of the nephron.
[4]pH of urine is on the acid side (4.5–6.9) when all bicarbonate is reabsorbed.
[5]Potassium ion is almost completely reabsorbed before it reaches the distal nephron. The potassium ion in the voided urine is actively secreted into the urine in the distal tubule in exchange for sodium ion.

account for the changes in the composition of the ultrafiltrate after it leaves Bowman's capsule. The selectivity of this solute movement is determined by the same principles that govern solute movement at other biologic barriers. And the availability of a huge absorptive surface area in close contact with the circulation provides the conditions essential for these transport processes to operate at maximum efficiency.

The transport processes that permit cells, in general, to accumulate vital substances against concentration gradients also allow the tubular epithelial cells to reclaim these same essential solutes from the tubular urine (cf. p. 72). Thus, nutrients such as glucose, amino acids and some vitamins are salvaged from the tubular urine by active transport, an indispensable mechanism since their physicochemical properties preclude effective passive diffusion (Fig. 7-2). Glucose, for example, under normal conditions is completely reclaimed from the urine in the proximal convoluted tubule. Glucose appears in the voided urine only when the quantity delivered to the kidneys is greater than that which saturates the active transport process, a situation that may occur following a meal rich in carbohydrates or in patients with diabetes mellitus.

The process of greatest consequence to the final composition of voided urine is the active transport of sodium ions (Na^+), which may take place along almost the entire length of the tubule and collecting duct (Fig. 7-2). Not only is this ion the principal solute of the ultrafiltrate (see Table 7-2), but its active removal from the filtrate is also largely responsible for the reabsorption of water and a number of other important urinary constituents, including chloride, bicarbonate, hydrogen and potassium ions (Figs 7-2 to 7-4).

THE PROXIMAL TUBULE. The active reabsorption of Na^+ begins in the proximal convoluted tubule. By the time the tubular urine reaches the loop of Henle, about two-thirds of the Na^+ originally filtered at the glomerulus has been returned to the circulation. The isotonicity of the filtrate is maintained through-

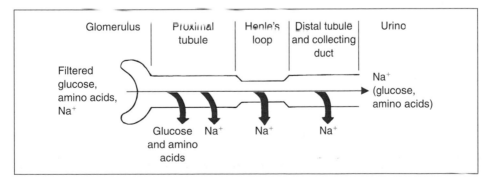

Figure 7-2. *Sites of active transport of glucose, amino acids and Na^+. Glucose and amino acids are excreted only when the amount filtered exceeds saturation levels of active transport mechanisms. Na^+ is excreted in direct proportion to intake. In this figure, as in Figures 7-3 and 7-5, the heavy arrows indicate active transport processes; in the later figures the light arrows indicate passive diffusion.*

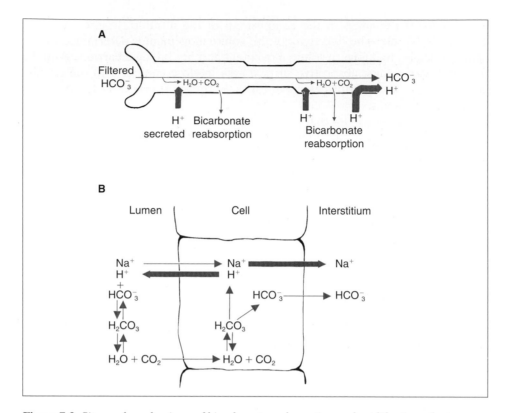

Figure 7-3. *Sites and mechanisms of bicarbonate reabsorption and acidification of urine. (A) Hydrogen ion secretion in exchange for Na^+ takes place in proximal and distal tubules. Under normal conditions urine is acidic, so all bicarbonate is reabsorbed and excess H^+ is excreted in urine. Bicarbonate ion is excreted only when the body has to readjust pH to account for excess of base. (B) Bicarbonate is reabsorbed as CO_2, which is formed from carbonic acid. In the tubular cell CO_2 is hydrated, catalyzed by carbonic anhydrase. This process yields additional H^+ for secretion into the tubular urine, while the HCO_3^- formed is returned to the circulation along with actively transported Na^+.*

out the proximal segment by the concomitant removal of water in proportion to the amount of solute reabsorbed.

The electroneutrality of the filtrate is also maintained. Therefore a major portion of the Na^+ reabsorbed is accompanied by an equivalent quantity of anion, principally Cl^- and also HCO_3^-. The renal epithelium is relatively impermeable to HCO_3^-. However, in the presence of hydrogen ion, HCO_3^- is readily converted to carbonic acid, which then forms water and carbon dioxide:

$$H^+ + HCO_3^- \rightleftharpoons H_2CO_3 \rightleftharpoons H_2O + CO_2$$

The H^+ is obtained from the tubular epithelial cell and is secreted into the

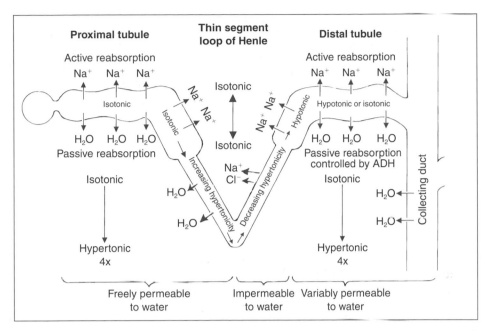

Figure 7-4. *Functional organization of the nephron in relation to reabsorption of Na$^+$ and water and to formation of hypotonic and hypertonic urine. (Modified and redrawn from R.F. Pitts.* The Physiological Basis of Diuretic Therapy. *Springfield, IL: Charles C. Thomas, 1959.)*

tubular urine in exchange for Na$^+$. The carbon dioxide that is liberated by the reaction of H$^+$ and HCO$_3^-$ readily diffuses into the renal epithelium. Within the tubular cell the reverse process occurs, and carbon dioxide is rapidly hydrated with the help of the enzyme *carbonic anhydrase,* which catalyzes this reaction. The carbonic acid formed then ionizes to yield HCO$_3^-$, which combines with Na$^+$ and is returned to the extracellular fluid and circulation. The overall result of these reactions is the reabsorption of Na$^+$ with an equivalent amount of HCO$_3^-$ (Fig. 7-3). The removal of HCO$_3^-$ is also responsible, in part, for the ultrafiltrate becoming more acid than the plasma from which it was derived.[2] Drugs that inhibit carbonic anhydrase, such as acetazolamide, produce diuresis because they inhibit the reabsorption of HCO$_3^-$ from the proximal tubule. Their ability to increase the excretion of bicarbonate, and therefore alkalinize the urine, is the basis for their use in poisoning with some acidic drugs, like salicylates, in order to increase their elimination into the urine.

Immediately after filtration, the concentration of each of the constituents of the ultrafiltrate is identical with its concentration in plasma. As water leaves the

---

[2] HCO$_3^-$ is considered a base by definition, since it can accept the proton H$^+$.

tubular urine, however, the constituents of the glomerular filtrate tend to become more concentrated. As higher concentration gradients are established between the tubular urine and the fluids of its surroundings, the newly formed gradients furnish the force necessary for passive diffusion of solutes (and drugs) across the tubular cell and back into the blood.   In addition to secreting H^+ (in exchange for Na^+), the cells of the proximal tubule are also capable of secreting endogenous organic compounds from the blood into the urine. There are at least three separate mechanisms, one for the transport of organic acids, such as uric acid, another for organic bases, such as histamine, and another for neutral compounds (see Table 7-3). Since this movement into urine is against the concentration gradients produced by the normal removal of water from the glomerular filtrate, these processes are active transport mechanisms, requiring cellular energy to perform work. The solutes remaining in the plasma after its passage through the glomerulus (only one-fifth of the blood entering the glomerulus is filtered) come to the tubule by way of the efferent arteriole. Passive diffusion along concentration gradients accounts for solute movement out of plasma into the interstitium and the tubular cells; the active component of secretion involves only the movement of solute from the tubular cells into the tubular urine. However, these secretory systems, unlike the system for H^+ secretion, play only a minor role in the formation of urine in healthy individuals, but as we shall see are important in the excretion of drugs.

Table 7-3. *Examples of organic acids and bases actively secreted into the proximal renal tubules*

Acids		Bases	
Drugs or drug metabolites	*Naturally occurring compounds*	*Drugs*	*Naturally occurring compounds*
Acetazolamide	Uric acid	Amiloride	Choline
p-Aminohippuric acid (PAH)	5-Hydroxyindoleacetic acid (5-HIAA)	Quaternary ammonium	Dopamine
Chlorothiazide	Glucuronide conjugates	compounds	Histamine
Furosemide	Glycine conjugates	Quinine	Serotonin
Glucuronic acid conjugates		Triamterene	Thiamine
Glycine conjugates			
Methotrexate			
Penicillins			
Phenolsulfonphthalein (PSP)			
Probenecid			
Salicylic acid			
Sulfate conjugates			
Thiazide diuretics			

THE LOOP OF HENLE. About one-third of the glomerular filtrate remains unabsorbed at the end of the proximal tubules and enters the loop of Henle. This hairpin-like structure is key to the ability to form a **hypertonic** urine. The essential factors in the ability to elaborate a urine hypertonic to the body fluids are (1) an anatomic arrangement of those loops of Henle with adjacent capillary loops that descend deep into the medulla which allows for a *countercurrent exchange* to maintain medullary hypertonicity; (2) the *permeability* of the descending limb to water and not sodium chloride; (3) the *impermeability* of the ascending limb to water despite its active transport of Na^+ and Cl^-; and (4) the concentration of total solutes in the interstitial fluids of the medulla, which makes this region hypertonic to normal plasma and other body fluids.

The epithelial lining of the entire loop of Henle contains only a single layer of cells; the structure and function of the cells in the descending limb differ from those in the ascending limb. The epithelial cells in the descending segment are flat and permit the passive diffusion of water through channel proteins called aqueporins in the luminal plasma membrane. In the ascending limb the cells are thicker, impermeable to water, and actively reabsorb Na^+ and Cl^- by a carrier protein.

In the kidney cortex, both the proximal and distal tubules are in contact with interstitial fluid that is isotonic with the plasma entering the kidney. In contrast, in the medulla the concentration of total solutes, mainly sodium chloride and urea, in the interstitial fluid progressively increases from the cortex to the pelvis.

At the deepest portion of the medullary tissue the sodium chloride concentration may be two to three times that in other body fluids. As a result, the loop of Henle and its parallel capillary are exposed to a gradually changing fluid environment as they course through the medullary tissue from the cortex to the end of the medulla and back again. The collecting duct, which passes through the medulla on its way to the ureter, is also subjected to progressively increasing hypertonic surroundings.

The tubular urine leaving the loop of Henle and entering the distal convoluted tubule is hypotonic to the plasma and fluids in the cortex. Moreover, the net loss of sodium, chloride and water from the urine during its passage through the loop accounts for only a small portion of their total reabsorption. One may well ask at this point, 'How can a loop of Henle be essential for the production of a hypertonic urine when the fluid that leaves it is hypotonic and only decreased by about 25% in volume and content of solute?' The answer is that Henle's loop serves the special purpose of establishing and maintaining the hypertonic gradient in the medullary interstitium that is essential for the final concentration of urine in the collecting duct.

Not surprisingly, the loop of Henle is the target for a class of diuretic drugs used in the treatment of edema, hypertension, and heart failure. These 'loop diuretics' include drugs such as furosemide (LASIX). They increase excretion of water from the body by blocking the reabsorption of Na^+, K^+, and Cl^- from the ascending portion of the loop of Henle. This effect results from an inhibitory action on a transporter protein (called NKCC2 or BSC1), inserted in the apical membrane of the epithelium in the ascending limb.

DISTAL CONVOLUTED TUBULE AND COLLECTING DUCT. Active reabsorption of Na^+ and Cl^- continues in the distal convoluted tubule through the action of another transport protein in the luminal plasma membrane (referred to as NCC or TSC, thiazide sensitive cotransporter). This transporter is inhibited by the thiazide class of diuretics, important agents in the treatment of hypertension. In the distal tubule some reabsorption of Na^+ exchanges for H^+, which determines the final pH of the voided urine. However, in the distal segment, unlike the situation in the proximal tubule, Na^+ can also exchange for another cation, K^+. Since a major portion of the latter is completely removed from the tubular urine before it reaches the distal tubule, this secretion of K^+ in exchange for Na^+ in the distal tubule accounts for most of the K^+ that is excreted. Also unlike the situation in the proximal tubule, the active reabsorption of Na^+ and the secretion of K^+ and H^+ in the distal convoluted tubule and collecting duct are modulated by aldosterone, a hormone synthesized by the adrenal cortex. Under normal conditions, the amount of Na^+ absorbed under the influence of aldosterone affects the quantity of the K^+ and H^+ excreted into the distal segments of the nephron. Sodium reabsorption by these mechanisms also can be inhibited by diuretic agents. These drugs are referred to as potassium-sparing diuretics, because by blocking sodium reabsorption in the distal tubule they indirectly reduce the amount of potassium secretion in this site. One type (e.g. amiloride) blocks the sodium channel protein in the apical membrane. The other type are analogs of aldosterone (e.g. spironolactone) and block the interaction of the hormone with its cytosolic receptor.

Unlike the proximal segment and loop of Henle, the permeability characteristics of the tubular epithelium in the distal tubule and the collecting duct are not constant with respect to water. Here the removal of water from the tubular fluid is dependent on the presence of a hormone, antidiuretic hormone (ADH; *anti,* 'against'; L. *diureticus,* 'to make water through'). This hormone, also referred to as vasopressin, is produced by the posterior lobe of the pituitary. In the absence of ADH, the epithelium of the distal segment and collecting ducts is relatively *impermeable* to water; as Na^+ and other solutes are removed, water is unable to follow passively along the established osmotic gradients. As a result, in the absence of ADH, the slightly hypotonic fluid delivered to the distal segment by the loop of Henle becomes more and more dilute as solutes unaccompanied by water are reabsorbed. Thus, when ADH secretion is completely suppressed, as it would be in overhydration, as much as 15% or more of the water of the original glomerular ultrafiltrate may escape reabsorption and be voided as hypotonic urine. A classic example of a drug that inhibits ADH action is alcohol. Alcohol inhibits the release of ADH from the pituitary, causing diuresis. However, it does not increase the excretion of alcohol in the urine, as alcohol is predominantly eliminated through metabolic processes.

As the levels of circulating ADH are increased, the distal tubule and collecting duct become increasingly permeable to water, and then water is reabsorbed together with solute. As the collecting duct courses through the medulla, water diffuses out of the tubular lumen in response both to the continued reabsorption of Na⁺ and to the steeper osmotic gradients established and maintained by the loop of Henle; a hypertonic urine will result. Although only one-fifth of the nephrons have long medullary loops, the urine formed in *every* nephron is affected by the medullary hypertonicity during its passage through the collecting ducts. Thus, three basic factors are necessary to convert the isotonic urine of the glomerular filtrate to a concentrated urine: (1) the active reabsorption of the major urinary solutes, particularly sodium and its attendant anions; (2) the presence of ADH; and (3) a hypertonic medullary interstitium maintained by the activities of the loop of Henle. And in normal individuals on a balanced diet, the voided urine is hypertonic; it is decreased in volume and content of essential solutes to less than 1% of what was originally filtered at the glomerulus.

Renal Excretion of Drugs

GLOMERULAR FILTRATION AND TUBULAR REABSORPTION. As blood flows through the glomerulus, any drug that is free in the plasma will be filtered together with other plasma constituents. Only drugs bound to protein or drugs of excessively large molecular size will be retained in the bloodstream. Since the epithelial lining of the renal tubules is like any other epithelial barrier, reabsorption of drugs from the glomerular filtrate is governed by the familiar principles of biotransport. As we have seen, the conservation and removal of water in the normal formation of urine create concentration gradients in favor of solute movement out of the tubular urine. Thus, drugs will passively diffuse back into the circulation in accordance with their lipid/water partition coefficients, degree of ionization and molecular size (Fig. 7-5).

When the glomerular filtrate enters the proximal tubule, its pH is the same as that of plasma, 7.4. However, the pH of the voided urine may vary from 4.5 to 8.0, depending on the amount of H⁺ secreted and the quantity of HCO₃⁻ reabsorbed. Normally the urine is somewhat more acidic than plasma as a result of the secretion of H⁺ into the distal tubule. This increased acidity of the tubular urine profoundly affects the rate of reabsorption of weak electrolytes (cf. pp. 65–69). The nonionized forms of weak electrolytes, being more lipid-soluble, may readily diffuse back (reabsorption) into the circulation, whereas the ionized or charged forms are 'trapped' in the tubular urine and excreted. Let us consider, for example, the weak electrolyte salicylic acid, which is a predominant metabolite of aspirin. In plasma, at pH 7.4, more than 99.9% of salicylic acid exists in the ionized, water-soluble form, with only a very small fraction as the nonionized, freely diffusible species:

$$\text{Undissociated}$$
$$\text{salicylic acid} \rightleftharpoons \text{Salicylate ion} + \text{H}^+$$
$$\text{At pH 7.4} \qquad 0.01\% \qquad\qquad 99.99\%$$

Both the salicylate ion and salicylic acid are filtered across the glomerulus. As water is removed from the glomerular filtrate, a concentration gradient is established

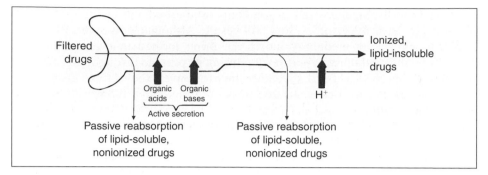

Figure 7-5. *Excretion of drugs. Lipid-soluble and nonionized drugs are passively reabsorbed throughout the tubule. In distal segments, the secretion of H⁺ favors reabsorption of weak acids (less ionized) and, conversely, excretion of weak bases (more ionized). Active secretion of organic acids and bases occurs only in the proximal segment.*

between the urine and plasma, and some salicylic acid diffuses back into the blood. Acidification of the urine depresses the ionization of salicylic acid, since

$$\frac{[\text{Salicylate ion}] \times [\text{H+}]}{[\text{Undissociated salicylic acid}]} = \text{a constant}$$

Thus the increase in H^+ concentration drives the equilibrium to the side of undissociated salicylic acid, thereby increasing the fraction of the more lipid-soluble, nonionized form. The higher concentration gradient of the undissociated species favors more rapid reabsorption, and consequently the rate of salicylic acid excretion is reduced. Conversely, an alkaline urine promotes the urinary excretion of salicylic acid. In fact, practical use is made of these effects of pH on drug excretion in the treatment of poisoning with certain weak acids, such as aspirin or phenobarbital. Sodium bicarbonate may be administered in order to produce an alkaline urine and hasten elimination of the drug (cf. p. 359). Conversely, for weak bases, such as cocaine, an alkaline urine retards excretion and an acidic urine formed by the administration of ammonium chloride enhances urinary elimination.

TUBULAR SECRETION. Whereas active reabsorption plays a significant part in the conservation of many essential endogenous compounds like glucose, carrier-mediated processes account for the reabsorption of only small quantities of a few drugs or nonessential substances. In contrast, the mechanisms responsible for active tubular secretion of organic compounds are of lesser consequence in the normal formation of urine, but are important processes for the excretion of a number of drugs and drug metabolites. The epithelial cells of the proximal tubules contain transport proteins that are inserted into the plasma membranes on the vascular (basolateral) and luminal (apical) side of the cells. These carriers bind drugs and facilitate their transport across the plasma membrane. Three major types of transporters have been identified in the proximal tubule and are expressed in other tissues as well. Two of these, the organic anion transporters (OAT) and the organic cation transporters (OCT) are named for their substrates. The third type, the multi-drug resistant (MDR) gene product or p-glycoprotein, derives its name from its first identification in tumor cells.

Examples of substrates for the organic anion transporters include a variety of acidic drugs such as penicillin and salicylic acid, and acidic drug metabolites such as glucuronide conjugates. The acid para-aminohippuric acid (PAH) is secreted so rapidly by this carrier type that it is entirely removed from the plasma in a single pass through the kidney. The substrates for the organic cation transporters include quaternary ammonium compounds. And the substrates for the multi-drug resistant transporters include both neutral and cationic compounds such as digoxin and quinolone antibiotics (Table 7-3).

There are limits to the capacity of these carrier mechanisms to actively secrete compounds from the blood into the urine. In addition, drugs may bind to the same carrier, share the same transport process, and compete with each other for binding sites on the same carrier. Consequently, when multiple compounds that share the same transport process are present in the blood coming to the tubule, one compound may inhibit the secretion of another. If the total quantity of drug or drug metabolite to be secreted is in excess of available carrier, the rates of secretion of the individual compounds will be decreased compared with their rates in the absence of each other. For example, the agent probenecid, used in the treatment of gout, binds avidly to the organic anion transporter and blocks the tubular secretion of penicillin. When penicillin was in short supply during the period after its introduction into therapeutics, co-administration of probenecid was used as an effective method for prolonging retention of the antibiotic in the body by blocking its tubular secretion.

The extent to which a drug or drug metabolite is eliminated in the urine following tubular secretion is dependent on the degree of its ionization within the tubular urine. Secretion of the quaternary ammonium compounds is tantamount to urinary elimination, since these agents are fully ionized regardless of the pH of the urine. Organic acids, such as penicillin, also are highly ionized in the urine and therefore undergo little reabsorption.

RATE OF DRUG EXCRETION. The rate at which a drug will be eliminated in the urine is the net result of the three renal processes: glomerular filtration, tubular secretion, and tubular reabsorption. The rates of glomerular filtration and tubular secretion are dependent on the rate at which a drug is presented to the kidney – on its concentration in plasma. The rate of reabsorption by the tubules is dependent on the concentration of drug in the urine. For glomerular filtration, it is the concentration of free drug in the plasma that is important, since protein-bound drug cannot be filtered. On the other hand, the extent of protein binding, as long as it is reversible, makes little difference in the rate of elimination of those agents that can be actively transported out of the renal tubular cell. The fraction of drug that is bound in plasma is in equilibrium with the fraction of drug that is free. As the latter is removed by secretion, the protein-drug complex dissociates, and more free drug becomes available to the active secretory process. Thus it is the concentration of both free and bound drug in plasma that is important in determining the rate of tubular secretion.

Determinations of the rates at which certain drugs are excreted by the kidney have proven to be useful procedures for diagnosing the functional status of this organ. For example, if we wish to assess the competence of the glomeruli, we need a means of measuring the volume of plasma that the glomeruli are capable of filtering in a given period. A simple way of obtaining this information is to determine the rate at which a foreign compound present in the plasma appears in the urine. The compound used as a yardstick of glomerular competence would have to satisfy the following requirements: (1) it must be freely filterable in the glomeruli, i.e. it must not be bound to plasma protein; (2) it must be neither reabsorbed nor actively secreted into the tubular urine; (3) it must be nontoxic and have no direct or indirect pharmacologic effect on renal function; (4) it must remain chemically unaltered during its passage through the kidney; and (5) it must be a chemical the concentration of which can be accurately determined in both urine and plasma. The polymeric carbohydrate inulin meets all these requirements. It is freely filterable by the glomeruli; it can reach the urine only by glomerular filtration; all the inulin filtered is excreted, since it is not reabsorbed in its passage through the tubules; and methods are available for its quantitative determination in body fluids. Therefore, following inulin administration, the amount recovered in the urine in a given interval is equal to the amount filtered by the glomeruli in that same period. For example, if 10 mg is the amount of inulin recovered in the voided urine in 10 minutes, then inulin is being filtered in the glomeruli at the rate of 1 mg/minute.

The next question we need to answer in order to determine the efficiency of the glomeruli is, 'How many milliliters – what volume – of plasma have to be filtered each minute to yield the amount recovered per minute in the urine?' The answer can be obtained very easily by taking a sample of blood during the time the urine is being collected and determining how much inulin is present per milliliter of plasma. If we find the plasma concentration to be 0.008 mg/ml, then 125 ml of plasma must be filtered each minute to provide the 1 mg excreted by the kidney per minute:

$$\frac{\text{Amount excreted in urine per minute}}{\text{Amount in plasma per milliliter}} = \frac{\text{Number of milliliters of plasma}}{\text{filtered per minute}}$$

(Equation 1)

$$\frac{1\,\text{mg/min inulin in urine}}{0.008\,\text{mg/ml inulin in plasma}} = 125\,\text{ml/min, volume of plasma filtered}$$

Quantitative data on kidney function obtained in this manner are termed a *renal plasma clearance study*. **Renal plasma clearance** is defined as the volume of plasma needed to supply the amount of a specific substance excreted in the urine in 1 minute. A substance like inulin, which not only is completely filter-able but is neither reabsorbed nor secreted by the tubular cells, has a renal plasma clearance identical to the rate at which it is filtered by the glomeruli. Thus the clearance of a substance such as inulin measures the *glomerular filtra-tion rate* (GFR), expressed in milliliters per minute. In a healthy 70-kg adult male the average GFR is about 130ml/min, indicating that 130ml of plasma are filtered by the glomeruli each minute. This value was established using the pro-cedures just described; similar procedures are used clinically to assess glomeru-lar function in patients.

Renal plasma clearance (Cl_R) is usually calculated as follows:

$$Cl_R \text{ (ml/min)} = \frac{U \times V}{P}$$

(Equation 2)

where U is the concentration of the test substance per milliliter of urine, V is the volume of urine excreted per minute and P is the concentration of test substance per milliliter of plasma. In our example above, the volume of urine collected in 10 minutes was 10ml. Thus V = 1 ml/min and U = 10mg/10ml, or 1mg/ml. Then:

$$Cl_R = \frac{1\,mg/ml \times 1\,ml/min}{0.008\,mg/ml} = 125\,ml/min$$

Whereas Equations 1 and 2 are mathematically identical, the latter indicates not only the functional capacity of the glomeruli but also the kidney's ability to con-centrate urine by removal of water. Comparison of the milliliters of plasma cleared with the milliliters of urine voided in 1 minute yields direct information of the amount of water reabsorbed during passage through the tubule. In our example, 124ml of each 125ml filtered was absorbed. And simple arithmetic shows that continued excretion at the rate of 1ml per minute will lead to a daily output of urine of 1440ml.

Certain organic acids, such as para-aminohippuric acid (PAH), are secreted so rapidly and efficiently by the renal epithelium that they are almost entirely removed from the plasma in a single passage through the kidney. (Obviously, this can occur only when the plasma levels are low enough to ensure that the carrier transport system is not overloaded.) These acids are also not reabsorbed to any significant degree. A substance like PAH can then be used in clearance studies to obtain information about the total amount of plasma flowing through the kidneys in a stated unit of time. The term *clearance* is used here to mean exactly what it did in the case of the clearance of inulin: the amount of plasma needed to supply the amount of a specific substance excreted in the urine in 1 minute. Then, if the kidneys extract all of a compound that is delivered to them by the blood during a single passage, the clearance of that substance is equal to the volume of plasma flowing through the kidneys per minute. By measuring the concentration of PAH per milliliter of urine (U), the volume of urine excreted per minute (V) and the concentration of PAH per milliliter of plasma (P), and then applying Equation 2, we obtain the renal clearance of PAH in milliliters per minute. This clearance of PAH represents the rate of plasma flow through the kidneys. The average renal plasma flow in a healthy 70-kg adult male is about 650 ml/min.

The determination of the renal plasma clearance of any drug can give some insight into the mechanisms by which the drug is excreted when this clearance is compared with the normal glomerular filtration rate, i.e. 130 ml/min as obtained with inulin. If the concentration of drug not bound to plasma proteins is used to calculate its renal plasma clearance, an expression of the *excretion ratio* is obtained:

$$\text{Excretion ratio} = \frac{\text{Renal plasma clearance of drug (ml/min)}}{\text{Normal GFR (ml/min)}}$$

A ratio of less than 1 indicates that the drug is filtered, perhaps also secreted, and then partially reabsorbed. A substance such as glucose has an excretion ratio of zero since it is completely reabsorbed in the healthy individual. A value greater than 1 indicates that secretion, in addition to filtration, is involved in the excretion. Obviously, the greatest excretion ratio, about 5, would be obtained with a substance like PAH.

Excretion of Drugs by the Liver

Each day the liver secretes 0.5–1.01 of bile into the duodenum through the common bile duct (Fig. 7-6). This secretion, which is rich in bile acids, is functionally important for the digestion and absorption of fats. Normally, about 80–90% of the bile acids secreted are reabsorbed from the intestine and transported through the portal blood back to the liver to be available again for secretion. Thus the major portion of the daily output of bile acids is conserved through this portobiliary circulation, or *enterohepatic cycle;* only a small daily deficit has to be replaced by the body.

Large quantities of bile are discharged into the duodenum in response to food intake, and the total quantity of bile acids available is recirculated twice during digestion of a single meal. During this digestion period, the concentration of bile acids in the bile duct or blood vessels draining the intestine is frequently higher than that in the hepatic fluids or intestinal contents, respectively. Also, the bile acids exist largely as ionized solutes. Therefore, passive diffusion alone could hardly account for their secretion into bile or their almost complete reabsorption from the intestine against high concentration gradients. But in both liver and intestinal epithelial cells there is an active transport system that ensures that adequate supplies of bile acids can be cycled between liver and intestine.

Many drugs and their metabolites are also excreted by the liver into bile. However, many agents reaching the small intestine in this way are not subse-

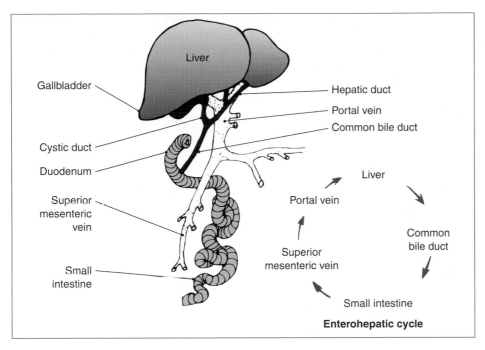

Figure 7-6. *Relationships of the biliary ducts and blood supply to the liver and intestine. Bile, containing bile acids, is discharged into the duodenum. The bile acids are reabsorbed from the small intestine and returned to the liver by way of the superior mesenteric and portal veins.*

quently excreted in the feces. They are almost completely reabsorbed because their physicochemical properties are favorable for passive diffusion across the intestinal barrier. These agents then remain in the enterohepatic cycle until they are eliminated by other means. For example, enterohepatic cycling was shown to be largely responsible for the persistence in the body of glutethimide (DORIDEN), a hypnotic used frequently in the past, but rarely today. Glutethimide is only slowly excreted by the normal kidney, but experimentally its urinary excretion was increased fourfold in animals whose bile duct was prevented from emptying into the small intestine. For drugs in current use, enterohepatic cycling is important for prolonging the action of the immunosuppressant agent mycophenolate mofetil, used to prevent transplant rejection, and of the contraceptive agent ethinylestradiol, as well as of other drugs.

Certain drugs, including organic acids and bases, are actively transported from liver into bile by mechanisms very similar to those that secrete these same substances into the tubular urine. Many of the same transporters are expressed in liver cells and in renal proximal tubules, as well as in other sites such as the choroid plexus of the brain. Protein-bound drug is fully accessible to this biliary active transport system, as it is to renal tubular secretion. Unlike the bile acids, however, the acidic and basic drugs do not recycle to any significant degree.

There is little evidence that active transport processes are available within the intestine for the absorption of foreign organic acids, and the physicochemical properties of both the acids and bases are not conducive to absorption by passive diffusion (cf. p. 90). Bases such as the quaternary ammonium compounds are fully ionized, and the organic acids are ionized to an even greater extent at intestinal pH than at urinary pH values. Thus the active transport of the acidic and basic drugs from the liver into bile becomes an effective means of eliminating them from the body by way of the feces. An exception may be the metabolite of a drug formed by a conjugation reaction. After active transport into the bile and emptying from the gall bladder into the small intestine, the conjugate may undergo enzymatic cleavage that releases the parent drug and the conjugating moiety. Enzymes of the normal intestinal bacterial population contribute to this process. Although the conjugate is likely to be too polar to undergo intestinal reabsorption, the parent drug, once released, may be sufficiently lipophilic to return to the circulation.

The active biliary transport of these foreign organic acids has found practical application in the past in diagnostic tests of liver function. The compound most frequently used for this purpose was the dye sulfobromophthalein which is predominantly excreted in the bile. In the average individual with a normally functioning liver, most of the dye is excreted into the intestine within 30 minutes after intravenous administration. Whether liver function is normal or depressed is indicated by the amount of dye remaining in a sample of blood withdrawn 30 minutes after the beginning of the test.

SYNOPSIS

The principal route for drug excretion is by way of the kidney, although drugs may be excreted in any media eliminated from the body. The renal mechanisms that account for the rate and extent of urinary excretion of drugs are identical with those that normally account for the formation and final composition of voided urine. Urinary excretion of drugs begins with glomerular filtration of any drug that is not bound to plasma proteins and has a sufficiently low molecular size. In most cases, the final concentration of the drug in the voided urine is determined by how much is passively reabsorbed in its passage through the renal tubule. The concentration gradient for passive back diffusion is created by the active reabsorption of Na^+ and the concomitant removal of water. The extent of reabsorption of the drug is dependent on its lipid solubility and degree of ionization at the pH of the tubular urine. Active secretory mechanisms in the proximal tubule account for the rapid elimination in the urine of certain drugs, including organic acids and bases. The excretion of a drug into urine is characterized by its renal plasma clearance. In a 70-kg healthy subject this value ranges from nearly 0 to a maximum of renal plasma flow (650 ml/min), depending upon the extent of glomerular filtration, tubular secretion, and reabsorption of the drug.

GUIDES FOR STUDY AND REVIEW

By what routes can drugs be excreted from the body? What is the principal route for drug excretion?

What are the renal mechanisms that normally account for the formation and final composition of voided urine? What single process is of greatest significance in determining the final composition of urine?

What kinds of material are filtered at the glomerulus? What special structural characteristics of Bowman's capsule are of great functional significance? How is the composition of the glomerular filtrate related to that of plasma?

How do the events taking place in the proximal tubule influence the composition, volume and tonicity of the urine delivered to the loop of Henle? What ions are actively absorbed in the proximal tubules? How do these active transport processes influence the reabsorption of water? of passively transferred solutes?

How is bicarbonate ion reabsorbed? What influences the rate at which H^+ is made available in the renal tubule cell? How would alteration in the rate of H^+ formation in the renal tubular cell influence the rate of reabsorption of bicarbonate ion from the tubular urine?

What special purpose does the loop of Henle serve? What are the structural and functional characteristics of the loop of Henle that account for its ability to influence markedly the tonicity of voided urine? What are the functional differences between the descending and ascending limbs? What are the differences in the volume and tonicity of the urine entering and leaving the loop of Henle?

What influences the reabsorption of water in the distal convoluted tubule and the collecting duct? What hormone plays a role in the reabsorption of water? How does the presence of this hormone influence the final tonicity of voided urine?

What are the three basic factors that are necessary to convert the isotonic urine of the glomerular filtrate to a concentrated urine? What percentage of the Na^+ filtered is normally reabsorbed? of the water? of bicarbonate ion? of glucose?

What are four mechanisms by which drugs can produce diuresis? Where in the nephron do they act?

What are the mechanisms responsible for urinary drug excretion?

What are the factors that determine the rate at which drugs are filtered at the glomerulus? How does binding to plasma proteins affect this rate? How can rates of glomerular filtration explain differences in the duration of action among sulfa drugs? Are there any unbound (free) drugs that cannot be filtered at the glomerulus?

How is glomerular filtration rate measured? What properties does a drug have to possess in order to be used to measure GFR? to measure total renal plasma flow?

What factors determine whether a drug will be reabsorbed from the tubular urine? How can the rate of reabsorption of a weak acid be decreased? of a weak base be decreased? How does the process of reabsorption affect the amount of drug in voided urine?

What general types of drugs are secreted into the tubular urine? How does this process affect the amount in the voided urine?

A total of 400 mg of drug X was found in a 10-minute urine sample collection from a healthy adult male. Midway during this 10-minute interval, the plasma concentration of drug X was 25 mg% (25 mg/100 ml plasma). What is the renal plasma clearance of this drug? What is the excretion ratio of this drug? How is drug X handled by the kidney and how do you know this?

What general types of drugs are secreted by the liver into the bile? For what general types of compounds does biliary secretion become a relatively effective means of elimination from the body? In what ways are biliary secretion into the intestine and renal secretion into the tubular urine similar?

SUGGESTED READING

Bennett, P.N. *Drugs and Human Lactation* (2nd ed). Amsterdam: Elsevier, 1996.

Berkhin, E.B. and Humphreys, M.H. Regulation of renal tubular secretion of organic compounds. *Kidney Int.* 59:17–30, 2001.

Inui, K.-I., Masuda, S. and Saito, H. Cellular and molecular aspects of drug transport in the kidney. *Kidney Int.* 58:944–958, 2000.

Koeppen, B.M. and Stanton, B.A. *Renal Physiology* (3rd ed). St Louis: Mosby, 2001.

Kusuhara, H., Suzuki, H. and Sugiyama, Y. The role of P-glycoprotein and canalicular multispecific organic anion transporter in the hepatobiliary excretion of drugs. *J. Pharm. Sci.* 87(9): 1025–1040, 1998.

Roberts, M.S., Magnusson, B.M., Burczynski, F.J., and Weiss, M. Enterohepatic circulation: physiological, pharmacokinetic and clinical implications. *Clin. Pharmacokinet.* 41(10):751–790, 2002.

Wilson, J.T. Determinants and consequences of drug excretion in breast milk. *Drug Metab. Rev.* 14:619, 1983.

8 How the Actions of Drugs are Terminated

II. Biotransformation

The interaction between a drug and the living organism in which the body brings about a chemical change in the drug molecule is variously referred to as *detoxification*, *drug metabolism* or *biotransformation*. The term *detoxification* has historical significance; the first foreign agents shown to be chemically altered by the body were indeed converted into substances of less potential toxicity. This term has been largely discarded since it is now apparent that the chemical reactions of the body can at times yield compounds of greater toxicity than the parent drugs. The term *metabolism*, as it was originally used, designated the process by which food, on the one hand, is built into living matter (anabolism) and living matter, on the other, is broken down into simple products within a cell or organism (catabolism). Metabolism is the sum of the chemical changes in living cells by which energy is provided for vital processes and activities and new materials are produced and assimilated for growth and maintenance. The chemical reactions that drugs undergo in the body do not ordinarily provide such energy or new materials. Thus the term *biotransformation* is preferable to drug metabolism for describing the chemical aspects of the fate of foreign compounds which are not normally considered under carbohydrate, protein, fat, vitamin, hormone or mineral metabolism.

Before considering the general aspects of the many reactions responsible for the chemical alterations of drugs and the pharmacologic significance of these biotransformations, let us briefly discuss the mechanisms by which they occur.

THE MEDIATORS OF BIOTRANSFORMATION

The chemical alterations of drugs, like the chemical changes taking place in normal metabolism, are not spontaneous reactions; they are catalyzed reactions. Drug biotransformation takes place in the presence of enzymes, the protein catalysts which accelerate the reaction but remain essentially unchanged in the process.

The word *enzyme* occasionally denotes more than just a catalytic protein. Many enzymes require nonprotein organic compounds called *prosthetic groups*, or *coenzymes*, which play an intimate and frequently essential role in catalysis. Ordinarily, the term *prosthetic groups* is reserved for groups which are bound firmly to the protein and cannot be readily removed without destroying the enzyme, whereas *coenzymes* refer to dissociable entities necessary for the reaction. Some enzymes also require small ions, such as Mg^{2+}, for full catalytic activity. We shall use the term *enzyme* to refer to the entire enzyme system, thereby including all the *cofactors* necessary for optimum activity.

Mode of Action of Enzymes

Enzymes, like receptors, produce their activity by combining reversibly with the substances on which they act – by combining with their *substrates*. Moreover, the forces responsible for this enzyme-substrate binding are the same as those which account for drug-receptor interactions: ionic bonds, hydrogen bonds and Van der Waals attractive forces. The consequence of this binding is also comparable to that of the drug-receptor interaction, since the combination of enzyme and substrate initiates a sequence of events that leads to the appearance of end products of the reaction.

$$\text{Enzyme} + \text{substrate} \rightleftharpoons \text{Enzyme-substrate complex}$$
(Equation 1)

$$\text{Enzyme-substrate complex} \rightleftharpoons \text{Enzyme} + \text{products of enzyme action}$$
(Equation 2)

Enzymes show specificity for the substances upon which they act, and this specificity is also akin to that of receptors and the drugs with which they combine. The specificity of both types of interaction arises from the number and kinds of bonds formed and the spatial configuration of the 'active sites' for bond formation on or within the macromolecule (Figs 8-1 and 8-2). In fact, the principle of the 'lock and key' fit between a chemical compound and the active sites of an enzyme was outlined by Emil Fischer several years before its adaptation by Ehrlich into his concept of receptors.

Although nearly all the individual reactions of normal metabolism are catalyzed by separate enzymes, few of the enzymes are absolutely specific for a particular substrate. Most can also act on structural analogs of their physiologic substrates – on drugs. For example, the enzyme in muscle or nervous tissue that acts on acetylcholine also acts on the drug methacholine, but at a slower rate. Methacholine differs from acetylcholine only by the addition of a methyl group:

$$
\begin{array}{c}
\qquad\quad CH_3 \\
\qquad\quad | \\
CH_3 - N^+ - CH_2 - CH - O - C = O \\
\qquad\quad | \qquad\qquad | \qquad\quad | \\
\qquad\quad CH_3 \qquad\quad CH_3 \qquad CH_3 \\
\qquad\qquad\qquad\qquad \uparrow
\end{array}
$$

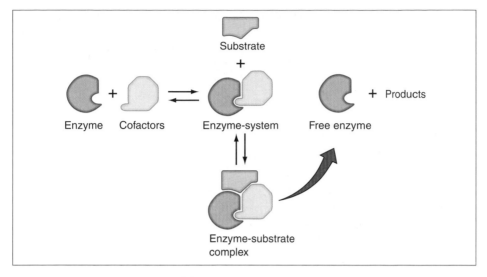

Figure 8-1. *Schematic diagram of the interaction of substrate with an enzyme requiring a cofactor. For some enzymes, the step involving the combination with cofactor or activating metal is not needed. (Modified from W.D. McElroy, Q. Rev. Biol. 22:25, 1947.)*

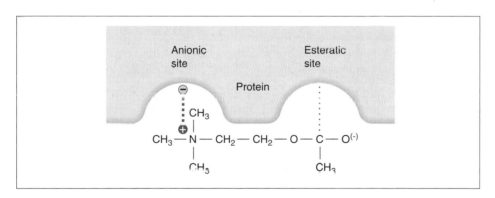

Figure 8-2. *Interaction of acetylcholine with the enzyme acetylcholinesterase. There are two active sites for binding on the enzyme: the anionic site and the esteratic site. At the anionic site an ionic bond is formed between the positively charged nitrogen and a negatively charged group of the enzyme. At the esteratic site the ester bond is actually split. (Modified from I.B. Wilson, Fed. Proc. 18:752, 1959.)*

Many other biotransformations are also carried out by enzymes of moderate specificity which catalyze similar reactions of normal metabolism. However, a few enzymes show less specificity by catalyzing reactions of a variety of physiologic substrates and drugs, whereas others lack true specificity and act on a diverse group of drugs but on few physiologic substrates.

Enzyme Kinetics

The rate of a chemical reaction is understood to mean the rate at which the concentrations of reacting substances vary with time. And according to the law of mass action, the rate of any reaction is proportional to the concentrations of the reactants present at any given time. It follows that the velocity of an enzymic process should be proportional to the concentrations of enzyme and substrate. In fact, when the concentration of substrate is held constant, it can be shown that within fairly wide limits the speed of an enzyme reaction is proportional to the enzyme concentration (Fig. 8-3). However, only in certain instances does the speed of an enzyme reaction parallel the substrate concentration when the enzyme concentration is held constant. This relationship exists at low and intermediate substrate concentration. But at higher levels of substrate, the rate of enzyme action stops increasing and becomes virtually independent of the concentration of substrate (Fig. 8-4).

The curve in Figure 8-4 is similar to the curve in Figure 4-7 (p. 70), which depicts the rate of facilitated diffusion as a function of the concentration of solute. The reason why the rate of enzyme action does not increase beyond a certain level of substrate is also very much like the reason for the limited capacity of the facilitated diffusion process. When a substrate molecule combines with a molecule of enzyme, there is an interval (even though this may be measured in milliseconds) before the enzyme-substrate complex dissociates and the reaction products are freed. Following this interval the enzyme molecule is ready to combine with another molecule of substrate. By the mass action interpretation, the more abundant the substrate molecules, the less time required to form the substrate-enzyme complex. But at constant temperature and other fixed

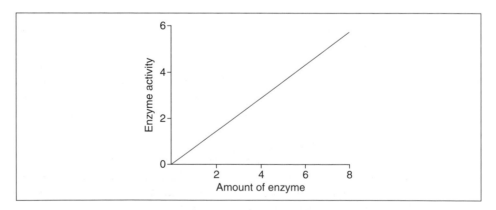

Figure 8-3. *Effect of enzyme concentration on enzyme activity when the substrate concentration remains constant. Units are arbitrary. Such data may be obtained* in vitro *by determining the quantity of end product formed per unit time in mixtures containing different amounts of enzyme, e.g. the amount of para-aminobenzoic acid (or diethyl-aminoethanol) formed by hydrolysis of the local anesthetic procaine, using varying amounts of plasma as the source of enzyme.*

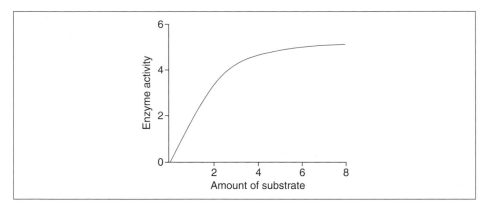

Figure 8-4. *Effect of substrate concentration on enzyme activity when the enzyme concentration remains constant. Such data may be obtained* in vitro *by determining the quantity of end product formed per unit time in mixtures containing different amounts of substrate.*

conditions, the *rate of dissociation* of the complex is independent of substrate concentration and is the same for all substrate concentrations. So at or above a certain substrate level, the enzyme is operating at maximum speed because the intervals when it is unused become negligible. On this basis, an additional rise in substrate levels does not lead to an increase in rate of reaction. The rate-limiting step is the rate of dissociation of the enzyme-substrate complex.

A reaction is said to be a *monomolecular* or *first-order reaction* when only one substance is reacting and when the reaction velocity is proportional to the concentration of this substance. In the intact organism the concentration of enzyme usually remains constant, so that only the changing substrate concentration influences the rate of metabolism or biotransformation. Therefore, when the substrate concentration is low and active sites on the enzyme are available for occupancy, the enzyme reaction is like a first-order reaction even though two reactants have to combine. At high substrate concentrations, when the enzyme is saturated, the velocity of the reaction becomes almost constant. Since it is no longer dependent on the concentration of reactants, it is said to be a *zero-order reaction.*

It will be recalled that the term *enzyme* refers to the complete enzyme system, i.e. the protein as well as any cofactors necessary for activity. Therefore the failure of a reaction to increase in rate with an increase in substrate concentration – zero-order kinetics – may occur not only when the enzyme is saturated, but also when the supply of a cofactor is insufficient.

Most drugs are administered therapeutically in amounts that lead to concentrations well below the saturation levels of their enzyme system; their rate of biotransformation is proportional to drug concentration. However, in later discussions we shall note a number of instances in which the rate of biotransformation may be constant and independent of the concentration of drug in the body.

CHEMICAL PATHWAYS OF BIOTRANSFORMATION

Most drugs are subject to chemical alteration by the body. The few that appear not to be, such as the diuretic agent chlorothiazide, are called *biochemically inert* although they are pharmacologically active. Chemical alterations can take place in many tissues and organs. In the intestine, for example, drugs may be biotransformed either within the epithelial cell or by digestive enzymes or enzymes of the symbiotic microorganisms present in the intestinal lumen. Biotransformation may also occur in the plasma, kidney and brain; but by far the greatest number of chemical reactions occurs in the liver with the rate of reaction often highest in this organ.

The reactions in which drugs are chemically altered by the body are many and varied. They can, however, be divided into two main categories: *synthetic (conjugation) reactions* and *nonsynthetic reactions*.

Synthetic Reactions or Conjugations

The synthetic reaction, or *conjugation*, involves the chemical combination of a compound with a *molecule provided by the body*. The latter, known as the conjugating agent, is usually a carbohydrate, an amino acid or a substance derived from these nutrients. The families of enzymes that catalyze these reactions are called transferases because they transfer the conjugating agent onto the compound. The tendency for a particular compound to combine with a given conjugating agent depends on its possessing an appropriate group or 'center for conjugation,' such as carboxyl (—COOH), hydroxyl (—OH), amino (—NH$_2$) or sulfhydryl (—SH).[1] Thus any compound, whether a drug, chemical from the environment, or a normal body constituent, may participate in a conjugating reaction as long as it possesses one of the necessary centers for conjugation. When the parent molecule does not possess such a functional group, it may acquire one as a result of a nonsynthetic reaction; the metabolite, or end product of the nonsynthetic reaction, then undergoes further biotransformation by conjugation. For example, benzene contains no center for conjugation but acquires one when it is converted by the body to phenol; phenol, by virtue of the hydroxyl group it has acquired, is then conjugated.

Since mere possession of a center for conjugation determines the occurrence of a particular synthetic reaction, it is obvious that a wide variety of compounds may act as substrates for the enzyme of a specific conjugation process. Thus all the enzymes of the synthetic reactions are specific only with regard to certain reactive groups in compounds; compounds with similar centers of conjugation may or may not be structurally related in other respects.

---

[1]Another conjugation reaction involves the addition of the amino acid cysteine to aromatic or halogenated hydrocarbons. The types of compounds undergoing this process are few in number, and therefore the process will not be considered further. The conversion of cyanides to thiocyanide is also considered a conjugation process.

The small number of chemical centers that can enter into conjugation places a limit on the number of synthetic reactions that are possible. Of the dozen or so that are known to occur in animals and insects, the following are the primary synthetic pathways of biotransformation in humans: glucuronide synthesis, glycine and glutamine conjugations, acetylation, sulfate conjugation, methylation, and glutathione conjugation (Table 8-1).

The features common to all the synthetic reactions are worthy of emphasis. First, these reactions require that energy and a conjugating agent be supplied by the body. Second, *none* of the reactions is confined to drugs; a number of substances formed in normal metabolic processes also undergo conjugation. Usually, these synthetic reactions change drugs and normal metabolites into compounds that are, respectively, pharmacologically and biologically *inactive*. Moreover, with the exception of methylated drug products, conjugated metabolites are usually less lipid-soluble than the parent compounds. Most conjugated compounds are relatively strong acids, because the conjugating moiety of the product is generally ionized at physiological pH. Thus, ordinarily the conjugation processes lead not only to inactivation of drugs but also to their more rapid elimination in the urine and feces, because the end products are less likely to be reabsorbed once they have reached the tubular urine or intestine. The limited number of conjugation reactions and the small number of chemical centers which can participate in them make it relatively easy to predict the reactions that will occur with given agents. If a drug carries one of the centers for conjugation, some conjugation can be expected to take place; only the extent of the reaction is unpredictable. Moreover, a compound may be excreted as several different conjugates if one or more of its groups can serve as the center for conjugation for more than one reaction, e.g. salicylic acid or acetaminophen (Table 8-1).

Glucuronide Conjugation

The synthesis of glucuronide conjugates is one of the most frequently occurring reactions because several of the chemical groups commonly encountered in the structure of drug molecules can act as centers for conjugation. Also, the general availability of the carbohydrate glucose provides an ample supply of the conjugating agent, glucuronic acid $C_6H_{10}O_6$. The functional groups may be an *amino* (—NH_2), a *carboxyl* (—COOH), a *sulfhydryl* (—SH) or a *hydroxyl* (—OH), either phenolic (attached to a ring structure) or alcoholic (attached to a straight-chain organic compound).

Salicylic acid, with both an hydroxyl and a carboxyl group, can combine with glucuronic acid in two ways[2]:

---

[2]Throughout this text, the diagrams of chemical reactions show only the overall process. All the chemical reactions involved in conjugation and in many of the nonsynthetic reactions are more complicated than the diagrams indicate.

Table 8-1. *Examples of conjugation, oxidation, reduction and hydrolysis of drugs in humans*

Reaction	Drugs biotransformed	Naturally occurring compound metabolized
Conjugation		
Glucuronide conjugation	Salicylic acid	Bilirubin
	Morphine	Thyroxine
	Ethinylestradiol	
	Acetaminophen	
Glycine conjugation	Salicylic acid	Bile acids
	Benzoic acid	
	Nicotinic acid	
Acetylation	Sulfonamide drugs	Choline
	Isoniazid	
Sulfate conjugation	Phenol	Steroids
	Acetaminophen	
Methylation	Nicotinamide	Histamine
	Methadone	Epinephrine
	Quinidine	Thyroxine
Glutathione conjugation	Oxidation product of acetaminophen	
Oxidation		
Microsomal enzymes	Phenobarbital	Steroids
	Phenytoin	
	Propranolol	
	Meperidine	
	Quinine	
	Codeine	
	Chlorpromazine	
	Parathion	
Nonmicrosomal enzymes	Ethanol	Vitamin A
	Methanol	Xanthine
	Acetaldehyde	Epinephrine
	Caffeine	Serotonin
	Isoproterenol	
Reduction		
Microsomal enzymes	Prednisolone	Cortisone
	Nitrobenzene	
Nonmicrosomal enzymes	Chloral hydrate	
Hydrolysis	Procaine	Acetylcholine
	Aspirin	
	Succinylcholine	

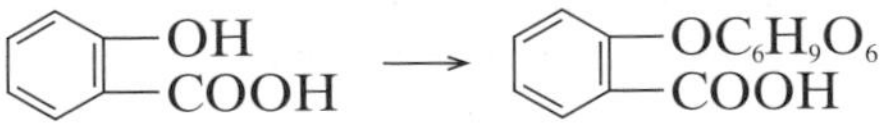

salicylic acid (SA)   ether glucuronide of SA

or

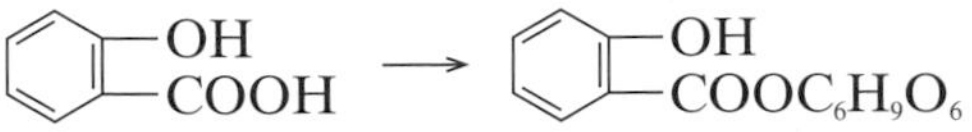

SA   ester glucuronide of SA

Other examples of compounds that undergo conjugation with glucuronic acid are given in Table 8–1. Some drugs, such as many of the anti-anxiety benzodiazepines, are also eliminated as glucuronides, but only after they have acquired a center for conjugation through nonsynthetic reactions. Aspirin is first rapidly biotransformed to salicylic acid and then is eliminated as conjugates of the latter.

The glucuronides are rapidly eliminated in the urine, being highly ionized and water soluble. They are also secreted in the bile; however, this action does not always lead to their elimination in the feces. The enzymes of the bacteria normally present in the intestine can remove the glucuronic acid from the parent compound, and if the latter is lipid soluble, it will be reabsorbed. The establishment of an enterohepatic cycle will of course prolong the presence of the drug in the body. The sedative drug glutethimide and phenolphthalein, a cathartic drug, show this type of behavior (cf. p. 149).

Glucuronide conjugates are generally pharmacologically inactive. A notable exception is one of the glucuronide conjugates of morphine. This metabolite may contribute to the overall analgesic effect of the drug, especially when elimination of the conjugate by the kidney is impaired by renal disease.

Amino Acid Conjugation

Several amino acids may serve as conjugating agents, but only in reactions with compounds that possess a *carboxyl group*, –COOH. In humans the amino acids utilized in these reactions are glycine and glutamine. We may again use salicylic acid to exemplify this type of conjugation:

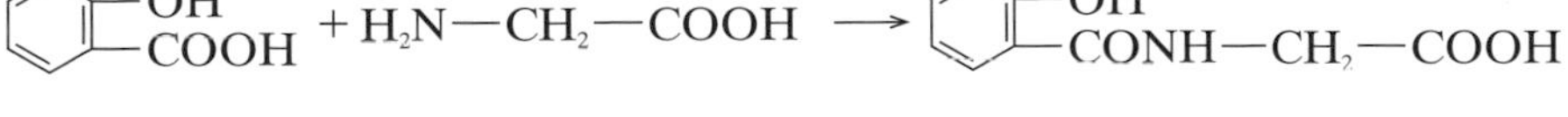

SA   glycine   salicyluric acid

The amino acid conjugates, like the glucuronides, are for the most part more water-soluble than their parent compounds and, therefore, are more readily excreted in the urine. They are not secreted into the bile to any significant extent.

Acetylation

This reaction is really the converse of amino acid conjugation; acetylation occurs when a compound containing an amino group is conjugated with an acid provided by the body. Acetylation is the primary route of biotransformation for the sulfonamide drugs, thus:

sulfanilamide   acetic acid   acetylsulfanilamide

The acetylation of sulfonamides exemplifies two important points: (1) a decrease in lipid solubility does not necessarily mean an increase in water solubility, and (2) biotransformation does not always lead to the production of a less toxic agent. The acetyl derivatives of a number of the first clinically useful sulfonamides are not only less lipid soluble, but also less water soluble than their parent compounds. For example, the solubility of sulfathiazole is 98 mg per 100 ml water at 37°C, whereas its acetylated compound is soluble to the extent of only 7 mg per 100 ml. The sulfonamides and their acetylated derivatives are also less soluble at acid pH. Therefore, injury to the urinary tract may result from the precipitation of the conjugated sulfonamide within renal passageways as the kidney concentrates the urine and it becomes more acid.

Sulfate Conjugation

The reaction of sulfate (derived from sulfur-containing amino acids such as cysteine) with hydroxyl groups and certain compounds containing an amino group is frequently called ethereal sulfate synthesis. A typical example is:

phenol   phenyl sulfate

The ethereal sulfates appear to be more water-soluble than their parent compounds and are readily excreted in the urine. Sulfate conjugation is an important pathway for a number of drugs including acetaminophen and estradiol.

Methylation

A methyl group, —CH_3, derived from the amino acid methionine can be transferred from the conjugating agent to a phenolic hydroxyl group (an –OH attached to a ring) or to various amines, and even to nitrogen contained within a ring structure. This reaction is an important physiologic process, accounting for the conversion of norepinephrine[3] to epinephrine.

norepinephrine   epinephrine

Methylation is also one of the major pathways of inactivation of either norepinephrine or epinephrine:

epinephrine   metanephrine

Two different enzymes catalyze these reactions, the former primarily in the adrenal medulla and the latter primarily in neuronal tissue and the liver. Other important endogenous compounds are also methylated, including histamine and the hormones estradiol and thyroxine.

The biotransformations of compounds such as nicotinamide are examples of the addition of the methyl group to a nitrogen contained within a ring, viz.:

nicotinamide   *N*-methylnicotinamide[4]

The attachment of a methyl group to the ring nitrogen creates a quaternary ammonium compound with a fixed positive charge, which is poorly reabsorbed from the tubular urine following glomerular filtration.

[3]The designation *nor* is from the German meaning 'nitrogen without a radical'; in this case, norepinephrine is epinephrine without the radical —CH_3 attached to the nitrogen atom.
[4]The *N* indicates that the methyl group is attached to the nitrogen.

Glutathione Conjugation

The tripeptide glutathione, consisting of the three amino acids glycine, cysteine, and glutamate, is conjugated by the enzymes, glutathione transferases, onto reactive sites of drug metabolites, generated by oxidative reactions. In many cases, glutathione conjugation inactivates xenobiotic metabolites that are toxic to cells such as the liver and kidney. The supply of glutathione is limited in tissues such as the liver, and when depleted by synthetic reactions (or liver disease) the toxicity of the metabolites is observed. A notable example is a toxic metabolite of acetaminophen, which is normally detoxified to glutathione conjugates. These conjugates undergo further changes to mercapturic acid derivatives that are excreted in the urine. In the case of alcoholism, when liver cirrhosis is present, limiting the supply of glutathione, the toxic acetaminophen metabolite accumulates, contributing additional injury to liver cells.

Nonsynthetic Reactions

In nonsynthetic reactions the parent drug itself is chemically altered by oxidation, reduction, hydrolysis[5] or a combination of these processes. Usually these nonsynthetic reactions represent only the first stage of biotransformation which explains why they are frequently termed phase 1 reactions. The second stage encompasses all the conjugation reactions[6] of the metabolites formed in the nonsynthetic processes (phase 2 reactions). Since most drugs undergo two-stage biotransformation, the end products of the nonsynthetic reactions are generally not eliminated from the body as such, even though they are usually less lipid-soluble than their parent drugs; they are usually excreted only after conjugation (Fig. 8-5). Again, unlike the products of the conjugation reactions, the products of the first stage of biotransformation are not always pharmacologically inactive. Indeed, instead of inactivating an agent, the nonsynthetic processes may *convert an inactive drug into an active agent or change an active drug into another pharmacologically active compound* (Fig. 8-5). If the latter change takes place, the metabolite may have (1) a qualitatively similar pharmacologic activity but be less, equally or more active[7]; (2) a qualitatively different type of pharmacologic activity; or (3) a greater toxicity. For instance, the opioid analgesic codeine is active only after biotransformation to its metabolite morphine. In contrast, sali-

---

[5]*Oxidation* is a chemical reaction in which oxygen is added to a compound or, by extension, the proportion of oxygen in a compound is increased by removal of other groups.
Reduction is the opposite of oxidation, i.e. the removal of oxygen or an alteration which leads to a decrease in the proportion of oxygen in a compound.
Hydrolysis refers to the cleavage of a compound by the addition of water.
[6]Conjugation reactions are frequently termed Phase 2 reactions whether they are reactions of the drug molecule or a product of a Phase 1 reaction with endogenous substances.
[7]Here, quantitative difference refers to the effects produced by equal amounts of drug, i.e. a more active drug produces a greater intensity of effect when given in the same amount as a less active agent.

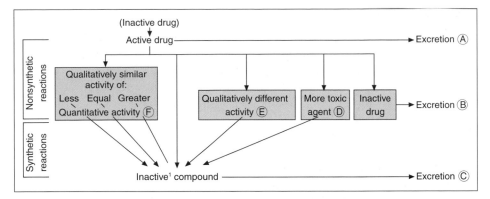

Figure 8-5. *Effect of biotransformation on the pharmacologic activity of a drug in the body. The original drug administered may be either an active or an inactive drug. The inactive drug is first converted to an active one. An active drug may be excreted unchanged (A) or biotransformed by a nonsynthetic reaction and excreted without additional chemical alteration (B). The active drug may also be conjugated directly and excreted as the conjugate (C).*

Alternatively, the active drug may undergo a nonsynthetic reaction, and the products of this reaction may be conjugated and excreted as the conjugate (C). The nonsynthetic reaction may yield a more toxic agent (D), an agent with qualitatively different activity (E) or an agent with quantitatively different activity either less, equal to or greater than that of the parent compound (F).

[1]*Almost without exception the products of synthetic reactions are pharmacologically inactive, but some few exceptions are known, e.g one of the glucuronide conjugates of the opioid analgesic morphine.*

cylic acid, the metabolite of aspirin, has analgesic activity both qualitatively similar to, and approximately equipotent to, that of its parent drug. Table 8-2 lists some of the many known examples of biotransformation that lead to changes in activity of the administered drug.

The rate of change of an active drug into another active drug has an important bearing on the resulting pharmacologic activity. If the biotransformation is rapid, the pharmacologic effect will be largely that of the metabolite. If the transformation is slow, the observed effect may be that of both the parent drug and the metabolite.

The term **prodrug** is used to describe a compound that is converted to the pharmacologically active agent *after administration*. Although many older drugs such as castor oil, cascara, and some antihistamines, are now known to be inactive until biotransformed, their utility as prodrugs was accidental rather than deliberate. Today, however, the prodrug approach is widely used to overcome problems of absorption, distribution, and biotransformation associated with certain drug molecules. The prodrug concept has been most successfully applied to facilitating absorption and distribution of drugs with poor lipid solubility, increasing the duration of action of drugs that are rapidly eliminated, overcoming

Table 8-2. *Changes in pharmacologic activity produced by biotransformation*

Drug	Activity of drug	Metabolic reaction	Activity of metabolite
Parathion	Inactive	Oxidation	Toxic agent (insecticide)
Codeine	Inactive	Oxidation	Potent analgesic
Aspirin	Analgesic	Hydrolysis	Similarly potent analgesic
Rifampin	Antituberculin	Oxidation	Equally potent antituberculin
Methanol	Depressant	Oxidation	Different activity and more toxic

problems of poor patient acceptance of a product, and promoting site-specific delivery of a drug. For example, levodopa, which is absorbed from the gastrointestinal tract and distributed to the central nervous system, is a precursor or prodrug of dopamine, an endogenous compound that is poorly, if at all, distributed to brain after oral administration. Dopamine is not only less readily absorbed and distributed into the brain, but it is also more rapidly metabolized than is levodopa. Levodopa is, therefore, the therapeutic agent used to treat patients suffering from Parkinson's disease, a disorder associated with a deficiency of brain dopamine. The way in which prodrugs can enhance patient compliance is illustrated by the use of hydrolyzable esters to mask the bitter taste of antibiotics such as erythromycin. The proton pump inhibitor omeprazole (PRILOSEC) is an example of a prodrug that enhances delivery of the active agent to its site of action. The prodrug is administered orally in an enteric-coated tablet to prevent its dissolution and nonspecific activation in the acidic gastric medium. Omeprazole is absorbed as such and diffuses into the gastric parietal cell which secretes hydrogen ions through the action of an enzyme, the proton pump. The acidic environment of the enzyme promotes the formation of a reactive metabolite from the prodrug that binds to and inhibits the proton pump.

Whether a particular compound is amenable to oxidation, reduction, or hydrolysis depends, as it does in the synthetic reactions, on the presence of an appropriate functional group or chemical structure. However, the mere presence of such a group in a drug does not mean that it will undergo one of the nonsynthetic reactions. Consequently, the reactions of the first stage of biotransformation are much less predictable than those occurring in the second stage. These similarities and differences between the synthetic and nonsynthetic reactions are summarized in Table 8-3.

The reactions classified as nonsynthetic are many and varied, but they may be categorized on the basis of the type of enzyme involved. One group consists of

Table 8-3. *Comparison of synthetic and nonsynthetic drug biotransformations*

	Synthetic reactions	Nonsynthetic reactions
Type of reaction	Determined by functional group	Determined by functional group
	Limited number	Wide variety
	Relatively predictable	Relatively unpredictable
Metabolite	Almost always less lipid-soluble	Usually less lipid-soluble
	Almost always pharmacologically inactive	May have less, equal, greater or different activity
Reactions catalyzed by nonmicrosomal enzymes	All except glucuronide conjugation	Most hydrolyses; some oxidations and reductions
	No stimulation of rate of biotransformation by other drugs	No stimulation of rate of biotransformation by other drugs
Reactions catalyzed by microsomal enzymes	Only glucuronide conjugation	Most oxidations and reductions; some hydrolyses
	Rate of reaction stimulated by drugs	Rate of reactions stimulated by many agents

reactions mediated by enzymes of moderate specificity whose substrates may be either foreign compounds or substances normally present in the body. Most hydrolyses and a few, but important, oxidations and reductions fall into this group. The vast majority of oxidations and reductions belong to the second category of reactions; these reactions are catalyzed by enzymes that *lack specificity* and which, with a few notable exceptions, are concerned *entirely with drug biotransformation* and not with normal metabolism. These remarkable enzymes of drug biotransformation are known as *microsomal enzymes.*

Microsomal Enzymes

Microsomal enzymes are located predominantly in liver cells, where they are associated with a subcellular component, the endoplasmic reticulum. This reticulum is a network of lipoprotein tubules extending throughout the cytoplasm and continuous with the cellular and nuclear membranes, but functionally different from both. Electron microscopy has revealed that part of the surface of this endoplasmic network is smooth and the remainder is 'rough', being studded with ribonucleoprotein granules called ribosomes (Fig. 8-6). The rough-surfaced cellular fraction contains the enzymes involved in protein synthesis. The

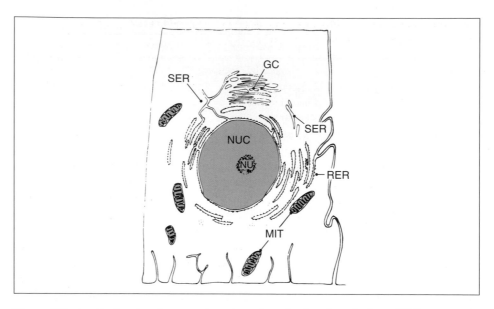

Figure 8-6. *A cell, showing the smooth and rough endoplasmic reticulum. (SER = smooth endoplasmic reticulum; GC = Golgi complex; RER = rough endoplasmic reticulum; MIT = mitochondria; NU = nucleolus; NUC = nucleus.)*

enzymes that can metabolize drugs are associated primarily with the smooth-surfaced endoplasmic reticulum. Experimentally, when liver (or other) cells are ruptured by homogenization, the endoplasmic reticulum is fragmented. The fragments can then be separated from other parts of the cell by differential centrifugation. The sediment obtained after very high-speed centrifugation is known as the microsomal fraction; it contains the smooth-surfaced fragments and their associated drug-metabolizing enzymes, or microsomal enzymes.

Microsomal enzymes lack specificity and are capable of metabolizing substances of widely different structure, but they appear *only to catalyze reactions of compounds that are lipid-soluble*. In fact, this requirement for lipid solubility may explain the apparent paradox of a component of living cells being able to biotransform foreign compounds but being largely unable to promote similar reactions of natural metabolites. For example, the lipid-soluble drug amphetamine is biotransformed by the microsomal enzyme system:

$$\text{amphetamine} \quad \bigcirc\!\!-\text{CH}-\underset{\underset{\displaystyle \text{CH}_3}{|}}{\text{CH}}-\text{NH}_2 \quad \longrightarrow \quad \bigcirc\!\!-\text{CH}_2-\underset{\underset{\displaystyle \text{CH}_3}{|}}{\text{C}}=\text{O} + \text{NH}_3$$

amphetamine   phenylacetone   ammonia

On the other hand, the less lipid-soluble natural amine tyramine is not altered by microsomal enzymes but undergoes a similar reaction in the presence of a nonmicrosomal enzyme, monoamine oxidase:

$$HO\!-\!\!\bigcirc\!\!-\!CH_2\!-\!CH_2\!-\!NH_2 \quad \longrightarrow \quad HO\!-\!\!\bigcirc\!\!-\!CH_2\!-\!\underset{\underset{H}{|}}{C}\!\!=\!\!O + NH_3$$

      tyramine   benzylaldehyde   ammonia

Like amphetamine, many drugs are lipid-soluble, whereas most natural substances are less lipid-soluble and more water-soluble than their foreign counterparts. It has been suggested, therefore, that the microsomal enzymes, associated as they are with a lipoprotein cellular component, are themselves protected by a lipid barrier which restricts diffusion of hydrophilic compounds.

One microsomal enzyme system has some additional properties that are noteworthy. First, this enzyme system mediates the glucuronic acid conjugation – the *only* synthetic reaction carried out by a microsomal enzyme system. Second, the microsomal enzymes involved in glucuronide syntheses are different from almost all the other microsomal enzymes in that they can form glucuronides with a wide range of *natural metabolites*, e.g. bilirubin, as well as with foreign substances (xenobiotics). All the other microsomal enzymes are concerned with oxidation and reduction, and with the important exception of steroid hormones and fatty acids, their substrates are almost exclusively drugs or other foreign substances (cf. Table 8-1).

The liver, the principal site of biotransformation of drugs, is also the main organ in which microsomal enzyme reactions are carried out. Similar reactions are also catalyzed by microsomal fractions of the lung, kidney, and intestinal mucosa, but generally at a lesser rate than in preparations from the liver. Reactions in the intestinal mucosa may be a significant factor in reducing the bioavailability of some orally administered drugs. You will recall that drugs absorbed from the small intestine pass through the liver before entering the systemic circulation (cf. p. 84). Thus biotransformation within the intestinal epithelium added to that in the liver may markedly decrease the amount of administered drug available for activity. The combined action of intestinal and hepatic drug metabolizing enzymes on a drug's bioavailability is known as the *first-pass effect*.

Oxidation

Oxidation is one of the most general biochemical reactions of foreign compounds because there are so many ways in which a compound can be oxidized (see Table 8-1). The oxidation transformations catalyzed by the microsomal enzyme systems include (1) the addition of a hydroxyl group to a ring structure or to a side-chain attached to a ring; (2) the removal of a methyl ($-CH_3$) or an ethyl ($-C_2H_5$) group from an oxygen, nitrogen or sulfur atom of a compound;

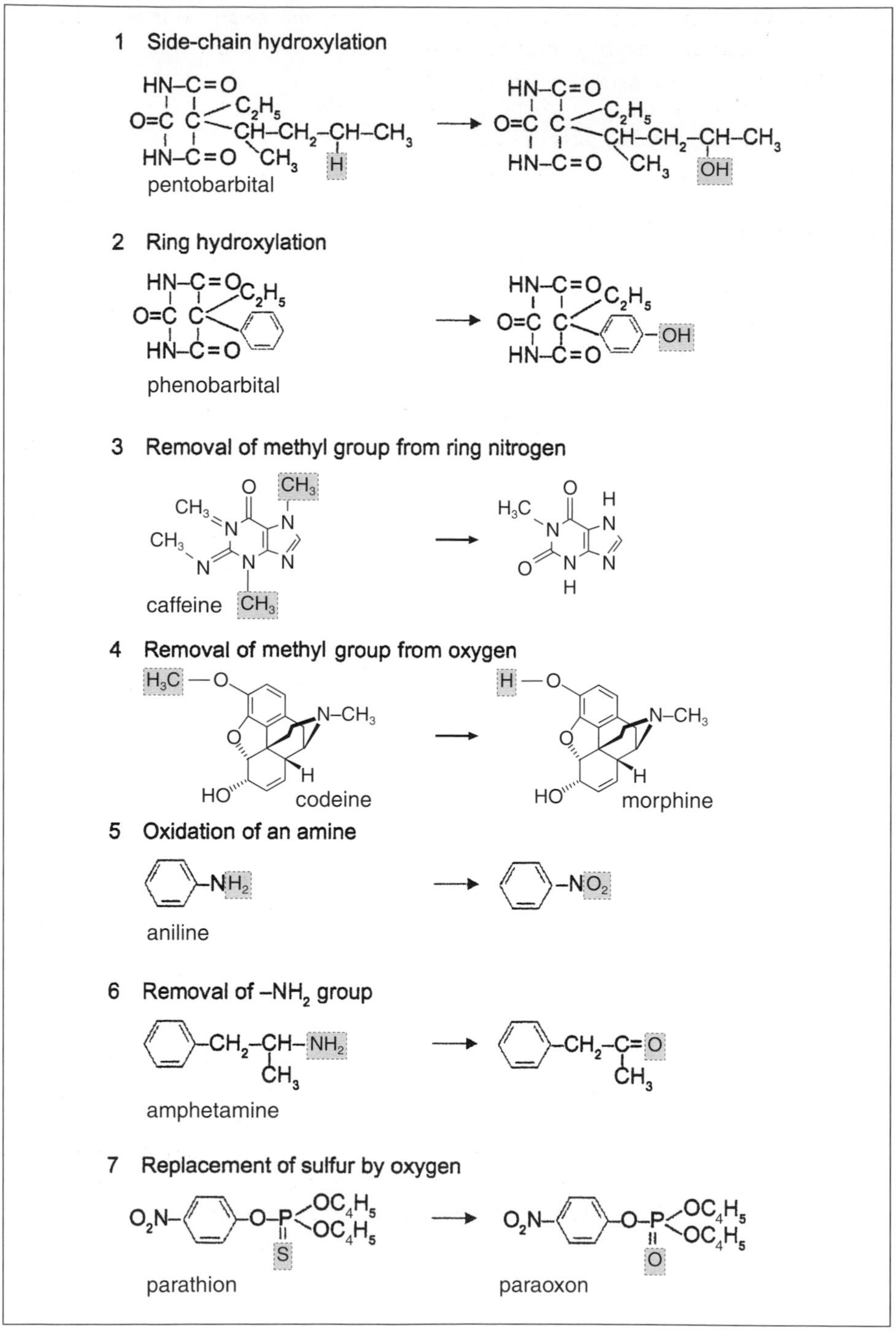

1   Side-chain hydroxylation

pentobarbital

2   Ring hydroxylation

phenobarbital

3   Removal of methyl group from ring nitrogen

caffeine

4   Removal of methyl group from oxygen

codeine   morphine

5   Oxidation of an amine

aniline

6   Removal of –NH₂ group

amphetamine

7   Replacement of sulfur by oxygen

parathion   paraoxon

Figure 8-7. *Oxidative reactions catalyzed by microsomal enzyme systems.*

(3) the replacement of an amine group (—NH$_2$) by oxygen; (4) the addition of oxygen to a sulfur or nitrogen atom; and a variety of other processes. Specific examples of these reactions are illustrated in Figure 8-7.

The microsomal enzymes that catalyze oxidative reactions consist of many structurally and biochemically related proteins encoded by at least 14 different gene families in humans. A common feature of this enzyme family is the presence of an iron-containing moiety, heme, present also in hemoglobin. The binding properties of the heme, detected using the tools of spectrophotometry, are the basis for the family name for these enzymes, *cytochrome P450s or CYP450s*. With identification of the genes that code for individual enzymes in this family and the elucidation of the amino acid sequences of each isozyme, a system of nomenclature has been adopted to identify individual proteins in this enzyme class. Among the most important drug-metabolizing enzymes in this family are CYP3A4 and CYP2D6. Because individual enzymes can now be expressed in artificial cell systems, their substrates and factors that affect their activity can be identified.

The oxidations catalyzed by nonmicrosomal enzymes are less varied than those of the microsomal fraction but are important reactions of many naturally occurring substances as well as of drugs. The enzymes that oxidize the nutritionally essential vitamin A also catalyze the reactions of various foreign alcohols and aldehydes:

$$CH_3OH \longrightarrow HCHO \longrightarrow HCOOH$$
$$\text{methyl} \quad \text{formaldehyde} \quad \text{formic}$$
$$\text{alcohol} \qquad\qquad\qquad\qquad \text{acid}$$

$$CH_3CH_2OH \longrightarrow CH_3CHO \longrightarrow CH_3COOH$$
$$\text{ethyl} \qquad \text{acetaldehyde} \qquad \text{acetic}$$
$$\text{alcohol} \qquad\qquad\qquad\qquad \text{acid}$$

In males, there is considerable nonmicrosomal enzyme alcohol dehydrogenase that resides in the intestinal mucosa as well as the liver; its activity in the intestines can contribute significantly to the first-pass effect of alcohol.

The oxidation of amines to aldehydes can also be catalyzed by nonmicrosomal soluble enzymes, such as monoamine oxidase (cf. p. 169) or diamine oxidase. Their substrates include compounds normally found in the body, e.g. epinephrine, tyramine and histamine, as well as drugs like isoproterenol. Xanthine oxidase, the nonmicrosomal enzyme responsible for converting the purine bases of nucleic acids into uric acid, also catalyzes the oxidation of caffeine and other foreign xanthines.

Reduction

Reduction reactions involve the addition of hydrogen to a nitrogen, oxygen, or carbon double bond. Examples include the conversion of a nitro ($-NO_2$) group to an amine ($-NH_2$), as occurs with the anti-anxiety agent clonazepam, and the change of a carbonyl ($-C=O$) to a hydroxyl ($-OH$), as occurs with the opioid analgesic methadone. The addition of hydrogen to double bonds, particularly in the metabolism of some steroid hormones, is another example of reduction carried out by nonmicrosomal enzymes. The enzymes of the microsomal fraction are concerned primarily with the addition of hydrogen to nitrogen atoms of foreign compounds, e.g.:

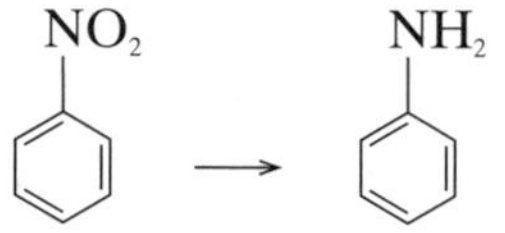

nitrobenzene   aniline

Hydrolysis

Hydrolysis as a mechanism of biotransformation of drugs occurs only in compounds with an ester linkage:

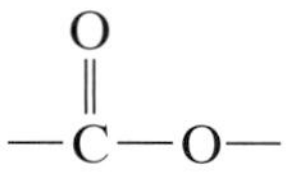

or an amide linkage:

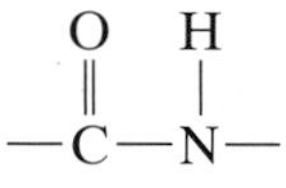

When an ester is hydrolyzed by an esterase, an alcohol (phenolic or straight chain) and an acid are formed; when an amide is acted upon by an amidase, the products are an amine and an acid. For example:

aspirin → salicylic acid + acetic acid

procaine → para-aminobenzoic acid (PABA) + diethylaminoethanol

procainamide → PABA + diethylaminoethylamine

The esterases are found in plasma, liver and many other tissues, primarily in the nonmicrosomal soluble fraction. They are responsible for hydrolyzing acetylcholine and other esters such as succinylcholine, used in surgery to paralyze muscles. The amidases are also nonmicrosomal enzymes and are found principally in the liver but not in plasma.

Major Pathways of Biotransformation

We have seen that a single compound such as salicylic acid can be conjugated in at least three different ways. Salicylic acid may also undergo several oxidative reactions, and these metabolites may be conjugated as well. Since so many drugs are similar to salicylic acid in possessing several groups that can be altered chemically by enzymic activity, they too give rise to a variety of end products. Usually, one or two pathways account for the major metabolic alterations. For salicylic acid, the conjugates with glycine and glucuronic acid are the major

Table 8-4. *Major route of biotransformation of some common functional groups*

Hydroxyl (—OH)
    Alcohols (straight chain, i.e. aliphatic): oxidation; glucuronide conjugation
    Phenols (ring structure, i.e. aromatic): glucuronide conjugation; sulfate conjugation; methylation

Carboxyl (—COOH)
    Aliphatic: oxidation; glucuronide conjugation
    Aromatic: glycine conjugation; glucuronide conjugation

Amino (—NH$_2$)
    Aliphatic: deamination (removal of amino group and formation of aldehyde); glucuronide conjugation
    Aromatic: acetylation; glucuronide conjugation; methylation
    Aromatic rings: hydroxylation

metabolites. Although it is not always possible to predict which reactions will take place, Table 8-4 lists the most probable major reactions of some important functional groups.

FACTORS AFFECTING DRUG BIOTRANSFORMATION

We saw earlier that the rate of biotransformation of drugs is influenced only by changing the substrate concentration since, under normal conditions, the concentration of enzyme is usually constant. However, there are several factors that alter the activity of enzymes, and these are tantamount to decreasing or increasing the concentration of enzyme available for drug biotransformation. These alterations in enzyme activity are pharmacologically important because the duration and intensity of action of many drugs are determined largely by the rate at which they are biotransformed.

Enzyme Inhibition

Enzymes are true catalysts – they are not changed appreciably during a reaction, but as proteins they are subject to decomposition in the body. Under normal conditions the rate of enzyme production equals its rate of degradation. Obviously, however, any abnormal condition, such as malnutrition or disease, that decreases the overall rate of protein synthesis may also result in decreased availability of enzymes. Since the liver plays such an important role in protein synthesis as well as in metabolism, malfunction of this organ may reduce the rate of drug biotransformation. In addition, there are many therapeutic agents, dietary components, and environmental chemicals that interact with enzymes of biotransformation and inhibit their activity. Examples include the antiulcer agent omeprazole, the antifungal agent ketoconazole, and a component of grapefruit juice, all documented CYP450 inhibitors.

To catalyze a reaction, an enzyme must be able to combine with its substrate. Therefore, any agent that interferes with a substrate's access to active binding sites will also decrease the rate of metabolism, even when the concentration of enzyme is normal. A decrease in metabolic rate of a given substrate is said to be *competitive inhibition* when the interfering agent is (1) a compound that is itself a substrate for the enzyme or (2) a compound that undergoes no catalytic change but combines reversibly with the active sites of the enzyme because of its structural similarity to the substrate. Methacholine is an example of a substrate that competes with acetylcholine for the active sites on the enzyme cholinesterase (cf. p. 154). The second type of competitive inhibition is exemplified by the action of amphetamine. As we have seen, amphetamine is not biotransformed by monoamine oxidase, but it can inhibit the metabolism of tyramine, a natural substrate of this enzyme. These competitive interactions may be represented as follows:

$$E + S_1 + S_2 \rightleftharpoons ES_1 + ES_2 \rightleftharpoons E + P_1 + P_2 \qquad \text{(Equation 3)}$$

$$E + S_1 + I \rightleftharpoons ES_1 + EI \rightleftharpoons E + P_1 + I \qquad \text{(Equation 4)}$$

where E is enzyme, S_1 and S_2 are substrates, I is a nonsubstrate and P_1 and P_2 are the end products of the metabolism of S_1 and S_2, respectively.

In Equation 3, S_1 may represent acetylcholine, the natural substrate of cholinesterase (E), and S_2 may be the drug substrate, methacholine, which can bind to the same active sites on the enzyme as acetylcholine. In Equation 4, S_1 may be tyramine, the endogenous substrate of monoamine oxidase, and the nonsubstrate, I, may be amphetamine, which combines with the active sites of this enzyme even though this combination does not lead to biotransformation of the drug.

In both cases, the effect of two agents *competing* for the same quantity of enzyme is to reduce the rate of metabolism of the primary substrate, S_1, as predicted by the law of mass action. First, the degree of inhibition produced is dependent on the concentration of the primary substrate, S_1, relative to the concentrations of either S_2 or I. The greater the number of molecules of S_1 present in the total number of molecules capable of combining with active sites, the greater the possibility that a molecule of S_1 will complete the binding reaction. Then, since the rate of metabolism is proportional to substrate concentration, increasing the ratio of S_1 to either S_2 or I will decrease inhibition. A sufficiently high ratio of S_1 to either S_2 or I will force almost complete occupancy of active sites by S_1 despite the presence of either S_2 or I (Fig. 8-8). Thus *competitive inhibition can be overcome by a large enough concentration of substrate*. Of course the extent of inhibition is also determined by the relative rates of dissociation of the complexes formed, i.e. on the rates of dissociation of ES_1, ES_2 or EI. The rates of dissociation of all three complexes must be sufficiently rapid to make free, unoccupied sites available for continuous combination with molecules of S_1.

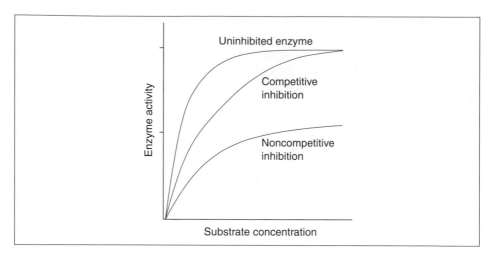

Figure 8-8. *Effect of inhibitors on enzyme activity. The rate of the catalyzed reaction is plotted as a function of substrate concentration when the amount of enzyme is constant and the concentration of each of the inhibitors is also constant.*

Inhibition of metabolism may also be brought about by an agent unrelated in structure to the substrate but capable of combining with the enzyme in such a way as to prevent the formation of an enzyme-substrate complex. This is termed *noncompetitive inhibition*. Many heavy metals, such as mercury, lead or arsenic, and the organic phosphate insecticides are typical noncompetitive inhibitors. Since noncompetitive inhibitors do not combine with the enzyme in the same manner as the substrate, an excess of substrate cannot displace the inhibitor from the enzyme surface. Noncompetitive inhibition may be reversible or irreversible; the important point is that the concentration of substrate does not influence the reversibility or the degree of inhibition (Fig. 8-8). When the action of a noncompetitive inhibitor is irreversible, the enzymatic activity is destroyed and new molecules of enzyme must be synthesized before full enzymatic activity is restored. For example, in the blood, aspirin inactivates cyclooxygenase irreversibly in platelets to prevent clotting; since the life of a platelet is only a few days, new platelets must be synthesized to restore cyclooxygenase activity. Chemicals that are substrates of an enzyme but reduce its activity irreversibly are referred to as suicide inhibitors.

The inhibition of enzyme activity has pharmacologic significance aside from decreasing the rate of drug biotransformation and prolonging the duration of drug action. In certain pathologic conditions, the inhibition of specific normal metabolic processes may be beneficial. Under these circumstances, a chemical that can inhibit the appropriate enzyme system is a useful therapeutic agent; its receptor is the enzyme and not an integral, macromolecular component of tissue. Enzyme inhibitors that are therapeutically useful drugs include inhibitors of cholinesterase, monoamine oxidase, carbonic anhydrase, and xanthine oxidase, mentioned previously in this text. There are many others as well, such as the aspirin family of drugs that inhibit the fatty-acid oxidizing enzyme cyclooxygenase (COX) and the antihypertensive ACE inhibitors that block the generation of a vasoconstrictor peptide by angiotensin-converting enzyme (ACE).

Enzyme Induction

The enzymes of the microsomal fraction of cells possess yet another important characteristic: their ability to metabolize certain compounds can be *stimulated* or *increased* by the prior administration of a large variety of chemical substances. Various therapeutic agents, herbal medicines, food additives, pesticides, herbicides, and carcinogenic compounds, numbering in the hundreds, have been shown to increase the rate of their own biotransformation or that of other foreign agents and even of normal body constituents. More compounds are constantly being added to the list. There is no predictable relationship between either pharmacologic activity or structure and the ability of this diverse group of agents to stimulate microsomal enzyme activity. One property that some of the stimulating compounds have in common is that they are themselves substrates for one or more of the reactions catalyzed by these enzymes. However, not all substrates of the microsomal enzymes are inducers. Table 8–5 lists some of the

Table 8-5. *Agents stimulating microsomal enzyme activity in humans and the compounds whose biotransformation is affected*

Stimulating agents	Compounds whose rate of biotransformation is increased
Phenobarbital and other barbiturates	Phenobarbital (sedative, anticonvulsant)
	Dicumarol (anticoagulant)
	Warfarin (anticoagulant)
	Phenytoin (antiepileptic)
	Griseofulvin (antifungal agent)
	Digitoxin (increases performance of the failing heart)
	Bilirubin (naturally occurring breakdown product)
	Cortisol (naturally occurring hormone)
	Testosterone (male sex hormone)
Rifampin	Oral contraceptives
	Cortisol
	Warfarin
Phenytoin	Cortisol
Griseofulvin	Warfarin
Cigarette smoke	3,4-Benzopyrene (carcinogenic compound)
	Theophylline (anti-asthmatic agent)
Alcohol	Alcohol
	Diazepam (anti-anxiety agent)

agents known to stimulate drug biotransformation in humans and some of the substances whose metabolism is affected.

How is this enhancement of enzymic activity brought about? The evidence from the first studies of this phenomenon revealed that it is usually the consequence of an augmented rate of *protein synthesis;* the agents act to *induce* enzyme production. The barbiturate drug phenobarbital was one of the first drugs identified as an inducing agent. When animals were treated with phenobarbital, electron microscopy was used to show that there was an increase in the quantity of smooth endoplasmic reticulum, the cellular fraction associated with microsomal enzymes. Also, treatment with phenobarbital in the presence of compounds like puromycin, which prevent protein synthesis, blocked the increase in enzyme activity or increase in quantities of endoplasmic reticulum. Moreover, the compounds that produce an increase in drug biotransformation could not be shown to enhance the activity of enzymes when added to an incubation mixture *in vitro*; the phenomenon was evoked only in the intact animal. And the elapsed time between the start of drug treatment and the appearance of stimulated drug metabolism corresponded to known rates of protein synthesis. When the administration of the compound that stimulated the production of enzyme was discontinued, the rate of enzyme synthesis slowly returned to its normal level. Thus, prior administration of a variety of foreign agents may accelerate drug biotransformation, as well as metabolism of normally occurring substances, by increasing the total quantity of microsomal enzymes.

The term **enzyme induction** is used to refer to this phenomenon. The mechanism is now known to involve interaction of the inducing agent with a cytosolic protein (a receptor). This complex translocates into the nucleus of the cell and binds to unique gene sequences in the promoter region of the gene that regulate the transcription rate of the coding region. Several classes of receptors have been identified that have some similarities with respect to their structure. The first receptor that was characterized is referred to as the aryl hydrocarbon receptor or AhR. Polycyclic aromatic hydrocarbons, such as benzopyrene and dioxins, bind to this protein and induce synthesis of the CYP450 (CYP1A1) that hydroxylates these compounds. The barbiturates bind a different receptor, the constitutive androstane receptor (CAR), and induce other CYP450 enzymes as well as glucuronide-conjugating enzymes. And a third cytosolic protein, referred to as the pregnane X receptor (PXR), mediates CYP450 induction by hormones in the glucocorticoid family.

An example of how a chemical may stimulate its own biotransformation is illustrated in Figure 8-9 for benzopyrene, an aryl hydrocarbon which is a major coal tar carcinogen found in tobacco smoke. Weanling rats were given a single injection of benzopyrene at two different doses. The animals were sacrificed at intervals over the course of 6 days, and the benzopyrene-metabolizing activity of their livers was determined *in vitro*. Stimulation of enzyme activity, now known to be mediated by the CYP450 isozyme 1A1, was evident for both doses at the earliest time of testing, the large dose producing a stimulation of greater intensity and longer duration. Benzopyrene becomes carcinogenic only *after* its

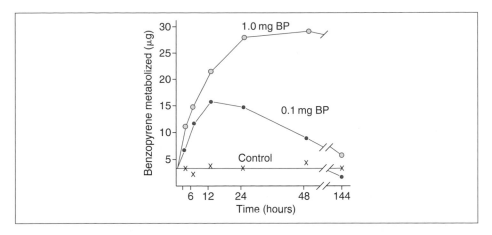

Figure 8-9. *Stimulation of the biotransformation of a drug produced by prior administration of the same drug. A single injection of benzopyrene (BP), either 0.1 mg or 1.0 mg, was administered to two groups of rats. Animals were sacrificed at intervals over the course of 6 days, and the benzopyrene-metabolizing activity of their livers was determined in vitro. Each point is the average from two rats. (From A.H. Conney, E.C. Miller and J.A. Miller,* J. Biol. Chem. *228:753, 1957.)*

biotransformation and cigarette smoking is known to increase its rate of bio-transformation in humans. Thus, the very source of the procarcinogen increases benzopyrene's potential for toxicity.

Phenobarbital has been shown to increase the rate of biotransformation of a wide variety of agents, metabolized by certain CYP450 isozymes and the glu-curonide-conjugating enzymes. One of the drugs affected by phenobarbital is dicumarol (bishydroxycoumarin), a drug used to decrease the clotting ability of blood in patients prone to form clots too readily. Dicumarol is itself a good example of a drug that produces its pharmacologic action by inhibition of an enzymatic process. It interferes with the liver's normal synthesis of clotting factors, particularly the synthesis of prothrombin. The dose of dicumarol needed to lower the clotting ability of blood to an appropriate level is adjusted for each patient according to his particular requirements. This is done by moni-toring the patient's blood prothrombin concentration, or *prothrombin time*, until a dose is found which yields the desired effects. Once established, the dose is maintained. Figure 8-10 illustrates what happens when phenobarbital is given to a patient who is receiving such a maintenance dose of the anticoagulant. In the presence of phenobarbital, the plasma concentration of dicumarol falls, indi-cating an increased rate of biotransformation of the latter, and the prothrombin time decreases (blood is clotting more rapidly), indicating a diminution of anti-coagulant activity. If additional dicumarol were given during phenobarbital administration, the concentration of the anticoagulant might become much too high were the barbiturate to be discontinued. Excessive dosage of an anticoagu-lant can lead to internal hemorrhage. On the other hand, if phenobarbital

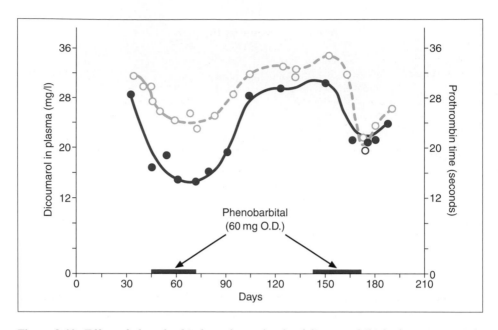

Figure 8-10. *Effect of phenobarbital on plasma levels of dicumarol (bishydroxycoumarin)* (●) *and on prothrombin time* (○) *in a human subject (dose of dicumarol: 75 mg per day). Phenobarbital was administered (60 mg once daily) during the period indicated by heavy marks on the abscissa. (Redrawn from S.A. Cucinell, A.H. Conney, M. Sansur and J.J. Burns, Drug interactions in man: I. Lowering effect of phenobarbital on plasma levels of bishydroxycoumarin [dicumarol] and diphenylhydantoin [DILANTIN]. Clin. Pharmacol. Ther. 6:420–429, 1965.)*

administration were continued and the dose of dicumarol were not increased to counteract the effect of enzyme induction, the value of the anticoagulant therapy might be nullified. These principles apply as well to the most frequently prescribed oral anticoagulant, warfarin (COUMADIN), which is primarily cleared by CYP2C9.

Whenever microsomal enzymes convert a drug to an inactive metabolite, the consequences of enzyme induction will be decreased therapeutic activity, as in the case of dicumarol. However, we have seen that an inactive drug, or prodrug, may be changed to an active agent or that an active drug may be converted to a compound of greater or different pharmacologic activity. In such cases the increase in microsomal enzyme activity by the concomitant use of another drug may lead to enhanced pharmacologic effect or even to toxicity. For example, the insecticide malathion is an inactive compound; its toxicity in insects as well as in humans is contingent on its conversion to the active metabolite malaoxon. Malathion's usefulness as an insecticide depends on the fact that malaoxon is more stable in insects than in mammals. In humans, the prodrug is not only activated by microsomal enzymes but is also rapidly inactivated by nonmicrosomal hydrolysis (Fig. 8-11). The latter process reduces the quantity of insecticide

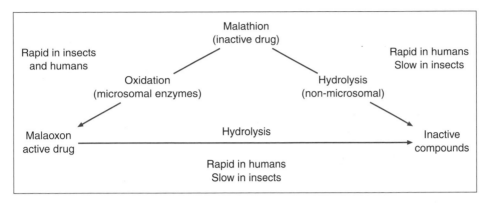

Figure 8-11. *Biotransformation of the insecticide malathion in human and insect hosts.* *(Modified from T.A. Loomis,* Essentials of Toxicology. *Philadelphia: Lea & Febiger, 1970.)*

available for oxidation to the toxic metabolite. The insecticide may become more harmful to humans, however, if microsomal enzyme activity has been stimulated.

Although the microsomal enzyme systems are largely confined to reactions involving foreign substances, they do participate in the metabolism of some important normal body constituents. The steroid hormones are normal substrates for nonsynthetic reactions, and substances like bilirubin and thyroxine are natural substrates for glucuronide conjugation, the one synthetic enzyme system catalyzed by the microsomal fraction of cells. Many experiments in animals and in human subjects indicate that the metabolism of normal body constituents can also be accelerated by various inducers of the microsomal enzymes. In addition, androgens, estrogens, progestational steroids and other hormones influence drug action by altering the activity of the microsomal enzyme systems. Clearly, the phenomenon of enzyme induction and the possibilities it creates for interactions among foreign agents and between drugs and naturally occurring substances have far-reaching significance.

SYNOPSIS

The actions of drugs in the body are terminated by biotransformation and by excretion primarily through the kidneys and liver. The elimination of most drugs depends on these processes acting in concert. The great majority of drugs are lipid-soluble chemicals which readily cross biologic barriers. This solubility characteristic permits their easy access to sites where they may produce a pharmacologic effect. It would lead equally to their indefinite retention in the body if means were not available to convert them into less lipid-soluble materials since lipid-soluble drugs are not excreted to any significant degree by the kidney or the liver. However, the reactions that drugs undergo during biotransformation yield products that are almost invariably less lipid-soluble than their parent compounds. It is significant, too, that the enzymes catalyzing the greatest number and variety of drug biotransformations – the microsomal enzymes – act almost exclusively on lipid-soluble substrates of exogenous origin.

Most drugs undergo chemical alteration by the body, being biotransformed by either a nonsynthetic reaction or a conjugation process or a combination of the two. Almost all these reactions are catalyzed by enzymes, many of which also catalyze normal metabolic processes. Among the most important enzymes of drug biotransformation are those of the smooth endoplasmic reticulum which contains the cytochrome P450 oxidative enzymes and the glucuronide conjugating enzymes. The activity of all enzymes involved in drug biotransformation may be decreased or inhibited by pathologic conditions or chemical agents. The stimulation of enzyme activity through chemical induction of gene transcription and new enzyme synthesis is an important phenomenon for microsomal enzyme systems.

Drugs may be biotransformed into inactive metabolites by either nonsynthetic (Phase 1) or synthetic (Phase 2) reactions. The nonsynthetic reactions can also convert an inactive drug into an active agent or an active agent into another compound with less, equal, greater or different pharmacologic activity. The consequences evoked by these potential changes in activity and by the phenomenon of enzyme induction warrant careful consideration in long-term therapy with single or multiple drugs.

GUIDES FOR STUDY AND REVIEW

How is the chemical alteration of a drug brought about in the body? What mediates these chemical reactions? In what ways are the reactions of drug biotransformations analogous to the reactions of drugs and receptors?

What is a first-order reaction? a zero-order reaction? How does the order of a reaction relate to the rate at which a drug is biotransformed? Does the rate of biotransformation of most drugs follow first-order kinetics or zero-order kinetics?

What are some of the features common to all synthetic or conjugation reactions? What functional groups of drugs act as centers for conjugation reactions? What are the most important synthetic pathways of biotransformation in humans? Which of the conjugation reactions of drug biotransformation is the most frequently occurring and why?

How do the two basic types of drug biotransformation reactions (synthetic and nonsynthetic) compare with respect to number of different reactions possible; the rapidity with which the metabolites formed are excreted in the urine or feces; the pharmacologic activity of the metabolites formed; the number of reactions catalyzed by microsomal enzyme systems?

How may the administration of one drug affect the biotransformation of another drug? What are the characteristics of competitive inhibition and how can the effects of this type of inhibition be overcome? How does competitive inhibition differ from noncompetitive inhibition? What are the potential pharmacologic consequences of the inhibition of biotransformation of a drug?

What types of drug biotransformation can be enhanced (stimulated) by the prior administration of drugs? How is this stimulation brought about? How does this phenomenon affect the onset and duration of drug action when the metabolite formed is an inactive drug? an active drug?

SUGGESTED READING

Anders, M.W. (ed.). *Bioactivation of Foreign Compounds*. New York: Academic, 1985.

Benford, D., Gibson, G.C. and Bridges, J.W. (eds). *Drug Metabolism from Molecules to Man*. Philadelphia: Taylor & Francis, 1987.

Bock, K.W. Vertebrate UDP-glucuronyltransferases: functional and evolutionary aspects. *Biochem. Pharmacol.* 66:691–696, 2003.

Conney, A.H. Induction of drug-metabolizing enzymes: a path to the discovery of multiple cytochromes P450. *Annu. Rev. Pharmacol. Toxicol.* 43:1–30, 2003.

Denison, M.S. and Nagy, S.R. Activation of the aryl hydrocarbon receptor by structurally diverse exogenous and endogenous chemicals. *Annu. Rev. Pharmacol. Toxicol.* 43:309–334, 2003.

Guengerich, F.P. Cytochrome P-450 3A4: regulation and role in drug metabolism. *Annu. Rev. Pharmacol. Toxicol.* 39:1–17, 1999.

Guengerich, F.P. Update information on human P450s. *Drug Metab. Rev.* 34:7–15, 2002.

Gillette, J.R. Metabolism of drugs and other foreign compounds by enzymatic mechanisms. *Prog. Drug Res.* 6:11, 1963.

Gorrod, J.W., Oelschlager, H. and Caldwell, J. (eds). *Metabolism of Xenobiotics*. Philadelphia: Taylor & Francis, 1988.

Lewis, D.F.V. *Guide to Cytochromes P450: Structure & Function*. London: Taylor & Francis, 2001.

Mandel, H.G. Pathways of Drug Biotransformation: Biochemical Conjugations. In: La Du, B.N., Mandel, H.G. and Way, E.L. (eds), *Fundamentals of Drug Metabolism and Drug Disposition*. Melbourne: Krieger Publishing Company, 1979, p.179

Ortiz de Montellano, P.R. (ed.) *Cytochrome P450: Structure, Mechanism and Biochemistry* (2nd ed.) New York: Plenum Press, 1995.

Sueyoshi, T. and Negishi, M. Phenobarbital response elements of cytochrome P450 genes and nuclear receptors. *Annu. Rev. Pharmacol. Toxicol.* 41:123–143, 2001.

Tukey, R.H. and Strassburg, C.P. Human UDP-glucuronyltransferases: metabolism, expression, and disease. *Annu. Rev. Pharmacol. Toxicol.* 40:581–616, 2000.

Willson, T.M. and Kliewer, S.A. PXR, CAR and drug metabolism. *Nat. Rev. Drug Discov.* 1:259, 2002.

9 General Principles of the Quantitative Aspects of Drug Action

I. Dose-Response Relationships

Up to this point we have considered some of the fundamental principles of pharmacology on rather qualitative grounds. These principles must find expression in quantitative terms as well; only then can they provide the basis for evaluation and comparison of drug safety and effectiveness and for the rational application of drug effects to therapeutics.

One of the most basic principles of pharmacology states that the degree of effect produced by a drug is a function of the quantity of drug administered. Even the word *dose*, the term used to quantitate drugs, has this relationship implicit in its definition, since dose is the *amount of drug needed at a given time to produce a particular biologic response*. We have seen that in the living system a drug is usually present as a solute and that it can produce its characteristic effect only if it reaches its site of action or its receptor. We ought more properly to define dose, then, as the amount of drug necessary to yield an appropriate *concentration* of material at the site in the system where the interaction occurs. Usually a drug does not reach its site of action instantaneously; its rate of accessibility is determined primarily by either or both the processes of absorption and distribution. Nor does the drug's presence at its locus of action continue indefinitely; redistribution, biotransformation and excretion operate separately or conjointly to remove it from the site and from the body. Thus, at any given moment, the concentration of drug at a site of action, and consequently the magnitude of drug effect, is a function not only of the *dose administered* but also of *time* – the time involved in getting the drug to and from its site of action (Fig. 9-1).

Although the three properties – dose, time and effect – are interdependent, it is more expedient to quantitate the response to the administration of a drug by treating the dose-response relationship separately from the time-response relationship. Time may be eliminated from consideration of the dose-response relationship by determining the effect produced by given doses only after the observed effect has attained its maximum level. Dose is eliminated as a variable in the time-response relationship by studying the appearance and disappearance

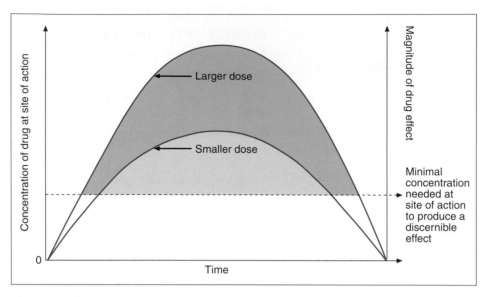

Figure 9-1. *Theoretical curves summarizing the interrelationships of dose, time and magnitude of drug effect. Two different doses of the same drug are given at time 0. Absorption and distribution account for increase in concentration and in magnitude of effect. Elimination – i.e. redistribution, biotransformation and excretion – accounts for decrease in concentration and in magnitude of effect. These idealized curves are seen only under special conditions of drug administration. The elimination curves usually obtained are hyperbolic with concavity upward. The resultant curve of the actual amount reaching the site of action is also nonsymmetric but is modified by many factors discussed in Chapters 11 and 12.*

of effects following the administration of a *single* dose. In this chapter we shall examine the magnitude of drug effect (or drug response) as a function of the dose administered. In Chapter 10, we shall turn our attention to the degree of drug effect as a function of time.

QUANTITATIVE ASPECTS OF DRUG-RECEPTOR INTERACTIONS

Application of the Law of Mass Action

As we have seen, a pharmacologic effect is considered to be the consequence of a reversible chemical, or physicochemical, reaction between a drug and a reactive entity of the living organism. The biologic reactant may be either a 'receptor' or some other component of equal functional importance; in most cases it is a receptor. The product of this reaction becomes the stimulus for the events leading to the effect, which is seen as a biochemical or physiologic change or as the disappearance or appearance of clinical symptoms:

$$\text{Drug} + \text{receptor} \rightleftharpoons \text{Drug-receptor complex} \xrightarrow{\quad\text{Stimulus}\quad} \text{Effect}$$

Enzymes, like receptors, produce their activity by combining reversibly with the substances upon which they act:

Enzyme + substrate $\rightleftharpoons$ Enzyme-substrate complex $\longrightarrow$ Products

As was previously noted, this enzyme reaction obeys the law of mass action, the degree of the chemical reaction between enzyme and substrate being proportional to the concentrations of these reacting substances present at any given time. The rate of appearance of metabolic products is then dependent on the extent and effectiveness of the combination of substrate and enzyme – on the rate of formation of the enzyme-substrate complex. Since the substrate-enzyme and drug-receptor interactions are so similar, it should also be possible to explain the quantitative aspects of the latter on the basis of the laws governing chemical equilibrium. Thus, by analogy, the occupancy of receptors by a drug should be proportional to the dose of drug and the number of free, unoccupied receptors. Or, more properly stated, the occupancy of receptors by a drug should be proportional to the *concentration* of the drug and the *concentration* of unoccupied receptors. In turn, the magnitude of a pharmacologic effect elicited by a drug should be dependent on the extent of the chemical reaction involved; i.e. it should be directly proportional to the number of receptors occupied by drug molecules.

A.J. Clark (1885–1941) is largely responsible for applying mass action principles to the concept of drug-receptor interactions and thereby providing a plausible, quantitative basis for the dose-effect phenomenon. In the simplest quantitation of the dose-effect relationship formulated by Clark, the following assumptions are made:

1. The law of mass action is applicable to a reversible reaction between one drug molecule and one receptor.
2. All receptors are identical and equally accessible to the drug.
3. The intensity of the response elicited by the drug is directly proportional to the number of receptors occupied by the drug and is a direct consequence of the drug-receptor interaction.
4. The amount of drug which combines with receptors is negligible compared to the amount of drug to which the receptors are exposed, so that the effective drug concentration does not change during the reaction.

The relationship between dose and effect may then be derived as follows. For the reaction:

$$\text{Drug} + \text{free receptor} \underset{k_2}{\overset{k_1}{\rightleftharpoons}} \text{Drug-receptor complex}$$
$$[C] \quad (100 - Y) \quad\quad Y$$

where [C] = the concentration of drug (C is actually the concentration of unbound drug, but by assumption 4 it is, for all practical purposes, equal to the original concentration of drug at the site of action); and Y = the percentage of the total number of receptors occupied by drug. Thus

$$(100 - Y) = \text{Percentage of unoccupied, free receptors}$$

Then the rate of combination of drug and unoccupied receptors is proportional to the product of the drug concentration, [C], and the concentration of unoccupied receptors, $(100 - Y)$:

$k_1[C] (100 - Y)$, where k_1 is a constant of proportionality specific for the given reaction of combination

The rate of dissociation of the drug-receptor complex is proportional to Y, the percentage of receptors occupied by drug:

k_2Y, where k_2 is the specific constant for the reverse reaction

At equilibrium, when the rate of combination is equal to the rate of dissociation,

$$k_1[C] (100 - Y) = k_2Y, \text{ or}$$

$$[C] = \frac{k_2Y}{k_1(100 - Y)} \qquad \text{(Equation 1)}$$

Since the ratio of two constants is itself a constant, we can substitute K for k_2/k_1 in Equation 1, and K is then the equilibrium dissociation constant of the particular reaction

$$[C] = \frac{K\,Y}{(100 - Y)} \qquad \text{(Equation 2)}$$

This mathematical expression of the relationship between dose and effect takes on more meaning and clarity when it is represented in its graphic form. Such graphic representations of the quantitative aspect of drug action are called *dose-effect* or *dose-response curves*. Figure 9-2A illustrates a characteristic shape of the dose-effect curve obtained for a system in which increasing amounts or concentrations of drug produce progressively increasing intensities of response. In this example, the contraction, or shortening, of the longitudinal muscle of a segment of small intestine is the response to either acetylcholine or propionylcholine, a drug structurally similar to acetylcholine.

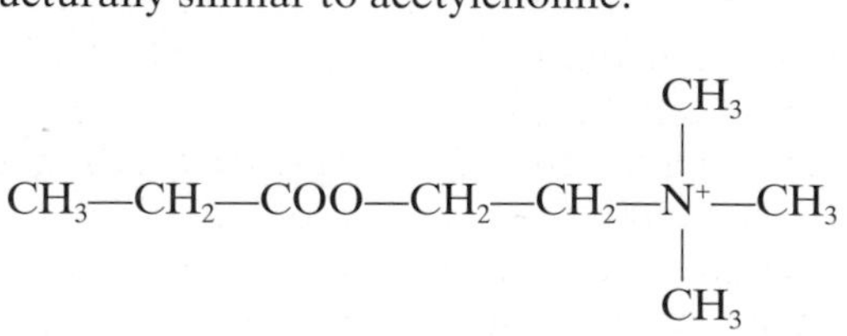

$$CH_3-CH_2-COO-CH_2-CH_2-\overset{\displaystyle CH_3}{\underset{\displaystyle CH_3}{\overset{|}{\underset{|}{N^+}}}}-CH_3$$

Propionylcholine

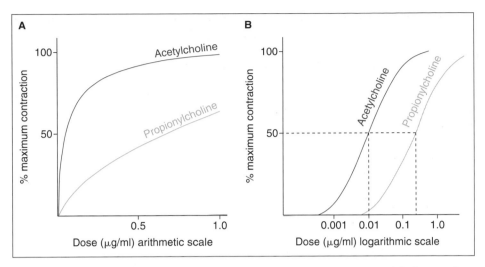

Figure 9-2. *Dose-effect curves for the action of acetylcholine and propionylcholine on the guinea pig ileum. The ordinate shows the response of the segment of small intestine as a percentage of the maximum contraction obtainable under the conditions of the experiment. The dose of the drugs is shown on the abscissa as concentration (micrograms per milliliter). In A, a linear scale is used; in B, a logarithmic scale. The horizontal* -------- *in B indicates the points at which 50% of the maximal effect is attained. The perpendiculars dropped from the intersections indicate the doses that produce the 50% maximal response. (Modified from* Gaddum's Pharmacology *[revised by A.S.V. Burgen and J.F. Mitchell]. London: Oxford University Press, 1968)*

The effect is elicited by adding solutions of the drug in varying concentrations, at different times, to the bath in which the isolated tissue is immersed (Fig. 9-3). The dose (expressed as concentration) is the independent variable and, by convention, is plotted on the horizontal scale, the abscissa; its value is not determined by any other variable and can be chosen or varied at will. The dependent variable, the effect, is plotted on the vertical scale, the ordinate. In Figure 9-2 the response to a dose of drug is expressed as the percentage of the maximum contraction which can be obtained under the conditions of the experiment.

Since the assumption has been made that the magnitude of response is a faithful indicator of the degree of receptor occupancy, the values on the ordinate are equivalent to Y of Equation 2, the percentage of total receptors occupied by drug. This assumption does not hold for many drug-receptor interactions, and more sophisticated equations describe the deviations from the simple case in which response is proportional to receptor occupancy. Only this simple case is discussed here. As the dose is increased, the pharmacologic effect (shortening of the muscle) increases in a gradual, continuous fashion. The increments in response to equal increases in dose become progressively smaller as a maximum value is approached, until further increases in dose produce no perceptibly greater effect. Obviously, the maximum response corresponds to the

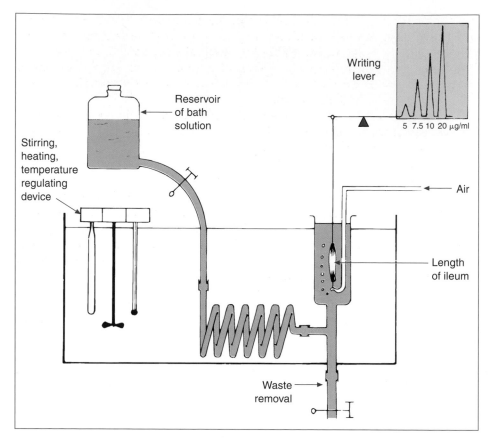

Figure 9-3. *Apparatus for recording contractions of the longitudinal muscle of a segment of small intestine (ileum) in response to drugs. Solutions containing drug may be added directly to the medium bathing the tissue and removed by flushing with several volumes of solution from the reservoir. Solution in tissue bath is aerated and usually kept at about 37°C.*

point at which receptor occupancy is approaching 100%. Thus the relationship between dose and effect describes a hyperbolic function with concavity downward. The term *graded* is applied to this type of relationship in which the *responding system is capable of showing progressively increasing effect with increasing concentration of drug.*

The Log Dose-Effect Curve

The initial portion of the curve in Figure 9-2A, particularly for acetylcholine, is so steep that it is virtually impossible to gauge the magnitude of increase in response that corresponds to small increments in dose. This huddling together of the smaller doses is inevitable when an arithmetic scale is used to display a dose range in which the largest dose is many times that of the smallest. On the other hand, when the effect is approaching maximum, large increments in dose produce changes in response which are now too small to evaluate accurately. What we need is a way of expanding the abscissal scale used to depict smaller doses that will still permit representation of a wide dose range. Both of these objectives can be achieved if the scale of doses is made logarithmic or if the doses are converted to their logarithms.

On a logarithmic scale, if each dose is double the preceding dose, the intervals between doses are equal, since the logarithmic transformation has the property of turning multiplication into addition. The curves resulting from such a transformation are illustrated in Figure 9-2B; the values of the independent variable – dose – are plotted on a logarithmic scale, whereas the values along the ordinate remain on an arithmetic scale as in Figure 9-2A. Inspection of the two methods of graphic representation makes it clear that the logarithmic scale permits presentation of not only more detailed data in the low dose range but also a wide range of doses in a single graph. Comparison of the linear and semilogarithmic dose-response curves in Figure 9-4 shows that this is advantageous even when the range of values is narrow.

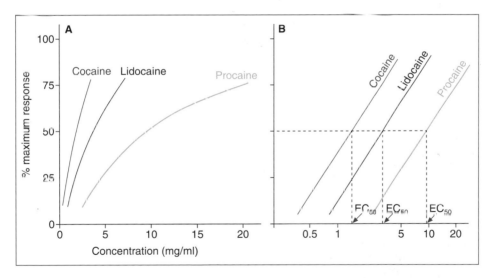

Figure 9-4. *Arithmetic and semilogarithmic dose-effect curves of three local anesthetics. Abscissa: concentration of drug – in A on arithmetic scale, in B on logarithmic scale. Ordinate: response expressed as percentage of the maximal response. Local anesthetic activity was determined in guinea pigs following intracutaneous injection of different concentrations of each local anesthetic. The degree of local anesthesia was measured by determining the number of times out of 40 that a pinprick (applied to a shaved area of the back) failed to elicit a response. The horizontal dashed line in B indicates the point of 50% maximal response. The perpendiculars dropped from intersections cut the abscissa at concentrations that produce the 50% maximal response, the EC_{50}s. The EC_{50}s are approximately equivalent to the reciprocal of the affinities of the drugs for the receptor binding site. Cocaine has the highest and procaine the lowest affinity.*

The shape of the curve obtained when the abscissal values are converted to the logarithmic scale also has certain features which are preferable to those of the hyperbola. The typical S-shaped log dose-effect curve has a center of symmetry. This midpoint represents the dose at which 50% of the maximum response is elicited (see Fig. 9-2B). Above the midpoint, the log dose-effect curve, like the hyperbola, slowly approaches a maximum value corresponding to the point at which the biologic system no longer has the capacity to respond. The lower end of the logarithmic curve also approaches zero asymptotically. (Reminder: there is no log value for zero.) But the middle segment of the curve is almost linear, a fact that is of practical importance since line segments lend themselves to mathematical analysis more readily than do curves. Figure 9-4 shows more clearly than Figure 9-2 how data points that represent the middle portion of the dose-effect curve can be fitted by straight lines when plotted logarithmically, but not when plotted arithmetically.

From our earlier considerations of drug-receptor interactions we know that a single receptor can react with a number of drugs, provided that each drug is structurally complementary to the receptor surface. Thus, drugs that possess similar chemical or physicochemical properties and that initiate the same selective pharmacologic response probably do so by acting on the same population of receptors. In a simple biologic system, such as the isolated small intestine, we would anticipate that drugs producing the same effect would also yield similar dose-effect curves if they acted by the same mechanism. Both graphic representations in Figure 9-2 show that about twenty times more propionylcholine than acetylcholine is required to produce a given contractile response. But only the semilogarithmic plot indicates that the dose-effect curves for the two drugs are almost identical in shape and approach the same maximal level of response. This evidence strongly supports the conclusion that both drugs act at the same receptor. Furthermore, drugs that produce the same effect by the same mechanism generally yield log dose-effect curves whose nearly linear middle segments parallel each other (see Fig. 9-4). The converse is also true, as a rule: two drugs that have nonparallel log dose-effect curves but which elicit qualitatively similar responses act by different mechanisms. Thus, aside from practical reasons, semilogarithmic dose-response curves are convenient devices for comparing the mechanisms by which two or more drugs produce the same end effect. And in pharmacology it is customary to use semilogarithmic dose-effect curves to evaluate the quantitative aspects of the action of a single drug or to compare the actions of several drugs.

Why do equal quantities of acetylcholine and propionylcholine produce different degrees of contraction of the isolated small intestine when both drugs act by the same mechanism and have identically shaped log dose-effect curves? And why does it require less lidocaine (XYLOCAINE) than procaine (NOVOCAIN), and even a smaller concentration of cocaine, to produce the same extent of local anesthesia when all three agents act at the same receptor site? These questions are readily answered by analyzing the equation for the interaction of a drug with its receptor. In deriving Equation 2, the assumption was made that the magnitude of response elicited by a drug is directly proportional to the number of receptors occupied by the drug. When effects of equal intensity are produced by several drugs acting at the same receptor, then Y – the percentage of the total number of receptors occupied – must be the same for each drug. It follows that the only way *unequal* concentrations of different drugs can produce effects of *equal* magnitude is for the constant, K, to have different values for each drug interacting with the receptor. This constant, which we said is the equilibrium dissociation constant for a given reaction, is then also a measure of the **affinity** of a drug for a particular receptor. The affinity indicates the strength of the interaction of a drug and receptor. The greater the affinity of a drug, the greater its propensity to bind with a given receptor and the smaller the value of the equilibrium dissociation constant, K. And further inspection of Equation 2 indicates that the smaller the value of K, the lower the concentration needed to produce the same intensity of response. Thus, when several drugs acting at the same receptor and yielding similarly shaped log dose-effect curves are compared, the position of their curves along the abscissa is indicative of their relative affinities. The curve for the drug with the greatest affinity (acting at the lowest concentration) will lie closest to the ordinate. Curves for drugs with lesser affinities for the receptor will lie farther to the right (see Fig. 9-4).

A numerical expression of the affinity of a drug is also easily obtained from its log dose-response curve. When the fraction $Y/(100 - Y)$ is equal to 1, then K is equal to the drug concentration and has the dimensions of concentration. Thus, since

$$[C] = \frac{K\,Y}{(100 - Y)}$$

when $Y/(100 - Y) = 1$, then $[C] = K$.

The fraction $Y/(100 - Y)$ is equal to 1 when Y = 50%, i.e. when one-half of the receptors are combined with drug, or one-half of the maximal effect is attained. The concentration of drug that produces 50% maximum effect is referred to as the EC_{50}. This value is estimated by drawing a horizontal from the point of 50% maximal response to intersect the dose-effect curve and then dropping a perpendicular from this intersection to cut the abscissa at the EC_{50} concentration. In the simplest model of drug-receptor interaction described above the EC_{50} is equal to the equilibrium dissociation constant, K. The reciprocal, 1/K, is a measure of the affinity of the drug for the receptor. Figure 9-4 shows that the affinity of cocaine is about twice that of lidocaine and about seven times greater than that of procaine.

Of course, statements about the affinity of a drug or the comparative affinities of several drugs have relevance only for a particular reaction with a given receptor. A single drug may have different affinities for different receptors, and the relative affinities among drugs may change from receptor to receptor. Moreover, the calculated values of the affinity of a drug for its receptor must be considered only as an approximation unless the receptor is an identified or isolated entity. When a drug produces its response by interacting with a known enzyme or other macromolecule, the concentration of all the reactants can be measured, i.e. the concentration of drug and macromolecule as well as that of the drug-macromolecule complex. And then the *observed response can be determined directly by the concentration of the drug-macromolecule complex.* Obviously, however, the majority of receptors do not exist as isolated entities but as integral components of living systems that are infinitely more complex than the simple systems for which the chemical laws were formulated. Even under these conditions, however, there are several methods for measuring the equilibrium dissociation constant of a drug and receptor, and by convention a subscript is appended to the K value, e.g., K_d, to indicate the method of determination.

Whereas the concentration of a drug applied to a system and the consequent biologic response can both be measured very accurately, the concentration of the complex formed between drug and a postulated receptor can only be approximated by currently available methods. We already know that drugs have to traverse various biologic barriers to reach their site of action and that they may combine with nonreceptor macromolecular tissue components as well as with receptors. Even in the relatively uncomplicated isolated tissue or organ preparation, there are many obstacles interposed between the drug and its site of action that may influence the quantity of drug actually entering into the combination leading to a response. Thus the quantity of drug that has produced the response can be analyzed only indirectly from the effect produced by the combination. But even though the affinity between drug and receptor cannot be accurately estimated when the receptor has not been isolated, there is no doubt that drug-macromolecule combinations obeying mass law kinetics are involved in a drug action. Thus the mass action interpretation of dose-effect curves is conceptually applicable and valid. Ligand binding studies of receptors that have been isolated have lent support to these principles.

Potency

Even though the log dose-effect curve yields only an approximation of the affinity of a drug, it nevertheless provides an accurate measure of another characteristic of a drug – its potency. Potency is determined simply by the dose needed to produce a particular effect of given intensity; like affinity, potency varies inversely with the magnitude of the dose required to produce the effect. As we have seen, the intensity of drug effect is determined by the inherent ability of a drug to combine with its receptor and by the concentration of drug at this site. Thus, potency embodies the conceptual aspects of drug-receptor interactions; it is influenced by the drug's affinity for its receptor and by factors regulating how much drug reaches the receptor, i.e. absorption, distribution, biotransformation and excretion.

Potency, unlike affinity, is a comparative rather than an absolute expression of drug activity; potency connotes the dose required to produce a particular effect *relative to a given or implied standard of reference.* For example, just knowing that 10 mg of morphine administered subcutaneously produces relief from the pain induced by a calibrated painful stimulus tells us little, by itself, about morphine's potency. It only tells us in absolute units the *dose* required to produce a given intensity of response. We find, however, that 1.5 mg of hydromorphone (DILAUDID) or 120 mg of codeine, administered by the same route, is as effective as 10 mg of morphine in relieving the pain induced by the same stimulus. We also find that the shapes of the log dose-effect curves for the three drugs are similar and reach the same maximum (Fig. 9-5). Now we can say that morphine is about seven times less potent than hydromorphone, but about twelve times more potent than codeine.

The position of the log dose-effect curves on the dose axis reflects these relative potencies. A great deal is known about the receptors for narcotic analgesics – for the opioids – and, although we now have a better understanding of how they produce their analgesic effects, no definitive explanation can be furnished for the observed differences in potencies. It is obvious, however, that differences in potencies between drugs can occur only as a result of differences in the

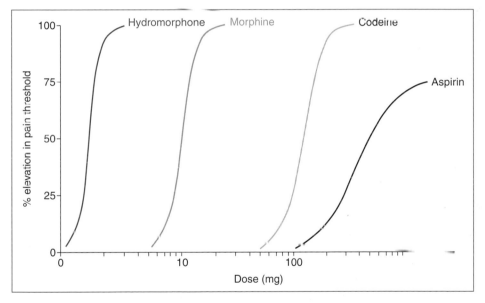

Figure 9-5. *Log dose-effect curves, typical of those that can be obtained in healthy human males, for the analgesic action of three opioid drugs – hydromorphone, morphine and codeine – and one non-opioid drug, aspirin. The ordinate shows the analgesic effect as the percentage of elevation of the pain threshold, i.e. the increase in magnitude of the painful stimulus required to elicit pain after drug administration as a percentage of the magnitude of the stimulus required to elicit the same degree of pain before drug administration. The position of the curves indicates that hydromorphone is more potent than morphine and the latter more potent than codeine, regardless of the response level at which they are compared. The different shape and maximum height of the curve for aspirin do not permit comparison with the opioid analgesics in terms of potency. More aspirin than opioid analgesics is required to produce the same degree of response; aspirin is incapable of producing more than a certain degree of analgesia, even at high doses.*

relative affinities of the drugs for the same group of receptors or differences in the proportion of a dose ultimately reaching the receptor site(s), or both factors.

It is inappropriate to express the relative activities of two drugs in terms of potency unless they both produce their effects by the same mechanism and can exert the same maximum effect. In many instances, for example, pain of low or moderate intensity, such as toothache, is as effectively relieved by aspirin as by codeine. However, it takes about five to ten times more aspirin than codeine to achieve the same effect. On the other hand, codeine is frequently useful in obtunding severe pain, whereas aspirin, even at the highest tolerated doses, is not (Fig. 9-5). Aspirin and codeine act at different sites and produce their analgesic effects by different mechanisms. Although codeine is often said to be more potent than aspirin, it would be better to state that codeine and aspirin are therapeutically equivalent in some applications but that codeine has the potential for exerting a greater maximum effect.

It is important to point out that the potency of a drug is in no way related to its value, efficacy or safety. The least potent drug among agents with similar actions may be no less effective than the most potent one as long as each agent is employed in its appropriate dosage. Low potency becomes a disadvantage only when the size of the effective dose makes it difficult or awkward to administer. From the therapeutic point of view, it matters little whether the dose is 1 mg or 1 g. The only real concern is that the dose, whatever its magnitude, be both effective and safe.

Drug Antagonism

A drug whose interaction with a receptor becomes the stimulus for a biologic response is known as an *agonist*. Drugs which act on the same receptor may differ, not only in their affinity but also in their maximum effect, or efficacy. A full agonist refers to a drug with the greatest maximum effect when compared to others in the same class. A partial agonist demonstrates significantly lower maximum effect. Furthermore, some drugs may have affinity but no efficacy. Drugs that interact with a receptor but do not trigger the sequence of events leading to an effect are known as *antagonists*. Antagonists act only to interfere with or prevent the formation of an agonist-receptor complex. Drug antagonism at the receptor level is analogous to enzyme inhibition and, like the latter, is readily analyzed within the framework of mass action kinetics.

Just as with enzyme inhibitors, antagonists can be classified as *competitive* or *noncompetitive* (cf. pp. 175–176). An antagonist is competitive when it combines reversibly with the same binding sites as the active drug and can be displaced from these sites by an excess of the agonist. Conversely, an antagonist is noncompetitive when its effects cannot be overcome by increasing concentrations of the agonist. The noncompetitive antagonist does not change the binding of the agonist but reduces its efficacy. Noncompetitive antagonists are generally presumed to bind to the receptor at a different site from the agonist. Even though noncompetitive antagonists cannot be influenced by increasing concentrations of the agonist, the effect of the antagonist may be reversible; in reversible, non-competitive antagonism, the removal of the antagonist restores the system to full activity. In irreversible, noncompetitive antagonism, the receptor is permanently altered and has to be resynthesized.

The quantitative aspects of drug antagonism are readily analyzed from log dose-effect curves. First let us consider the contractile response of the isolated guinea pig ileum to acetylcholine in the absence and presence of a competitive antagonist, atropine. In Figure 9-6, the curve at the left is for acetylcholine alone and that at the right for acetylcholine when a constant amount of atropine is present in the medium bathing the isolated tissue. The two curves are identical in shape and attain the same maximum. But when atropine is present, it is as if acetylcholine had become a less potent drug, since much more is required to produce responses equal in magnitude to those elicited before the addition of the antagonist. Atropine has affinity for the acetylcholine receptor and is able to combine with it. But the atropine-receptor combination by itself produces no biologic response; atropine merely decreases the number of receptors available for occupancy by acetylcholine. Hence the response to a particular dose of acetylcholine is reduced. As the dose of acetylcholine is increased, the agonist

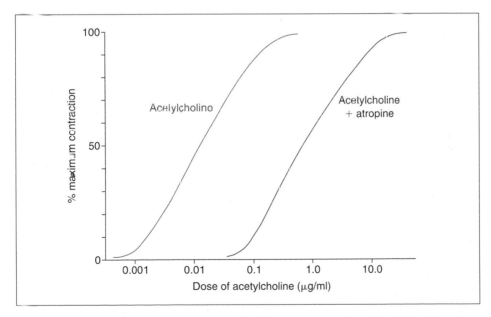

Figure 9-6. *Log dose-effect curves depicting competitive antagonism. The effect of acetylcholine on the guinea pig ileum is shown in the absence and presence of the competitive antagonist atropine (see Figs 9-2 and 9-3). The ordinate shows the response as percentage of the maximum contraction obtainable under the conditions of the experiment. The abscissa shows the dose of acetylcholine as concentration. The curve on the left is for acetylcholine alone; that on the right, for acetylcholine in the presence of a constant concentration of atropine (0.0002 µg/ml).*

displaces atropine from the receptor until, at a sufficiently large dose, all receptors are occupied by acetylcholine and a maximal contractile response is obtained. Thus the log dose-effect curve for an agonist in the presence of a competitive antagonist will be shifted to the right, indicating a reduction in the effective affinity of the agonist for its receptor; the shape of the curve and the maximal response, however, are not altered by the competitive antagonist.

Competitive antagonism can also be demonstrated in the intact animal. In the experiments illustrated in Figure 9-7, the response to the agonist – intravenously administered histamine – was measured as a prompt but transient fall in blood pressure. Administration of the antagonist diphenhydramine (BENADRYL) produced no change in blood pressure. When diphenhydramine was administered prior to the injection of histamine, the dose-effect curves for histamine were shifted farther and farther to the right as the dose of the

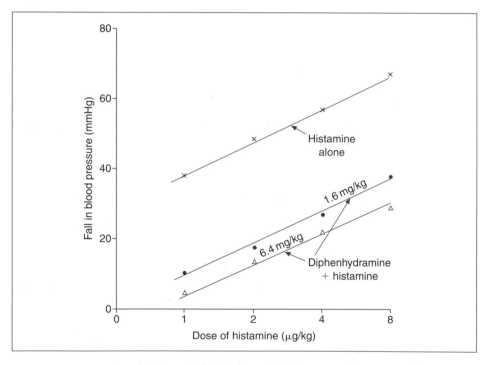

Figure 9-7. *Log dose-effect curves depicting competitive antagonism in the intact animal. Abscissa: Dose of histamine (µg/kg) administered intravenously to an anesthetized dog. Ordinate: Fall in blood pressure (mmHg) determined by difference in measurements just before and immediately after injections of histamine. The effect of increasing doses of histamine (×) was first determined. The antagonist diphenhydramine was then given, followed by the same series of challenging doses of histamine. Two doses of diphenhydramine (1.6 [●] and 6.4 [△] mg/kg of body weight, respectively) were used. (Data from G. Chen and D. Russell,* J. Pharmacol. Exp. Ther. *99:401, 1950. Copyright © 1950, American Society for Pharmacology & Experimental Therapeutics.)*

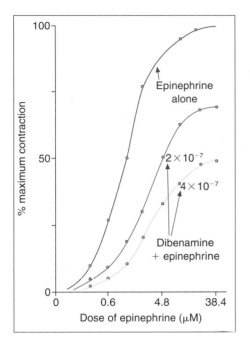

Figure 9-8. *Log dose-effect curves depicting noncompetitive antagonism. The effect of epinephrine on the isolated cat spleen preparation is shown in the absence and presence of the noncompetitive antagonist dibenamine. The ordinate shows the response as percentage of the maximum contraction obtainable under the conditions of the experiment. The abscissa shows the dose of epinephrine as micromolar concentrations. The curve on the left is for epinephrine alone, and the middle and right-hand curves are for epinephrine in the presence of 2 and 4 × 10⁻⁷ molar concentrations of dibenamine, respectively. (Modified from R.K. Bickerton, J. Pharmacol. Exp. Ther. 142:99, 1963. Copyright © 1963, American Society for Pharmacology & Experimental Therapeutics.)*

antagonist was increased. Since similarly shaped curves with the same potential maximum were obtained, diphenhydramine is a competitive antagonist of histamine — an *antihistamine* whose antagonism can be completely overcome by the administration of sufficient histamine.

We would anticipate that a noncompetitive antagonist influences the log dose-response curve very differently from a competitive antagonist. First, there is a decrease in the maximal height of the response curve. This follows from the fact that even a large excess of agonist cannot overcome the effect of the noncompetitive antagonist. The agonist-antagonist curve will be shifted to the right somewhat, since the response to a particular dose of agonist will be reduced. But the apparent affinity of the agonist is unchanged because the two agents do not interact at the same binding site. The slope of the curve is also reduced in proportion to the degree of non-competitive antagonism produced. All these characteristics of noncompetitive antagonism are illustrated in Figure 9-8 for the effect of two concentrations of the antagonist dibenamine[1] on the contraction of an isolated animal spleen in response to the agonist epinephrine.

The noncompetitive antagonism exemplified by dibenamine may be considered reversible. As dibenamine is eliminated from the body or from the biologic system, the response of the receptor to the agonist is slowly restored. The pharmacologic effect produced by an organic phosphate insecticide, such as

---

[1]Dibenamine is an experimental drug, the forerunner of adrenergic antagonists that have clinical use in the treatment of hypertension.

parathion, is an example of irreversible, noncompetitive antagonism. Parathion produces its effect by inhibiting the enzyme cholinesterase. The product formed by the interaction of the insecticide and the enzyme is so stable that the restoration of enzyme activity depends on the synthesis of new enzyme.

The type of drug antagonism we have been discussing is termed *pharmacologic antagonism* since the antagonist interferes with the mechanism by which most pharmacologic effects are produced – it interferes with the formation of an agonist-receptor complex. There are, however, other ways in which one drug may decrease the observed response to another without directly interfering with receptor occupancy. We shall discuss these other types of drug antagonism in Chapter 12 together with the many ways in which the prior or concurrent administration of one drug modifies the effects of another drug.

THE QUANTAL DOSE-RESPONSE RELATIONSHIP

So far, we have examined the relationship between dose and effect only in the system of a single biologic unit capable of graded response, i.e. capable of showing a progressively increasing magnitude of effect with progressively increasing concentration of a drug. We saw that graded dose-effect curves could be obtained in a simple system, such as the isolated small intestine, as well as in the complex system of the intact animal. The response elicited – in our examples, contraction of muscle (Fig. 9-2) and lowering of blood pressure (Fig. 9-7), respectively – was measurable on a *continuous scale* – and this is the important point. For there are many pharmacologic effects which cannot be measured as graded responses on a continuous scale; instead, they either occur or do not occur. For example, if one were determining the relationship between the dose of a barbiturate and its propensity to induce sleep, the effect could be measured only as an all-or-none response – either sleep was induced by a particular dose, or the subject was still awake. Another, yet obvious, example is the determination of the relationship between dose and the ultimate toxicity of a drug; here the criterion of response is whether the experimental animal is dead or alive after a particular dose is administered. The all-or-none response is known as the quantal response.

In the graded type of dose-effect relationship, it is assumed that the response of an individual biologic unit increases measurably with increasing concentration of drug. In the quantal type, the assumption is made that the individual units of the system respond to a given criterion or not at all. To examine the graded dose-effect relationship, we obtain quantitative data of response at each of several doses administered to a single biologic system. To explore the relationship between dose and quantal response, however, we must use many subjects and obtain *enumerative* data of the *number* either responding or not responding to each given dose. The quantal dose-response curve, then, does not relate dose to an expression of intensity of effect, but rather to an expression of the *frequency* with which any dose of a drug produces an all-or-none pharmacologic effect. In toxicity tests in animals, the quantal response may be death or the appearance of a particular adverse effect, such as convulsions. In clinical trials, the quantal response may be the abrupt disappearance of a symptom, such as pain or irregular heartbeat, or the appearance of an unwanted effect, e.g. nausea or vomiting.

The Normal Distribution Curve

Let us examine a quantal dose-response curve for a group of animals when the observed response is death, as measured by cessation of respiration. We will use a large group composed of members of a single species. To ensure uniformity within the group, all members will be of the same strain, sex, age and approximate weight and will have been bred and kept in the same environmental conditions. Each animal will receive drug X in progressively larger doses (calculated on the basis of body weight) until a dose is reached that is just sufficient to cause death. Such a minimally effective dose of any drug that evokes a stated all-or-none pharmacologic response is called the *threshold* dose.

One of the first observations we would make in our experiment is that not all the animals died at the same threshold dose. In fact, even though we chose an apparently uniform group of animals, we find that it is necessary to use a wide range of doses in order to affect all the individuals. If we tally the number of animals for which any given dose is lethal and plot these numbers in order of uniformly increasing threshold doses, we obtain a bar gram, or histogram, of the distribution of frequencies of response. This is illustrated in Figure 9-9, not for our hypothetical drug X, but for ethyl alcohol administered in a carefully controlled experiment to a group of rats. Now we can clearly see that only a few animals respond at the lowest doses and another small number at the highest doses. Larger numbers of animals respond to any given threshold dose lying between these extremes. But the maximum frequency of response occurs in the middle portion of the dose range.

The larger the number of subjects studied, the greater will be the range of doses between the extremes. With an infinitely large number of animals we arrive at the smooth, symmetric, bell shaped curve known as the *normal frequency distribution* (Fig. 9-10). The curve is called *normal* because it is very common of natural distribution found almost everywhere. We could obtain normal distribution curves for data of such items as the IQs of thousands of people, or the variations in a dimension of a part which is manufactured in large quantities, or even the probability of possible outcomes on the throws of two dice. And in pharmacology the quantal curve describing the distribution of minimal doses of a drug that produce a given effect in a group of biologic subjects fits the normal curve reasonably well, whether the effect observed is therapeutic, adverse or even lethal. In other words, the drug doses required to produce a quantitatively identical response in a large number of test subjects are distributed in the normal pattern.

Since the normal distribution expresses the frequency of occurrence of random values of different magnitude, we may well ask, 'Why does the quantal

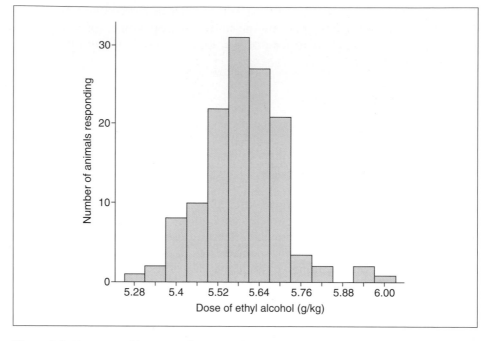

Figure 9-9. *Frequency histogram showing relationship between dose and effect. Progressively larger amounts of ethyl alcohol were injected into each of 130 rats until respiratory failure occurred. The dose (in grams per kilogram of body weight) that killed each particular animal was recorded. All animals dying following a dose increment of 0.06 g/kg of body weight were grouped together.*

dose-effect curve obtained in an apparently homogeneous group of animals so closely resemble the normal distribution curve?' The only answer is that our initial assumption of homogeneity was incorrect. Differences *do* exist among individuals, even when we minimize errors of measurement and eliminate the variables of species, strain, age, sex, weight and other factors under our control. But the nature of these differences becomes apparent only when a *group* of individuals is challenged, as by the administration of a drug. The graded dose-effect curve, constructed from data relating intensity of response to drug dosage in a single or average individual, obscures the biologic variation. The quantal curve, made up of the all-or-none responses of single individuals, readily discloses the variability that normally exists within a seemingly uniform group.

It is not surprising that there is wide variation in the quantity of a drug required to produce a given response in a group of test subjects. Rather, it is to be expected in view of the innate complexity of the biologic system and the many intercoupled processes involved in getting a drug to and from its site(s) of action. In Chapter 11 we shall discuss in some detail the more important factors known to contribute to and account for biologic variation. For the variables that may affect drug response in individuals (or even in a particular individual at dif-

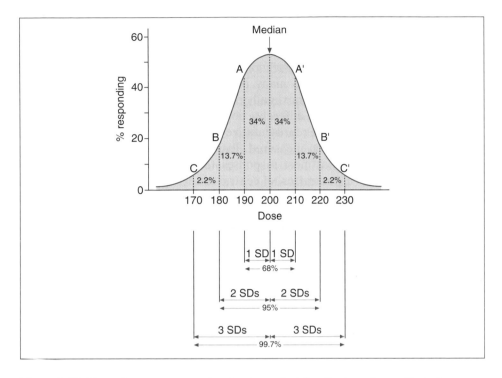

Figure 9-10. *Normal curve representing the theoretical distribution of quantitatively identical responses of individual animals following administration of drug X to a uniform population.*

ferent times) must be taken into account if drugs are to be used successfully as therapeutic agents. But even though individuals are not alike in their response to drugs and may require personalized adjustment of dosage, general guidelines for the intelligent use of any drug are still needed. The methods devised to quantitate the phenomenon of pharmacologic variation provide these guidelines and help to minimize errors of prediction.

Concepts Statistically Derived from the Quantal Dose-Effect Curve

It is never possible to examine an infinitely large group of subjects experimentally. To obtain the desired information, we must resort to studying samples taken from the population – the collection of items defined by a common characteristic. Then, with the use of appropriate statistics, we can reach general conclusions from the fragmentary data. Since the doses for quantal responses to drugs are so often distributed normally, the statistical procedures applicable to the normal curve can also be applied to the quantal dose-response curve.

The normal distribution curve (see Fig. 9-10) extends to infinity in both directions, never quite reaching zero. Theoretically, this means that a few individuals

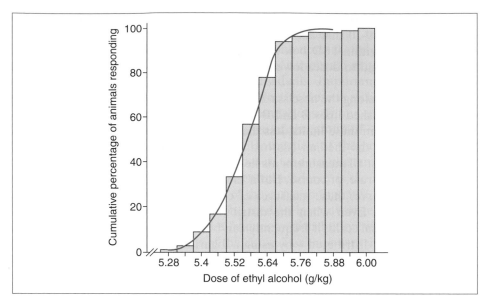

Figure 9-11. *Quantal dose-response curve (summation of the frequency histogram, Fig. 9-9). Every bar of Figure 9–9 is added to all preceding bars as dose is increased. The total number of animals responding at each dose and to those below is converted to the percentage of total animals (130). (The curve is drawn through the midpoints of the summated bars.) For example, a total of 21 rats, or 16.2% of the total, died by the time the fourth dose was administered. At doses up to 5.52 g/kg 22 more died, giving a total of 43 rats, or 33.1% of the total number.*

those of the group for which the dose is threshold or *above* threshold; the number of animals responding in each group will increase with increasing size of dose. For example, the data in Figure 9-12 were obtained by administering phenobarbital to 11 groups of 20 mice, each group receiving a different dose. Loss of the righting reflex was taken as the indication that an animal was asleep, and cessation of respiration, that an animal was dead. The number of animals responding at each dose level was recorded. When the percentage of animals responding was plotted against the corresponding dose level, S-shaped curves were obtained just like those for the distribution of the threshold doses of individual animals in the groups. The reason for this, of course, is that in both methods, any dose along the curve gives the percentage of animals responding to that dose and to all lower doses.

The statistical methods applicable to the quantal dose-effect curve can also be applied to the graded type of response if the measured response is made all-or-none. To do this, an arbitrary intensity of effect is selected and the response is called positive whenever the threshold or level is either reached or exceeded. For example, a 40–50% reduction in heart rate might be used as the criterion of therapeutic response to a drug which slows the heartbeat (Fig. 9-13). In the same manner, any effect of a drug may be treated as a quantal response.

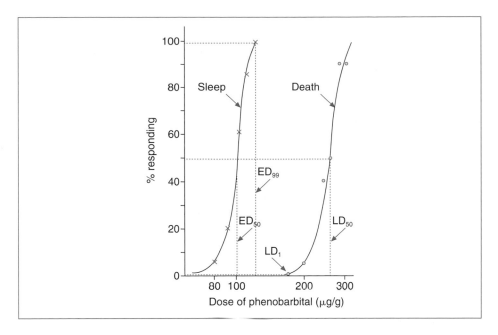

Figure 9-12. *Quantal dose-response curves representing the cumulative number of animals responding as the dose is increased. Groups of 20 mice were injected with different doses of phenobarbital. The following results were obtained:*

% Animals asleep	Dose (µg/g)	% Animals dead	Dose (µg/g)
5	80	5	200
20	90	15	220
60	103	40	240
85	110	50	260
100	120	90	280
		90	300

Evaluation of Drug Safety

The data in Figure 9-12 are for a single agent administered in various doses to groups of animals of the same species. As dose was increased, two separate curves were obtained, one for the hypnotic effect of the barbiturate and one for its lethal effect. These curves illustrate an important principle of pharmacology: there is no *single* dose-response relationship that can adequately characterize a drug in terms of its full spectrum of activity. The ideal drug would produce its desired effect – its therapeutically useful effect – in all biologic systems without inducing any side-effect, i.e. an effect other than that for which the drug is administered. But there is no ideal drug. Most drugs produce many effects, and

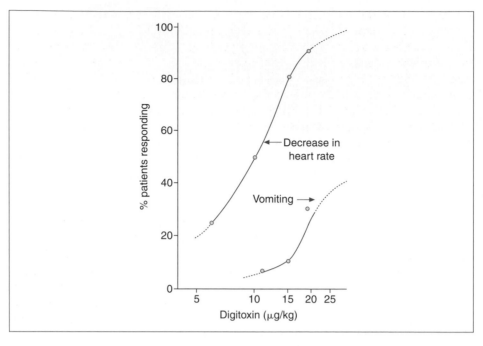

Figure 9-13. *Quantal dose-response curve of a graded response. Ten patients with cardiac irregularities were given single oral doses of digitoxin at intervals of 1 week. The desired response was made quantal by determining the dose that produced a 40–50% decrease in heart rate. The undesired effects were nausea and vomiting. The curve at the left shows the per cent of patients responding with the desired effect, and that at the right, with the undesired effect (dashed curves indicate theoretical responses to doses above and below those actually used). The overlap of the curves is so great that even at ED_{50} a few patients would be expected to show an adverse effect. For individual patients this type of relationship may be even more critical. For example, one patient required 15 µg/kg of body weight for the desired effect and vomited at a dose of 18 µg/kg, an increase in dose of only 20%. (Redrawn from D.F. Marsh,* Outline of Fundamental Pharmacology, *1951. Courtesy of Charles C Thomas, Publisher, Springfield, Illinois.)*

all drugs produce at least two effects. And it is also a truism that no chemical agent can be considered entirely safe. For every drug, there is some dose that will produce a *toxic effect* – one deleterious to the subject or even life-threatening.

Given the fact that any chemical can be expected to produce toxic effects, the risks entailed in its use must be weighed against its effectiveness before it can be considered a salutary agent. In Chapter 13 we will discuss the specific ways in which the use of drugs may be harmful. At this point, we shall consider only the general principles involved in the quantitative evaluation of drug safety.

The safety of a drug depends on the degree of separation between the doses producing a desirable effect and the doses at which adverse effects are elicited. Since both the therapeutic and undesirable effects of a drug can be characterized by quantal dose-response curves, we can use these curves to obtain a statement of the **margin of safety** of the drug. For example, we can calculate the median lethal dose and the median therapeutic dose and express these as a fraction. Such an expression is known as a *therapeutic index*. The LD_{50}/ED_{50} for the data in Figure 9-12 is about 2.6. This ratio tells us that about two and one-half times as much barbiturate is required to produce a lethal effect in 50% of the animals as is needed to induce sleep in the same proportion of animals.

The aim of drug therapy, however, is *to achieve the desired therapeutic effect in all individuals without the risk of producing a hazardous effect in any*. Obviously, a measure of drug safety based on the doses at the lowest toxic and highest therapeutic levels of response, such as LD_1/ED_{99}, is more realistic and more consistent with this aim than is the ratio LD_{50}/ED_{50}. Even the term applied to the therapeutic ratio LD_1/ED_{99} connotes this idea of relative safety; it is called the *certain safety factor* (CSF). The CSF for phenobarbital is about 1.34 (see Fig. 9-12). A CSF greater than 1.0 indicates that the dose effective in 99% of the population is less than that which would be lethal in 1% of the population. A CSF less than unity is indicative of overlap between the maximally effective and minimally toxic doses.

An alternative expression of drug safety, *the standard safety margin*, is also calculated from the extremes of the quantal dose-response curves. The standard safety margin has the dimension of per cent; it is the percentage by which the ED_{99} has to be increased before the LD_1 is reached:

$$\text{Standard safety margin} = \frac{LD_1 - ED_{99}}{ED_{99}} \times 100$$

Thus the dose of phenobarbital, which is predicted to be effective in all but 1% of individuals needs to be increased by 34% before the drug would be lethal to 1% of the population.

We saw earlier that the values at the ends of the dose-effect curve depend on the size of the population being measured. These values are less precise than the median dose, which is derived independently of the number of observations and is unaffected by the extremes. However, the advantages of using measures of drug safety based on the LD_1/ED_{99} far outweigh the imprecision of this ratio. This can be more fully appreciated when we examine how the interpretation of therapeutic indices is affected by the slopes of the dose-response curves.

Let us consider the case in which the curves for desirable and undesirable effects parallel each other, as illustrated in Figure 9-14 for phenobarbital (Ph) and drug A. Theoretically, this would be the relationship whenever the lethal or toxic effects are a continuation, or the result of a continuation of the therapeutic effect. If the therapeutic ratio LD_{50}/ED_{50} were the criterion of drug safety, drug A and phenobarbital would be judged equally safe since the ratio is numerically the same for both drugs. An entirely different evaluation of relative safety is reached, however, if we compare these agents on the basis of their respective CSFs. The slopes of the curves for phenobarbital are sufficiently steep that there is a separation between the maximally effective dose and the minimally toxic

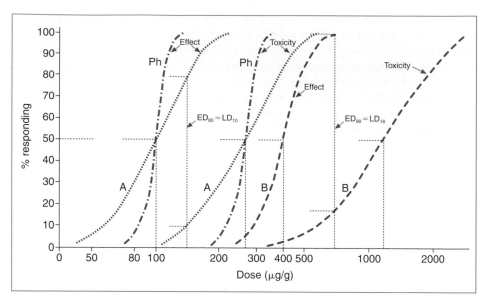

Figure 9-14. *Quantal dose-response curves for effect and toxicity of phenobarbital (Ph), drug A and drug B. The ordinate represents the per cent of animals responding and the abscissa shows dose (μg/g of body weight) on a logarithmic scale. Groups of 20 mice were injected with different doses of each of the three drugs. The responses observed were loss of righting reflex (effect) and cessation of respiration (toxicity). The LD_{50}/ED_{50} of phenobarbital and drug A is 2.6; the LD_{50}/ED_{50} of drug B is 3.0.*

dose. This margin of safety of phenobarbital is denoted by a CSF greater than 1.0. The slopes of the dose-response curves for drug A are much flatter than those for the barbiturate. As a consequence, the efficacy of drug A overlaps its toxicity. For example, the dose of drug A effective in 99% of the population corresponds to the dose at which toxicity may be anticipated in 30% of the individuals. Even at a dose effective in 80% of the population, 10% may show toxicity. When the CSF for drug A is calculated, it is found to be far less than unity, and its standard safety margin has a negative value. Thus, when the safety of drug A is measured by methods utilizing the extremes of the dose-response curves, drug A is shown to be not at all safe.

Death or toxicity may result from any of several mechanisms unrelated to that producing the desired effect. In this event the dose-response curves usually do not parallel each other, and the ratio between efficacy and toxicity is different at different levels of responses. The curves for drug B in Figure 9-14 illustrate the situation when the slope of the toxicity curve is flatter than that for the therapeutic effect. Again, whereas the ratio derived from the median doses is rather large, this index is misleading and gives a false assessment of the relative safety of the drug. Thus, for considerations of drug safety it is not enough to know only how the median doses are related. What must be known as well is how the *slopes* of the curves are related, and this is reflected by the ratio

LD_1/ED_{99}. Whether or not the curve for toxicity parallels that for efficacy, the flatter the curves, the greater the likelihood of undesirable effects occurring within the therapeutic range of doses, and the smaller the value of the CSF.

It was previously pointed out that whereas all drugs are capable of eliciting at least two responses, most drugs can and do produce many more effects. Since almost all drug effects are dose-dependent, the methods used to relate mortality and efficacy can also be employed in assessing the relationship between the desired effect and any other effect. Thus a drug may have as many therapeutic indices as it has side-effects.

Some side-effects, such as nausea or dizziness, may be merely unpleasant and uncomfortable. Even when the dose-response curves for such nontoxic effects fall well within the range of therapeutic doses, this does not ordinarily become a deterrent to the use of the drug. For example, the use of digitoxin or other digitalis preparations is frequently associated with nausea and vomiting, as would be anticipated from the large overlap in the curves for desired and undesired effects (see Fig. 9-13). The appearance of these unpleasant effects is taken as the criterion of the beginning of toxicity when digitalis dosage is being adjusted for a particular patient. However, the therapeutic value of digitalis justifies its continued use in congestive heart failure. But there are other side-effects of drugs which, though not necessarily lethal, may nevertheless seriously impair normal function. The gastrointestinal bleeding frequently associated with the use of aspirin or ibuprofen in the treatment of arthritis and the hearing deficit occasionally induced by the antibiotic streptomycin are cases in point. Whether a drug with unavoidable toxic effects is safe enough to be used under any condition depends on the availability of safer drugs and the prognosis were the drug to be withheld. Judgments of therapeutic usefulness can be made only when the severity of the illness and the potential benefit of the drug are weighed against the risks of serious toxicity. For example, most anticancer drugs are highly toxic since they affect rapidly growing normal cells as well as cancer cells; but the nature of the disease frequently warrants drug treatment despite the many adverse effects the drug may cause.

THE SPECIFICITY AND SELECTIVITY OF DRUG ACTION

In our discussions of drug-receptor interactions we indicated that the majority of drugs show a remarkable degree of selectivity. They act at some sites to produce their characteristic effect, whereas their presence at other cells, tissues or organs does not lead to any measurable response. How can this be reconciled with the statement that most drugs produce many effects? The fact that a drug may produce a multiplicity of effects does not contradict the earlier statement about selectivity. Nor does this fact challenge the receptor concept of the specificity of drug action, i.e. that interactions occur only when the chemical structure and configuration of drug and receptor are complementary. On the contrary, the dose-effect relationships help to clarify what is meant by selectivity and specificity of drug action.

First of all, let us consider how, within the framework of receptor theory, a drug can produce more than one effect and still be a special key fitting only a specific, preexisting lock. The answer is actually very simple: a specific receptor may be *located at more than one site* in the intact organism. At each site, the response triggered by the combination of the drug with the specific biologic entity is observed as an alteration in the *physiologic function of that particular anatomic region.* Let us take the acetylcholine receptor, for example. Earlier in this chapter we saw that the muscles of the isolated small intestine contract in response to acetylcholine. Atropine inhibits this contractile response by competing with acetylcholine for certain receptor sites. However, this acetylcholine receptor type, the muscarinic receptor, is widely distributed and is present in many tissues and organs in addition to the intestinal muscle (cf. Chapter 14, Drug Actions Influencing the Autonomic Nervous System). Thus, when atropine is administered orally or parenterally so that it can be distributed throughout the body, many other effects of its inhibitory activity at the acetylcholine receptor become evident. In the stomach, the effect of atropine is to decrease the hydrochloric acid secreted in response to acetylcholine. In the oral mucosa, the action of atropine leads to the production of 'dry mouth' by interfering with the flow of saliva stimulated by acetylcholine. In the eye the antagonistic effect of atropine is observed as an increase in the diameter of the pupil. Yet atropine is a very *specific* drug – it antagonizes only the actions of acetylcholine or drugs that closely resemble acetylcholine. The several effects produced by atropine are the consequence of a *single mechanism of action,* due to its affinity for the muscarinic receptor, but its lack of selectivity results from a multiplicity of sites where its antimuscarinic effects occur.

The spectrum of effects produced by the antihistaminic drug diphenhydramine contrasts sharply with that of atropine. As Figure 9-7 indicates, diphenhydramine can competitively antagonize the effects of histamine by vying with the agonist for binding sites on the receptor. Histamine receptors, like those for acetylcholine, are widely distributed, so that many effects result from the antihistaminic action of diphenhydramine, e.g. prevention of the vasodilator activity of histamine on small blood vessels or antagonism of the constrictor action of histamine on smooth muscles of the respiratory tract. The action of diphenhydramine is not limited, however, to histamine receptors. Because of structural similarities to atropine, diphenhydramine can also antagonize the actions of acetylcholine and produce many of the effects of atropine. This drug also gains access to the brain, where it interacts with histaminic and muscarinic receptors and produces a state of somnolence. Diphenhydramine is a *nonspecific* drug – not because it produces many effects, but because the effects it produces are the consequence of *more than one mechanism of action.*

We may well ask, then, why is diphenhydramine called an antihistaminic drug? The answer to this question clarifies what we mean by selectivity of drug action. A drug is usually described by its most characteristic effect or by the action thought to be responsible for the effect. From a consideration of the dose-effect relationship, the most characteristic or prominent effect is the one produced at doses *lower* than those required to elicit other responses. A drug is considered *selective* when the effect for which it is being administered can be produced in nearly all individuals at doses which produce its other effects in only a few individuals. Thus, selectivity of drug action is measured by the therapeutic indices – certain safety factor or standard safety margin. Since diphenhydramine is called an antihistaminic drug, we anticipate that the curve for its antihistaminic activity would lie to the left of curves for all its other effects. This is indeed the case. But diphenhydramine is not an especially selective drug: there is a great deal of overlap between the curve for histamine antagonism and the curves for other effects. In particular, the overlap of the curve for the desired effect and that for drowsiness is so great that this side effect would be expected to occur in a large segment of the population receiving the drug; calculation of the standard safety margin with respect to inhibition of salivation also yields a relatively large negative value.

Clinically, diphenhydramine causes somnolence in about half of those who take the drug, and about one in four persons also experiences other side effects like dry mouth. Whereas the occurrence of dry mouth would be a nuisance, the drowsiness so often encountered might be a desirable, adjunctive effect in patients about to retire for the night. If an individual had to remain alert in order to operate an automobile, however, sleepiness would be an undesirable accompaniment of therapy. Thus, because diphenhydramine is neither a specific or selective drug, newer, more selective antihistamines, e.g. loratidine (CLARITIN) and fexofenadine (ALLEGRA), have been developed that do not produce drowsiness in most people.

Although atropine is a specific drug, it too is not selective; inhibition of the action of acetylcholine at a number of different sites is produced by about the same dose of the antagonist. For example, if atropine were administered to decrease gastric acidity, dry mouth would be expected to occur almost routinely as a side effect of therapy. In contrast, the pharmacologic effects of the anticoagulant heparin are almost entirely confined to the blood and, as such, are both specific and selective. We have mentioned previously that heparin prevents the coagulation of blood by combining with macromolecules essential to this process. Its toxic effect is the result of a continuation of its therapeutic effect – too much anticoagulant activity leading to spontaneous bleeding. The limitation in the number of effects heparin may produce is related to the fact that the biologic entity with which heparin combines has a limited physiologic role and anatomic distribution.

The choice of the route of drug administration may sometimes confer selectivity of action on a drug that is ordinarily nonselective. For example, if the ophthalmologist applies atropine directly to the surface of the eye in order to dilate the pupil, the other pharmacologic effects of atropine may be largely averted. The quantity administered to achieve the local effect on the pupil is usually too small to yield a concentration, after absorption, that would be sufficient to elicit responses at sites other than the eye.

Differences in distribution of drug within the intact organism can also make one drug more selective than another acting by the same mechanism. This type of selectivity usually results from differences in an agent's ability to traverse certain biologic barriers. Drugs with structures similar to the structure of atropine (some of the quaternary ammonium compounds referred to previously) are examples of chemicals with selectivity of action through selective biologic permeability. These atropine-like compounds may decrease gastric acidity or salivary secretions or have effects similar to those of atropine on the eye and the small intestine. However, the water-soluble quaternary ammonium compounds do not traverse the so-called blood-brain barrier as readily as does lipid-soluble atropine. Consequently, when administered at sites outside the central nervous system, the quaternary ammonium compounds, unlike atropine, do not have activity within the brain. Atropine and the atropine-like quaternary ammonium compounds combine specifically with the acetylcholine receptor, but the latter drugs show fewer effects than does atropine because they cannot reach as many receptor sites.

Very few drugs are as selective as heparin. And not all drugs that produce multiple effects are as specific as atropine – more than one mechanism of action may be involved. But it is clear that selectivity and specificity are the most important characteristics of a drug in determining its therapeutic usefulness. The greater the selectivity and specificity, the less the likelihood of undesirable effects and the greater the margin of safety.

SYNOPSIS

One of the most fundamental principles of pharmacology states that the intensity of response elicited by a drug is a function of the dose administered. In one sense we can take this to mean simply that as the dose of a drug is increased, the magnitude of effect is also increased. Or we can say that as the dose of a drug is increased, the number or proportion of individuals exhibiting a particular, stated response is also increased. These two fundamental relationships between dose and response have been termed *graded* and *quantal*, respectively. The graded and quantal dose-response relationships are examined by different techniques, and each type provides different information about the quantitative aspects of drug action. Both types can be clearly and precisely defined with the use of special descriptive forms called *dose-effect* or *dose-response* curves, which are graphic representations of mathematical expressions.

The graded response is examined by administering increasing amounts of drug to a single subject, or to a specific organ or tissue. As dose is increased, the pharmacologic response increases in a continuous fashion, first in large and then in progressively smaller increments, until additional increases in dose elicit no further increase in effect.

The graphic representation of the typical relationship between graded response and dose takes the form of a hyperbola with concavity downward when effect (the dependent variable) and dose (the independent variable) are expressed in arithmetic units. When the units of measure of either the dose or the response, or both, are transformed mathematically from arithmetic units to other units, the form of the curve is also altered. In the transformation most frequently used, the dose is changed to the logarithm of the dose or, alternatively, the abscissal scale is made logarithmic. Such a transformation converts the hyperbola into an S-shaped curve with a central segment that is practically linear. The midpoint of the log dose-effect curve is identified with the dose, the ED_{50}, at which 50% of the maximum response is elicited. Drugs that produce similar effects by acting at the same receptor generally have similarly shaped log dose-effect curves with the same maximum. Their linear middle segments also are usually parallel.

The receptor concept and the reversibility of drug-receptor interaction permit us to explain the graded type of dose-effect relationship on the basis of the laws governing chemical equilibrium. In the drug-receptor reaction, the reacting substances are the drug and the unoccupied receptors and the product is the drug-receptor complex. However, in order to apply the law of mass action to the dose-response phenomenon, two important assumptions are made. First, the response to the drug is directly proportional to the percentage of the total receptors occupied by the drug, so that the latter is estimated in terms of the response observed. Second, the amount of drug combined with receptors is negligible, and thus the concentration of free drug remains essentially unchanged during the reaction. At equilibrium (the point at which the response to a given concentration of drug has attained its full level), the percentage of total occupied receptors is proportional to the product of the drug concentration times the percentage of unoccupied receptors. The drug concentration does not change during the reaction; only the proportion of free and occupied receptors changes. This means, then, that the ratio of the percentage of occupied receptors to that of unoccupied receptors is proportional to the dose of drug administered. The mathematical expression of this statement is the equation for a hyperbola. It is thus possible to explain the graded dose-response relationship in terms of the percentage of total receptors occupied; a maximum response would be equivalent to 100% occupancy of receptors (although, in reality, there are numerous exceptions to this relationship).

From the mass action interpretation of dose-effect curves, it follows that when several drugs acting at the same receptor produce effects of equal magnitude, the percentage of total receptors occupied must be the same for each drug. It does not follow, however, that equal concentrations of each drug at the receptor lead to effects of equal intensity. The intensity of effect produced is *directly* proportional to the percentage of total receptors occupied by a drug. But the percentage of the total receptors occupied by a drug is a function of drug concentration as well as of the drug's ability to combine with its receptor. The ability of a given drug to combine with a particular receptor is a constant; it is known as the *affinity* constant. Different drugs have different affinities for the same receptor site. The concentration of drug needed to produce a stated intensity of effect at a given receptor varies inversely with its affinity. Therefore, to produce effects of equal intensity requires a lower concentration of a drug with a higher affinity than of a drug with a lesser affinity. And it follows that the position of the log dose-effect curve on the abscissa reflects the affinity of a drug for its receptor; i.e. the greater the affinity, the closer the curve to the ordinate.

The positions of the dose-effect curves of several drugs along the abscissa also provide an expression of the relative potencies of the drugs – potency being the dose of a drug required to produce a standard effect. The closer the dose-effect curve to the ordinate, the smaller the dose required to produce a given effect and the more potent the drug. Only drugs that act at the same group of receptors and that are capable of eliciting the same maximal response can be compared with respect to potency. However, potency is determined only in part by a drug's affinity for the receptor; it is also influenced by absorption, distribution, biotransformation and excretion, the factors that determine how much drug will reach the receptor. The potency of a drug tells us nothing about its effectiveness or safety and is, therefore, a relatively unimportant characteristic for therapeutic purposes; it is important only for decisions about drug dosage.

Drugs are called antagonists when they interact with a receptor and produce no response of their own but impair the receptor's capacity to combine with or respond to an active drug – an agonist. An antagonist is said to be competitive when its inhibitory effects can be surmounted by excess agonist. In this type of antagonism there is parallel displacement of the log dose-effect curve to the right, indicating a reduction in the apparent affinity of the agonist for the receptor but no change in the maximum effect. An antagonist is said to be noncompetitive when it does not compete with the agonist for the same sites on the receptor or inactivates the receptor in such a way as to prevent its effective combination with an agonist. The effect of the noncompetitive antagonists cannot be prevented by excess agonist. As a consequence the log dose-effect curve of the agonist is shifted to the right with no change in the apparent affinity and a reduction in the the maximum response.

The graded dose-effect curve gives us information about the dose required to produce a specified intensity of effect in an individual. But individuals are not alike; each is the product of his inheritance and the environmental conditions to which he has been exposed from conception. Since the general principles of pharmacology are formulated for the 'average' but hypothetical person, we need some means of evaluating the 'average' dose-response relationship that will be representative of a group of individual values. We also need to know the variability about this average, so that we can get a broad picture of the relationship between dose and effect among all individuals. The quantal dose-response relationship provides this information.

The concept of averageness indicates a tendency for a group or 'sample' of items to distribute themselves equally on both sides of a dividing line. To determine this central value dividing the sample into two groups of equal numbers requires the enumeration of all the individual values of the sample and then the calculation of the point of equal division – the *median*. Thus the quantal dose-response relationship is determined by noting the *frequency* with which any dose of a drug evokes a stated, fixed (all-or-none) pharmacologic effect. The quantal curve describes the distribution of minimal (or threshold) doses that produce a predetermined effect in a population of individual organisms. The median of the quantal curve is the dose at which 50% of the population manifests the given effect and 50% does not. Hence the term *median effective dose*, ED_{50}, or median lethal dose, LD_{50}, is used to express the smallest dose required to produce the stated or lethal effect, respectively, in 50% of the population.

The quantal dose-effect curve takes on a bell shape like that of the normal distribution when the frequency of occurrence of threshold doses is plotted against the actual doses needed to elicit the stated quantal response. This means that, whereas the great majority of individual effective doses differ relatively little from the median, very marked departures from the median dose are not at all infrequent. In order to measure this variability about the average value in the most meaningful way, we use the parameter *standard deviation* (SD). We find, with very little error, that about 16% of the population responds to doses up to 1 SD below and 84% to doses 1 SD above the median. About 95% of the distribution lies less than 2 SDs away from the median, and less than 1% of the total population lies beyond 3 SDs from the median.

The quantal dose-response curve takes on an S-shape when the number of individuals responding at each dose level is integrated from the lowest to the highest doses. This cumulative curve can be more conveniently used for the analysis of data, such as in the assessment of drug safety or drug selectivity.

Every drug has at least two quantal dose-response curves, one for the desired therapeutic effect and one for a toxic effect. It is imperative, then, to assess the relative safety of a drug in terms of its potential danger relative to its potential usefulness. An approximate statement of relative safety may be obtained by comparing the LD_{50} with the ED_{50}. The larger this therapeutic index, the greater the relative safety. However, this index alone is not sufficient for a true assessment of drug safety, since median doses tell nothing about the slopes of the dose-response curves for therapeutic and toxic effects. If the slopes are flat, there may be a great deal of overlap between the curves even when the median doses are widely separated. Since the aim in therapy is to achieve a salutary response in 100% of the patients and a toxic effect in none, drug safety can be better assessed by using a ratio derived from the extremes of the respective quantal curves, such as LD_1/ED_{99}. This ratio is known as the certain safety factor (CSF). Another useful measure of safety is the standard safety margin: the percentage increase in the ED_{99} (the dose effective in 99% of the population) needed to produce a lethal or toxic effect in 1% of the population.

Few drugs are so specific that they manifest only two effects. Most drugs have many effects and thus many dose-effect curves. If all the effects produced by a single drug are due to a single mechanism of action, then the drug is still said to be specific. If the effects are due to several mechanisms of action, the drug is nonspecific. However, a drug's selectivity depends on its capacity to produce one particular effect in preference to others – to act in lower doses at one site than those required to produce effects at other sites. Thus the relationship of the curves for different effects of a single drug determines its selectivity. Selectivity can be measured by the same ratios used to assess drug safety, and these indices may express selectivity of drug action with respect to two potentially beneficial or two potentially toxic effects. Certainly, selectivity of action is one of the more important characteristics of a drug.

GUIDES FOR STUDY AND REVIEW

What factors determine how much of the quantity of drug administered reaches a site of action? How does one go about studying the relationship between the dose of drug administered and the magnitude of effect produced?

What are dose-response curves? In dose-response curves what is the independent variable? the dependent variable? By convention on which scale is each of these variables plotted? What is the typical form of the curve representing the relationship between graded response and dose when both variables are plotted on an arithmetic scale? What is the typical shape of the curve when the dose is expressed on a logarithmic scale? What are the advantages of using semilogarithmic graphic representations of dose-effect relationships?

How does the graded dose-effect relationship differ from the quantal dose-response relationship? How is each type of dose-response relationship examined? What information does the graded dose-effect relationship give us? the quantal dose-response relationship?

How can you explain the graded type of dose-effect relationship in terms of the laws governing chemical equilibrium? In the drug-receptor interaction what are the reacting substances? what is the product? What assumptions must be made about a drug-receptor interaction in order to apply the law of mass action?

How are the dose-effect curves of two drugs related to one another when the two drugs produce the same pharmacologic response by acting at the same receptor? What can you infer about the mechanisms of action of two drugs that elicit qualitatively similar pharmacologic responses but which have nonparallel log dose-effect curves?

What is the magnitude of the effect produced by a drug when it occupies 100% of its receptor? According to the mass action interpretation, when two drugs acting at the same receptor produce effects of equal magnitude, what must be true about the total receptors occupied by each drug?

When two drugs produce the same response by the same mechanism, what determines the concentration of each drug that is required to produce effects of equal intensity? What is the relationship between affinity and concentration of drug needed to produce a stated intensity of effect at a given receptor? How can apparent and relative affinities be determined from log dose-effect curves?

How is potency defined? How does potency differ from affinity? How can the relative potencies of several drugs be determined from their log dose-effect curves?

What is an antagonist? an agonist? a partial agonist? How can a competitive antagonist be distinguished from a noncompetitive antagonist? How does the log dose-effect curve of an agonist in the absence of an antagonist compare with its log dose-effect curve in the presence of a competitive antagonist? in the presence of a noncompetitive antagonist? How is the maximum response of an agonist affected by a competitive antagonist? a noncompetitive antagonist?

How do you define median? What is a median effective dose? an ED_{50}? an LD_{50}? What is a threshold dose?

What is the shape of the quantal dose-response curve when the frequency of occurrence of threshold doses is plotted against the actual dose needed to elicit the stated quantal response? when the number of individuals responding to each dose level is integrated from the lowest to the highest doses?

How do you define standard deviation? What does the standard deviation tell you about the variability of a population? What percentage of a population is included within 1 SD on either side of the median? within 2 SDs on either side of the median? 3 SDs?

What is the term given to the ratio LD_{50}/ED_{50}? What does this ratio tell you about the relative safety of a drug? Does this ratio give any indication of the relative slopes of the dose-response curves for therapeutic and toxic effects? Why is knowledge of the relative slopes of the curves for therapeutic and toxic effects important for the assessment of the safety of a drug? What expressions of drug safety are more realistic and consistent with the aim of drug therapy? How do you calculate the certain safety factor (CSF)? the standard safety margin? How are these measures useful in evaluating the relationship between therapeutic effect and any other effect of a drug?

What is meant by 'specificity' of drug action? by 'selectivity' of drug action?

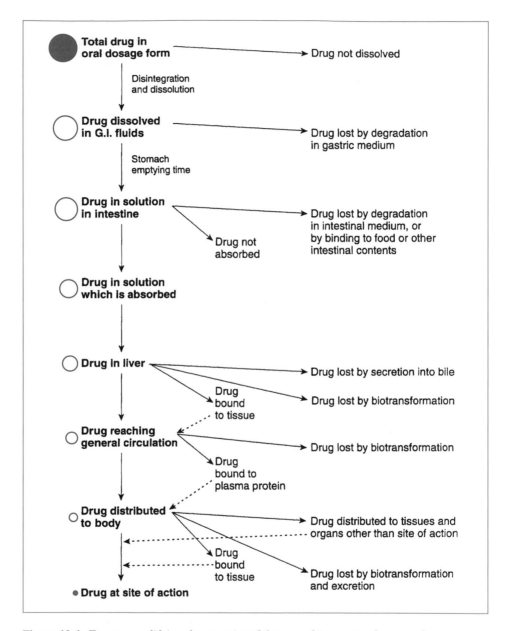

Figure 10-1. *Factors modifying the quantity of drug reaching a site of action after a single oral dose.*

measurable signs of response. Although modified indirectly by the processes of elimination, it is determined largely by the rate of accessibility of the drug to its site of action. This includes the rates of absorption, distribution and localization within the target organ or tissue. The time for onset of action may in some cases

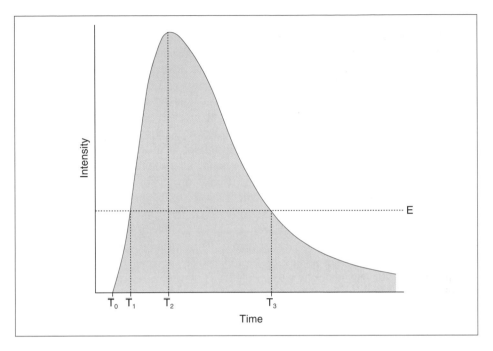

Figure 10-2. *Intensity of effect as a function of time. Drug administered at Time 0 (T_0).*
E = minimum level of measurable response; T_0 to T_1 = time for onset of drug effect; T_0 to
T_2 = time to peak effect; T_1 to T_3 = duration of action.

include the delay occasioned by the need for biotransformation of the drug from
an inactive to an active form.

The peak effect for most drugs occurs when the drug concentration at a site
of action has reached its maximum level. The time needed to reach this point is
determined by the balance between the rate processes operating to deliver the
drug to its site of action and those responsible for removing the agent from the
site and from the body.

The duration of action of a drug extends from the time of onset of an effect
to the time when the response is no longer perceptible. This phase of the temporal course of drug action is affected primarily by the rates of the elimination
processes but is also modified by continuing absorption from the site of administration. In addition, compensating physiologic reflexes set in motion by the
response to the drug itself may contribute to the termination of drug effect. (For
example, nitroglycerin used in the treatment of coronary artery disease produces a fall in blood pressure. This fall induces compensatory reflexes that
attempt to correct the disturbance and return the blood pressure to normal
levels.)

The time course of drug action is frequently studied by correlating the amplitude of effect with the concentration of drug present in the blood at various
times after administration. We have seen that the blood circulation occupies a

central position with regard to absorption, distribution and excretion. A drug is absorbed from its site of administration (or administered directly) into the blood before it is distributed to the organs and tissues; and in the process of excretion, the movement of drug occurs in the reverse direction. Generally, levels of drug are determined in plasma or serum rather than in whole blood, which also contains red blood cells, white blood cells, and platelets. The conventional use of plasma levels as the correlates of intensity of drug effect is based on the assumption that the concentration of a drug in the plasma is a valid indicator of its concentration at the site of action. This is indeed the case when the equilibrium between plasma and tissues occurs at a rapid rate. But when the movement of a drug from the plasma to its site of action is slow, the intensity and duration of effect may not be synchronous with the changes in plasma levels. For example, when an anesthetic dose of the poorly lipid-soluble drug phenobarbital is administered intravenously, 10–15 minutes elapse before any effects are seen, and anesthesia takes about 30 minutes to appear. During this latency period, the plasma level falls rapidly while the concentration of phenobarbital within the brain slowly rises (Fig. 10-3). The time course of the changes in brain concentration coincides with the onset of action, but there is a lack of correspondence between changes in plasma levels of phenobarbital and the time course of effects produced.

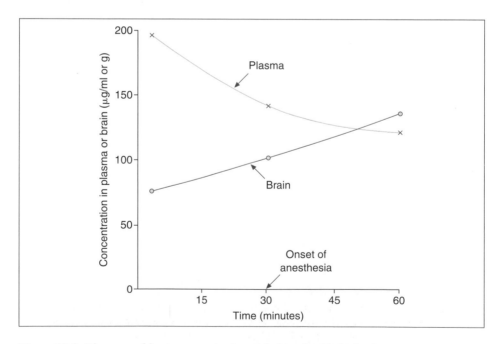

Figure 10-3. *Plasma and brain concentrations of phenobarbital after intravenous administration to animals. The dose was 100 mg/kg. Onset of anesthesia was at 30 minutes after administration. (Data from L.C. Mark et al.,* J. Pharmacol. Exp. Ther. *123:70, 1958. Copyright © 1958, American Society for Pharmacology & Experimental Therapeutics.)*

There may also be a temporal difference between the plasma concentrations of a drug and the time course of its effect when there is a delay between interaction with a target site and onset of a measurable change in the biological system. This phenomenon may be observed with drugs such as enzyme inhibitors that block synthesis of an essential protein. In this case, the onset of drug effect will not occur until the protein product is depleted by normal degradative processes. A notable example of this phenomenon is illustrated with the anticoagulant effect of warfarin. This drug acts as an inhibitor of an enzyme involved in synthesis of clotting factors. The time course of its inhibitory effect on this enzyme can be expected to mirror its plasma concentrations. But the time course of its anticoagulant effect is dependent on the levels of these clotting factors. Upon initial drug treatment these factors are depleted relatively slowly, and therefore there is a delay in onset of drug effect.

However, for many drugs the changes in concentration in plasma *do* mirror the changes in concentration at the effector site and the intensity of drug response. This relationship is illustrated in Figure 10-4 for the opioid analgesic pentazocine, a partial agonist. It is obvious that plasma levels of drugs can be conveniently measured in humans as well as in experimental animals, whereas drug concentrations at sites of action can be determined only in animals, and even then only with much difficulty. As is conventional in pharmacology, therefore, we shall use plasma level data in our considerations of the time course of drug action.

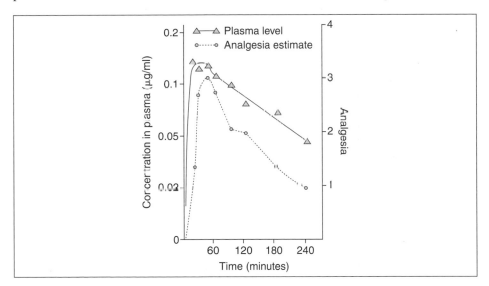

Figure 10-4. *Plasma concentrations of pentazocine and its effect on relief of pain in humans at various times after intramuscular administration of 45 mg per 70 kg of body weight. Pain evaluation or analgesia: 0 = no pain relief; 1 = some relief; 2 = moderate relief; 3 = high degree of relief; 4 = complete relief or no pain. The results represent the average of eight patients. (Redrawn from A.B. Berkowitz, J.H. Asling, S.M. Shnider and E.L. Way, Relationship of pentazocine plasma levels to pharmacologic activity in man. Clin. Pharmacol. Ther. 10:320, 1969.)*

We shall begin by examining separately (1) the rate and extent of entry of a drug into the blood circulation, i.e. its rate of absorption into the body and bioavailability, and (2) its rate of elimination from the blood and from the body. We shall then see how the kinetics of the rise and fall in plasma levels of a drug affect the duration of action of a single dose of the drug and delineate the frequency with which multiple doses may be given.

RATE OF DRUG ABSORPTION

Most drugs move across biologic barriers in accordance with the principles of passive diffusion and at a rate proportional to the concentration gradient. This means, of course, that as absorption proceeds, the total amount of drug available at the site of administration diminishes and the concentration gradient becomes progressively smaller. Since the rate of diffusion is always proportional to the gradient produced by the amount of drug still to be absorbed, the rate of absorption also decreases with time (first-order kinetics). The rate of absorption is constant and independent of the amount of drug available for absorption, i.e. exhibits zero-order kinetics, only when facilitated diffusion or active transport is involved, and then only at drug concentrations that saturate the carrier mechanism. At concentrations below saturation, the rates of the specialized transport processes and passive diffusion can be similarly characterized, i.e. *a constant fraction of the total amount of drug present is transported in equal units of time* (cf. pp. 70–72). Thus, most drug absorption follows the kinetics of a *first-order* reaction, a reaction whose velocity is proportional to the concentration of a single reactant (cf. pp. 156–157). The rate of absorption can therefore be characterized by an *absorption half-life*, the time it takes to absorb 50% of the amount of drug that is available for absorption.

The time course of absorption of phenobarbital (Fig. 10-5) is typical of drugs showing first-order absorption kinetics. These data were obtained by determining the amount of drug remaining in the intestine at various times after administration. If no biotransformation takes place at the site of administration, then the amount of drug that has disappeared from the depot directly represents the amount of drug absorbed. Such techniques of obtaining information about the isolated process of absorption are, by and large, applicable only to experimental animals. However, very good approximations of the rate of drug absorption in humans have been made indirectly by mathematical analyses of plasma levels of the drug, corrected for the portion lost through elimination.

Although constant-rate absorption (i.e. zero order) is the exception rather than the rule for most drugs, the rate of entry into blood can be made independent of the amount of drug available for absorption. Constant-rate absorption can be achieved whenever conditions of administration provide a supply or reservoir of drug to replenish the quantity removed from the site. A good example is seen in the case of the administration of gaseous anesthetics. The apparatus used by the anesthetist constantly supplies drug to be mixed with the air inhaled and, thus, replaces the quantity of drug removed during each breath

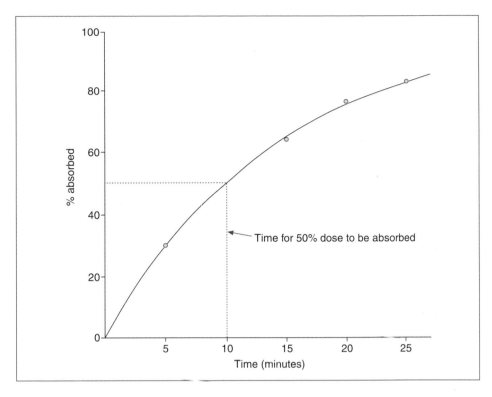

Figure 10-5. *Absorption of phenobarbital from the small intestine of the rat. Each point on the curve represents the mean absorption in four to six rats calculated from the amount of drug remaining in the intestine at the end of the particular interval.*

the patient takes. However, the more usual way of making drug absorption proceed at a rate that approaches a constant is through the preparation of special dosage forms (cf. pp. 96, 99–100). Solid pellets of hormones for subcutaneous implantation provide a remarkable example of such sustained-release preparations. As Figure 10-6 shows, about 1% of the total amount of administered testosterone is absorbed each day for at least 40 days. After this time, the absorption rate ceases to be practically constant and gradually diminishes. Now contraceptives are available for subcutaneous implantation that slowly release their progestogen content over 5 years. Other types of sustained-release medications, such as oral preparations of antihistamines (cf. p. 96) or special solutions of insulin for subcutaneous injection (cf. p. 106), are also designed to achieve a constant rate of absorption, but obviously for shorter periods. Unfortunately, these dosage forms do not always attain their objective; they do not exhibit true zero-order kinetics or maintain drug concentrations in body tissues at a constant level, since, in many cases, the release rate of drug is rapid initially and then declines continually over several hours.

In each of the examples of special dosage forms cited above, the more or less

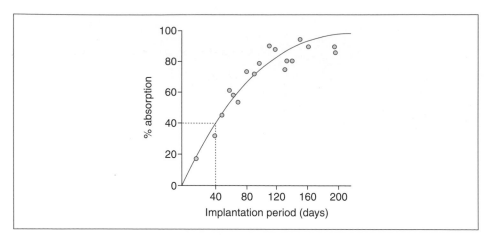

Figure 10-6. *Rate of absorption of testosterone pellets in the human. Pellets were accurately weighed and then implanted subcutaneously and allowed to remain in these depots for varying intervals. After removal, each pellet was reweighed. Each point represents the percentage absorbed from a single pellet in a single subject. (From P.M.F. Bishop and S.J. Folley,* Lancet *I:434, 1944.)*

constant rate of drug entry into blood is accomplished by making the disintegration or dissolution of drug from the dosage form the rate-limiting process for absorption. With these sustained-release preparations (cf. pp. 99–100; Fig. 5-9), the rate-limiting factor is not the chemical-physical character of the drug molecule but rather that of the drug delivery system itself. Therefore, the absorption of even highly soluble drugs can be made to follow zero-order kinetics. Controlled, continuous drug release enhances selectivity of action not only by reducing the frequency of drug administration and eliminating the 'peaks' and 'valleys' in the plasma level and effect of drug following conventional drug administration methods (Fig. 10-7) but also by minimizing the daily dose needed to maintain the desired therapeutic effect while reducing the likelihood of unwanted effects. These therapeutic systems also increase patient compliance by decreasing the number of times a patient must remember to take medication.

The extent of absorption of a drug following its administration will also affect the plasma levels and therefore the time-response relationship. As described earlier (Chapter 5), numerous factors can affect the extent of absorption, the bioavailability, of a drug given by its various routes and in various formulations. Only the intravenous route assures that the entire drug dose enters the systemic circulation. By other routes the bioavailability may be less than 100%. As we have described, for example, drugs with poor lipophilicity due to fixed charges, with high molecular weights, or with extensive first-pass biotransformation may have very low bioavailability by the oral route.

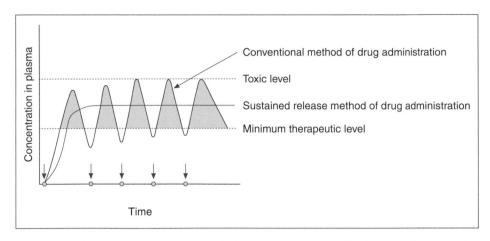

Figure 10-7. *Schematic representation of plasma concentration of a drug as a function of time after multiple doses administered by conventional method (↓) and after drug delivery by means of a sustained release therapeutic system. (Modified from J.E. Shaw, Drug delivery systems,* Annu. Rep. Med. Chem. *15:302, 1980.)*

RATE OF DRUG ELIMINATION

The rate at which a drug disappears from the body is dependent on the rate of its biotransformation and on the rates of its excretion by one or more routes. Collectively, these processes are called *elimination*. We stated previously that, for many drugs, the changes in concentration in plasma reflect the changes in the amount of drug in the body. Thus the net rate of all the processes involved in terminating the presence of a drug in the organism may be determined by following the rate of decrease of plasma levels of the agent. And when the drug is administered intravenously, the rate of decline directly represents the overall rate of drug elimination uncomplicated by the kinetics of drug absorption. The rate of elimination of a given agent determined after its intravenous administration is a property characteristic of the drug. It is a constant for a particular individual, provided that other agents or conditions do not change the rate of biotransformation or excretion.

As a general rule, elimination, like absorption, follows first-order kinetics. Most drugs disappear from the body and the plasma at a rate that is dependent upon the plasma concentration at any given moment. When the concentration is high, the rate of disappearance (amount of drug per unit time) is rapid; when the plasma level is low, the rate of elimination is slow. Ideally, the concentration of drug in the body will decline with time in the form of the typical 'decay' curve shown in Figure 10-8A for the elimination of ethanol in the dog following administration of a small dose. Since it is a constant fraction of the alcohol present in the body that is eliminated in each equal time interval, conversion of concentration to the logarithmic scale yields a straight line, as in Figure 10-8B.

When the elimination of a drug follows first-order kinetics, the rate of

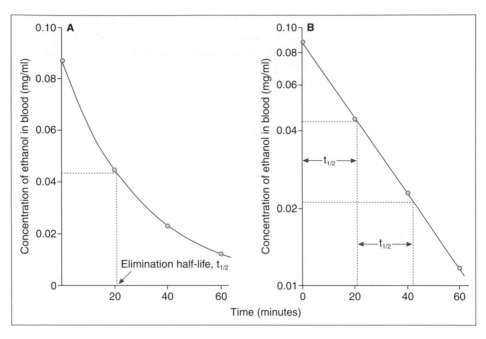

Figure 10-8. *First-order rate of elimination; decline of ethanol content in blood following intravenous administration of a small dose to a dog. The abscissa represents time after the first point. In A, the ordinate is concentration in blood (mg/ml) on an arithmetic scale; in B, on a logarithmic scale. Elimination half-life, $t_{1/2}$, is about 20 minutes. (Modified from E.K. Marshall, Jr., and W.F. Fritz, J. Pharmacol. Exp. Ther. 109:431, 1953. Copyright © 1953, American Society for Pharmacology & Experimental Therapeutics.)*

elimination can be described by a pharmacokinetic parameter called the *elimination half-life*, or half-time for elimination, $t_{1/2}$. This term describes the time required to eliminate one-half of the quantity of drug that was present in the system at the point *when the measurement was begun.* For example, the elimination half-life of a small dose of ethanol is determined by measuring the time needed for a given blood ethanol level to decline by 50%. From Figure 10-8 this is seen to be about 20 minutes, whether we use the blood level obtained immediately after administration or an intermediate one as our point of reference. The information conveyed by knowledge of the elimination half-life is useful because it permits comparison of the elimination rates of several drugs, provided that they all follow first-order kinetics. But from the practical standpoint, as we shall see below, its greatest utility is in calculating the frequency with which multiple doses of a drug can be safely administered.

   The elimination half-life of a drug is dependent on two independent parameters (see Table 10-1). One is the speed at which the drug undergoes biotransformation and excretion, or its **total plasma clearance (Cl$_T$)**. This term is analogous to the one addressed earlier with respect to the kidney, the renal plasma clearance (Chapter 5), but includes all mechanisms and routes of elimination. The total plasma clearance of a drug indicates the volume of plasma cleared by all routes and mechanisms per unit time. It represents the sum of the renal plasma clearance and clearance by biotransformation and other routes. The second parameter that governs the elimination half-life is the size of the distributional space of the drug in the body, or its **apparent volume of distribution (V$_D$)** (see Chapter 6). This value can be determined experimentally in several ways. One approach is to estimate the plasma concentration after intravenous administration when the drug has been distributed but not yet eliminated. In practice, a plasma concentration at time 0 (Cp$_0$) is estimated by extrapolation from the plasma decay curve. Then:

$$V_D = \frac{Dose}{Cp_0}$$

When the rates of biotransformation and excretion are proportional to the amount of drug remaining in the body, the overall rate of elimination will also be first order, and the total plasma clearance will be constant. We would anticipate an exception to the rule of first-order elimination, however, if either biotransformation or excretion proceeds at a constant rate, i.e. follows zero-order kinetics. The effect on the overall rate of elimination will depend on which process – biotransformation or excretion – plays the major role in elimination and which is the zero-order process. A few examples in which one of the processes involved in elimination is governed by zero-order kinetics will illustrate the general phenomenon.

Rate of Biotransformation

Since almost all drug biotransformation is mediated by enzymes, the factors determining the kinetics of biotransformation are those that determine the velocity of an enzymic reaction (cf. pp. 156–157). When the substrate concentration is low and active sites on the enzyme are available for occupancy, the rate of biotransformation will be first order. However, zero-order kinetics are obtained at substrate concentrations that are high enough to saturate the enzyme, overtax the supply of a cofactor, or deplete the levels of a conjugating moiety. As the substrate or drug concentration falls below saturation levels, the rate of reaction ceases to be constant and reverts to first order. While it is theoretically possible for *any* drug to be biotransformed at a constant rate, most drugs are administered for therapeutic purposes in amounts that lead to concentrations well below the saturation levels of their enzyme systems. Thus, zero-order biotransformation is generally not a factor in drug elimination. However, there are a number of drugs whose elimination is known to depend on a metabolic reaction that can be saturated at drug concentrations commonly reached after ordinary doses. And many drugs, when taken in overdose, may achieve concentrations in the liver that saturate enzymes of biotransformation. Similarly, if one has liver disease, there may be a reduction in the levels of biotransforming enzymes, increasing the likelihood that they will become saturated.

The fate of ethanol in humans and other animals provides a good example of how a zero-order mechanism of biotransformation affects the overall rate of drug elimination. It is of practical as well as theoretical importance, since this biotransformation process exhibits zero-order kinetics at a drug concentration produced by the ingestion of a very small quantity of alcohol – about one average-sized drink of whiskey. This 'dose' of ethanol produces blood levels considerably higher than that found in the experiment shown in Figure 10-8. In that case, a very small dose of ethanol was eliminated with first-order kinetics.

Ethanol undergoes a series of oxidative reactions yielding the end products, carbon dioxide and water:

$$C_2H_5OH \rightarrow CH_3CHO \rightarrow CH_3COOH \rightarrow CO_2 + H_2O$$

The enzyme system responsible for the conversion of alcohol to acetaldehyde – the first metabolic step mediated by alcohol dehydrogenase – is saturated at low concentrations of substrate. Hence, the rate of metabolism of ethanol in humans is very often constant, irrespective of the quantity of alcohol present in the body.

The rate of elimination of ethanol also is almost constant, since biotransformation is the primary pathway for its removal from the body. Normally less than 2% of the total alcohol administered or ingested is excreted in the urine, exhaled through the lungs or lost in perspiration. Consequently, the decline in blood levels after intravenous administration of alcohol closely follows zero-order kinetics until very low blood concentrations are reached. This is clearly evident from a comparison of the data in Figure 10-9 with those in Figure 10-8A. (Note that the data in both figures are for the same animal.) Even 20 hours after the administration of a very large dose, the blood alcohol level is seen to decrease linearly, indicating that the rate of disappearance is constant and independent of the substrate concentration (Fig. 10-9). For example, the blood level declines from 0.62 to 0.46 mg/ml between 20 and 21 hours, and in the next hour the decrease is also 0.16 mg/ml. Only when the blood level has fallen below 0.1 mg/ml does the rate become first order. In contrast, elimination starts out as a first-order process when the dose administered is small enough so that the initial blood concentration does not exceed saturation levels (Fig. 10-8).

The average human adult metabolizes about 8 g (10 ml) of pure ethanol per hour, although there is considerable variation in the rate of ethanol elimination (cf. Fig. 9-9). [Remember, the concept of metabolizing a quantity per unit time (g/hour) describes zero-order kinetics.] This quantity is equivalent to about 20–25 ml of liquor (40–50% ethanol), less than 1 ounce of whiskey or one 12-ounce bottle of beer. The slow rate of ethanol elimination and its independence of the quantity present in the body are, obviously, the cause of the well-known effects associated with repeated dosing at a rapid rate (Fig. 10-10). Alcohol is distributed throughout the total body water, which in a 70-kg person is about 40 liters. If the body contained 1 fluid ounce of whiskey, the calculated blood level of alcohol would be about 0.25 mg/ml (or 0.025%); at 2 fluid ounces the blood

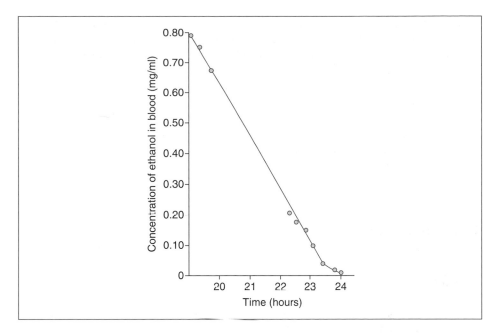

Figure 10-9. *Zero-order rate of elimination; curve illustrating decline of ethanol content in blood following intravenous administration of a large dose to the same dog as in Figure 10-8. The abscissa represents the time beginning 19 hours after administration. The plotted data show the change from zero-order to first-order kinetics when low concentrations are reached between 23 and 24 hours after administration. (From E.K. Marshall, Jr., and W.F. Fritz,* J. Pharmacol. Exp. Ther. *109:431,1953. Copyright © 1953, American Society for Pharmacology & Experimental Therapeutics.)*

would contain 0.5 mg/ml (or 0.05%)[1]. To arrive at these figures, the assumption has to be made that the entire dose was instantly available for distribution. In actuality, it would take the ingestion of more than 1 ounce to produce this level because absorption is not instantaneous, and some elimination takes place before absorption is complete. Objectively measurable effects of alcohol, such as impairment of visual acuity, have an onset at blood levels between 0.15 and 0.55 mg/ml, whereas mild intoxication is associated with blood levels of 1 mg/ml (or 0.1%), a body content of about 4 ounces of whiskey (Fig. 10-11). In the mildly intoxicated individual, the duration of effective blood concentrations would be about 3 hours, and about 5 hours would be needed to eliminate the dose taken at the outset.

Aspirin is another commonly used drug that shows unusual characteristics of elimination. Again, this is of practical importance since the effects of enzyme

---

[1]The blood alcohol percent is defined as g/ml, multiplied by 100. Concentrations of ethanol in blood are also frequently expressed in terms of mg%; mg% is defined as the number of milligrams per 100 ml.

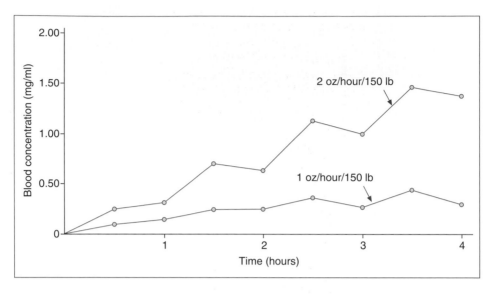

Figure 10-10. *Accumulation of ethanol in blood of human subjects following ingestion of 1 or 2 ounces of 100-proof whiskey (50% ethanol) every hour. First drink at time 0 and one drink each hour thereafter. Lower curve: dose, 1 ounce per hour; each point is the mean of samples from 25 males. Upper curve: dose, 2 ounces per hour; each point is the mean of samples from 10 males. (Redrawn from R.B. Forney and F.W. Hughes, Alcohol accumulation in humans after prolonged drinking.* Clin. Pharmacol. Ther. *4:619, 1963.)*

saturation become evident at blood levels attained with the ordinary analgesic dose of aspirin: two tablets, or 600 mg. As a consequence of zero-order kinetics, the relative rate of elimination of aspirin diminishes as the dose increases. From Figure 10-12 it can be seen that it takes longer to eliminate 50% of the quantity administered as the dose increases from 0.25 to 1.5 g. Note that in Figure 10-12 the rate of aspirin elimination is depicted in terms of the amount remaining in the body, instead of the plasma concentration of aspirin. This is in accordance with the assumption that the concentration of drug in plasma is indicative of the amount in the body, and vice versa (based on conversion using the apparent volume of distribution).

A number of processes are involved in the biotransformation of aspirin, two of which are saturable under the conditions of its clinical use. Aspirin is first hydrolyzed to salicylic acid, a rapid reaction with a half-time of 15 minutes. Salicylic acid, in turn, is conjugated partly with glucuronic acid and partly with glycine. These conjugates, together with some minor metabolites and free salicylic acid, are excreted almost exclusively in the urine (Fig. 10-13). All the processes of biotransformation and excretion are first order with the exception of the conjugation of salicylic acid with glycine to form salicyluric acid and with glucuronic acid to form the ether glucuronide (cf. p. 161). Salicyluric acid formation has been found to change from first-order to near zero-order kinetics when the amount of salicylic acid in the body exceeds the quantity derived from the

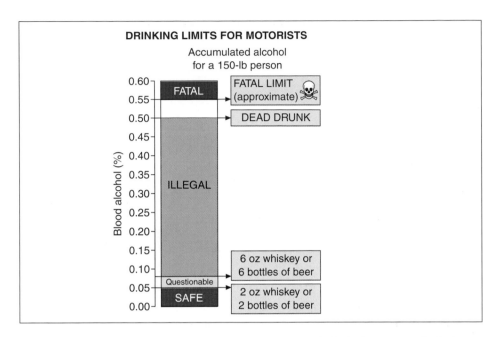

Figure 10-11. *Relationships between ingestion of various alcoholic beverages, alcohol levels in the blood and the ability of an individual to drive an automobile after consuming alcohol. (N.B. Blood alcohol % equals the number of grams of ethanol per 100 ml of blood; e.g. 0.1 alcohol % = 0.1 g per 100 ml blood, or 100 mg per 100 ml blood, or 100 mg%). (From R.N. Harger, in J.P. Economos and F.M. Kreml [eds.],* Judge and Prosecutor in Traffic Court. *Chicago: American Bar Association and the Traffic Institute, Northwestern University, 1951.) (Legal limits are different for different states in the USA, and are frequently changed. However, the legal limit, the limit at which the individual is declared to be 'operating under the influence' of alcohol, is 0.08% for many parts of the US.)*

biotransformation of less than 1 g of aspirin; the glucuronide conjugating system is saturated at somewhat higher levels of salicylic acid. When conventional dosage forms are administered and the aspirin is absorbed normally, it would take only two tablets to reach the level at which salicyluric acid formation ceases to be a first-order phenomenon.

When the salicylic acid derived from aspirin in the body is below saturation levels, the overall rate of elimination of salicylate follows first-order kinetics because all the elimination processes are first order, as shown in Figure 10-12 for the elimination of the 0.25-g dose of aspirin. The salicylate elimination half-life under first-order conditions is about 3.1 hours. At these low doses the major process responsible for salicylate elimination is its conjugation with glycine, since the first-order rate of salicyluric acid formation is much faster than the rates of glucuronide synthesis. When doses of aspirin of 1 g or more are administered, the glycine conjugation reaction becomes practically zero order and the glucuronide conjugation with the phenolic group of salicylate also approaches the limit of its capacity. As a consequence, the overall rate of elimination of the

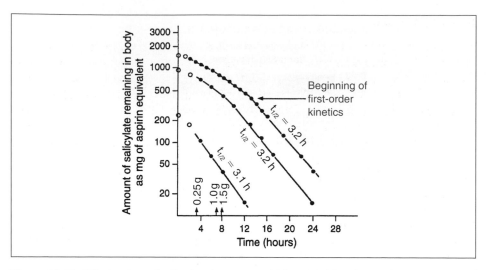

Figure 10-12. *Elimination of salicylate by a normal 22-year-old male as a function of dose. Doses taken were 0.25, 1.0 and 1.5 g aspirin, respectively. Vertical arrows on the time axis indicate the time necessary to eliminate 50% of the dose. Half-times ($t_{1/2}$) are for straight-line portion of curves where rate is first order. (Modified from G. Levy, J. Pharm. Sci. 54:959, 1965. Reproduced with permission of the copyright owner.)*

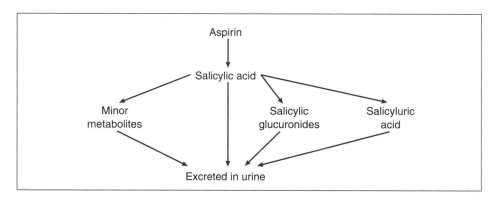

Figure 10-13. *Biotransformation of aspirin in man.*

salicylate derived from large doses of aspirin displays complex kinetics, indicative of a mixture of apparent zero-order and first-order processes. As Figure 10-12 shows, the curves for the 1.0- and 1.5-g doses of aspirin do not become linear until the salicylic acid remaining in the body drops to the quantity equivalent to about 300 mg of aspirin. This indicates a lack of conformity with first-order kinetics. Below 300 mg the curves for all three doses are linear and first order. Moreover, the time required to eliminate 50% of the salicylate in the body lengthens as the dose of aspirin increases, because less of the more rapidly formed salicyluric acid is contributing to the overall elimination process.

Rate of Excretion

The kidney plays the major role in excretion of drugs, and as has been seen, urinary excretion begins with glomerular filtration of any drug that is not bound to plasma proteins. The rate of appearance of drug in the glomerular filtrate is dependent on the rate at which the drug is presented to the kidney. This rate is always proportional to the levels of drug in plasma, since a constant fraction, one-fifth, of the volume of blood coming to the glomerulus is filtered per unit of time. Thus, glomerular filtration is a first-order rate process with respect to the free (non-protein-bound) drug. The final concentration of drug in voided urine is determined by how much of the filtrate is passively reabsorbed after filtration as the urine travels through the tubule. The rate of passive reabsorption is also first order because it is proportional to the concentration gradient established between the tubular urine and blood. Since glomerular filtration and passive reabsorption represent the mechanisms by which most drugs are excreted, it follows that the excretion of most drugs is usually first order.

Active tubular secretion is an important mechanism of urinary elimination primarily for certain organic acids and bases (cf. Chapter 7). Since the rate of active transport is limited by availability of carrier, secretion could become zero order at blood levels of drug that saturate the carrier mechanism. (The same principle applies to those drugs that are actively secreted by the liver into bile.) Although the potential exists for the establishment of zero-order kinetics for those drugs actively secreted by the tubules, their maximal secretory capacity appears rarely, if ever, to be exceeded in drug therapy. Penicillin is a case in point. The secretory capacity for penicillin in a person with normal kidneys is so high that even massive doses – greater than those ordinarily needed even in intensive therapy – do not yield blood levels that saturate the process. Indeed, this rapid elimination is one of the drawbacks of penicillin therapy. If it were possible to saturate the renal secretory process with extremely large doses of penicillin, it would perhaps be unnecessary to use special dosage forms to prolong its residence in the body.

In summary, the kinetics of urinary excretion of drugs are almost always first-order phenomenon with the rate proportional to the plasma concentration. The proportionality constant, the renal plasma clearance, is independent of the administered dose and ranges from a negligible value (for highly lipophilic agents and those with molecular weights greater than albumin or highly bound to albumin) to the value for renal plasma flow (for those cleared by glomerular filtration and tubular secretion in one pass through the kidneys).

In using plasma concentration data to evaluate the kinetics of drug elimination, the assumption is made that the rate of decline of plasma levels after intravenous injection reflects the rate at which the drug is leaving the entire body. This means that the rate of decrease in plasma levels is also a reflection of changes in the *amount of drug remaining in the body* (cf. Fig. 10-12). We have just said that the rate of urinary excretion of drug is predictably proportional to plasma levels under most conditions, i.e. the rate of urinary excretion is usually first order. Consequently, the rate of appearance of drug in the urine also represents the rate at which the amount of drug remaining in the body changes with time (Fig. 10-14). Urinary excretion data can serve, then, as another means of determining kinetics of drug elimination. All we need to know is the amount of drug *not excreted* at any time after administration. When the drug is not metabolized and is excreted only in the urine, the amount of drug remaining in the body can be calculated directly from the total dose administered and the quantity of drug excreted in the given interval. Thus:

Total dose administered − Amount excreted = Quantity of drug remaining in body

When urinary excretion represents the mechanism by which most of a drug is removed from the body, the overall rate of elimination generally follows first-order kinetics. A constant fraction of the drug still in the body will be excreted per unit time. Therefore, a straight line is obtained when the amount of drug not excreted is plotted on a logarithmic scale against time on an arithmetic scale. This is illustrated in Figure 10-14 for penicillin, whose elimination is primarily the result of urinary excretion. Under these conditions, the elimination half-life, about 25 minutes, can be read directly from the graph.

When a drug is biotransformed as well as excreted, the kinetics of its elimina-

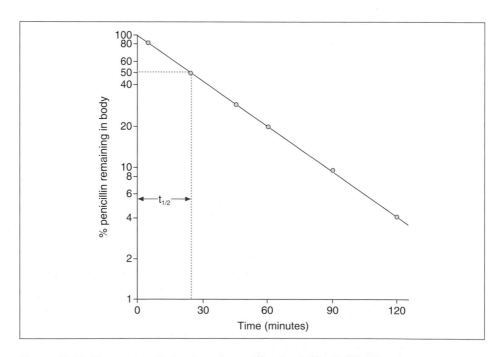

Figure 10-14. *First-order elimination of penicillin. Penicillin G (50,000 units, 30 mg) was injected intravenously in a dog at 0 time. (Modified from H. K. Beyer et al.,* Am. J. Physiol. *166:625, 1951.)*

tion can also be interpolated from urinary excretion data, provided that the products of biotransformation appear in the urine. In this situation, the amount of drug not excreted is calculated from the difference between the total urinary content of unchanged drug plus its metabolites and the quantity of drug originally administered. This is how the data of Figure 10-15 for 'amphetamine remaining to be excreted' were obtained. The total quantity of unchanged amphetamine plus its metabolites (expressed as amphetamine) was determined in the urine for each given interval. The amount of amphetamine remaining in the body was then calculated for each point of the graph by subtracting from the dose administered the cumulative sum of amphetamine plus its metabolites excreted up to that point. As Figure 10-15 indicates, the kinetics of amphetamine elimination is shown to be first order whether evaluated from blood level or urinary excretion data.

The data in Figure 10-12 for aspirin were also obtained by determining the rate of urinary excretion of its metabolites. The urinary output of unchanged salicylic acid (there is almost no unchanged aspirin excreted), salicyluric acid and the glucuronide conjugates was measured at various times after aspirin administration. The total amount of aspirin eliminated in the given interval is then equal to the quantity that has to be biotransformed to yield the sum of the

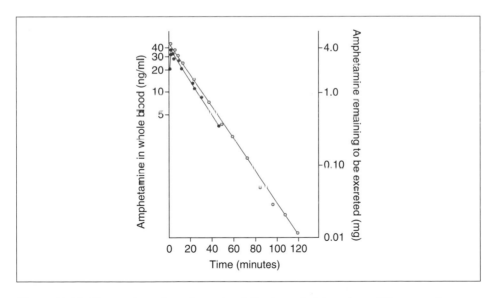

Figure 10-15. *Elimination of amphetamine following administration of 10 mg to a human subject. Total urinary content of unchanged amphetamine plus its metabolites (expressed as amphetamine) was determined for each given interval. The amount of amphetamine remaining in the body was then calculated for each point of the graph by subtracting the cumulative urinary content of amphetamine and its metabolites from the dose administered. (● = concentration in whole blood in ng/ml [1 ng = 0.001 μg]; ○ = amount of amphetamine, in milligrams, remaining to be excreted.) (From M. Rowland, J. Pharm. Sci. 58:508, 1969. Reproduced with permission of the copyright owner.)*

voided metabolites. In turn, the amount of aspirin not excreted can easily be determined from the difference. Thus the ordinate of Figure 10-12 represents the amount of aspirin remaining in the body, calculated from the total excretion of its metabolites at various times after administration. That the elimination of aspirin in doses of 1 g or more does not conform to first-order kinetics is readily ascertained from this semilogarithmic plot of amount remaining in the body versus time. Under appropriate conditions, then, the rate of excretion of a drug can be used to determine not only its overall rate of elimination but also the type of kinetics this elimination follows.

The elimination half-lives of chemical agents may vary widely when urinary excretion is the primary mechanism of elimination, e.g. about 30 minutes for penicillin to 1 week for digitoxin to more than 9 years for the metal strontium. Since the rate of passage into urine is generally proportional to the blood level, these enormous differences in half-lives of elimination can arise only from differences in the rates at which free drug is presented to the kidney and in the extent of glomerular filtration, tubular secretion and reabsorption. A major source of the differences in the elimination half-lives of drugs cleared primarily by the kidney arise from their distribution within the body. The elimination half-life is directly proportional to the volume of distribution. The greater the volume of distribution of a drug, the smaller the amount of the administered dose remaining in the blood, the lower the concentration of drug presented to the kidney per unit time, and the longer the half-life (see Fig. 6-1). For agents not biotransformed and not bound to plasma protein, the shortest half-lives are associated with drugs distributed only within the plasma-water, the intermediate ones with those distributed to the extracellular fluid compartment and the longest with those distributed in the entire content of body water. Drugs belonging to the last category are usually lipid-soluble, and this property is conducive to extensive reabsorption from the tubular urine as well. The theoretical relationships between elimination half-life and apparent volume of distribution are shown in Table 10-1 for drugs cleared by glomerular filtration and tubular secretion (cf. pp. 143–145). The actual half-life of elimination determined experimentally for penicillin, between 25 and 30 minutes (Fig. 10-14), is entirely consistent with the theoretical value. Penicillin is secreted by the renal tubules and has an apparent volume of distribution greater than that of extracellular fluid but less than that of total body water. As would be predicted from Table 10-1, its half-life should lie between 13 and 44 minutes, as it does.

The theoretical half-lives in Table 10-1 were calculated by assuming that the movement of drug into the fluid compartments of the body is readily reversible. That is to say, when the concentration gradient within extravascular fluid compartments favors movement in the opposite direction, drug moves back into the blood. However, no limits can be set for how long a drug may remain in the body when it is strongly bound to tissue components and, thus, restricted in its outward movement. The long half-lives of digitoxin and strontium, as well as many other agents, are due to sequestration within tissues or organs.

Table 10-1. *Theoretical relationship between elimination half-life and volume of distribution in a 70-kg subject*

Mechanisms of urinary excretion	Drug distributed in[1]		
	Plasma water (3000 ml)	Extracellular fluid (12,000 ml)	Body water (41,000 ml)
Glomerular filtration – 130 ml/min	16 min	64 min	219 min
Tubular secretion – 650 ml/min	3 min	13 min	44 min

[1]Entries in each column are values of the fastest possible elimination half-life. Elimination half-lives have no upper limit; renal clearance may be extremely low (near zero) if a drug is extensively reabsorbed or protein-bound, or has an apparent volume of distribution greater than total body water due to extensive tissue binding. Source: Modified from W.B. Pratt and P. Taylor, *Principles of Drug Action* (3rd ed.), New York: Churchill Livingstone, 1990, p. 279.

THE TIME COURSE OF DRUG ACTION AFTER SINGLE DOSES

So far, we have considered the temporal course of drug action only in a piece-meal fashion. We have examined the factors that influence the ascending portion of the time-response curve separately from those that determine its descending portion. Now we shall consider how all these factors acting in concert affect the overall time course as well as the separate phases of drug action.

Relationship of Elimination Half-life and Duration of Action

First, we will consider the case in which a drug is administered intravenously, equilibrates rapidly into its entire volume of distribution, acts reversibly on a site to produce its effect, and is eliminated by first-order kinetics. Under these conditions, the *duration of action increases as the logarithm of the dose increases.* The reason for this relationship can be easily deduced from the following example. Suppose that drug X has an elimination half-life of 4 hours and that its just-effective concentration in the body corresponds to 1 unit/ml of plasma. A dose is given that will establish a plasma concentration of 8 units/ml. The duration of action will then be 12 hours, or three half-lives (Fig. 10-16). When the dose is doubled, i.e. sufficient to yield 16 units/ml of plasma, the duration of action is extended by only 4 hours, or one elimination half-life, since in the first 4 hours the plasma level will fall to 8 units/ml. Redoubling the dose so that the initial plasma level is 32 units/ml again increases the duration of action by only 4 hours. Thus, geometric increases in dose produce linear increases in duration of action. This relationship implies that, for a drug that is eliminated rapidly, it is in practice almost impossible to produce a prolonged action by giving massive doses intravenously. Moreover, the quantity of drug that can be safely administered at one time is limited by its dose-related toxicity. Because of this, the

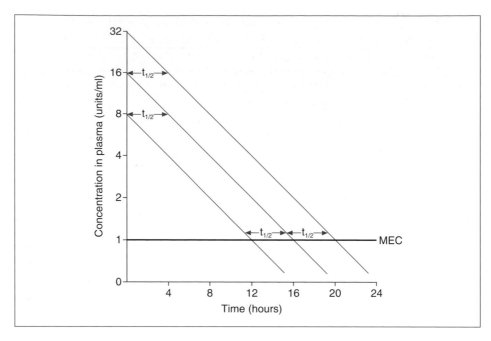

Figure 10-16. *Relation between duration of action and dose for a drug eliminated by first-order kinetics. Elimination half-life is 4 hours. If action lasts until the drug remaining in the body is reduced to the minimal effective concentration (MEC, shown in graph as 1 unit), then the duration of action increases as the logarithm of the dose increases. (Note that the units along the ordinate are on a geometric scale.)*

duration of action of many drugs with short elimination half-lives must instead be increased through alternative routes of administration or infusions rather than bolus injections.

The duration of action is not always predicted by the elimination half-life of a drug. The duration of action may outlast its presence in the organism because of an irreversible effect on the target site. For example, aspirin has an elimination half-life of only 15 minutes, but a single dose prolongs bleeding time for 7 days. The prolonged duration results from an irreversible effect on an enzyme in platelets (cyclooxygenase), which prevents clotting. Another reason may be bio-transformation of the drug to an active metabolite that has a much longer elimination half-life. A number of the benzodiazepine anti-anxiety agents exemplify this phenomenon.

The duration of action of a drug may also be much shorter than predicted for drugs with long elimination half-lives. One reason may be that the drug redistributes from its site of action into a tissue reservoir where it produces no effect. An important example of this phenomenon is illustrated by many highly lipophilic drugs. These drugs rapidly gain access to the brain where they act but also quickly leave the brain as the drug more slowly accumulates in tissues such as muscle and fat. For example, the drug thiopental, used for induction of general anesthesia, is extremely lipid-soluble and diffuses rapidly across biologic barriers. Thus the rate at which it reaches various parts of the body is directly dependent on the rate of blood flow through the particular organ or tissue. The brain, liver, kidney and heart are perfused by blood more rapidly in proportion to their mass than are other body masses (cf. Table 6-1). Together, these organs, which constitute only about 4.8% of body weight, receive almost 50% of the cardiac output, or about 2.55 l of blood per minute in the average 70-kg individual. It is for these reasons that thiopental reaches its maximum concentration at its site of action in the brain within 1–2 minutes after intravenous administration (see Fig. 10-17). At this time the concentration in brain is similar to that in the plasma. Because thiopental is about 100 times more lipid-soluble than phenobarbital and is also less ionized in body fluids, it penetrates much more rapidly into the brain than phenobarbital and produces a much more rapid onset of anesthetic effect (Fig. 10-3).

The more slowly perfused areas of the body, such as muscle and skin, acquire the drug at a much slower rate; it takes 15–30 minutes for thiopental to reach its maximum level in these lean tissues (Fig. 10-18). Several hours may be required before thiopental reaches its peak concentration in fat, an even more poorly perfused tissue. But as the thiopental enters lean tissues first and then the fat,

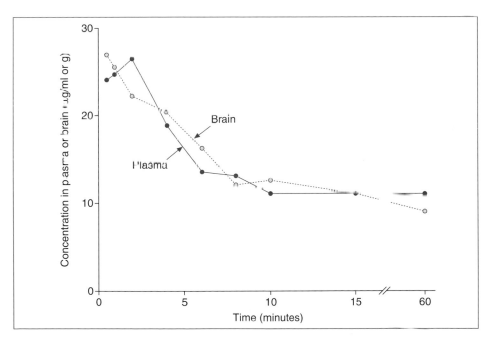

Figure 10-17. *Plasma and brain concentration of thiopental after intravenous administration (15 mg per kg of body weight) to rats. Onset of anesthesia was between 1 and 2 minutes. (●——● = plasma; ●----● = brain.) (Modified from A. Goldstein and L. Aronow, J. Pharmacol. Exp. Ther. 128:1, 1960. Copyright © 1960, American Society for Pharmacology & Experimental Therapeutics.)*

the circulation increase in number. Since transfer of drug across the gastrointestinal epithelium is slower than movement from interstitial space into the circulation, the delay in onset of action is longest by the oral route.

The penicillin data (Fig. 10-19) also point out how the route of administration can alter the duration of action, the amplitude of the peak concentration and the time to this maximum level. Our points of reference for comparison are the data obtained following intravenous administration of penicillin. This route yields the highest and most rapidly attainable serum concentrations because the entire dose is placed directly into the bloodstream. The duration of action of an intravenous dose also reflects the rate of elimination unmodified by absorption. Figure 10-19 shows that, even though the dose is sufficient to establish an initial concentration 100-fold greater than the minimum effective level, the action of intravenously administered penicillin lasts only 5 hours.

When an aqueous solution of penicillin is given intramuscularly, the amplitude of the peak concentration attained is not much lower, and the duration of action not much longer, than after intravenous injection. Moreover, the peak blood level is reached soon after the drug is deposited in the muscle. Together, these facts signify that the rate of absorption from the intramuscular site during activity is extremely rapid – so rapid, in fact, that the major portion of the dose reaches the blood before very much elimination has taken place. The rate of decline of serum levels then approaches that following intravenous injection, since little influence is exerted by continued absorption. In contrast, after subcutaneous administration, a much lower peak is reached at a later time, yet the duration of effective concentrations is somewhat longer. The lower and later peak indicates that the rate of absorption is insufficient to keep up with the rate at which penicillin is being eliminated. But continued absorption even at a rate slower than elimination is sufficient to compensate partially for the drug that is being lost. As a result, the duration of action of the subcutaneous dose is longer than that given intramuscularly. The lowest and latest peak is associated with oral administration, the route with the slowest rate of absorption. Again, continued entry of drug into the body provides for a duration of action of orally administered penicillin longer than that given intravenously. Because only about one-third of an oral dose is absorbed, the serum concentrations are considerably lower than after subcutaneous administration, which provides much higher bioavailability.

Generally, the total clearance and volume of distribution of a drug, and therefore its elimination half-life, are independent of the route of administration. As a consequence, for equal doses of a given drug given by different routes, it is a change in the *rate of absorption* that produces a change in its time course of action. The slower the rate of absorption relative to elimination, the later are the minimally effective and peak concentrations attained and the lower is the value of the latter. The duration of action will also become longer with a slower rate of absorption provided that (1) the rate of absorption is sufficiently rapid relative to elimination to yield levels above the minimal effective concentration, and (2) the entire dose at a site of application is absorbed.

The duration of action of a drug that is rapidly eliminated, such as penicillin, is not altered very much, as we have just seen, by changing its rate of absorption *as long as absorption remains first order*. The duration of action, however, can be markedly prolonged when the kinetics of absorption approach zero order. The administration of special dosage forms achieves this because the drug is released at a rate slower than its rate of absorption. For example, penicillin combines with procaine to form a salt that goes into aqueous solution very slowly compared with the potassium salt of penicillin. The rate of dissolution of procaine-penicillin in body fluids is even further reduced when it is administered in oil. As a result, absorption proceeds at a nearly constant rate for a considerable period. A single intramuscular injection of procaine-penicillin in oil provides therapeutic drug levels for more than 24 hours (curve P-IM in Fig. 10-19), whereas the same dose of penicillin in water is effective for little more than 5 or 6 hours.

THE KINETICS OF DRUG ACCUMULATION FOLLOWING MULTIPLE DOSES

Multiple-dose Schedules

The aim in most therapeutic situations is to produce an alteration in a particular function of an organism and to maintain this change for an adequate period. This calls initially for attaining an effective concentration of drug in the body and then for keeping this level relatively constant. Achieving an initial effective concentration is a simple matter if an appropriate route and dose are used. It is the maintenance of this effective level that poses problems. We have seen that increasing the size of the dose is not only ineffective in prolonging drug action but also limited by considerations of dose-related toxicity. However, the duration of drug action can be safely prolonged by continually delivering drug into the body to counterbalance what is lost through biotransformation or excretion or both. Sustained-release preparations, if available, represent one way of doing this, but the more usual procedure is to give repeated doses of drug at regular intervals.

It is obvious, since the rates at which different drugs are eliminated from the body vary widely, that no single schedule for repeated dosage would be appropriate for each and every drug. But the development of a rational dosage schedule for any drug is governed by principles applicable to all agents and is a relatively simple procedure for drugs that are eliminated by first-order kinetics. For any given agent we need to know: (1) what concentration will produce the desired effect; (2) what dose will yield this concentration; and (3) how long the level of drug in the body will remain effective after the selected dose is administered. What constitutes an effective concentration of drug in the body is determined by the dose-response relationships of the therapeutic agent. The magnitude of the dose required to produce this particular drug level depends on the route of administration and the volume of distribution of the given drug.

And the elimination half-life of the drug tells us how long an effective level of drug will remain in the body. In addition, there may be a concentration that should not be exceeded in order to avoid toxicity. The range between the minimal effective level and the maximal allowable is referred to as the therapeutic window.

Let us suppose that drug X, with an elimination half-life of 4 hours, produces its desired effect when the total quantity of drug in the body is at least 1 g but not greater than 2 g. If we administer an initial dose of 2 g, we would immediately achieve this goal (assuming instantaneous absorption and distribution). After 4 hours, however, the level in the body would have fallen to half this amount, or 1 g. We could then replace the quantity of drug lost by giving an additional 1-g dose. If we continued giving 1 g every 4 hours, the drug level in the body would never exceed 2 g since the quantity lost between doses equals the quantity replaced at the next dosing interval. The rate of drug administration that just establishes, but does not exceed, the desired drug level in the body is the *maintenance dose rate*. In our example, where the body content of between 1 and 2 g represents the required effective range, then 1 g every 4 hours is the maintenance dose rate, and 1 g is the maintenance dose of drug X. The larger initial dose of 2 g, which was used to achieve the desired drug level quickly, is called a *loading dose* or *priming dose*.

What would happen if we began therapy with drug X by administering the maintenance dose of 1 g from the start? Or, alternatively, if we continued administering the loading dose of 2 g every 4 hours? If we administer the maintenance dose from the outset, the amount of drug X in the body would rise until a maximum of 2 g were present. This is so because more drug is being given every 4 hours than is being eliminated in the dosing intervals up to the point at which the body content reaches 2 g. At a body content of 2 g, however, the rate of elimination – 1 g every 4 hours – would equal the rate of drug entry into the body. No further accumulation would occur, and so a *steady-state condition* has been achieved. Simple arithmetic shows that it takes seven doses to just about reach this point (Table 10-2). If we administer the loading dose every 4 hours, the amount of drug in the body will also increase until the rate of elimination equals the rate of drug entry into the body, and it would again take about seven doses to approximate this point (Table 10-2). But since the rate of administration is 2 g every 4 hours, the level of drug in the body has to be 4 g before the rate of elimination will be 2 g every 4 hours. Thus, if a drug is given at regular intervals and if a constant fraction of what is present in the body is eliminated in the interval, *the amount of drug in the body will accumulate until the quantity cleared in the interval between doses is equal to a single dose.*

If the assumption is made that each single dose is absorbed instantaneously, marked fluctuations in the level of drug in the body will occur due to elimination during the intervals between doses. In the example cited, just before the second 1-g dose is administered, only 0.5 g would be present. Just after the instantaneous absorption of the second dose, the body content would be 1.5 g. There would be ever-greater fluctuation if 2 g were administered every 4 hours.

Table 10–2. *Accumulation of drug X in the body*[1]

Dosing interval														
	1		*2*		*3*		*4*		*5*		*6*		*7*	
	A[2]	*B*[3]	*A*	*B*	*A*	*B*	*A*	*B*	*A*	*B*	*A*	*B*	*A*	
Administration of 1 g of drug X:														
Body content (g)	1.0	0.5	1.5	0.75	1.75	0.88	1.88	0.94	1.94	0.97	1.97	0.99	1.99	
Administration of 2 g of drug X:														
Body content (g)	2.0	1.0	3.0	1.5	3.5	1.75	3.75	1.88	3.88	1.94	3.94	1.97	3.97	

[1]Elimination half-life of drug X = 4 hours. Dosing interval = 4 hours.
[2]Figures in columns headed A represent the amount of drug X in body immediately after a dose is given.
[3]Figures in columns headed B represent amount of drug X in body just before dose is given.

It can be readily appreciated that after oral administration the fluctuation in the body content of drug would be less severe, provided that the entire oral dose were absorbed well within the dosing interval. Continued absorption of drug tends to flatten out the fluctuations due to drug elimination in the intervals between doses. When the rate of drug entry into the body becomes constant, i.e. when it is near zero order, as in the case of a continuous intravenous infusion, there will no longer be fluctuations.

The extent to which the drug content in the body rises and falls can also be minimized by shortening the interval between doses. However, the amount of drug administered per dose must also be reduced to match the amount eliminated in the new interval. For example, if drug X were given every 2 instead of every 4 hours, less than one-half of the amount present in the body would be eliminated in the 2-hour interval. Were the maintenance dose to remain 1 g, drug X would continue to accumulate beyond the desired level, since more drug was being put into the system than was being eliminated in the interval between doses. To avoid this accumulation, the maintenance dose must also be reduced so that the ratio of the maintenance dose to the dosing interval (the dosing rate) is unchanged.

For any given interval between doses, the slower the rate of elimination, the smaller the degree of fluctuation in drug levels, since a smaller fraction of drug is lost from the body during the interval. By the same token, the maintenance dose will represent a progressively smaller fraction of drug present in the body as the rate of elimination becomes slower. Take, for example, drug Y with an elimination half-life of 24 hours. In a 4-hour interval only about one-tenth of the drug in the body is cleared, whereas one-half of drug X, with an elimination half-life of 4 hours, is eliminated in an equal period. Thus, if we wished to maintain drug Y at a body content of 2 g, we would require a maintenance dose of only one-tenth this amount, or 0.2 g, once the desired level had been established. As in the case of drug X, we could establish this 2-g level quickly by administering a primary dose of 2 g and then continuing at 4-hour intervals with the small main-tenance dose. But if we started with the maintenance dose rate of 0.2 g every 4 hours, how long would it take to reach the 2-g level for drug Y in the body? The lower curve of Figure 10-20 indicates that even after 3 days, only about 90% of the desired body content could be reached on this schedule. To obtain the full 2-g level would require almost 6 days. The upper curve of Figure 10-20 shows that when a dose of 0.4 g of drug Y is given every 4 hours, it requires only 24 hours to attain a level greater than 90% of the desired body content. If adminis-tration at this higher dose rate were continued beyond 24 hours, the body content of drug Y would climb until a 4-g level was reached (dashed line in Fig. 10-20). Once the desired body content of 2 g was reached with the higher dose, however, institution of the maintenance dose rate would prevent further accu-mulation. We may conclude from these data that when administration starts with the maintenance dose (the quantity of drug lost in the interval between doses), the slower the rate of elimination, the smaller the maintenance dose and the longer it takes to establish a desired level of drug. Thus, drugs that are elimi-nated slowly from the body also accumulate slowly compared with drugs having short half-lives. Generally, when a drug is administered at a constant rate, either by maintenance doses at a fixed dosing interval or as a continuous infusion, 50% of the steady state condition is achieved in one elimination half-life, 93% in four half-lives, and 99% in seven half-lives (illustrated in Table 10-2).

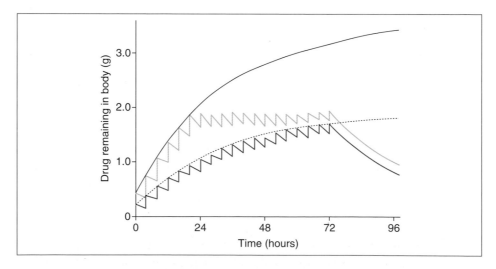

Figure 10-20. *Accumulation of drug with repeated dosage at regular intervals. Elimination half-life = 24 hours. Dosage intervals = 4 hours. In lower curve, dose is 0.2 g; in upper curve, dose is 0.4 g for the first six doses, then 0.2 g. Zigzag solid lines represent fluctuations in blood level in intervals between doses. Dosage was stopped at 72 hours. Dashed lines indicate course of continued accumulation if dosage were continued at original dosage level. (After J.H. Gaddum,* Nature *[Lond.] 153:494, 1944. Reprinted by permission. Copyright © 1944 Macmillan Journals Ltd.)*

When circumstances call for drug therapy, it is often imperative to produce an effective concentration in the body as quickly as possible, certainly within a few hours. For drugs with slow rates of elimination, which preclude the rapid build-up of effective drug concentrations through administration of the maintenance dose, the obvious solution is to increase the magnitude of the initial doses. Thus, the initial use of loading doses followed by maintenance doses to establish an effective drug concentration quickly and maintain it indefinitely is the usual procedure for drugs with very long half-lives. The dosage schedules for digitalis glycosides, used in the treatment of patients with congestive heart failure, is a case in point. For example, the elimination half-life of digitoxin is about 7 days; about 10% of the drug present in the body is eliminated daily. It would take weeks to establish a therapeutic drug concentration if the maintenance dose were administered from the start. Clearly, this would constitute improper therapy for a patient whose life may depend on how rapidly the abnormal condition can be brought under control. Ordinarily, in *digitalization*, the entire quantity of drug needed to produce an effective drug concentration is given, in divided doses, during a single day. This is followed by much smaller daily maintenance doses – doses just sufficient to replace what is lost during the dosing interval. The loading dose of digitoxin needed to establish appropriate therapeutic drug levels is not given as a single dose because this drug has a very narrow margin of safety (cf. Fig. 9-13). By giving divided doses, the physician can stop further administration if the patient manifests toxic reactions at doses corresponding to the lower end of the dose-toxicity curve. The same principles apply for regimens of digoxin, the more commonly used digitalis glycoside.

Another example of the need for loading doses of a slowly eliminated drug is provided in the treatment of malaria with chloroquine. This drug has an elimination half life of about 1–2 months, largely attributable to an extraordinarily high volume of distribution (about 200 liters/kg), associated with extensive binding to tissues such as the liver. Without loading doses the necessary drug concentration cannot be attained quickly enough to be effective in terminating acute attacks of the disease. Typical regimens call for a loading dose of 30 mg/kg in the first 2 days and 5 mg/kg repeated on days 7 and 14 thereafter.

Ideally, the laws governing the accumulation of drugs in the body should be applied to the administration of every agent, since no single fixed schedule is appropriate for all drugs. Although the method of administration of many drugs is soundly based, convenience and patient comfort frequently dictate less rational procedures. Adherence to principles is of particular importance, however, for drugs that are rapidly eliminated as well as for those that are slowly removed from the body. In the former case, it is easy to produce an effective concentration quickly but difficult to maintain this level without marked fluctuations. For drugs that are slowly eliminated, it is difficult to attain effective levels rapidly without loading doses, but toxic amounts can accumulate easily unless attention is paid to this possibility.

Accumulation and Toxicity

Any chemical agent that gains access to the body has the potential for producing a toxic or deleterious effect. However, the risk on repeated or chronic exposure is increased by accumulation resulting from a long elimination half-life. As we have discussed, a long elimination half-life is attributable to slow clearance and/or a large volume of distribution.

The cumulative toxicity of slowly eliminated chemicals is well exemplified by certain metals like lead that bind to various components of tissues. Binding to bone is responsible for the very long half-life of lead, in excess of 2 months. In turn, the slow rate of elimination results in a slow rate of accumulation upon chronic exposure. The banning of leaded gasoline and removal of lead-containing paints from older housing has led to a marked decrease in the exposure to lead, from sources such as air and dust, and in the blood lead levels in the US population. However, blood lead screening continues to reveal excessive accumulation in some children, especially in urban centers. The toxicity of lead includes neurological effects, especially in infants and children, and damage to the kidneys. What is so insidious is that toxic symptoms may appear before there is awareness that chronic exposure to a dangerous environmental pollutant has occurred.

The insidious way in which toxicity can result from drug accumulation is also illustrated by an agent like the bromide ion, which was once widely utilized as a sedative and in the treatment of epilepsy. It was supplanted decades ago by agents that were safer and more efficacious, but its use by the general public for a variety of ailments continued, and preparations containing bromides were freely available without prescription in the US until the late 1980s. The bromide ion has a volume of distribution somewhat greater than extracellular fluid. Since it is not bound to tissue components, one might anticipate that its sojourn in the body would be relatively short. Nevertheless, it has a half-life of about 12 days. Its rate of excretion is slow because it is handled by the kidney in much the same way as chloride ion, i.e. it is filtered at the glomerulus and largely reabsorbed in the tubules. The maintenance dose of bromide ion, about 0.9 g per day, if taken from the start, would produce no ill effects, because almost 6 weeks would elapse before effective concentrations would be attained in the body fluids. This rate of accumulation, inevitable as it is, is much too slow, since no one taking the drug voluntarily would wait so long for an effect. Thus, large doses were taken to produce an effect rapidly. And, when dosage continued at the same loading dose rate (a common practice), cumulative poisoning often occurred. Table 10-3 shows how bromide accumulates when what appears to be a moderate dose, 1 g three times a day, is taken for a prolonged period. The minimal effective blood concentration is about 50 mg per 100 ml, and this level is only attained after a week. After 3 weeks of continuous administration at the same rate, the blood level rises to 110 mg per 100 ml, a blood concentration that may well produce toxic effects. Drug manufacturers in the United States apparently heeded the conclusions published in the *AMA Drug Evaluations* that bro-

Table 10-3. *Accumulation of bromide when 1 g potassium bromide is taken 3 times a day by an adult[1]*

Bromide content	Duration of administration (weeks)					
	3 days	1	2	3	4	5
In body (g)	5.6	11	19	22	24	25
In plasma (mg/100ml)	28	55	95	110	120	125

[1]Body weight, 60 kg.

mides are 'useless as hypnotics' and that 'their use is deemed inadvisable' and they are now omitted from OTC formulations.

The role which tissue redistribution plays in toxicity upon repeated exposure is clearly seen in the case of agents like thiopental (Fig. 10-18). If thiopental is readministered before the large fraction of a previous dose has been removed from lean tissues and fat, the effect of the second dose is to prolong the duration of action of thiopental. The concentration gradients between plasma and lean tissues, and between these tissues and fat, would be decreased by the concentrations of drug still present in the less rapidly perfused areas. As a result, the initial plasma concentration falls more slowly. And in turn, the rate of outflow of thiopental from the brain to plasma is slowed and the duration of drug action becomes longer. The persistence of thiopental in tissues unrelated to its pharmacologic effect explains its cumulative effects upon repeated administration.

Under the usual circumstances of its administration, the accumulation of thiopental in adipose tissue presents a problem only to the anesthetist. However, the same principles that account for rapid redistribution of this highly lipid-soluble drug also account for the slow accumulation of other lipid-soluble drugs and poisons in the fat depots of the body. Among such chemicals is the insecticide DDT (chlorophenothane); its former widespread use to combat malaria afforded many opportunities for humans and animals to come in contact with it over an extended period[2]. The quantity necessary to produce even minimal signs of toxicity is large. With judicious use, this quantity would almost never be ingested by animals or by human beings eating plants or the flesh of animals exposed to the environmental contaminant. But once in the body, DDT is very slowly eliminated, primarily by biotransformation. Thus, DDT accumulates in the fat depots if the rate of elimination is slower than the rate of ingestion. While the chemical remains in the adipose tissue, it is harmless. It is only when sufficiently large amounts are mobilized from these fat stores (as in food deprivation or marked weight loss) that toxicity may result.

[2]The use of DDT is now restricted by law in most countries.

SYNOPSIS

The time course of drug action is delineated in terms of the effective drug concentration that is attained in the body following drug administration. The time to a minimally effective concentration denotes the onset of drug action, the first measurable response; the total time an effective concentration is present in the body defines the duration of drug action.

The time course of drug action is determined by the rates of absorption, distribution and elimination of the drug and is dependent on the dose administered. The concentration of a drug in the blood at various times after administration may be used to describe the temporal course of drug action if the assumption is made that there is a correlation between the pharmacologic response and the concentration of the drug in blood. For many drugs this assumption is sufficiently valid to yield approximations of their time course of action. This relationship does not hold for drugs that act irreversibly, since their effects may persist long after the drugs have left the body.

Most drugs are absorbed at a rate proportional to the amount present at the site of application at any given moment; i.e. the rate of absorption usually follows first-order kinetics. When a supply of drug is available to replace that removed by absorption, a constant amount of drug, rather than a constant fraction of the quantity present, is absorbed per unit time. This zero-order rate of absorption has usually been approached through the use of sustained-release medications, which makes dissolution or disintegration of the preparation the rate-limiting factor in the drug's absorption. Zero-order absorption kinetics is more easily and consistently realized, however, by the use of sustained-release drug delivery devices.

The faster the rate of absorption, the sooner the onset of action. (This is true even for prodrugs, which are inactive until they are biotransformed.) The faster the rate of absorption relative to elimination, the sooner the maximum drug concentration is attained and the higher is the actual value of this peak. And for any given rate of absorption, the larger the dose administered, the faster the onset of action, the higher the peak concentration and the longer the duration of action.

The rate of absorption of a given agent is determined by its physicochemical properties and by the number and kind of biologic barriers which it must traverse to reach the bloodstream. Thus different drugs may have different rates of absorption from the same site of application, but a single agent will have different rates of absorption only when administered by different routes or in different dosage forms. Ordinarily, absorption of drugs given orally is slower than by the other common routes of administration. However, this slower rate of absorption leads to less fluctuation in the levels of drug present in the body as they change with time after administration. When a completely absorbable drug is absorbed at a rate relative to elimination that provides for effective drug levels, the duration of action may be longer after oral than after other routes of administration.

The overall rate of elimination of most drugs is also proportional to the amount of drug present or remaining in the body, since each of the elimination processes (biotransformation and excretion) usually follows first-order kinetics. The excretion of drugs by glomerular filtration is usually first order. Renal tubular secretion and biotransformation are the only processes with the potential for proceeding at constant rates, independent of the amount of drug remaining to be eliminated. The organic anionic, cationic, and other drugs secreted by the renal tubule are rarely given in doses large enough to saturate the carrier mechanisms. Therefore apparent zero-order kinetics of excretion is the exception rather than the rule. Any drug biotransformation can become zero order at levels that saturate the enzyme system. This does not occur frequently. However, it is a factor in the rates of elimination of some drugs, including the common agents, ethyl alcohol and aspirin, even when these are taken in small quantities.

The rate of urinary excretion is dependent on the rate at which drug is presented to the kidney. The rate of filtration is further dependent on the amount of unbound drug coming to the glomerulus. The greater the volume of distribution, the smaller the concentration of free drug in blood. Therefore the greater the volume of distribution, the slower the rate of excretion. Also, the more extensive the reabsorption of drug from the tubular urine, the slower the rate of excretion. Moreover, since urinary excretion is usually first order, the time course and overall rate of drug elimination may be determined by following the rate of appearance in urine of unchanged drug and its metabolites (provided that the kidney is the organ of drug excretion).

Information concerning the rate of elimination of a drug can be summarized in a parameter called the elimination half-life. This index is the time needed to reduce the amount of unchanged drug in the body to one-half its value. It is measured under postabsorption and postdistribution conditions, i.e. when the amount of drug in the body is not modified by continuing absorption. Therefore, the elimination half-life is most conveniently determined from the rate of decline of blood levels following intravenous administration. The elimination half-lives of different agents vary over a wide range from minutes to years. Generally, the elimination half-life of an agent is determined by its apparent volume of distribution (V_D) and its total plasma clearance (Cl_T), such that $t_{1/2}$ is proportional to V_D/Cl_T.

If all the elimination processes are first order, the elimination half-life of the drug does not change with dose; it will always take the same amount of time to eliminate one-half of the drug present in the body. In the case of intravenously administered drugs, this means that doubling the dose does not double the duration of action, but increases it only by one elimination half-life. Thus, for drugs eliminated by first-order kinetics, increasing the dose is not an effective way of increasing duration of action and, furthermore, is limited by dose-related toxicity. When a zero-order process is involved in the elimination of a drug, the time to eliminate 50% of the drug becomes progressively longer as the dose increases; the amount of drug eliminated per unit time ceases to be a constant fraction of that remaining in the body and approaches a constant amount of drug.

Most therapeutic situations call for the administration of more than one dose of a drug. Decisions concerning the frequency with which multiple doses should be administered are particularly important for two classes of drugs: (1) those that are so rapidly eliminated that effective concentrations are difficult to maintain and (2) those that are so slowly eliminated that accumulation to toxic levels may occur easily. The principles governing the selection of appropriate dosing schedules apply equally to both classes. These principles involve (1) giving an initial dose that will establish but not exceed the desired drug concentration in the body and (2) continuing to administer drug in an amount equal to that lost from the system. If a drug is given at regular intervals and if the dose given at the beginning of an interval equals the amount of drug eliminated during the previous interval, the drug will not accumulate in the body. In other words, when the quantity of drug administered into the body equals the quantity of drug removed from the body in the interval between doses, no accumulation will occur. This quantity of drug is called the maintenance dose. If the maintenance dose is administered at regular intervals from the outset of therapy, the amount of drug in the body will rise until the amount eliminated in the interval between doses is equal to the maintenance dose. Thus, for a given dosing interval, the shorter the half-life of a drug, the more rapidly will the desired level of the drug be attained; the longer the half-life, the more slowly will the content of drug in the body rise when the maintenance dose is given from the start. Since in most cases it is necessary to produce an effective drug concentration rapidly, large doses, called loading doses, are given initially. When the desired level of drug in the body has been achieved, therapy is continued with the smaller maintenance dose.

Knowledge of the time course of drug action is important in determining how rapidly and for how long a drug may be expected to act, as well as in determining the relative dosage by different routes of administration. Knowledge of the relationship between rates of drug entry into and elimination from the body is fundamental to understanding the rationale of dosage schedules and of drug accumulation in the body.

GUIDES FOR STUDY AND REVIEW

What do we mean by latency or time for onset of action? by duration of drug action? When can changes in concentration of a drug in the plasma be used to describe the time course of drug action?

How does the rate of absorption change with time for a drug that is absorbed by a process of passive diffusion? What does this mean in terms of the amount absorbed in equal units of time? how is the amount absorbed per unit time related to the amount remaining to be absorbed?

How does the rate of absorption change with time when the kinetics of absorption approaches zero order? How can the rate of absorption be made to approach zero order? How and when do rates of disintegration and dissolution affect the kinetics of absorption? When would it be desirable to have absorption governed by zero-order kinetics?

Does a change in the absorption half-life or bioavailability of a drug influence the onset of drug action? the duration of drug action? the maximum effect produced by a given dose? How does an increase in the rate of absorption affect the time course of drug action? How does the route of drug administration affect the time course of drug action? Does a decrease in the rate of absorption always lead to an increase in duration of drug action? Under what circumstances may a decrease in the rate of absorption lead to a decrease in duration of action?

What processes determine the rate of drug elimination? If the overall rate of drug elimination is proportional to the amount of drug remaining in the body, what does this tell you about the kinetics of biotransformation and excretion?

When is the rate of drug biotransformation zero order? What is the relationship between the rate of biotransformation and the amount of drug remaining in the body when biotransformation is zero order? when biotransformation is first order? What common drugs are biotransformed by metabolic reactions that are zero order following the administration of ordinary or small doses? How does this zero-order biotransformation affect the duration of action of the drug after a single small dose? a single large dose? multiple doses?

What is the only process of urinary excretion that can display zero-order kinetics? Is this an important factor in the urinary excretion of any drug? What is usually true concerning the kinetics of elimination for drugs that are eliminated primarily by the urinary route?

What does the index *elimination half-life*, $t_{1/2}$, describe? How is this index measured? Does the elimination half-life change with the dose or route of drug administration? Under what condition is the $t_{1/2}$ the same as the time required to eliminate 50% of an administered dose? when is it different? How is the elimination half-life of a compound related to its total plasma clearance and volume of distribution?

When urinary excretion is the primary mechanism of elimination, how does volume of drug distribution, plasma protein binding or lipid solubility influence the renal plasma clearances and the elimination half-lives of drugs?

Drug X is eliminated by first-order kinetics. If an intravenous dose of drug X is doubled, how much will its duration of action be extended? Why? For a drug rapidly eliminated, is it practical to try to produce a prolonged action by giving massive doses?

How is the elimination half-life of a drug useful in calculating the frequency with which multiple doses of a drug can be safely administered? How does the elimination half-life of a drug affect the time required to reach a steady-state condition upon repeated dosing? Will there be drug accumulation in the body if a drug is given in a dose equal to the amount of drug eliminated during the interval between doses?

What is meant by maintenance dose? by loading dose? When is the use of loading doses essential for effective drug therapy?

Why may toxicity occur upon repeated exposure to agents whose residence time in the body far outlasts their duration of effective concentration? Why do small doses of lead compounds (which in themselves are ineffective) produce cumulative toxicity with chronic exposure? How does tissue redistribution explain the potential toxicity of lipophilic compounds such as thiopental or DDT?

SUGGESTED READING

Atkinson, A.J., Jr. and Kushner, W. Clinical pharmacokinetics. *Annu. Rev. Pharmacol. Toxicol.* 19:105, 1979.

AMA Drug Evaluation, 6th Edition, Chicago: American Medical Association, 1987.

Benet, L.Z. Effect of route of administration and distribution on drug action. *J. Pharmacokinet. Biopharm.* 6:559, 1978.

Gabrielsson, J. and Weiner, D. *Pharmacokinetic/Pharmacodynamic Data Analysis: Concepts and Applications.* Stockholm: Swedish Pharmaceutical Press, 1994.

Gaddum, J.H. Repeated doses of drugs. *Nature (Lond.)* 153:994,1949.

Levy, G. Relationship between elimination rate of drugs and rate of decline of their pharmacologic effects. J. *Pharm. Sci.* 53:342, 1964.

Levy, G. and Tsuchiya, T. Salicylate accumulation kinetics in man. *N. Engl. J. Med.* 287:430, 1972.

Nelson, E. Kinetics of drug absorption, distribution, metabolism and excretion. *J. Pharm. Sci.* 50:181, 1961.

Rowland, M., Tozer, T.N. and Rowland, R. *Clinical Pharmacokinetics: Concepts and Applications* (3rd ed.). Baltimore: Lippincott, Williams, and Wilkins, 1995.

Shargel, L. and Yu, A.B.C. *Applied Biopharmaceutics and Pharmacokinetics* (4th ed.). New York: McGraw-Hill/Appleton & Lange, 1999.

Van Boxtel, C.J., Holford, N.H.G. and Danhof, M. (eds). *The In Vivo Study of Drug Action: Principles and Applications of Kinetic-Dynamic Modelling.* Amsterdam: Elsevier Science, 1992.

Wagner, J.G. Pharmacokinetics. *Annu. Rev. Pharmacol.* 8:67, 1968.

Yacobi, A., Skelly, J. P., Shah, V.P. and Benet, L.Z. (ed.). *Integration of Pharmacokinetics, Pharmacodynamics and Toxicokinetics in Rational Drug Development.* New York: Plenum, 1993.

11   Factors Modifying the Effects of Drugs in Individuals

I. Variability in Response
Attributable to the Biologic System

Our considerations thus far have made it obvious that many factors play a role in determining the biologic effects observed when a chemical agent interacts with a living organism. The more complex the biologic system, the greater the number of variables that may affect the ultimate response. Some factors influence the *nature,* or *pharmacodynamics,* of the drug response. Sometimes these result in effects such as allergic responses that are qualitatively different from those for which the drug is usually administered. Most factors that modify the effects of drugs, however, do so by altering their *pharmacokinetics* and, thereby, the *intensity* of the response. Once recognized, these quantitative changes in the usual effects of drugs can be corrected by appropriate dosage adjustment. We have already discussed the most important factor in determining the intensity of a biologic effect in any individual – the dose of drug administered. But the intensity of drug effect is also dependent on how much of a dose reaches a site of action at any one time and how long the drug remains there in effective concentrations. Thus it follows that even for a single dose of a single agent, the variability in the intensity of response among different individuals may result from the influence of the many factors that affect absorption, distribution, biotransformation and excretion.

Most of the factors known to influence the nature or intensity of the response to drugs can be conveniently categorized on the basis of the source of the variability. The variables attributable to the biologic system account for differences in response to drugs among individuals of the same species as well as different species. This category includes body weight and size, age, gender, other inherited characteristics, and the general state of health. The second category includes the variables attributable to the conditions of administration, such as the dose, dosage form, route, and previous administration of the same or a different drug. These factors largely account for the differences in response observed in a single individual on different occasions. In this chapter we shall identify the major biologic sources of variability which make an individual respond to a drug in an unusual manner – unusual in the sense that the response is different from that anticipated in the 'average' subject or in the majority of a population. In Chapter 12 we shall deal with the ways in which the repeated administration of a single drug and the interactions of drugs concurrently administered modify the effects produced.

BODY WEIGHT AND SIZE

The magnitude of drug response is a function of the concentration of drug attained at a site of action, and this concentration is related to the volume of distribution of the drug. For a given dose, the greater the volume of distribution, the lower the concentration of drug reached in the various fluid compartments of the body. Since the volume of interstitial and intracellular water is related to body mass, weight has a marked influence on the quantitative effects produced by drugs. In general, the apparent volume of distribution is directly proportional to body weight. Therefore, one would anticipate that a particular quantity of drug might be more effective in lighter subjects than in heavier ones, and in general small persons require lower amounts of drugs than large persons in order to produce effects of equal intensity.

The average adult dose of a drug is calculated on the basis of the quantity that will produce a particular effect in 50% of a population between 18 and 65 years of age and weighing about 70 kg (150 lb). Since the dose required is roughly proportional to body size, the variation in effects produced by a drug can be minimized when the dose is determined on the basis of a certain amount per kilogram of body weight. Thus:

$$\text{Dose required} = \frac{\text{Average dose}}{70\,\text{kg}} \times \text{Weight of individual (kg)}$$

This method of adjusting dosage to eliminate a source of biologic variation may be quite suitable for those persons whose weights are within the limits considered normal for their height and age. For abnormally lean or obese individuals, dosage adjustments must also take into account the changes in ratios of body water to body mass. In the obese subject, the total volume of body water is about 50% of the body weight, whereas the value is closer to 70% for the lean individual (Table 11-1). It is for this reason that body surface area, which is based on both height and weight, is often a more discriminative index than weight alone for adjustment of drug dosage over a wide range of body sizes. (Nomograms are available to estimate surface area from the weight and height of an individual.) It should be recognized, however, that the effect of an unusual body composition such as obesity may differ for a highly lipophilic drug which accumulates in fat from that of a drug which does not distribute into fat tissue.

AGE

Some effects of age on the quantitative aspects of drug activity are inseparable from those attributable to size, since the two variables are directly related

Table 11-1. *Effect of age, gender and body type on body composition*

	Age (years)	Mean body weight (kg)	Total body water (% body weight)	Fat (% body weight)
Infant	Less than 3 months	3.5–8.3	70	
Infant	1	10	57	
Male	20–30	72	58	19
	40–50	77	56	25
	60–70	77	54	25
Female	16–30	58	52	29
	40–50	62	49	35
	60–70	64	42	45
Obese male	31	100	49	33
Lean male	26	69	70	7

during the early part of life. However, age, not size, is the more dominant factor in the variability of drug action in the infant and young child. And the elderly also frequently respond to drugs in a manner that cannot be imputed merely to differences in body weight. These individuals at the extremes of the lifespan are often unusually sensitive to drugs; their responses occur at the far left of the normal distribution and quantal dose-response curves. This apparent increase in sensitivity is associated with changes in rates of absorption, distribution, bio-transformation and/or excretion.

In the elderly, several factors increase the likelihood of a different response to drugs from that in healthy young adults. The incidence of disease is higher, which, depending on the pathological process, may affect the response to some drugs. The use of therapeutic agents is greater, which increases the risk of drug interactions. In addition, the aging process leads to changes in some organ systems that can influence the pharmacokinetics of some drugs. The most common and predictable change is a linear decline in renal function that begins at around age 30 years and reaches 50% by age 90 years. This change is reflected in the lower renal clearance of the endogenous substance creatinine, primarily a marker of glomerular filtration rate. Consequently, the renal plasma clearance for many drugs declines linearly with age. Since the elderly are likely to respond to drugs in a manner quantitatively different from the way the average adult responds, cautious estimates of drug dosage are always indicated.

At the other end of the age scale, in newborn infants, particularly premature infants, many of the enzyme systems responsible for normal metabolic conversions and drug biotransformations are underdeveloped. For example, many of the important microsomal enzymes concerned with oxidation and glucuronide conjugation are either lacking or present in very low quantities. As a consequence, natural metabolites such as bilirubin (Table 8-1) or drugs such as

Table 11-2. *Effect of age on biotransformation*

| | Drug biotransformed ($\mu mol/g$)[1] at age | | |
Drug	2 Weeks	3 Weeks	Adult
Hexobarbital	4.2	10.3	16.6
l-Amphetamine	1.9	15.1	21.1
Chlorpromazine	11.4	31.5	32.3
p-Nitrobenzoic acid	1.76	5.28	8.1

[1]Micromoles of drug metabolized or metabolite formed per gram of protein of liver.
Data from J.F. Fouts and R.H. Adamson, *Science* 129:897, 1959.

hexobarbital are biotransformed very slowly (or not at all) in the young of humans and other animals (Table 11-2). However, these enzyme systems develop quickly. Most of them increase to adult levels within 1–8 weeks after birth, and within the first year of life they reach maximal activity. Recent studies have shown that even within a given enzyme family such as the cytochrome P450 isozymes the age when adult enzyme activity is achieved in human liver varies remarkably and for some isozymes is higher in the fetus than the adult.

The renal excretion of drugs is also depressed in the very young, primarily as a result of a decreased rate of presentation of drug to the kidney. As Table 11-1 indicates, water constitutes a greater percentage of the total body weight of the infant than of individuals in other age groups. The greater volume available for distribution lowers the concentration of drug in the blood coming to the kidneys. In addition, the volume of blood flowing through the kidney per unit time is smaller in the infant in proportion to this total body water content. Because of the greater volume of distribution and the lower rate of blood flow, the rate at which drugs are filtered by the neonatal glomerulus is relatively slow. For example, the elimination half-life of inulin is three times longer in the average infant than in the average adult, despite the corrections that are made for differences in relative body water content. Drugs that are secreted by the renal tubular cells, such as para-aminohippuric acid (PAH), are also eliminated more slowly in infants than in adults (cf. pp. 147–148). This deficiency in all likelihood is traceable to the incomplete development of the active transport processes.

The relatively slow clearance of some drugs in the infant has important therapeutic implications. Depending on the route and frequency of administration, drug action tends to be either heightened or prolonged, or both, even when dosage is adjusted according to body size. If the appropriate dose is given intravenously or by a route in which absorption is rapid, the concentration attainable at a site of action – and therefore the intensity of response – is likely to be no different from usual. Effective drug levels, however, will persist for longer periods (Fig. 11-1A). An increase in the duration of action of a single dose of a drug is not in itself harmful and may even be salutary. Rather, the danger lies in the accumulation to toxic levels if the spacing between doses does not take into account the higher residual drug level in the infant's body prior to each successive dose (cf. pp. 247–251).

Ordinarily, the rate of passive diffusion is unaltered in the infant. If anything, it may be increased because of incomplete development of the anatomic barrier. This is certainly true for the blood-brain barrier, which is unusually permeable in the newborn. The newborn can also absorb large molecules, such as proteins, from the gastrointestinal tract, and this increased permeability may extend to still other chemical entities. A decreased rate of absorption is likely only for those few agents that are actively transported; these transport mechanisms may be deficient at other barriers as they are in the renal tubular epithelium. Since most drugs are absorbed by passive diffusion, it follows that the rate of absorption of drugs is, for the most part, the same in the very young as in the adult. Nevertheless, when drugs are administered by slow-absorption routes, the ensuing changes in the time course of action may be more deleterious to the infant than if administration were by fast-absorption routes. When a dose of a drug is rapidly absorbed, the rate of elimination has little effect on the maximum concentration reached in the body (cf. Fig. 10-18). But when the rate of absorption is slow, the peak drug concentration attained is determined by the rate of absorption *relative* to elimination. For a given rate of absorption, the slower the rate of elimination, the higher the peak drug level and the greater the magnitude of drug effect following equivalent dosage. Thus a drug given by a slow-absorption route in a dosage calculated by weight will yield higher peak levels in the infant than in the adult because of the reduced elimination rate in the infant (Fig. 11-1B). Under these circumstances of administration, the likeli-

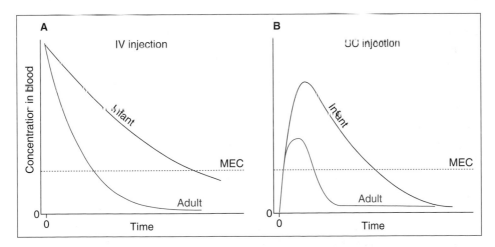

Figure 11-1. *Effect of age on the maximum blood concentration and duration of action of a drug. (A) Drug A given by intravenous route to an adult and a 3-month-old infant in equivalent doses based on milligrams of drug per kilogram of body weight. (B) Drug given by subcutaneous injection to an adult and a 3-month-old infant in equivalent doses based on milligrams of drug per kilogram of body weight. MEC = minimum effective concentration in blood.*

hood of cumulative toxicity with repeated administration is also greater than by fast-absorption routes; not only does a single dose yield a higher drug level in the infant compared with the adult but the higher level also prevails for a longer period (Fig. 11-1B).

The combination of depressed renal function and decreased rates of drug biotransformation accounts for many drug toxicities in the newborn infant. For example, the antibiotic chloramphenicol (CHLOROMYCETIN) is conjugated with glucuronic acid to the extent of about 90% in the adult with an elmination half-life of about 3–4 hours. The conjugated antibiotic is excreted rapidly by renal tubular secretion as well as by glomerular filtration. The important hepatic enzymes that are involved in glucuronide conjugation are not fully developed until after 3 or 4 weeks of extrauterine life. Consequently, in the newborn infant, when chloramphenicol is administered, most of it remains as the free, unconjugated drug. Not only is the free drug poorly eliminated in the urine due to reabsorption from the glomerular filtrate, but glomerular filtration in the neonate is itself relatively inefficient. Therefore, a dose adjusted from the conventional adult dose only on the basis of body weight leads to high and prolonged levels of free chloramphenicol in the newborn, with an elimination half-life of about 24 hours. Successive dosage on the usual schedules only aggravates the situation and produces free drug levels associated with severe toxicity. A number of deaths resulted from this routine adaptation of adult dosage to use in infants before it was recognized that the newborn baby is different from the adult in more than just size. Once the reasons for the neonate's vulnerability to chloramphenicol-induced toxicity were disclosed, the potential adverse effects were avoided by modified dosage regimens. More recently, prolonged elimination half-lives of other drugs cleared by glucuronide conjugation have been observed in the neonate, such as the value for the antiviral agent zidovudine (AZT), used to prevent maternal to fetal transmission of the HIV virus.

The deficiency of enzymes in infants as well as other factors involved in their growth and development also renders them more susceptible than older children to nontherapeutic chemicals in their environment. For example, infants less than 6 months old are extraordinarily sensitive to agents that convert hemoglobin, the oxygen-carrying protein of red blood cells, to methemoglobin, which cannot carry oxygen. Two factors are responsible. First, fetal hemoglobin is oxidized to methemoglobin more readily than is the adult form of the protein; fetal hemoglobin is only slowly replaced by adult hemoglobin during the first 5 or 6 months of life. Second, the young infant – but not the older child – is deficient in the enzyme necessary to reduce methemoglobin to hemoglobin. Consequently, it takes only very small quantities of a chemical, such as an aniline dye, to produce methemoglobinemia in an infant. Even the amount of aniline dye formerly used in inks for marking laundry at times proved sufficient to cause this toxicity.

These two factors plus a third developmental variable also account for the severe, sometimes fatal, methemoglobinemia seen when formulas for infants are prepared with water that contains inorganic nitrates. (Water from wells is a particularly insidious source of this potentially toxic chemical in rural communities because of the extensive use of nitrate-containing fertilizers.) This represents a qualitatively different effect in very young infants, since inorganic nitrates do not lead to methemoglobin formation in older children and adults. Hemoglobin is not oxidized to methemoglobin by inorganic nitrates; the nitrates must first be reduced to inorganic nitrites. In infants, but not in older individuals, ingested inorganic nitrates are converted to nitrites by the enzymatic activity of bacteria present in the upper gastrointestinal tract. It is the nitrites that are absorbed and that oxidize hemoglobin, causing toxicity in infants. Nitrate-reducing bacteria require a near-neutral or only slightly acidic environment to grow. In older individuals, bacteria do not normally invade or multiply in the upper intestine since the entering stomach contents produce an unfavorable acidic environment. Consequently, in older subjects, ingested nitrates are not chemically altered within the intestine, but are absorbed as such before reaching an area where bacterial action can affect them. In contrast, the less acidic stomach contents of infants provide conditions of pH conducive to bacterial growth within the upper small intestine. Thus it is the decreased acidity of the upper intestinal tract of infants compared with that of older individuals which is the factor responsible for the qualitatively different response to ingested nitrates (Fig. 11-2).

GENDER

Simply on the basis of weight, women may require smaller doses of drugs than men to manifest the same magnitude of response. For drugs with a narrow margin of safety, these differences may necessitate a dosage reduction for women. There also may be gender differences in response to drugs because of the unequal ratios of lean body mass to fat mass. In the adult female, adipose tissue represents a greater and water a smaller percentage of total body weight than in the adult male (see Table 11-1).

Whereas differences in drug effects attributable to gender appear to be of only minor consequence, in pregnant women the use of all drugs except those essential to maintain pregnancy should be approached with caution. As was mentioned earlier (see Chapter 6, Distribution from Mother to Fetus) almost any agent in maternal blood may cross the placental barrier, and drugs with little potential for producing adverse effects in the mother may be harmful to the developing embryo or fetus. Drugs given to the mother at parturition may also have long-lasting effects in the newborn; the latter not only may lack the mechanisms necessary for terminating the action of many drugs, but also loses those of the mother as soon as contact with the maternal circulation is severed.

GENETIC FACTORS

A few members of a supposedly homogeneous population respond to drugs in an entirely unusual and highly unpredictable fashion. These responses may take

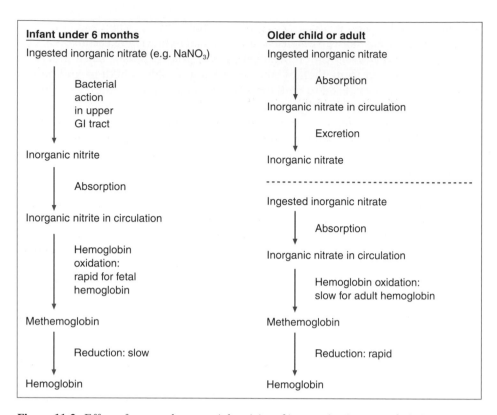

Figure 11-2. *Effect of age on the potential toxicity of inorganic nitrates and nitrites.*

the form of extreme sensitivity to small doses or insensitivity to high doses of a drug whose administration normally produces qualitatively similar effects only at much higher or lower doses. The drug reactions may also be qualitatively different from the effects usually observed in the majority of subjects. The term idiosyncrasy (Gk *idios,* 'one's own,' 'peculiar,' 'distinct'; *synkrasis,* 'a mixing together') has long been used to denote both quantitatively and qualitatively abnormal drug response. Although this terminology recognized that the exceptional responses were not explicable in the same terms as other commonly encountered biologic variations, the reasons for their occurrence remained relatively obscure until advances in biochemical genetics provided the knowledge necessary to seek plausible explanations for these phenomena. The mechanisms underlying the unusual responses to several drugs have now been elucidated and shown to be of genetic origin; it is quite likely that all drug idiosyncrasies will turn out to be genetically conditioned abnormalities. Thus the term *idiosyncrasy,* as it applies to drug reactivity, has taken on a more satisfactory meaning; it may now be more precisely defined as a *genetically* determined, abnormal response to a drug. And the increasingly important branch of pharmacology that deals with the study of genetic modifications of drug response is known as *pharmacogenetics.* Before considering the abnormal drug responses that have been shown to be idiosyncratic, we shall discuss briefly the basic genetic mechanisms involved and how idiosyncrasies can be recognized.

The Genetic Basis of Abnormal Drug Responses

The structure, function and development of each entity of a biologic system are determined by heredity. All the genetic information transmitted from generation to generation is contained in genes, the submicroscopic chemical entities located at various areas on chromosomes. Chromosomes always exist in pairs, each species having its own characteristic number. There are 23 pairs of chromosomes in humans, only one pair of which carries the X or *sex-determining gene.* In the female, each of the two sex chromosomes has the X gene. In the male, only one of the sex chromosomes carries the sex-determining gene; the chromosome lacking the X gene is represented by Y. The term *sex-linked* describes any inherited trait carried on the X chromosomes; a trait located on any of the other 22 pairs of chromosomes (in humans) is referred to as an *autosomal* trait.

An inherited trait is controlled by either a single gene, a pair of genes or many genes. If many genes are involved in the transmission of a specific trait, the inherited characteristic shows continuous variation within the species. In other words, if multigenetic or multifactorial inheritance is involved, the specific trait shows a normal distribution within a population, i.e. it follows a normal, bell-shaped distribution curve (cf. Fig. 9-10). The distribution of height in humans is a typical example of an inherited trait whose magnitude is continuously variable (Fig. 11-3A). In contrast, if an inherited trait is determined by a single gene, there can be no continuous variation; the individual either possesses the characteristic or lacks it. Maleness or femaleness is a good example of such *discontinuous* variation.

The biotransformation of atropine in rabbits furnishes a model of discontinuous variation that is more pertinent to our discussion. Certain members of this species possess an enzyme atropine esterase, which hydrolyzes atropine, whereas the enzyme is completely lacking in other rabbits. A single gene or pair of genes controls the production of atropine esterase, and the enzyme appears to be completely absent in animals that have not inherited this autosomal trait. The enzyme is also absent in most mammalian species, including the human. Rabbits capable of hydrolyzing atropine are much more resistant to the drug's effects than those which lack this mechanism for eliminating the drug. If progressively larger doses of atropine were administered to a substantial number of rabbits and the frequency with which a certain dose produced death were determined, the frequency could not be expressed as a normal distribution. Rather, the studied population would be found to be divided into two distinct groups – there would be discontinuous variation, such as illustrated by the bimodal distribution in Figure 11-3B. The bell-shaped curve at the left in B may be considered representative of the group lacking atropine esterase and responding to lower

the mechanisms responsible for idiosyncratic drug reactions, in the instances in which they have been elucidated, have been traced to genetic modification of specific proteins. In fact, such genetic alterations may go undetected until the abnormal system is suitably challenged by a drug. Some of the important discoveries of inheritable abnormalities have been made when the responses to some drug, or the biotransformation of a drug, indicated a discontinuous variation. The term **pharmacogenomics** has been given to the study of the manner in which variability in response of patients to drugs results from genetic differences in pharmacodynamics.

Hence, the various mechanisms involved in idiosyncratic responses may be categorized according to the role which the altered protein usually plays in drug activity. The alteration of an enzyme normally responsible for drug biotransformation may prolong or shorten the duration of action if this reaction is the principal mechanism for the drug's elimination. Abnormalities of proteins of other systems may either result in a prolonged effect of a drug or be manifest as a novel drug response. Modifications that change the functional activity of a drug transporter may lead either to decreased responsiveness if an agent is unable to reach its target site or to unusual responses if a chemical reaches extraordinary sites of distribution. Finally, alteration of a receptor protein may lead to increased or decreased intensity of drug effect. Examples of each type of idiosyncrasy are listed in Table 11-3 and briefly discussed below.

Abnormalities in Biotransformation Processes

Within many families of Phase 1 and Phase 2 enzymes, variant forms have been identified based on *in vitro* and *in vivo* assessment of enzyme activity. Once techniques were available for genomic analysis, the nucleotide sequences in the genes coding for enzymes of biotransformation were determined. With this approach many variant forms have been characterized with respect to gene mutations and the functional significance of the mutations with respect to transcription and translation of the gene into the enzyme protein. Three examples will serve to illustrate the impact of genetic variants in enzymes of biotransformation on the duration of action of drugs cleared by those pathways.

One of the earliest documented genetic abnormalities of a drug-inactivating enzyme markedly prolonged the effect of the muscle-relaxing drug succinylcholine. This drug is widely used in surgical procedures in which relaxation of muscles is desirable for a short period. Normally, succinylcholine is so rapidly hydrolyzed by the cholinesterases of plasma and liver that its action persists for only a few minutes after its administration is completed. In a few patients, however, the drug was found to produce muscular relaxation and apnea (partial or complete suspension of respiration) of several hours' duration. Subsequent investigations of cholinesterase activity in the affected patients and their families revealed the presence of atypical cholinesterase as a genetically determined trait. The frequency of occurrence of this genetic abnormality in the population as a whole is about 1 in 3000[1].

---

[1]Genetic variants leading to increased cholinesterase activity are also known but are rare.

Another well-documented case of genetic variation in the biotransformation of drugs in humans is that of isoniazid, an agent useful in the treatment of tuberculosis. Here, it is an enzyme of a conjugation process, acetylation, which is affected. Figure 11-4 shows the frequency distribution of the rate of biotransformation of isoniazid (as measured by the plasma concentration of free drug 6 hours after administration) in 267 individuals belonging to 53 families. The discontinuous variation is clearly seen: one group of individuals may be classified as 'rapid inactivators,' the other as 'slow inactivators.' Acetylation is the major pathway of elimination of isoniazid; slow inactivators have been found to possess a reduced quantity of the enzyme, N-acetyltransferase, which acetylates the drug. In this case, then, the genetic abnormality is a difference in the amount of available enzyme rather than an alteration in the enzyme protein itself. The individuals with the enzyme deficiency are more prone than normal persons to develop serious toxic effects on the usual dosage schedule. This has practical significance, since the incidence of slow inactivators is very high among certain geographic groups: 44–54% in American Caucasians and African Americans; 60% in Europeans; only 5% in Eskimos.

More recently, extensive studies have characterized genetic variants among the cytochrome P450 family of enzymes. For example, variants of the CYP2D6 enzyme result in both unusually fast and unusually slow rates of biotransformation of drugs that are substrates for this enzyme. The functional significance in an individual with a variant form of the enzyme depends on whether the biotransformation by this pathway is an activating or inactivating process. For example, individuals with low CYP2D6 activity, so-called poor metabolizers,

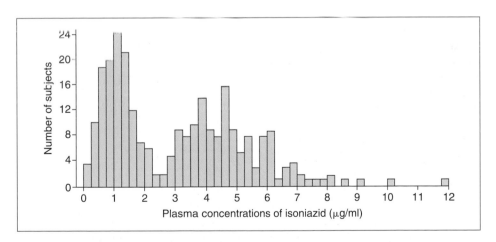

Figure 11-4. *Plasma concentration of isoniazid determined 6 hours after its oral administration (9.8 mg/kg of body weight) to 267 members of 53 families. The frequency distribution shows a bimodality, with the mean plasma concentration for one subpopulation at about 1 µg/ml and for the other subpopulation, between 4 and 5 µg/ml. The subpopulations were designated 'rapid inactivators' and 'slow inactivators'. (From D.A.P. Evans, K.A. Manley and V.C. McKusick,* Br. Med. J. *2:485, 1960.)*

Table 11-3. *Drug idiosyncrasies classified according to the role of the genetically altered protein in drug activity*

Genetic abnormality of protein involved in	Type of alteration	Chemicals whose activity is affected	Manifestation of abnormality
Drug biotransformations			
Plasma cholinesterase	Decreased activity	Succinylcholine	Prolonged drug effect
Plasma cholinesterase	Increased activity	Succinylcholine	Decreased responsiveness to drug
Acetylation	Reduced quantity of enzyme	Isoniazid	Increased toxicity due to accumulation
Cytochrome P4502C9	Decreased activity	Warfarin (COUMADIN)	Increased toxicity due to accumulation
Cytochrome P4502D6	Decreased activity	Codeine (a prodrug)	Decreased analgesic effect
Thiopurine methyltransferase	Decreased activity	Thiopurine	Increased hematologic toxicity
Atropine esterase	Presence in some rabbits	Atropine	Decreased responsiveness to drug
Production of endogenous substances			
Methemoglobin-reducing enzyme	Markedly decreased activity in erythrocytes	Nitrites, sulfa drugs and other drugs that oxidize hemoglobin	Prolonged methemoglobinemia; decreased oxygen-carrying capacity of hemoglobin
Blood clotting factors	Decreased affinity for drug	Warfarin (anticoagulant)	Marked decrease in response to drug

Hemoglobin	More easily oxidized to methemoglobin	Nitrites and other drugs that oxidize hemoglobin Nitrates (reduced to nitrites by intestinal bacteria)	Propensity to develop methemoglobinemia; erythrocytes rupture due to methemoglobin accumulation
Glucose metabolism	Reduced quantity of enzyme in erythrocytes	Primaquine, quinine, sulfa drugs, aspirin	Novel drug effect, hemolytic anemia; decreased number of circulating red blood cells due to lysis
Acetaldehyde metabolism[1]	Decreased affinity for metabolite	Ethanol	Toxicity due to accumulation of acetaldehyde (metabolite of ethanol)
Distribution			
Hepatic transporter protein ATP7B gene product	Deficient transport	Copper in diet	Excessive copper accumulates in liver, brain and other tissues
Intrinsic factor	Deficiency leading to poor absorption	Vitamin B_{12} in diet	Depressed formation of new erythrocytes
Drug transporters			
MDR1	Increased activity	Anti-epileptic agents	Greater likelihood of drug-resistant epilepsy, possibly due to decreased drug access to brain
Receptors			
Taste receptors	Altered combining capacity	Phenylthiourea	Inability to taste bitterness
B-1 adrenergic receptors	Gain of function	Beta blockers	Increased risk of heart failure

[1]Genetic defect occurs in 50% of Asian populations.

have been shown to exhibit a reduced analgesic response to the prodrug drug, codeine, which is activated by CYP2D6-catalyzed conversion to morphine.

Abnormalities in Functional Proteins and Enzyme Systems Other Than Those of Biotransformation

We have already discussed how the low level of an enzyme system that is essential for reducing methemoglobin to hemoglobin partially accounts for the infant's sensitivity to chemical agents producing methemoglobinemia (cf. pp. 264–265). Fortunately, in normal infants the deficiency is usually corrected within a few months after birth. There are, however, individuals who, at any age, show an abnormally prolonged duration of methemoglobinemia following exposure to nitrites, sulfa drugs or other agents capable of oxidizing hemoglobin to methemoglobin. This prolonged drug action is due to a genetic defect, the lack of the methemoglobin-reducing enzyme. In the normal person, a small amount of methemoglobin (about 1% of the total hemoglobin) is always present in the circulating blood as a result of the spontaneous oxidation of hemoglobin. Physiologically, the amount of methemoglobin is held in check primarily by the normal activity of the reducing enzyme. In individuals afflicted with hereditary methemoglobinemia and lacking the normal defense mechanism, the quantity of methemoglobin may rise to as much as 30–50% of the total hemoglobin. Such a decrease in available hemoglobin seriously impairs the capacity of erythrocytes to carry oxygen to the cells. But this level of methemoglobin is not incompatible with life. A decrease in the oxygen-carrying capacity of red blood cells does not become lethal until methemoglobin concentration reaches about 70% of the total hemoglobin. It can be readily appreciated, however, that in individuals with hereditary methemoglobinemia, the use of drugs which form additional methemoglobin may be extremely hazardous.

Another genetic defect in an enzyme system of the red blood cell is manifest as a novel drug effect in some individuals, particularly Black African and Mediterranean males[2]. In these genetically abnormal subjects the administration of the usual daily doses of the antimalarial drug primaquine produces a profound, acute reduction in the number of circulating red blood cells. The novelty of this effect is evidenced by the fact that no comparable hemolytic anemia can be provoked in nonsusceptible individuals even at doses many times greater than the usual dose. The susceptible individuals differ from normal subjects in having red blood cells that are deficient in an important enzyme involved in glucose metabolism[3]. The activity of this enzyme system is essential for mainte-

---

[2]At least 200 million are affected worldwide.

[3]The deficient enzyme is glucose-6-phosphate dehydrogenase (G6PD), just one of many enzymes involved in the process by which glucose is metabolized ultimately to carbon dioxide and water. Cells deficient in G6PD are unable to maintain normal levels of another compound, glutathione. Glutathione is a reducing agent which, by combining with oxidizing agents in the cell, prevents the oxidizing agents from damaging cellular components. In the absence of sufficient glutathione, these oxidizing agents in the red blood cells can produce hemolysis.

nance of cellular integrity. The trait is carried on the X chromosome and is, therefore, sex-linked. Persons with this trait can also develop hemolytic anemia in response to many other agents, e.g. quinine, sulfanilamide, aspirin and compounds present in fava beans. The sensitive individuals appear to be adversely affected, however, only when challenged by these drugs.

Abnormalities in Drug Absorption and Distribution

Another type of anemia, juvenile pernicious anemia, also has its origin in the inherited lack of a protein. In this instance the protein is one essential for the intestinal absorption of vitamin B_{12}, cyanocobalamin, a nutrient indispensable for the normal formation of red blood cells. In the absence of sufficient quantities of the vitamin, the number of circulating red blood cells is reduced as a result of a decreased rate of formation. The protein needed for vitamin B_{12} absorption, called *intrinsic factor,* is synthesized in the gastric mucosa and secreted into the stomach. When intrinsic factor is present, vitamin B_{12} combines with it and is carried to the ileum, where the complex attaches to the ileal surface. The vitamin is then transported across the intestinal mucosal cells and absorbed directly into the bloodstream. In the absence of intrinsic factor, the small quantities of vitamin B_{12} present in the normal diet escape absorption. Vitamin B_{12} absorption not mediated by intrinsic factor occurs only in the presence of quantities of the vitamin much greater than those made available from the usual dietary intake. Pernicious anemia also develops in adults, but unlike the juvenile form of the disease, it has not yet had a genetic basis clearly established.

According to the definition of a drug, the effects produced by the absence of intrinsic factor cannot truly be considered a *drug* idiosyncrasy. Even though vitamin B_{12} is administered as a drug to correct the abnormality, it is ordinarily regarded as a food constituent vital to normal development and nutrition.

Antithetically, the genetically determined deficiency of a specific transport protein converts a normal dietary constituent, copper, into a toxic chemical agent. This abnormality, known as Wilson's disease, results from mutations in the gene ATP7B which codes for a copper-transporting ATPase protein in the liver. More than two hundred mutations in the gene for this protein have been identified in the human population and are associated with this disease. Deficiency in the function of this intracellular transporter leads to the slow accumulation and deposition of copper, particularly in liver and brain, which produces the toxicity and clinical manifestations of the disease.

Genetic abnormalities of the drug transporter ABCB1, also called MDR1 or p-glycoprotein, have been found to influence the efficacy of several types of drugs that are substrates for this carrier protein. The most well characterized phenomenon is the amplification of the gene coding for the protein in tumor cells. The increase in gene copies leads to abnormally high production of the protein and greater functional activity. Since this transporter acts as an efflux pump for many chemotherapeutic agents, the tumor cells are relatively resistant to the drugs due to the decrease in intracellular concentrations at target sites.

More recently, polymorphisms in the gene have been identified in the human population. One variant, resulting in increased expression of the transporter, is associated with drug-resistant epilepsy. This phenomenon may be related to impaired distribution of some anti-epileptic agents into the brain, as a result of increased activity of the transporter in the vascular endothelium in the brain. It is likely that variants in the genes of other transporters will be discovered that contribute to the variability in drug absorption, distribution and excretion.

Abnormalities in Drug Receptor Proteins

Almost all the well-known genetically determined abnormalities in drug responses fall into the three categories discussed above. As drug receptors and their proteins have been isolated and their genes characterized, variant forms are being discovered that affect drug response. The first drug idiosyncrasies that could be directly linked to genetic alteration of receptors were those mediated by receptors controlling calcium movement in skeletal muscle and the senses of taste and smell. For example, a few people are unable to taste the compound phenylthiourea, even in concentrations 100 times greater than those at which most people find it an extremely bitter substance. When various populations were studied to determine their taste thresholds for phenylthiourea, the frequency of response was found to have a bimodal distribution, i.e. the subjects could be divided into two distinct groups, one of 'tasters,' the other of 'non-tasters.' The results of one such investigation are shown in Figure 11-5. More recently, the list of receptor polymorphisms with functional significance to drug response has grown rapidly. For example, variant forms have been found in the

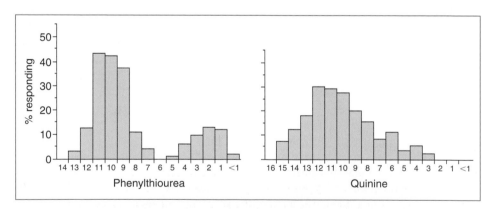

Figure 11-5. *Distribution of taste thresholds for phenylthiourea and quinine. Tests were performed in 200 Belgian women. Values on the abscissa are for increasing concentrations, left to right; each concentration differed by a factor of 2 from the one before. Subjects unable to taste even the most concentrated solutions are included in the category labeled <1. The normal distribution of the ability to taste quinine indicates that subjects unable to taste phenylthiourea were not deficient in the ability to taste all bitter substances. (Modified from A. Leguebe,* Bull. Inst. R. Sci. Nat. Belg. *36:1, 1960.)*

B-1 adrenergic receptor that affect the risk of disease and the response to adrenergic drugs. One polymorphism, resulting from a single amino acid substitution, leads to a receptor with enhanced coupling to its G-protein and greater response to adrenergic agonists ('gain of function'). Subjects who are homozygous with two alleles for the altered receptor are at increased risk of hypertension, an expected outcome of the receptor-induced increase in heart rate and contractility. Interestingly, these subjects demonstrate greater reduction in heart rate in response to B-1 adrenergic antagonists ('beta blockers'). Identification by genotyping of individuals homozygous for this receptor variant might well lead to the choice of this type of antihypertensive agent, in preference to other classes, and earlier use for prophylaxis against cardiovascular disease.

The Importance of Pharmacogenetics

The objectives of pharmacogenetics are twofold: (1) the investigation and identification of the genetic basis for unusual drug responses and (2) the development of methods for predicting those individuals who will react abnormally to drugs. Although routine investigations of large populations may not be justified considering the rarity of some idiosyncratic responses, thorough investigations are warranted in relatives of individuals in whom the diagnosis of a drug idiosyncrasy has been made. Thus the practical value of pharmacogenetic studies lies in their use to predict and prevent a potentially deleterious response to a drug *before* the drug is administered. The development of technology such as microarray gene chips, which permits rapid identification of multiple genetic polymorphisms in the human genome, is anticipated to lead to major innovations in the prediction of drug response in individual subjects. Despite the now well-known importance of pharmacogenetic factors, currently there are limited genetic or functional assays used to determine appropriate dosage regimens. One example is the analysis of thiopurine methyltransferase activity in patients undergoing cancer chemotherapy with drugs cleared by that enzyme. Genotyping and phenotyping of individual subjects for the genes and their products of importance to drug therapy can be expected as a major advance in clinical pharmacology in the near future.

Interspecies Variation

So far we have considered genetically controlled differences in drug responses only as observed among individuals of the same species, primarily human. However, genetic factors that influence the pharmacologic action of drugs are even more apparent when comparisons of drug responses are made between species. These interspecies differences in reactions to drugs, often remarkable, also have a direct bearing on the use of drugs in the human. The initial investigations of the pharmacologic properties of a drug are carried out in a variety of laboratory animals. Typically, the apparent volume of distribution of a drug is relatively predictable from species to species, because it is often directly proportional to body weight.

Because of other sources of interspecies variations, however, neither the efficacy nor toxicity of a compound in the human can be predicted solely from results obtained in other species. Thus, on the one hand, interspecies differences preclude the automatic transfer to human subjects of knowledge gained in animal experimentation. This means that the value of a drug can be ultimately ascertained only in the species in which it is to be used. (We shall deal more fully with this topic in Chapter 16.) On the other hand, without species variation in the response to drugs, there could be no drug therapy of organisms causing disease; the very success of the drug depends on its ability to cause selective injury to invading organisms, such as bacteria, without injuring the host.

Interspecies variations in response to drugs, both quantitative and qualitative, have their origins in differences in absorption, distribution or biotransformation of the drugs, as well as in dissimilarities in integral functions or organization of the living matter. There are countless known examples of these species differences. We shall cite only a few to illustrate how they complicate the development of therapeutic agents for human use.

Variation in Drug Biotransformation

Variation in drug biotransformation among species, even among closely related species such as mammals, is the rule rather than the exception. Thus the most probable cause of species differences in the response to drugs is the variability in the proportion of an administered dose of a drug that remains available to sites of drug action. These variations in drug biotransformation may be expressed qualitatively, as species differences in the pathways of metabolism, or quantitatively, as differences in the rate of biotransformation by reactions that are common to several species.

Differences in the pathway of biotransformation may appear as an inability of a particular species to carry out a given reaction due to the absence of an enzyme system generally found in other species. For example, glucuronide conjugation does not occur to any great extent in cats, although the reaction is a very common pathway of biotransformation for many drugs in dogs, rats and rabbits as well as humans. Again, dogs are unable to carry out some acetic acid conjugations that represent the principal routes of biotransformation in humans, rats and rabbits of agents such as the antitubercular agent isoniazid and the sulfa drugs. But even when there are no species differences in the occurrence of one or more enzyme systems, a single drug may be biotransformed by different reactions or at entirely different rates in various species. Amphetamine, for example, is biotransformed in humans, dogs and mice by similar mechanisms. In mice, however, the degree of biotransformation is more extensive than in the other species. Amphetamine is biotransformed in the rat by processes different not only from those in the mouse but also from those in yet another species, the guinea pig. The pathway of biotransformation of ephedrine, a drug closely resembling amphetamine in structure and pharmacologic activity, is entirely different in rabbits from that in rats, dogs and humans. But, in the case of ephedrine, almost no biotransformation takes place in the human, whereas the dog converts most of the drug into an equally active agent. Yet the microsomal enzyme systems responsible for the metabolism of amphetamine or ephedrine in any one of these species are present in all the species examined, as evidenced by their activity in the biotransformation of other drugs. Thus, even though a particular reaction occurs in many species, there appears to be no rationale for predicting the extent of the reaction with different compounds in the same species or with a given drug in different species. The data in Table 11-4 emphasize not only how great may be the species differences in rates of biotransformation of a single drug, but also that these differences display no consistent pattern.

The projection to humans of data obtained in animals can have serious consequences when a chemical produces toxic effects in the human that were unanticipated from the initial studies in animals. This may occur when biotransformation in humans is much slower than in other species or yields a toxic metabolite that is not formed by the species originally studied. Although the quest continues for an animal species that closely resembles the human in its handling of all drugs, the hope of finding the ideal specimen appears remote. Even studies in primates, the species closest to humans on the evolutionary scale, appear to have no better predictive value in humans than have studies carried out in the dog (see Table 11-4). Since animal studies must always serve as a guide, and since the vast species differences in drug response are well recognized, how can the dilemma be resolved so that translation of results to humans is less uncertain? There are no simple answers to this question as yet. However, much better animal and laboratory models are already available as a result of our increased basic understanding of many diseases and the tremendous advances made in molecular biology. For example, drug biotransformation studies of human enzymes can now be carried out in bacteria following the insertion of human genes into these organisms. Improved procedures such as this will not only promote the efficiency of drug screening processes but will also decrease the use of animals in preclinical development.

Table 11-4. *Comparative half-lives[1] of biotransformation of drugs in various species*

Drug	Human	Rhesus monkey	Dog	Mouse	Rat	Rabbit	Cat
Hexobarbital	6		4.3	0.3	2.3	1	
Meperidine	5.5	1.2	0.9				
Phenylbutazone	72	8	6		6	3	
Antipyrine	12	1.8	1.7				
Digitoxin	216		14		18		60
Digoxin	44		27		9		27

[1]Values in hours required to biotransform 50% of a dose of drug.

complex mechanisms, including for instance a significant reduction in the lipoprotein content of plasma or changes in the number of certain circulating blood cells (eosinophils). Thus it bears emphasizing that placebo effects are not imaginary. And just because they are real phenomena, they must be taken into account in pharmacology. First, the placebo may, under appropriate but limited circumstances, be used as a therapeutic aid. However, this is indicated only when a physician, after careful diagnosis, decides that there is no better form of drug or other therapy and that the administration of a placebo may elicit some beneficial results. Another justifiable and important place of placebos in pharmacology is in evaluating the pharmacologic efficacy of drugs. The results of many investigations indicate that the administration of a placebo produces a variety of positive responses in about 30–35% of the population. Studies also show that there is *no specific group* of individuals who can be classified as 'placebo responders'; at one time or another, all subjects may respond to placebos. Moreover, there is a lack of consistency, not only in the frequency of placebo responses from study to study, but also in the kind of response observed. Since all drugs may produce placebo effects, the placebo response obviously represents a complicating factor in the study of drugs, particularly in human subjects. In Chapter 16, in discussing the development of a new drug, we shall see how the placebo response is evaluated within each experiment to ensure that the information obtained about drug action is meaningful.

REMARKS

We shall postpone summarizing the contents of this chapter until we have discussed the factors modifying drug response that are associated with the conditions of drug administration. Then at the conclusion of Chapter 12, having viewed modification in drug response from the perspective of the variability attributable both to the biologic system and to the conditions of drug administration, we can summarize the many contributory factors from another point of view.

GUIDES FOR STUDY AND REVIEW

How may differences in body weight and size affect the intensity of response to a given dose of drug? On what basis is the average adult dose of a drug calculated? Why would body surface area be a more discriminative index than body weight for adjustment of drug dosage?

In which population groups would age be most likely to influence the response to a given drug dosage? What factors are responsible for variability in drug response in the elderly? in the very young?

In the very young, what factors account for changes in rates of drug absorption? for changes in rates of drug elimination? How do changes in the rate of drug absorption or rate of elimination affect the quantitative response to a drug in the very young? How does a decrease in the rate of elimination affect the *maximum concentration* in the body of a drug that is rapidly absorbed? slowly absorbed? How does a decrease in the rate of elimination affect the duration of action of a drug that is rapidly absorbed? slowly absorbed? When is it necessary to adjust the size of a single dose of a drug? the frequency of administration of a drug?

How do we now define the term *idiosyncrasy* with respect to response to a drug? How does the quantal (frequency) dose-response relationship distinguish between the normal variability in response to a drug and the variability due to an idiosyncratic response? The normal frequency distribution (continuous variability) is associated with which type of inheritance? The bimodal (discontinuous) biologic variation is associated with which type of inheritance?

Why are idiosyncratic responses to drugs usually attributable to genetic modifications of specific proteins? What is an example of an abnormal drug response that is brought about by a genetic modification in an enzyme of biotransformation? in a drug transporter? in a drug receptor?

How does interspecies variation in drug response complicate the development and testing of therapeutic agents to be used in humans? What are the most important factors (or sources) of species variation in response to drugs? For what general types of drugs is a marked difference between species a desirable and indeed an essential circumstance?

What are some of the physiologic variables, other than age, body weight and size, that may modify the response of an individual to a given dose of drug? How can severe liver or kidney disease influence the maximum effect and duration of action of a single dose of a drug? of multiple doses of a single drug? In the presence of liver disease, what dosage adjustments are necessary with respect to a drug eliminated primarily by biotransformation? In the presence of kidney disease, what dosage adjustments are necessary with respect to a drug eliminated primarily by urinary excretion?

How do psychologic factors influence the response to a drug? What is a placebo effect? What is a placebo?

What percentage of a population may be expected to display a 'placebo response'? What form may a placebo response take? Are 'placebo responders' always the same group of individuals or may anyone at some time respond to a placebo? How does the placebo response affect the determination of a drug's efficacy? In the development of a new drug, how is the placebo response evaluated to ensure accurate information about a drug's potential efficacy?

SUGGESTED READING

Alcorn, J. and McNamara, P.J. Ontogeny of hepatic and renal systemic clearance pathways in infants: part I. *Clin. Pharmacokinet.* 41:959–998, 2002.

Alcorn, J. and McNamara, P.J. Ontogeny of hepatic and renal systemic clearance pathways in infants: part II. *Clin Pharmacokinet.* 41:1077–1094, 2002.

Alcorn, J. and McNamara, P.J. Pharmacokinetics in the newborn. *Adv. Drug Delivery Reviews* 55: 667–686, 2003.

Beecher, H.K. *Measurement of Subjective Responses: Quantitative Effects of Drugs.* New York: Oxford University Press, 1959.

Beierle, I., Meibohm, B. and Derendorf, H. Gender differences in pharmacokinetics and pharmaco-dynamics. *Int. J. Clin. Pharmacol. Ther.* 37:529–547, 1999.

Bourne, H.R. The placebo: a poorly understood and neglected therapeutic agent. *Ration. Drug Ther.* 5:1, 1971.

Bressler, R. and Bahl, J.J. Principles of drug therapy for the elderly patient. *Mayo Clin. Proc.* 78:1564–1577, 2003.

Evans, W.E. and Johnson, J.A. Pharmacogenomics: the inherited basis for interindividual differ-ences in drug response. *Annual Review of Genomics & Human Genetics* 2:9–39, 2001.

Evans, W.E. Pharmacogenomics: marshalling the human genome to individualise drug therapy. *Gut* 52(Suppl II):ii10-ii18, 2003.

Goldstein, D.B., Tate, S. and Sisodiya, S.M. Pharmacogenetics goes genomic. *Nature Reviews Genet-ics* 4: 937–947, 2003.

Hrobjartsson, A. and Gotzsche, P.C. Is the placebo powerless? An analysis of clinical trials compar-ing placebo with no treatment. *N. Engl. J. Med.* 344:1594–1602, 2001.

Kearns, G.L., Abdel-Rahman, S.M., Alander, S.W., Blowey, D.L., Leeder, J.S. and Kauffman, R.E. Drug therapy: developmental pharmacology – drug disposition, action, and therapy in infants and children. *N. Engl. J. Med.* 349:1157–1167, 2003.

Lennard, M.S. Genetically determined adverse drug reactions involving metabolism. *Drug Safety* 9:60, 1993.

McLeod, H.L. and Evans, W.E. Pharmacogenomics: unlocking the human genome for better drug therapy. *Annu. Rev. Pharmacol. Toxicol.* 41:101–121, 2001.

Meibohm, B., Beierle, I. and Derendorf, H. How important are gender differences in pharmacoki-netics? *Clin. Pharmacokinet* 41:329–342, 2002.

Price-Evans, D.A. *Genetic Factors in Drug Therapy, Clinical and Molecular Pharmacogenetics.* Cambridge: Cambridge University Press, 1993.

Reidenberg, M.M. Evolving ways that drug therapy is individualized. *Clin. Pharmacol Ther.* 74:197–202, 2003.

Sakaeda, T., Nakamura, T. and Okumura, K. Pharmacogenetics of MDR1 and its impact on the pharmacokinetics and pharmacodynamics of drugs. *Pharmacogenomics* 4:397–410, 2003.

Small, K.M., McGraw, D.W. and Liggett, S.B. Pharmacology and physiology of human adrenergic receptor polymorphisms. *Annu. Rev. Pharmacol. Toxicol.* 43:381–411, 2003.

Xie, H.G., Kim, R.B. Wood, A.J. and Stein, C.M. Molecular basis of ethnic differences in drug dis-position and response. *Annu. Rev. Pharmacol. Toxicol.* 41:815–850, 2001.

12

Factors Modifying the Effects of Drugs in Individuals

II. Variability in Response Attributable to the Conditions of Administration

We have already discussed in detail how the size of the dose administered, the pharmaceutical formulation, and the route and frequency of administration modify the effects produced by a drug. Although these four factors are the most important variables attributable to the conditions of administration, several others may also profoundly affect the response to a drug. All these other factors have one condition in common: *the effects they produce are dependent on the previous administration of the same or a different drug*. We shall discuss first the modified drug effects that may be seen following the repeated administration of a single agent and then how the sequential or concurrent administration of two different drugs may enhance or diminish the effects of either or both.

MODIFIED DRUG EFFECTS AFTER REPEATED ADMINISTRATION OF A SINGLE DRUG

Drug Resistance

The term *drug resistance* describes a state of decreased responsiveness, or complete lack of responsiveness, to drugs that ordinarily inhibit growth or cause cell death. Drug resistance is therefore a phenomenon which, by definition, may be associated only with drugs used to eliminate (1) an uneconomic species such as insects, bacteria, viruses or other parasites or (2) rapidly replicating cells such as cancer cells in higher organisms.

Origin of Drug Resistance

The sequence of events leading to the emergence of a strain of bacteria with altered drug response is typical of the general phenomenon of the development of drug resistance. When a strain of bacteria is exposed for the first time to an antibacterial agent, the effect produced is what is anticipated: retardation of the normal growth rate or reduction in the size of the bacterial population. As drug therapy continues, however, bacterial growth resumes, indicating that the organisms now present are unaffected by the same concentration of drug that was inhibitory or lethal to the original population. Thus a bacterial population that was initially sensitive to a drug has become insensitive; it has *acquired* resistance. The clinical consequences of this acquired resistance in a patient under treatment for an infection can readily be appreciated. If the pathogenic organism is one that would normally respond to the drug being used, the patient would at first show improvement. Then when resistance developed, the patient would suffer a relapse as the infecting organism became refractory to the previously used drug.

How do organisms such as bacteria acquire this resistance to the toxic effects of drugs? The answer lies partly in the fact that some species of microorganisms undergo spontaneous mutation. Populations of many bacteria do not consist solely of genetically identical cells; they are normally composed of individuals with different degrees of inherited susceptibility to an antibacterial drug, including some genetically altered cells that are completely drug-resistant. The number of spontaneous mutants that are drug-resistant may be as few as one in ten billion cells. In the presence of an antibacterial agent, the mutants that are insensitive to the drug survive and multiply, giving rise eventually to an entirely new drug-resistant population. Thus the drug permits survival of the least susceptible organisms. And the appearance of drug resistance during therapy merely represents selective multiplication of those insensitive mutants that were present *from the beginning of the infection*. The only role that the drug plays is to select out the resistant cells at the expense of the sensitive strain.

The fact that it is the microorganism, and not the patient, that becomes resistant to the drug also accounts for the increase and spread of drug-resistant strains of bacteria within a human or animal population. Extensive and prolonged use of a particular antibacterial agent provides the opportunity for eliminating the bulk of sensitive microorganisms while sparing the resistant mutants. The latter become the predominant strain and spread from infected patients to uninfected individuals and from them to the community. For example, in the United States in 1940 to 1941, over 70% of patients with gonorrhea were rapidly cured by the use of various sulfa drugs. Four years later these same drugs failed in 70% of the patients, since many strains of the gonococcus had become resistant to sulfonamides. Fortunately, penicillin became available for use at this time and proved to be successful in treating the sulfonamide-refractory gonococcal infections. As a rule, microorganisms resistant to a particular drug like sulfanilamide tend to be equally insensitive to other chemically related agents, such as other sulfonamides. However, they remain sensitive to chemically dissimilar agents such as penicillins, which act by other mechanisms.

The genetic determinant of drug resistance may also be transferred from insensitive organisms to other organisms that are not direct offspring of the resistant cells. Cell-to-cell contact is necessary for this phenomenon, called *infectious drug resistance* (Fig. 12-1). Drug resistance may be acquired by a sen-

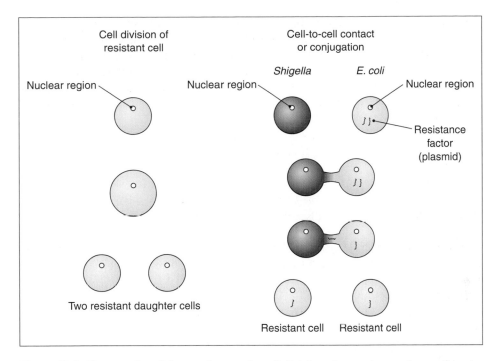

Figure 12-1. *The transfer of drug resistance. In cell division, drug resistance is transferred from the parent cell to daughter cells together with all the other genetic information contained on the chromosomes of the parent cell. This type of transfer retains the resistance to a drug within the particular strain and species of bacteria. In conjugation, the carrier of the genetic determinant for drug resistance, the plasmid, is independent of the chromosomes of the host bacterium. This extrachromosomal fragment, found in the cytoplasm and not in the nucleus, is self replicating. When a resistant cell conjugates with (or contacts) a nonresistant cell of the same or different strain or species, the resistance factor is passed to the nonresistant cell. In the figure this is shown as the transfer of drug resistance from the usually harmless, nonpathogenic* Escherichia coli *to* Shigella, *a pathogenic bacterium which causes dysentery.*

sitive organism in contact with an insensitive organism of the same or a different strain of the same species, or even of a different species. This has considerable clinical significance since it means that the genetic determinants of drug resistance may be transferred from a nonpathogenic to a pathogenic bacterial species. Reports from many areas of the world indicate that an increasing number of diseases are caused by microorganisms that have acquired resistance to several drugs by infectious transferral. The widespread use of antibacterial agents not only in medicine but in agriculture (livestock feed) is a contributory factor. Again, by preventing the growth of drug-sensitive organisms, the drug promotes the survival of those bacteria that can spread the infectious drug resistance.

The best means of overcoming drug resistance is to prevent its emergence in the first place. This can be accomplished most effectively by avoiding unnecessary, promiscuous use of antibacterial agents. Once it has been established that a particular agent can reasonably be expected to have a salutary effect, adequate doses should be given to stop the multiplication of micro-organisms as quickly as possible. Drug treatment should begin early and continue for a sufficiently long period to ensure that all the infectious organisms are eradicated before treatment is discontinued.

Mechanisms of Drug Resistance

There are a number of mechanisms that can account for the drug resistance of the genetically altered organisms, but we shall consider only those that have been shown to be most frequently responsible for the phenomenon (Table 12-1).

ELABORATION OF SPECIFIC INACTIVATING ENZYMES. This is one of the best-documented mechanisms by which mutants resist the activity of antibacterial agents. For example, the main basis for the bacterial resistance to penicillins and cephalosporins is the production of the enzyme penicillinase, which hydrolyzes the antibiotics to inactive metabolites. This enzyme is also referred to as β-lactamase because it breaks open the four-carbon lactam ring that is key to the antibacterial activity of these drugs. The production of this enzyme (as well as that of all enzymes) is genetically controlled; a microbial cell must possess the necessary genetic information in order to synthesize the active penicillinase molecule. Entire populations of some species of bacteria are natural producers of penicillinase and have always been penicillin-resistant because of the presence of large amounts of the enzyme. In such normally resistant bacteria, penicillinase is a constitutive enzyme, i.e. an enzyme that is an integral part of the normal organization of the cell.

Organisms that are initially sensitive may acquire resistance to penicillin in one of two ways. Some bacterial species have the genetic potential to synthesize penicillinase but produce it only in amounts too meager to protect the cells even against low concentrations of penicillin. However, penicillinase is also an *inducible* enzyme, and in the presence of an inducer (usually one of the penicillins), the enzyme is elaborated in increasingly greater quantities. Whereas trace amounts of penicillinase in an entire population, or large amounts in a few cells, are insufficient to protect the bacteria, an entire population producing penicillinase can cooperatively provide the means for survival. This is the type of penicillin resistance that can best be prevented by early use of large enough doses of penicillin to eradicate the organism before the emergence of increased enzyme activity.

The second way that mutants of normally sensitive bacteria can acquire resistance to penicillin is by penicillinase becoming a constitutive rather than an inducible enzyme. These mutants become the dominant forms by the mechanisms previously described: (1) selective multiplication in the presence of the drug of those insensitive variants arising from random mutations, and (2) infec-

Table 12-1. *Mechanisms and examples of drug resistance*

Mechanism	Resistant species	Drug to which resistance acquired
Elaboration of specific inactivating enzymes	Bacteria	Penicillins
		Cephalosporins
		Chloramphenicol
		Kanamycin
	Insects	DDT
		Malathion
Decreased intracellular availability	Bacteria	Tetracycline
		Sulfonamides
		Isoniazid
	Cancer cells	6-Mercaptopurine
		Methotrexate
	Parasites:	
	Malarial	Chloroquine
	Trypanosomes	Organic arsenic containing drugs
Decreased affinity of drug for its target site	Bacteria	Sulfonamides
		Streptomycin
	HIV	Reverse transcriptase inhibitors
		Protease inhibitors
	Cancer cells	6-Mercaptopurine
	Rats	Warfarin (used as rodenticide)

tious transfer of drug resistance. Mutants possessing constitutive enzymes produce large quantities of penicillinase even in the absence of the drug. Individuals infected by these insensitive organisms manifest an immediate rather than a delayed appearance of drug resistance at first exposure to penicillin.

Insect populations may also acquire resistance to various insecticides by producing specific inactivating enzymes. For example, insects that have become insensitive to malathion have been found to possess a greatly increased capacity to convert the insecticide to a nontoxic metabolite before its conversion to the toxic metabolite malaoxon (cf. Fig. 8-11).

DECREASED INTRACELLULAR AVAILABILITY. When a drug acts intracellularly, any change that significantly decreases its rate of entry renders the cell resistant to the action of the drug. Changes in the permeability characteristics of the cell membrane may decrease the rate of passive diffusion, whereas changes in a carrier system may diminish the rate of facilitated diffusion or active transport into a cell or accelerate its transport out. In either case the result is a lowered concentration of drug within the cell.

Malarial parasites that have become resistant to the antimalarial drug chloroquine have been found to accumulate less drug than sensitive plasmodia. The drug resistance to arsenic-containing organic compounds acquired by trypanosomes (the organisms causing sleeping sickness) has also been attributed to decreased intracellular concentrations of drug. And the resistance developed in certain malignancies to a number of drugs has been shown to involve a decrease in their accumulation in the cancer cells. For example, the resistance to methotrexate, a drug actively transported into cells, is due to a change in the affinity of the carrier for the drug. In other cases the resistance results from too rapid efflux out of the tumor cell, mediated for example by the multi-drug resistance transporter.

DECREASED AFFINITY OF DRUG FOR ITS TARGET SITE. We have seen that genetic modifications of specific proteins are responsible for idiosyncratic drug responses. The altered protein or enzyme, originating as an error in the normal replication process, becomes permanently encoded in the gene if the alteration is compatible with life. Analogously, genetic modification may be responsible for drug resistance when an alteration occurs in a protein that is the specific target of the drug causing growth inhibition or cell death. If the drug cannot interact with the altered protein as readily as with the normal protein, the cells containing the former will survive at the expense of those containing the latter. For example, sulfa drugs inhibit the growth of sensitive bacteria by competing with para-aminobenzoic acid (PABA) for binding sites on the enzyme catalyzing the first step in the synthesis of folic acid (cf. Fig. 11-6). In resistant bacteria the sulfa drugs can no longer interact effectively with this enzyme and, consequently, do not inhibit the incorporation of PABA into the essential vitamin. The enzyme is altered only with respect to the drug and can still combine effectively with its normal substrate. Thus, genetically determined alterations in enzymes of microorganisms are responsible for their resistance to the action of sulfa drugs as well as of other drugs. This mechanism accounts for the problem of resistance to antiviral agents, such as those used in HIV infections. The high mutation rate in viruses has led to many altered forms of the target enzymes of drug therapy. For HIV infection these targets include viral reverse transcriptase and viral protease with discoveries in the 1990s of many effective inhibitors of these enzymes. However, resistant viruses quickly emerged. Typically, mutant forms of the enzymes were found to have altered structures that result in decreased affinity of the drugs for these targets.

The Distinguishing Characteristics of Drug Resistance

Drug resistance and idiosyncratic drug response are both genetically based abnormal drug responses. They are readily distinguished from each other, however, in other respects: (1) the phenomenon of drug resistance is limited to those agents that ordinarily inhibit growth or cause cell death; (2) only the development of drug resistance is dependent on previous administration of the same or structurally related drug; and (3) drug resistance is seen only as a decreased responsiveness. The anticoagulant warfarin provides an excellent example, however, of a genetically determined abnormal reactivity classified as drug resistance or idiosyncrasy depending on the species involved. Warfarin, one of the most frequently used rodenticides, leads to selective cumulative toxicity and death in rats because of its slow rate of elimination in this species. A strain of rats has developed that is resistant to the lethal effects of the anticoagulant, and this acquired resistance is the result of genetic modification in an essential protein of the blood-clotting system. In contrast, the decreased anticoagulant activity of warfarin in some humans is an idiosyncratic response, since it is evident with the first administration in the genetically abnormal individual.

Drug Allergy

Allergy is an adverse response to a foreign chemical resulting from a previous exposure to the substance; it is manifested only after a second or subsequent exposure and then as a reaction *different from the usual pharmacologic effects of the chemical*. Since drug allergy occurs in susceptible individuals who usually constitute only a small fraction of all people receiving the particular drug, it could be classified as a cause of variability in drug response attributable to the biologic system. It is discussed here, however, to emphasize the fact that a drug can produce an allergic reaction only after a previous sensitizing contact with the agent or with one closely related in chemical structure. Since a minute amount of an otherwise safe drug may elicit the allergic response, the term *hypersensitivity*, although somewhat misleading, is used commonly to describe the sensitization reaction. Because the allergic response is unusual, it is sometimes confused with the idiosyncratic response. The inappropriateness of both these terms is readily revealed by considering the mechanism involved in the production of the allergic response and the characteristics of the reaction itself.

The Mechanism of the Allergic Reaction

Drug allergies are produced by essentially the same mechanisms as other allergies such as hay fever or food allergy. As far back as 1913, the Englishman Sir Henry H. Dale, who won the Nobel Prize in Medicine in 1936 for research in other areas, suggested that an allergic response involves a typical immunologic reaction.

The immune response is a normal defense mechanism that is set in motion when a foreign agent like bacteria is introduced into the body for the first time. The invasive organism stimulates the formation of specific proteins called *antibodies*. By definition, any substance which induces the synthesis of antibodies is an antigen. After the period required for their production, usually from several days to more than a week, the newly formed antibodies, or *immunoglobulins*, are found in blood plasma and other body fluids as well as in various tissues. The appearance of the antibodies signals the development of immunity to the particular antigenic bacteria (or other antigen); i.e. the antibodies react with the antigen that stimulated their production to form antigen-antibody complexes. It is the formation of such complexes that normally confers protection against the further development of disease by nullifying the otherwise damaging invading agents. Thus the immune system is the body's conventional way of safeguarding itself from harmful foreign substances such as bacteria or viruses.

These antigen-antibody interactions show a remarkable degree of physico-chemical specificity. It is the antigen itself that is responsible for this; antigens are also macromolecules, usually proteins, with a large number of determinant chemical groups, or 'antigenic sites'. Indeed, the action of an antibody upon the antigen that stimulated its production is usually compared to that of a lock and its key. However, the lock-and-key concept of the antigen-antibody reaction is somewhat different from the analogous interpretation of the interaction of a drug and its receptor. In the latter, the drug is the key that must fit the preexisting lock, the receptor, in order to open the way for the events that follow. In the antigen-antibody reaction there is a prefabricated key, the antigen, for which a specific lock, the antibody, must be fashioned. After the specific lock (antibody) has been installed, only the original key (antigen), or one very similar, can release what lies behind the locked door.

Allergic reactions, like the immune responses to bacteria, also begin with the formation of rather specific antibody proteins capable of complexing with their corresponding antigens. Since the substances responsible for hay fever or food allergy are either proteins or complex macromolecules, it is understandable in the classic immunologic context how these materials may act as antigens. But if antigens must be proteins or other large molecules with specific regions that can act as antigenic determinants, how can simple compounds like penicillin take part in the allergic reaction? Drugs that are small molecules and that are relatively simple in structure do not become antigenic until they combine with body proteins. It is the relatively stable complex formed between a drug and a conjugate protein that is the active antigen. Simple chemicals capable of binding with a protein to form a product that has antigenic properties are termed haptens; the structure of the hapten in the hapten-protein complex determines the specificity of the induced antibody.

The initial contact of an individual with a foreign material having potentially antigenic properties and the ensuing formation of a specific antibody comprise the sensitizing portion of the immune mechanism. The reaction part of the total phenomenon is seen only when the sensitized individual is reexposed to the antigen or hapten. The problem in allergy is that the formation of the antigen-antibody complex triggers a series of events that can be highly damaging. Thus, in the allergic individual, a normally protective and essential mechanism goes awry. The antibodies induced by bacteria or viruses act to neutralize these organisms on subsequent invasions. But the antibodies produced in response to haptens convert drugs that are harmless, if used properly, into noxious substances.

It is important to stress that the manifestations of drug allergy are the consequences of antigen-antibody actions and are unrelated to the pharmacologic activity of the eliciting drug. In some cases, the allergic response may be manifest as tissue damage or cell destruction resulting from the antibody forming a complex with the antigen bound to the tissue or cell. In other cases, the antibody is present in the circulation and when bound to antigen the complex deposits in a site such as the blood vessel wall and elicits an inflammatory response. And in many allergic reactions, the antigen interacts with a type of antibody bound to the surface of specialized cells containing inflammatory mediators (Fig. 12-2). These *mediators* are present as inactive precursors or stored within cellular vesicles and become pharmacologically active only when released. One of the chief mediators of allergy in humans is histamine, a natural amine widely distributed throughout the body and stored in high concentrations in mast cells and in basophils. It is because the allergic response is due to the

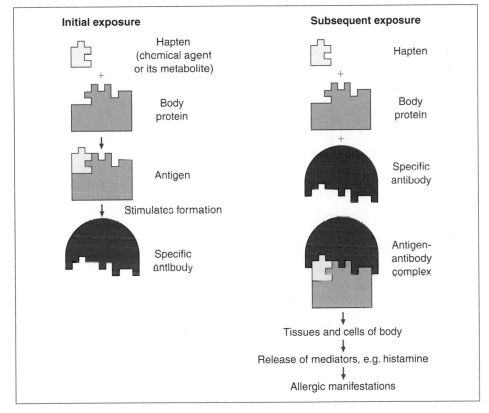

Figure 12-2. *Mechanism of the allergic response. In the initial exposure, the drug (hapten) combines with a body protein to form the antigen, which then stimulates the formation of specific antibodies. The present concept of the immunopathogenesis of histamine release from mast cells upon subsequent exposure to the hapten involves the following sequence of events: (1) the specific antibodies bind at one end to mast cells, leaving antigen-binding sites free to react; (2) the antigen binds to antibody at antigen-binding sites; and (3) the antigen-antibody complex triggers the release of histamine.*

release of one or more of these mediators, including leukotrienes, prostaglandins, platelet activating factor, bradykinin, and others, that various *allergic manifestations are effects characteristic of the mediators* and not the allergenic drugs.

Manifestations of the Allergic Reaction

Allergic reactions to drugs manifest themselves as a variety of symptoms involving various organ systems and ranging from minor skin rashes to a potentially fatal loss of blood pressure (Table 12–2). Reactions may be localized or widespread, and the symptoms may appear immediately or within hours to days following administration of the eliciting drug to the sensitized individual.

The immediate response is due in part to the release of histamine by the antigen-antibody complex. The reaction may involve the respiratory and gastrointestinal tracts, the blood vessels, the skin or all of these. Characteristic symptoms include difficulty in breathing due to constriction of the airways of the upper respiratory tract (bronchial asthma), swelling of the mucous membranes and a fall in blood pressure. *Anaphylaxis* is the most serious immediate type of allergic response. In its severest form – anaphylactic shock – death may occur within a few minutes as a result of complete obstruction of respiratory passages and the precipitous lowering of blood pressure.

Inflammation and excessive secretions of the nose and eyes (as in hay fever)

Table 12-2. *Common manifestations of allergic reactions in the human[1]*

Tissue or organ	Symptom	Hapten commonly involved
Skin	Hives (urticaria) and generalized itching	Penicillins
	Rashes	Cephalosporins
		Sulfonamides
		Allopurinol
	Exfoliative dermatitis (loss of superficial skin layers)	Tetracycline
		Sulfonamides
Mucous membranes (particularly of nose and eye)	Inflammation, swelling and excessive secretions	Sulfonamides
		Barbiturates
Respiratory tract	Difficulty in breathing	Penicillins
		Local anesthetics (esters)
Vascular system	Fall in blood pressure	Penicillins
Blood cells	Reduction in the number of one or more types of circulating blood cells	Penicillins
		Cephalosporins

[1]The presence of an antibody that reacts specifically with the sensitizing drug has been demonstrated in the case of each of the drugs cited as well as for a number of other drugs.

and generalized hives and itching may also be manifest as immediate allergic responses. But they are not typical of the immediate response, since their appearance is sometimes delayed. The severity of the delayed allergic responses may vary from trivial skin eruptions to destruction of red blood cells and blood-forming tissues and even to fatal loss of superficial layers of skin *(exfoliative dermatitis)*.

The pattern of allergic response to an agent is not entirely predictable in different individuals or in the same individual at different times. On the other hand, one or more allergic symptoms may be more commonly associated with a particular drug than are others from among the entire gamut of possible responses. For example, hives and generalized itching are the symptoms most frequently seen when individuals sensitized to penicillin are re-exposed to the antibiotic. In contrast, fatal anaphylactic reactions, which may follow the administration of as little as 1 μg of penicillin, are relatively rare. The important point is that the pattern of allergic response is dependent on the kind and amount of mediator(s) liberated, or the tissue or cell damage caused by the antigen-antibody reaction; it is independent of the chemical structure or pharmacologic effects of the eliciting drug.

Incidence of Allergic Reactions to Drugs

So many different drugs have haptenic qualities that allergic responses represent the largest single group of adverse drug reactions. However, the frequency of allergic reactions to most drugs appears to be low. For example, one of the most common offenders is penicillin. Yet the incidence of allergic responses may be not greater than 5–10% among the patients receiving the antibiotic. On the other hand, some drugs, such as caffeine, have no known incidence of allergic response; and some, such as phenylethylhydantoin (NIRVANOL), led to allergic manifestations in virtually everyone. The latter agent, designed for use in epilepsy, was withdrawn after a brief trial because of its allergenic propensity.

These estimates of the frequency of allergic drug responses are based, of course, on the number of such occurrences that have been reported and recorded. They do not ordinarily include the frequency of occurrence of mild allergic reactions. Nor do they take into account all those individuals who have received a particular drug and have not manifested adverse effects. Moreover, it is often difficult to prove that the response is indeed the result of an antigen-antibody reaction. The only unequivocal evidence that a drug has produced an allergic reaction is the presence of specific antibodies in plasma or tissues. Thus the best available estimates of potential allergenicity do not really assess the attendant risk to the patient using a particular drug. Even if valid estimates of the frequency of allergic responses to a given drug were available, they could be used only to predict the fraction of a population that might be expected to be allergic. They would have no predictive value for the response in a single individual, and at present there are no generally reliable and safe procedures by which sensitization to a drug in an individual can be ascertained before drug administration. Skin patch tests or skin injection tests may themselves be hazardous, since the small quantity of drug used in these diagnostic procedures may be sufficient to induce an allergic response. It is for these reasons that drugs known to be haptens, such as many of the antibiotics, should be reserved for use only in those illnesses in which they may be lifesaving.

In some instances, the hapten is not the drug administered but is a product of its biotransformation. For example, the allergic response to the local anesthetic procaine is caused by the antigenicity of one of its metabolites, para-aminobenzoic acid (PABA). Occasionally, too, the antigen-antibody reaction is not entirely specific for the hapten that induces the formation of the antibody. Thus, individuals sensitized to procaine may show an allergic response to other local anesthetics whose biotransformation yields either PABA or a compound closely related to PABA in structure. We saw earlier that sulfanilamide is sufficiently similar in structure to PABA to be able to inhibit its enzymatic incorporation into folic acid. This structural similarity is also characteristic of other antibacterial sulfa drugs. And in some individuals allergic to procaine, the first administration of a sulfonamide will also elicit the antigen-antibody reaction. The term *cross-sensitization* denotes this lack of absolute antibody specificity for the hapten that induces its formation. It is not possible to predict whether an individual will manifest cross-sensitization to agents other than the original eliciting hapten. Thus in patients with a known history of allergic responses to a drug, it is safest to avoid using any agent that may substitute for that drug in the antigen-antibody reaction.

The Distinguishing Characteristics of Drug Allergy

Drug allergy, toxicity, and idiosyncrasy are adverse effects which, fortunately, may be considered unusual because they occur infrequently. It is important to distinguish these three effects from each other, however, since the differences among them influence the subsequent use of a drug that produces any one of them. A sharp differentiation can be made on the basis of occurrence, dose-response relationships, the mechanism by which they are produced, and the particular manifestations of the adverse effects (Table 12-3).

The occurrence of toxicity as an adverse effect can be considered unusual only in the context of quantal dose-response curves and therapeutic indices. First, toxic responses to any drug may be produced in every individual exposed to the agent simply by increasing the size of the dose. Also, if considerable overlap exists between the curves for desirable and undesirable effects (cf. Fig. 9-13), the toxic effects would not be regarded as unusual since a sizable fraction of the total population may show adverse effects at doses that are well within the therapeutic range. On the other hand, given a drug with a certain safety factor of 1 or greater (cf. Fig. 9-12), the appearance of toxicity would be infrequent. Toxicity would be evident only in the few individuals who require a maximum dose to elicit the desired effect and who also show adverse effects at doses lying at the lowest extreme of the toxicity curve. (Individuals showing

Table 12-3. Distinguishing characteristics of toxic, idiosyncratic and allergic responses to drugs

	Toxic response	Idiosyncratic response	Allergic response
Occurrence			
Incidence in population	In all subjects, if dose high enough	Only in genetically abnormal subjects	From a few per cent to 100%, depending on drug
Incidence among drugs	All drugs	Few drugs	Many drugs
Circumstance	Prior exposure unnecessary	Prior exposure unnecessary	Prior exposure essential
Dose-response relationship	Dose-related	Dose-related	Independent of dose
Mechanism	Drug-receptor interaction	Drug-receptor interaction	Through antigen-antibody reaction; specific antibody formed in response to prior dose of antigen
Effect produced	Determined by drug-receptor interaction; depends on eliciting drug	Determined by drug-receptor interaction; depends on eliciting drug	Independent of eliciting drug; determined by mediators released by or direct action of antigen-antibody complex
Effect antagonized	By specific antagonists	By specific antagonists	By antihistamines, epinephrine or anti-inflammatory steroids like cortisone

such extreme sensitivity to an action of a drug could be called hypersensitive; hence the confusion in using the term *hypersensitivity* in referring to the allergic state.) A simple reduction in the dose may be sufficient to eliminate this type of adverse effect of any drug.

The size of the dose, however, does not determine whether an individual will have an idiosyncratic or allergic response to a drug. Idiosyncratic responses occur infrequently and only in genetically abnormal subjects. Heredity may also play a role in determining whether an individual is susceptible to one or more antigenic substances. But only in allergy is prior exposure to the offending drug an absolute requirement for the subsequent development of the adverse response. That prior exposure has occurred may not always be known. It may occur inadvertently through environmental contact or dietary intake. For example, moldy foods, such as bread or certain cheeses, or milk from penicillin-treated cows, may be the source of sensitization to this antibiotic.

Both toxic and idiosyncratic effects are the result of drug-receptor interactions and consequently show the usual dose-response relationships. Thus the pharmacologic effects observed are determined by both the physicochemical properties of the drugs and their ability to combine with specific receptor sites. In contrast, the manifestations of the allergic reaction are unrelated to the structure or pharmacologic activity of the particular eliciting drug; they are mediated through endogenous substances released by the antigen-antibody complex. There is, therefore, no predictable dose-response relationship between the hapten and the allergic effects. A minute amount of an otherwise safe drug may not only sensitize an individual but also elicit a severe allergic reaction. Conversely, an ordinary therapeutic dose may elicit only mild allergic symptoms in the sensitized patient. Moreover, since the effects seen in allergy do not result from the interaction of the antigenic drug and its normal receptor, the allergic response cannot be overcome by agents antagonizing the actions of the eliciting drug. Indeed, drugs which antagonize the allergic responses to one drug may be useful against similar effects of any antigenic drug. For example, nalorphine can abolish the toxic effects of an overdose of morphine or counteract the rare idiosyncratic response to the opioid analgesic. Nalorphine is useless, however, in treating allergic-like responses to morphine, whereas an antihistaminic drug may have ameliorative effects.

Drug Tolerance

Tolerance is a condition of *decreased responsiveness* acquired after prior or repeated exposure to a given drug or to one closely allied to it in pharmacologic activity. Tolerance is characterized by the necessity of increasing the size of successive doses in order to produce effects of equal magnitude or duration. Alternatively, it is an inability of the subsequent administration of the same dose of a drug to be as effective as the preceding dose.

Tolerance may be acquired to various effects of many drugs, especially those of opioid analgesics, barbiturates, alcohol and other agents depressing the

Table 12-4. *Mechanisms and examples of drug tolerance*

Drug disposition tolerance	*Pharmacodynamic tolerance*
Barbiturates	Barbiturates
Alcohol	Alcohol
Benzopyrene	Morphine and other opioid analgesics
	Nalorphine (antagonist of opioid analgesics)
	Amphetamine
	Methylphenidate
	Lysergic acid diethylamide
	Caffeine
	Nicotine
Tachyphylaxis	*Tachyphylaxis*
Ephedrine	Nitrates
Tyramine	Atropine
Morphine	

central nervous system such as benzodiazepines, nitrates, atropine, and central nervous system stimulants like amphetamine, nicotine, and caffeine (Table 12-4). The tolerance developed to drugs that profoundly affect mood, thought and behavior is frequently associated with either physical or psychologic dependence, or both. The interrelationship of tolerance and these other factors is discussed separately in Chapter 15. Here we are concerned only with the general aspects of the phenomenon of drug tolerance and the mechanisms responsible for its development.

Given that the quantitative effect of a drug is determined by its concentration and extent of chemical reaction at an effector site, there are several ways whereby an individual can become tolerant to a drug. Tolerance may be the consequence of conditions that produce a decrease in the effective concentration of the agonist at the site of action or a reduction in the normal reactivity of the receptor. Tolerance developed by the first mechanism is called *drug-disposition or biochemical tolerance*; that by the second is *cellular* or *pharmaco-dynamic tolerance.*

Drug-disposition tolerance may occur when a drug reduces its own absorption or its rate of transfer across any biologic barrier, or when it increases its own rate of elimination. The best examples of tolerance produced by this mechanism are provided by drugs like phenobarbital and ethanol, which are capable of increasing their own rates of biotransformation through stimulation of microsomal enzyme systems (cf. Table 8-5 and Fig. 8-9). However, drug-disposition tolerance accounts for only a small part of the total tolerance developed to these and other agents acting on the central nervous system; a reduction in the normal reactivity of receptors plays the principal role (see below).

Whether drug-disposition tolerance is exhibited as a decrease in peak effect and duration of action, or only as the latter, strongly depends on the route of drug administration. When a drug is given intravenously, the initial concentration at the target site – and hence the magnitude of effect observed – will be the same in tolerant and nontolerant subjects. In both, the entire dose will be distributed before differences in rates of biotransformation can significantly influence drug availability. However, as a result of the increased rate of drug elimination, the duration of action will be shorter in the tolerant state than it was before tolerance was developed. This means, of course, that the intravenous dose producing a toxic or lethal effect is essentially the same for both the nontolerant individual and the subject made tolerant to the drug by this mechanism. In contrast, when a drug is given to the tolerant subject by a slow-absorption route, both the duration of action and the peak effect observed will be reduced. This is so because, for any given drug, the faster the rate of elimination relative to absorption, the lower the peak concentration attained and the shorter the duration of action. Whereas the rate of absorption remains the same in the tolerant and intolerant state, the rate of elimination is increased in the tolerant individual.

Tolerance is sometimes the indirect effect of the administered drug, even though it develops as the consequence of a reduced effective concentration of an agonist at its target site. For a number of drugs do not produce all their effects by direct combination with a receptor. Instead, they act at other cellular sites to release endogenous, physiologically active substances like histamine, which are inactive in their bound form (see Chapter 14 for full discussion). Once released from their storage sites, these endogenous substances become agonists and combine with receptors to initiate an action-effects sequence (Fig. 12-3). (This is analogous to the antigen-antibody complex giving rise to the symptoms of allergy.) These stores of endogenous, active substances may be gradually depleted if the interval between doses of a drug that releases them is too short to permit their replenishment. As the stored quantity of the physiologic agonist is diminished, the effect elicited on repeated administration of the same or larger doses of the releasing agent is correspondingly reduced. For example, the histamine stored in various cells and tissues can be released by morphine. One of the effects produced by the released histamine is a dilatation of cutaneous blood vessels, readily observed in humans as flushing of the face, neck, and upper thorax. If small doses of morphine are given to an animal over a period of several weeks, there is little attenuation of this peripheral vasodilatation. However, with large doses, tolerance develops rapidly, due mainly to the unavailability of adequate stores of histamine. The term *tachyphylaxis* (cf. Table 12-4) is used to describe the acute development of tolerance to the rapid, repeated administration of a drug.

Tachyphylaxis may also occur as a result of a change in the sensitivity of the target cells. A case in point is the tolerance to nitroglycerin observed among

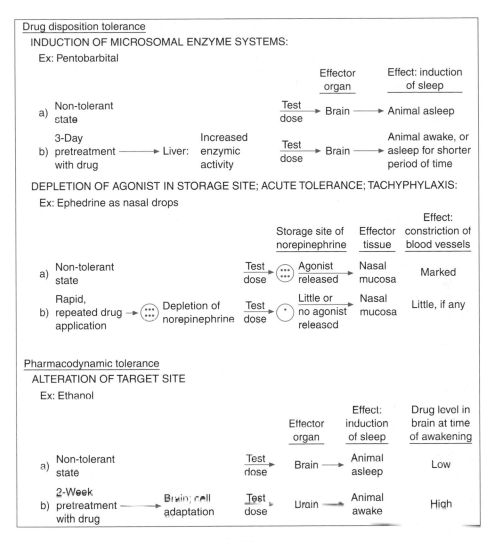

Figure 12-3. *Mechanisms of development of drug tolerance.*

workers exposed to this drug in the manufacture of explosives. During the first few days of their exposure, new employees frequently suffer severe headaches, dizziness and nausea. These symptoms quickly disappear as pharmacodynamic tolerance develops. But they may reappear if the worker returns to his job after a few days' absence; hence the term *Monday disease* to describe the return of symptoms after a weekend away from work. When nitroglycerin is used to treat angina pectoris, tolerance rarely develops, since continuous exposure to the drug is not customary. Transdermal patches containing nitroglycerin must be removed at night to avoid this problem (cf. p. 99). Although the mechanism of tolerance to nitrates is not clearly understood, it does not result from more rapid elimination of drug or decreased availability of drug to sites of action.

Another example of acute tolerance can be observed in the case of alcohol. The level of brain impairment or degree of intoxication is greater during the rising phase of the blood alcohol curve compared to the descending portion of the blood alcohol curve. Thus, a particular blood alcohol concentration will produce two different levels of intoxification in the same individual over a few hours, depending on whether their blood levels of alcohol are rising or falling. Two phenomena underlie this tolerance. First, the brain levels of alcohol are higher during the rising phase of the blood alcohol curve than during the falling phase. Second, the target receptors for alcohol (i.e. GABA receptors) become less sensitive to alcohol with continued exposure, even during acute exposure.

Pharmacodynamic or cellular tolerance is usually observed as a slowly developed phenomenon rather than acute tolerance or tachyphylaxis. Various mechanisms are involved in cellular tolerance, such as a decrease in the availability of receptors for binding to drugs, a decrease in receptor sensitivity, or a decrease in the ability of the bound receptors to produce a response. Much progress has been made in elucidating the molecular events that underlie these changes in ligand-gated ion channels and in G-protein-coupled receptors. With the former, continued exposure to the drug ligand may change the receptor composition through synthesis of different subunits that have lower affinity for the drug. With the latter, continued drug exposure may cause biochemical modification of the receptors, such as phosphorylation, that leads to their internalization by endocytosis and loss of availability for drug binding. And for some G-protein-coupled receptors, such as those activated by opioids, continued drug exposure leads to a change in the type of G-protein coupled to the receptors and therefore a change in signal transduction.

Tolerance of this type is seen with some classes of drugs acting on the central nervous system to produce changes in mood and behavior, including the opioids and the benzodiazepines. Altered reactivity of target sites within the brain is also the primary mechanism for the development of tolerance for those central nervous system depressants, the barbiturates and ethanol, which can also increase their own rate of biotransformation. The tolerance developed to ethanol provides an example of the evidence available to support this view. With chronic use, alcohol can induce microsomal enzymes to increase its metabolism, but this is a small component of the biotransformation pathway for alcohol. When the relationship between sleeping time and drug concentrations within the brain is determined, animals made tolerant to ethanol are found to awaken at brain levels of ethanol significantly higher than those at which nontolerant animals are still asleep. Even when chronic drinkers drink enough alcohol to produce high blood levels, they still exhibit tolerance. This is due to a reduced sensitivity of the cellular targets of alcohol, such as GABA receptors. Drug tolerance should not be confused with drug resistance, which involves a separate population of insensitive targets, such as bacteria.

It is apparent from what has been said that the development of tolerance may proceed by a number of mechanisms and that more than one of these may be operative in any given case. Tolerance to morphine, for example, may involve a decreased sensitivity of target cells within the brain as well as tachyphylaxis due to depletion of a physiologically active substance. And stimulation of microsomal enzyme systems in addition to a change in the reactivity of brain cells may account for the development of tolerance to ethanol. The degree of tolerance produced also varies widely from one group of drugs to another. For example, the habitual user of morphine may tolerate doses many times greater than the dose that would be lethal for a nontolerant person. In contrast, whereas individuals tolerant to alcohol or barbiturates have fewer and less marked effects from moderate doses of these agents than do abstainers, both tolerant and nontolerant subjects are affected almost equally by high or near-lethal doses of these depressants. Tolerance also does not develop uniformly to all the pharmacologic effects of a drug. In the case of morphine, for example, the highly tolerant individual exhibits tolerance to the depressant effects on the central nervous system but continues to have 'pinpoint' pupils and constipation.

Another characteristic of the tolerant state is that of cross-tolerance among drugs belonging to the same group of agents, acting by similar mechanisms. For instance, individuals made tolerant to morphine are also tolerant to heroin, methadone, and other opioids, but not to alcohol or barbiturates, which act on different receptors. On the other hand, the alcoholic may have some degree of tolerance to barbiturates, which act by similar mechanisms, but has none to the opioids. Tolerance disappears when administration of the drug that produced the phenomenon is discontinued. The rate of disappearance may be rapid, as in the case of nitrates, or prolonged, as for morphine. The special features associated with discontinuance of the use of drugs that act on the central nervous system are discussed in Chapter 15.

DRUG INTERACTIONS

It has been estimated that the average hospitalized patient may receive as many as six to ten different drugs during their confinement. In chronic disease states such as epilepsy, diabetes, and heart disease, when the patient contracts another illness, the concomitant administration of many drugs may be necessary. There are also other therapeutic situations in which multiple-drug therapy may constitute good practice. But there are many occasions when more than one drug is given to an individual, regardless of whether this is warranted. Whatever the rationale for administering several drugs concurrently, the question arises of how these drugs may affect each other's actions.

Two drugs administered at the same time may act wholly independently. For example, aspirin may lower the body temperature of the fevered patient while an appropriate antibacterial agent is eliminating the organism responsible for the disease as well as the fever. The effect of aspirin is apparently unaltered by the presence of the antibacterial agent, and vice versa. On the other hand, there are many known instances – and more come to light continually – of the concurrent use of two drugs changing the effects of one or both. The results may be a response greater than was anticipated, a decrease in effectiveness of one or both drugs, or an unanticipated toxicity. Many of the adverse effects are dose-dependent and occur only when sufficiently large doses of the interacting drugs are used. Some of the interactions may be trivial in nature, while others have proved disastrous. For example, the combination of a monoamine oxidase inhibitor, such as tranylcypromine, with another antidepressant agent like imipramine may produce convulsions, delirium, and death. To ensure the effectiveness and safety of multiple-drug therapy, the potential for drug interaction must be evaluated. In many cases newer agents in a drug class or a new class for the same therapeutic indication have replaced older drugs when interactions are less likely and therefore the use of the newer drug or drug class is safer.

We are not concerned here with the ways in which the prior administration of one drug may influence the subsequent administration of another in connection with the development of drug resistance, allergy, or tolerance. We shall limit our discussion to the interactions that occur when one agent alters the absorption, distribution, biotransformation, or excretion – or enhances or opposes the action or effects – of another drug.

Some of these interactions, such as the inhibition or induction by one drug of enzymes required for the biotransformation of other drugs, have already been discussed (cf. pp. 174–181) and will be mentioned again only briefly. To avoid ambiguity, however, we will begin by defining the terms used to describe the combined effects of drugs.

Terminology

Summation, Additive Effect, and Synergism

Summation, additive effect, and synergism refer to different situations in which the combined effect of two (or more) drugs acting simultaneously is either equal to or greater than the effect of each agent given alone (Fig. 12-4). When two drugs elicit the same overt response, regardless of the mechanism of action, and the combined effect is the algebraic sum of their individual effects, the drugs are said to exhibit *summation*. The term *additive effect* is usually used in those cases in which the combined effect of two drugs acting by the *same* mechanism is equal to that expected by simple addition. (Of course the magnitude of the combined effect must be within the capacity of the system to respond.) Thus, when small doses of codeine and aspirin are concurrently administered for the relief of pain, the combined effect is called summation since the two drugs act by different mechanisms. However, aspirin and acetaminophen act by the same mechanism to produce analgesia, and their combined effect is additive.

In *synergism*, the joint effect of two drugs is greater than the algebraic sum of their individual effects. The term is usually reserved for cases in which two drugs act at different sites and one drug, the synergist, increases the effect of the second drug by altering its biotransformation, distribution, or excretion. Thus in synergism the intensity of the effect may be potentiated or the duration of action prolonged. Inhibitors of drug biotransformation by the cytochrome P450 enzymes act as synergists of the drugs whose clearance is reduced; an example is the adverse effect of the antibiotic erythromycin to increase the risk of skeletal muscle toxicity of some of the statin-type cholesterol-lowering agents.

Antagonism

Any time the concomitant effect of two drugs is *less* than the sum of the effects of the drugs acting separately, the phenomenon is called *drug antagonism*. There are four mechanisms by which one drug may oppose the action of another, and different terminology is used to distinguish among them. The four types are *pharmacologic antagonism, physiologic antagonism, biochemical antagonism* and *chemical antagonism* (Fig. 12-4).

We have seen earlier (cf. pp. 196–200) that some drug-receptor combinations manifest themselves only as interactions that interfere with the formation of an agonist-receptor complex. When an antagonist like the antihistamine diphenhydramine reduces the effect of an agonist like histamine by preventing it from combining with its receptor, the interaction of the two drugs is known as *pharmacologic antagonism*.

Physiologic or *functional antagonism* is observed when two agonists, acting at different sites, counterbalance each other by producing opposite effects on the same physiologic function. For example, the effect of ibuprofen on promoting stomach irritation can be reduced by a histamine receptor antagonist (H_2 antagonist) such as ranitidine (XANTAC). Ibuprofen (or aspirin) increases gastric HCl secretion by inhibiting cyclooxygenase, preventing the synthesis of prostaglandin E_2 (PGE_2). When PGE_2 binds to its receptor, it inhibits adenylate cyclase, preventing HCl secretion from the parietal cells in the gastric mucosa. PGE_2 also facilitates bicarbonate secretion and helps make more protective mucous. Histamine acts at an H_2 receptor to stimulate adenylate cyclase and HCl secretion; the use of an H_2 antagonist prevents this. Thus, each agent acts at its own target, the ibuprofen acts at the cyclooxygenase enzyme, and the ranitidine acts at an H_2 receptor; their combined effect on gastric HCl secretion is the net result of the two opposing actions. The essential point about physiologic antagonism is that the effects produced by the two drugs counteract each other, but each drug is unhindered in its ability to elicit its own characteristic response.

Biochemical antagonism can be thought of as the opposite of synergism. This type of antagonism occurs whenever one drug indirectly decreases the amount of a second drug that would otherwise be available to its site of action in the absence of the antagonist. Thus a drug that increases the rate of biotransformation or excretion of an agonist, or competes with the agonist's transport to its site of action, is termed a biochemical antagonist. The best examples of biochemical antagonists are the many agents, such as phenobarbital or rifampin, which induce the microsomal enzyme activity responsible for the biotransformation of other drugs (cf. Table 8-5).

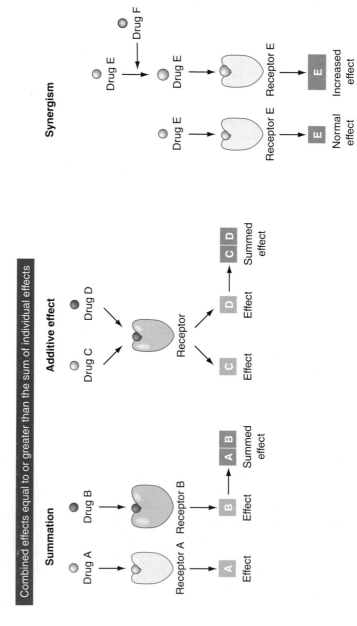

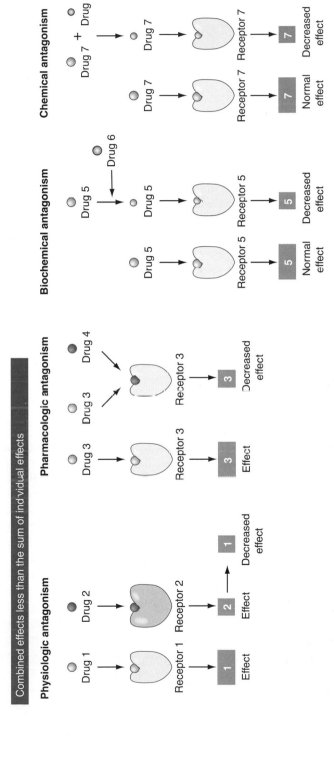

Figure 12-4. *Classification of drug interactions.*

The fourth kind of antagonism, *chemical antagonism*, is simply the reaction between an agonist and an antagonist to form an inactive product. The agonist is inactivated in direct proportion to the extent of chemical interaction with the antagonist. For instance, the anticoagulant effect of the negatively charged macromolecule heparin is antagonized when the drug combines with strongly basic dyes (toluidine blue) or basic proteins (protamine). This is analogous to the neutralization of excess gastric acid by any of the antacid drugs such as aluminum hydroxide or sodium bicarbonate.

Mechanisms Responsible for Adverse Effects Resulting from Drug Interaction

The word *adverse* applies not only to drug interactions that lead to a toxic manifestation, but also to those in which the combined drug action results in less than desired effectiveness. Examples of the major adverse interactions of commonly used drugs are listed in Table 12-5. Ordinarily, such adverse responses do not emanate from the additive effects of drugs acting at the same receptor site or from pharmacologic or physiologic antagonisms. The combined effects produced by such drug interactions may be readily predicted from the known pharmacology of the agents involved and can be taken into account before multiple-drug administration. Generally, drugs exhibiting summation do not cause problems when used concomitantly, since their combined effects also may be anticipated on the basis of available pharmacologic knowledge. Adverse reactions of combined medication are commonly associated with drugs that act synergistically or are chemically or biochemically antagonistic. Thus the mechanisms usually responsible for the adverse effects associated with drug interactions are those in which one drug affects the absorption, distribution, biotransformation or excretion of another.

Intestinal Absorption

Since the oral route is the one most frequently used for drug administration, drug interactions influencing absorption are most likely to occur within the gastrointestinal tract. One drug affects the absorption of another primarily by altering the amount of drug available for absorption, rather than by influencing the absorptive mechanism per se. A good example of such interaction is provided by cholestyramine, a drug used to lower plasma levels of cholesterol. Cholestyramine, a nonabsorbable resin, indirectly lowers plasma cholesterol levels by binding bile acids and preventing their reabsorption from the intestine and their enterohepatic cycling (cf. pp. 148–149). Plasma cholesterol levels fall in response to decreased enterohepatic cycling of bile acids because there is increased hepatic conversion of cholesterol to bile acids, increased hepatic uptake of cholesterol from the plasma, and decreased bile acids available to facilitate the intestinal absorption of cholesterol. The same binding characteristics that make cholestyramine useful in the treatment of hypercholesterolemia also account for the resin's interference in the absorption of a variety of drugs

Table 12–5. *Adverse interactions of some commonly used drugs*

| Interacting drugs | | Type or mechanism of | Adverse effects |
A with	B	interaction	
Alcohol (acute intoxication)	Antihistamines Barbiturates Benzodiazepines	Summation Synergistic; biotransformation of B inhibited by A	Increased depression of central nervous system
Alcohol (chronic abuse)	Barbiturates Anticoagulants	Biochemical antagonism of B by A through enzyme induction	Decreased effect of B
Anticoagulants, like warfarin	Salicylates (high doses) Quinidine	Summation	Increased bleeding tendency
Erythromycin Cyclosporine	HMG CoA reductase inhibitors	Synergistic; biotransformation of B inhibited by A	Increased muscle toxicity
Sulfonamides	Warfarin	Synergistic; displacement of B by A from plasma proteins	Increased bleeding tendency
Carbamazepine Rifampin St John's wort	Warfarin	Biochemical antagonism of B by A through enzyme induction	Decreased effect of B
Laxatives (prolonged use) Diuretics, like chlorothiazide	Digoxin	Excessive loss of potassium ion from body produced by A	Increased toxicity of B
Antacids	Tetracycline Isoniazid	Chemical antagonism; decreased absorption of B	Decreased effect of B
Cholestyramine	Warfarin Digoxin Thyroxine	Chemical antagonism; decreased absorption of B	Decreased effect of B
Probenecid	Methotrexate	Synergistic; inhibition of urinary excretion of B	Increased toxicity of B

such as chlorothiazide, thyroxine, anticoagulants, and various digitalis preparations.

Reduced absorption of drugs may also result from interactions with preparations used to neutralize excess gastric acid. For example, antacids containing calcium or magnesium form nonabsorbable complexes with tetracycline, thereby decreasing the amount of the antibiotic absorbed. This example of chemical antagonism also illustrates how a patient, through self-medication with antacids to relieve gastrointestinal distress, may inadvertently decrease the effectiveness of an agent prescribed by a physician. Antacids may enhance the absorption of a basic drug like diazepam by increasing the fraction of drug present in the nonionized and more absorbable form. Although changes in the alkalinity or acidity of the gastrointestinal tract affect the rate of absorption of ionizable drugs, this usually does not produce significant alterations in drug effectiveness or safety. However, drugs that decrease the rate at which the stomach empties its contents into the small intestine may markedly affect the absorption of drugs concomitantly administered. For example, codeine, morphine, atropine, and chloroquine are known to delay gastric emptying and to depress the rate of absorption of other drugs as well as of foodstuffs. On the whole, there is more evidence for drug interactions resulting in decreased effectiveness through diminished absorption than for increased toxicity due to enhanced absorption. However, there are examples of drugs that inhibit cytochrome P450 enzymes or efflux transporters in the intestinal mucosa and therefore cause increased oral bioavailability of agents that are substrates of these proteins. One example of that phenomenon occurred in a small number of patients receiving the CYP450 inhibitor erythromycin with certain antihistamines. The consequence of the greater bioavailability of the antihistamine was increased risk of fatal cardiac arrhythmia. This adverse effect led to removal of some antihistamines from the market.

Distribution

We have seen that many drugs bind to nonreceptor tissue components, such as plasma proteins (cf. pp. 118–121). Since the drug that is bound to non-receptor macromolecules is free neither to move to its site of action nor to produce a biologic effect, the binding sites represent sites of drug loss. These secondary binding sites also represent a reservoir of drug which may be made available to exert its pharmacologic effect. Certain drugs compete for binding sites on plasma or other proteins; a drug which binds more strongly may displace the drug forming weaker bonds. In this way, one drug may have a synergistic effect on another. For example, phenylbutazone can displace a number of other agents from proteins, including salicylates, penicillin, sulfonamides, the oral anticoagulant warfarin. In most instances the increased effectiveness of the displaced drug is not very significant. However, this type of interaction may have serious consequences for agents with high plasma protein binding and a low therapeutic index such as warfarin. This anticoagulant in plasma is 99% bound to albumin. The dosage of this drug must be very carefully adjusted for individual patients, because excessive concentrations can produce a dangerous increase in bleeding tendency. Phenylbutazone is now rarely used clinically for its anti-inflammatory effects, in part because of the excessive risk of drug interactions.

Biotransformation

There are many examples of enhanced drug activity brought about by the inhibition of the biotransformation of one drug by another. This phenomenon is usually so well recognized that it rarely results in unanticipated events following prescribed, combined medication with well-established drugs. For new drugs, methods are now available to identify the major enzymes involved in the drug biotransformation. From this information predictions can be made of possible drug interactions, based on the known inhibitors of the relevant enzymes. Inhibitors may exhibit selectivity with respect to their inhibitory actions on enzymes, even isozymes within an enzyme family. For example, some of the selective serotonin reuptake inhibitors (SSRIs) like fluoxetine (PROZAC) are primarily inhibitors of CYP2D6, whereas the immunosuppressant drug cyclosporine and the antibacterial agent erythromycin target CYP3A4. In many drug classes, newer agents have been developed to replace older drugs that cause drug interactions because of their actions as inhibitors of enzymes of drug biotransformation. An example is the development of the H_2 receptor blocker ranitidine (XANTAC) to improve upon the older drug cimetidine (TAGAMET) that inhibited the activity of certain cytochrome P450 isozymes.

There are also many examples of decreased drug activity brought about by the acceleration of the biotransformation of one drug by another; this type of biochemical antagonism results from the induction of drug metabolizing enzymes (cf. Table 8-5). Since the data obtained in laboratory animals are not always applicable to humans (cf. pp. 278–280), drug interactions involving enzyme induction were not always predictable. Indeed, some cases in which the effectiveness of one agent was unexpectedly reduced by concomitant administration of a second drug remained unexplained until subsequent investigation revealed the second drug to be an enzyme inducer. Many drugs have been identified that increase the synthesis rate of enzymes of biotransformation. Among the CYP450 inducers are barbiturates, anti-epileptic agents such as carbamazepine and phenytoin, the antibiotic rifampin, and some steroids. Chronic use of these drugs may lead to shortened duration of action of other agents that are substrates for an induced enzyme.

Some drugs such as ethanol can either inhibit or enhance the activity of certain cytochrome P450 isozymes, depending on the circumstances of drug administration. For instance, during acute ingestion of an intoxicating amount of alcohol, cytochrome P450 isozyme activity may be inhibited, but after chronic ingestion of alcohol for a prolonged period, there may be enzyme induction. These effects of ethanol on microsomal enzymes are of little consequence in the metabolism of ethanol itself, since the nonmicrosomal enzyme, alcohol dehydrogenase, accounts for most of the conversion of ethanol to acetaldehyde. However, the opposing effects of ethanol on microsomal enzymes help explain why interactions of alcohol with other drugs biotransformed by these enzymes vary with the amount of alcohol consumed and with the duration of alcohol use (see Table 12-5). It is well known, for example, that the usual hypnotic dose of barbiturates is relatively ineffective in the sober alcoholic, but produces a greater than expected effect in the inebriated alcoholic. Enzyme induction and an increased rate of biotransformation can account for the diminished effect of barbiturates in the sober alcoholic and inhibition of barbiturate biotransformation for the increased response in the intoxicated.

Renal Excretion

The quantity of a drug excreted in the urine depends in the first place on how much is presented to the kidney. This, in turn, is determined by extrarenal factors: the amount of drug remaining in the body; the degree of protein binding; and the volume of drug distribution. Once a drug reaches the glomerular filtrate, only reabsorption from or active tubular secretion into the urine will affect the amount ultimately voided. For ionizable drugs the rate of reabsorption can be markedly influenced by changes in the pH of the glomerular filtrate (cf. pp. 143–144). Thus, any drug that produces an alkaline urine enhances the excretion of weakly acidic drugs, whereas an agent that leads to an acidic urine increases the urinary elimination of a weakly basic drug. Many of the drugs given specifically to increase the volume of voided urine – diuretics – affect the excretion of other drugs by altering urinary pH. And we cited earlier how the administration of sodium bicarbonate can increase the excretion and shorten the duration of action of phenobarbital, a procedure useful in the treatment of poisoning by this agent.

We have seen that a number of drugs which are organic acids or bases, as well as some neutral compounds, are actively secreted by the renal epithelial cells, and it is the availability of carrier which limits the rate of active transport (cf. p. 144). Hence a drug that uses the same transport system as another agent will reduce the secretion of the second agent when the system is saturated by the simultaneous presence of the two substances. There are several therapeutic situations that call for the concurrent administration of two drugs known to share the same renal tubular secretory process. Such combined therapy may be important, for example, in the treatment of resistant infections that require the administration of enormous doses of penicillin. Here probenecid may be coadministered to decrease the rate of elimination of the antibiotic. Probenecid may also be administered with the cancer chemotherapeutic agent methotrexate to decrease the risk of gout associated with this drug. However, unless the dose of methotrexate is reduced, the probenecid may increase other toxicities of the chemotherapeutic agent, as a consequence of the inhibition of its tubular secretion.

The fact that organic anionic drugs are secreted by the same transport process as uric acid, a normal waste product of the body, is of practical significance. For example, blood levels of uric acid may be increased above normal as a side-effect of therapy with some diuretic agents like chlorothiazide which are also actively secreted by the renal tubule. In some susceptible individuals this inhibition of uric acid secretion contributes to the appearance of gout, a disease associated with excessive uric acid content of the body.

A change in the rate of drug elimination is, of course, reflected as a change in duration of action: an increase in the rate of excretion will shorten the duration of action, and vice versa. Whether a change in the rate of urinary excretion also alters the intensity of drug effect depends on the rate of absorption. For drugs rapidly absorbed, there will be little change in the maximum drug level attained in the body, since most of the drug is available for distribution before much excretion occurs. When a drug is slowly absorbed, however, changes in rates of elimination may have considerable influence on the levels of drug in the body. A decreased rate of excretion may permit drug concentrations to rise to toxic levels, whereas an increased rate may prevent the attainment of effective drug concentrations.

Drug Mixtures

The type of multiple-drug therapy we have been discussing involves the concurrent but separate administration of more than one drug. This is quite different from the simultaneous administration of several drugs mixed in a single pharmaceutical preparation. Conjoint but separate administration permits manipulation of the dosage of individual drugs so that the greatest benefit can be attained with the least possibility of undesirable effects. The timing of the administration can also be adjusted as required. Neither individual dosage nor timing is possible in the case of the single multiple-drug preparation. The fixed-dose drug mixture has another disadvantage when toxic effects occur: it is frequently impossible to ascertain which drug was responsible. Because of the disadvantages and possible risks associated with fixed-dose mixtures, there are only a few occasions when their use is justified. One notable example, marketed as AUGMENTIN, is the combination of a penicillin with an inhibitor of the bacterial enzyme that inactivates the antibiotic.

INTERACTIONS WITH DIETARY AND INHALED SUBSTANCES

The principles of variability in drug response due to the effect of one drug on another apply as well to the interaction of a drug with chemicals in the diet or in the ambient air. Numerous examples exist of the modification of drug response by dietary components. Typically an orally administered drug binds in the gastrointestinal lumen to a dietary substance that reduces its bioavailability, such as the effect of calcium in dairy products on the intestinal absorption of the antibiotic tetracycline. Chemical constituents in the diet have also been discovered to inhibit enzymes within the intestinal mucosa and therefore increase the bioavailability of drugs cleared by those enzymes. A notable example of this phenomenon occurs with the consumption of grapefruit juice, which contains an inhibitor of CYP3A4 and substantially increases the oral bioavailability of drugs such as warfarin (COUMADIN) and the cholesterol-lowering agent atorvastatin (LIPITOR). In both these examples the dietary component modifies the drug response by changing its pharmacokinetics.

An interaction can also result from a drug changing the response to a component of the diet. For example, use of a class of antidepressant drugs, the monamine oxidase inhibitors, can cause sharp rises in blood pressure and even fatal cerebral hemorrhage when the drugs are taken in combination with certain foods, These foods, such as some cheeses, red wine, and chicken liver, are rich in tyramine, a dietary constituent normally metabolized in the liver by monoamine oxidase. When the enzyme is inhibited by drug therapy, tyramine levels in the body rise excessively, cause release of norepinephrine from nerve terminals, and induce a hypertensive response. Warnings of this drug-diet interaction are provided on the labels and package inserts of all such drugs. Newer classes of antidepressant drugs such as SSRIs are preferred, in part because they avoid this type of safety problem.

As described earlier (Chapter 8), chemicals in the inspired air can also interact with drugs and modify their responses. Cigarette smoking, for example, results in exposures to chemicals, such as the aromatic hydrocarbon benzopyrene, that induce some CYP450 isozymes. Drugs cleared by those enzymes may have shortened elimination half-lives in chronic smokers. This mechanism explains why smokers exhibit a shorter duration of action with the drug theophylline, used as an airway dilator in certain pulmonary diseases.

SYNOPSIS

Drug effects are never identical in all individuals, or even in the same individual at different times. Yet the majority of people respond to most drugs in a fashion similar enough to permit the calculation of a standard therapeutic dose for a drug. However, this 'average' dose merely represents a starting point from which to estimate the appropriate dose for a given subject. The many variables contributing to the individuality of a complex living organism, or associated with the conditions present at the time of drug administration, must also be considered as factors potentially capable of modifying the usually observed drug effect.

In the past two chapters, we have considered the many factors contributing to individual variability in drug response from the perspective of the origin of the variability. Now we can summarize their influence on drug effects from the point of view of whether they produce quantitative or qualitative changes as a result of modifications in (1) absorption, (2) distribution, (3) biotransformation, (4) excretion, (5) receptors or target sites or (6) interactions unrelated to the normal pharmacodynamics of the drug.

Absorption. Differences in the rate and extent of absorption account in large part for the quantitative differences in an individual's response to drugs after administration by different routes. It is likely that differences in absorption, particularly after oral administration, also account for much of the commonly observed biologic variation in the responsiveness to drugs.

The rate of stomach emptying is one of the principal factors influencing rate of absorption, since the largest portion of the oral dose of most drugs is absorbed in the upper part of the small intestine. The rate at which the stomach empties its contents into the intestine is influenced by many factors, including the presence of food or of drugs which alter gastric motility. Occasionally, the interaction of the drug with certain food components or chemical agents results in a large fraction of the dose becoming unavailable for absorption. The more usual event is a decrease in the rate of drug absorption with but little change in the total amount of drug absorbed over a longer period.

Genetic abnormalities in drug absorption are relatively rare. The best-documented example is the inherited lack of intrinsic factor, a biologic entity secreted by the gastric mucosa and essential for the normal absorption of vitamin B_{12}.

Distribution. Changes in the response to drugs attributable to modifications in drug distribution may be brought about by differences in (1) the ratios of total body water or fat to body mass, (2) the binding capacity of nonreceptor proteins or (3) the permeability of a biologic barrier.

The average dose of a drug is calculated for the individual whose total content of body water is about 58% of body mass. Even after dosage is adjusted according to body weight, very young infants or very lean individuals may be less responsive than the average adult male to drugs distributed in body water, since their body water content is a larger percentage of their body weight. Conversely, the average woman or the obese individual might show a greater response. Pathologic conditions in which the normal body content of water is depleted (dehydration) or excessive (edema) may also alter the drug response. For drugs that are highly lipid-soluble, the differences in body fat content between males and females, and between lean and obese individuals, may influence the intensity of drug effect.

Many drugs bind to plasma or other proteins in varying degrees, and the fraction bound does not exert a pharmacologic effect until it is dissociated from the protein complex. Because many drugs compete for the same binding sites on plasma proteins, one drug may displace another when both are administered concurrently. The displaced drug is then free to leave the plasma and to act in concentrations higher than are ordinarily attained after the same dose given in the absence of the second drug. Whether the displaced drug will produce a large enough change in drug concentration at receptors to result in significant increases in response depends on its volume of distribution; the smaller the volume of distribution, the greater the increase in concentration.

A decrease in the quantity of available plasma proteins as the result of disease, malnutrition or genetic abnormality may also lead to an increased intensity of drug effect. In a few cases the inherited lack of a particular plasma protein may result in a novel effect, if the chemical is ordinarily bound and thus confined to plasma. In the genetically deficient individual, the unbound chemical is free to leave plasma and exert effects at sites to which it is normally not distributed.

Genetic alterations in the permeability or transport characteristics of parasitic and cancer cells can alter the ability of these cells to take up drugs that cause growth inhibition or cell death. This is one of the mechanisms by which resistance develops to antibacterial, antimalarial or anticancer drugs.

Biotransformation. Changes in the rate of drug biotransformation play a major role in variability in drug response because so many factors can affect the activity as well as the quantity of enzymes participating in these chemical reactions. Differences in pathways of biotransformation as well as in rates also account in large part for the differences in drug response between individuals of different species.

A decrease in the rate of biotransformation results in an increased duration of action or a greater magnitude of drug effect, or both. Conversely, an increase in the rate of enzymic activity leads to a decreased responsiveness or to a shorter duration of effective drug levels in the body, or both. When biotransformation converts an inactive agent to an active metabolite, an increased rate of biotransformation produces more rapid onset of drug effect.

The inhibition of the biotransformation of one drug by another is the most common mechanism of enhancing drug effect. But other factors such as age, genetic abnormalities and pathologic conditions may also make some individuals more sensitive than others to low doses of drugs. In the very young infant, the immaturity of some enzyme systems for drug inactivation, such as the glucuronide conjugating enzymes, is responsible. In genetically abnormal individuals, the altered enzyme may be unable to combine effectively with its drug substrate, or there may be an altered ability to synthesize the enzymes that catalyze specific drug biotransformations. Drug biotransformation also may be depressed in certain types of liver disease that affect the microsomal enzyme systems or impair hepatic blood flow.

Many drugs increase the activity of the microsomal enzymes involved in drug biotransformation by stimulating their synthesis. The concurrent use of a drug that enhances the rate of biotransformation of a second drug necessitates an increase in dosage of the latter to produce effects equal to those in the absence of the inducer. If the enzyme-inducing drug is suddenly withdrawn, severe toxic effects may occur unless the dosage of the second drug is suitably lowered. The decreased responsiveness to subsequent doses of a drug such as phenobarbital, which increases its own biotransformation, is one of the mechanisms for the development of tolerance to this drug.

The elaboration and induction of specific inactivating enzymes are also important mechanisms for the development of drug resistance in certain uneconomic species, such as bacteria and insects. The strains which have acquired specific enzymes or increased the quantity of these enzymes are capable of inactivating drugs that are lethal or inhibitory in the strains not possessing the enzyme activity.

Excretion. Modifications which influence the excretion of a drug or its metabolites ordinarily produce only quantitative changes in the effects of drugs, since it is only the rate of removal from the body which is affected. The kidney, as the principal organ for drug excretion, is also the site where most of these changes in rate of drug removal take place. Some factors decrease the rate of urinary excretion which, in turn, leads to an increased duration of drug action. Other factors increase the rate of drug presentation to the kidney and its clearance which decreases the duration of drug action.

Alterations in the renal clearance of a drug may be the result of changes in the rate of either glomerular filtration, tubular reabsorption or tubular secretion. In infants, the decrease in rates of both glomerular filtration and tubular secretion is primarily responsible for the impaired ability to excrete drugs. In infants the filtration rate is decreased because there is less blood flowing through the immature kidney and the volume of distribution of drug is greater than in the adult. Incomplete development of active transport processes accounts for the decrease in rate of tubular secretion in the infant. Renal function declines linearly with age after about age 30, so in the elderly renal clearance of drugs is predictably lower than in younger adults.

For drugs not extensively reabsorbed, any pathologic condition that decreases the rate of drug presentation to the glomerulus decreases the rate of drug removal from the body. A decreased rate of glomerular filtration may result from decreased glomerular blood flow, diseased glomeruli or an increased volume of drug distribution (as in edema). Conversely, an increased rate of glomerular filtration may result from increased glomerular blood flow, a decreased volume of drug distribution or a decrease in the amount of drug normally bound to plasma proteins.

Changes in the pH of the tubular urine will affect the rate of reabsorption of ionizable drugs. The rate of reabsorption will be decreased by a pH which favors the ionization of a drug, since the passive reabsorption of ions is so much slower than that of nonionized substances. The converse is equally true. Changes in urinary pH may be brought about by disease, by drugs which influence the normal formation of urine, by the intake of large quantities of acids or bases, or by foods which give rise to acidic or alkaline excretory products.

Alterations in the rate of the renal tubular secretory mechanisms affect the excretion of only those organic acids or bases, either normal metabolic products or drugs, which are transported by these processes. Decreased tubular secretion may be the consequence of interaction of drugs competing for the same secretory mechanism or of pathologic conditions which decrease renal blood flow or impair the function of the secretory processes themselves.

Drug receptors or target sites. Alterations in a receptor or a target site of a drug may be manifested as either an idiosyncratic response, drug resistance or drug tolerance. In the genetically abnormal individual, the receptor for the drug may be entirely absent or altered to such a degree that even extremely high concentrations of drug cannot produce effective interaction.

In drug resistance an enzyme or protein of an uneconomic species is altered in such a way that the drug can no longer combine with it to produce its lethal or inhibitory effect. The altered enzyme retains its capacity to bind with its normal substrate, however. The strains which possess the normal enzyme or protein are not resistant to the action of the drug and are inhibited or destroyed. As a consequence, the mutant strains, possessing the altered protein, survive and multiply and eventually become the predominant strains. This mechanism has been shown to account, in part, for the resistance developed to some antibacterial, antiviral, and anticancer drugs.

The development of tolerance is characterized by decreased responsiveness to a drug upon repeated administration. Tolerance is developed to many drugs which act in the central nervous system such as opioids and barbiturates. There is ample evidence to indicate that the mechanism of this tolerance involves changes in the receptor targets of these drugs and their ability to transmit signals in the nerve fibers where they are located. This kind of development of tolerance through cellular adaptation also occurs outside the central nervous system with respect to the action of drugs such as the nitrates.

Interactions unrelated to the normal pharmacodynamics of the drug. Factors which modify the pharmacokinetics of a drug, with few exceptions, produce an alteration only in the intensity of an anticipated pharmacologic effect. Qualitatively different responses as a result of modified pharmacokinetics occur only when drug biotransformation yields unusual products or when altered patterns of distribution permit a chemical to reach extraordinary sites of action. But when the administration of a drug elicits effects unrelated to its normal pharmacodynamic activity, then the intensity, the nature or the occurrence of the response cannot be predicted beforehand. This certainly is true for allergic or psychologic (placebo) responses to drugs. It is also true for most idiosyncratic responses unless the mechanisms of the specific genetic defect and its patterns of inheritance are known and the patient's family history is available.

The allergic response has a number of important characteristics which distinguish it from a toxic or idiosyncratic effect. The allergic response (1) requires prior exposure to the chemical and a primary sensitizing period before the individual manifests the response to subsequent exposures; (2) is a consequence of antigen-antibody interaction; (3) is unrelated to the usual pharmacologic effects of the eliciting drug; (4) is determined by the activity of the mediators released or the tissues or cells damaged by the antigen-antibody complex; (5) shows no consistent relationship between the severity of symptoms elicited and the size of the dose of eliciting drug; and (6) is antagonized by drugs like antihistamines, epinephrine or cortisone, but not by specific antagonists of the drug which produces the allergy.

Since many drugs may produce allergic responses, allergy is one of the most frequent side-effects of drug therapy. The incidence within the population of an allergic response to a given drug, however, is usually very low. Unfortunately, one cannot predict which patient will manifest an allergic reaction to what drug or which of the many possible allergic symptoms will constitute the response.

The placebo response is not a pharmacologic effect of a drug, since it is unrelated to the physicochemical properties of the eliciting drug. It is a psychologic response to drug administration induced by the circumstances of the administration and by the wish of patient and physician for a successful outcome. The intensity and nature of a placebo response following the administration of either an active drug or a material masquerading as an active drug vary widely and are completely unpredictable. All drugs may produce placebo effects, and any individual at some time may be a 'placebo responder.'

Idiosyncratic reactions are seen as novel drug effects when an inborn error affects the constitution of cells in such a way that they become susceptible to unusual interactions with certain drugs. Under ordinary circumstances the cell can compensate for the inherited abnormality. Indeed, frequently the abnormality is revealed first when an affected individual is exposed to a drug and has an unexpected response.

GUIDES FOR STUDY AND REVIEW

What are the general types of altered drug response that can occur only after repeated administration of a single drug (or of a drug closely related in structure)?

How is the phenomenon of drug resistance distinguished from that of drug tolerance? With what types of drugs is the phenomenon of drug resistance associated? What do we mean by 'economic species'? 'uneconomic species'?

What are the origins of drug resistance? What is infectious drug resistance? Why is infectious drug resistance of such great clinical significance? What is one of the most common mechanisms by which an uneconomic species acquires drug resistance, for example, the bacterial resistance developed to penicillin?

What is drug allergy? Why does an allergic response to a particular drug require prior exposure to that drug or to one very similar in structure? Does the allergic response show the usual dose-response relationship? How does this differ from the relationship between the dose and a toxic response to a drug? between the dose and an idiosyncratic response to a drug? What is the incidence of the allergic response in a population? the toxic response? the idiosyncratic response?

How is the allergic response related to the structure or pharmacologic activity of the drug eliciting the allergic response? What are some mediators of the allergic response? What types of drugs can be used to counteract the allergic response? How is this different from the way in which toxic or idiosyncratic responses to drugs are antagonized?

What is drug tolerance? Experimentally how would you determine whether an individual has acquired tolerance to a particular drug? To what types of drugs is tolerance usually acquired?

What do we mean by 'drug-disposition tolerance'? What is the mechanism by which drug-disposition tolerance is produced to a drug such as phenobarbital? How does drug-disposition tolerance affect the duration of action of a given dose of a drug compared to the duration of action of the same dose in the nontolerant state? Why is the intravenous dose producing a toxic or lethal effect essentially the same for both the nontolerant individual and the subject made tolerant to the drug by the mechanism of increased rate of drug elimination? Why is the peak effect of a drug reduced in the latter tolerant individual when the drug is given by a slow-absorption route?

What is tachyphylaxis? What is an example of a drug that produces tachyphylaxis?

What do we mean by pharmacodynamic or cellular tolerance? The repeated use of what types of drugs usually produces pharmacodynamic tolerance? What do we mean by cross-tolerance among drugs? What kinds of drugs exhibit cross-tolerance?

How does the tolerance developed to opioid analgesics like morphine differ from that developed to alcohol or barbiturates? Does tolerance develop uniformly to all the pharmacologic effects of a drug? To which of the characteristic pharmacologic effects of morphine does tolerance develop? not develop?

What are the terms that are used to describe the combined effect of two or more drugs acting simultaneously? What is the term used to refer to the situation in which two drugs elicit the same pharmacologic response and the combined effect is the algebraic sum of these individual effects? What is the special term used when both drugs act by the same mechanism? What do we mean by synergism? How does a synergist increase the effect of another drug?

What do we mean by the term *drug antagonism*? What are the four types of drug antagonism, and how are they distinguished from one another? What is an example of each type of drug antagonism?

The decreased bioavailability of orally administered tetracycline in the presence of a magnesium-containing antacid is an example of what type of drug interaction?

The increased bleeding tendency produced when an anticoagulant drug is displaced from protein-binding sites by another drug is an example of what type of drug interaction?

The decreased effectiveness of an anticoagulant drug in a patient who starts taking phenobarbital is an example of what type of drug interaction?

The action of an antihistaminic drug to alleviate some of the symptoms of an allergic response is an example of what type of drug interaction?

The use of epinephrine in preparations of local anesthetics is an example of what type of drug interaction?

What other types of chemicals, in addition to drugs, may interact with therapeutic agents to alter their pharmacokinetic and pharmacodynamic properties and cause variability in drug response?

SUGGESTED READING

Claing, A., Laporte, S.A., Caron, M.G. and Lefkowitz, R.J. Endocytosis of G protein-coupled receptors: roles of G protein-coupled receptor kinases and B-arrestin proteins. *Prog. Neurobiol.* 66:61–79, 2002.

Clavel, F. and Hance, A.J. HIV drug resistance. *N. Engl. J. Med.* 350:1023–1035, 2004.

deShazo, R.D. and Kemp, S.F. Allergic reactions to drugs and biologic agents. *JAMA* 278:1895–1906, 1997.

Gaddum, J.H. and Schild, H.O. Drug antagonism. *Pharmacol. Rev* 9:211, 1957.

Gintzler, A.R. and Chakrabarti, S. Opioid tolerance and the emergence of new opioid receptor-coupled signaling. *Mol. Neurobiol.* 21:21–33, 2000.

Gori, T. and Parker, J.D. Nitrate tolerance A unifying hypothesis. *Circulation* 106:2510–2513, 2002.

Hansten, P.D. and Horn, J.R. *Drug Interactions, Analysis and Management.* St Louis: Facts and Comparisons, quarterly.

Kim, R.B. *The Medical Letter Handbook of Adverse Drug Interactions.* Medical Letter, Annual.

Koch-Weser, J. and Greenblatt, D.J. Drug interactions in clinical perspective. *Eur. J. Clin Pharmacol.* 11:405, 1977.

McGrath, K.G., Zeiss, C.R. and Patterson, R. Allergic reactions to industrial chemicals. *Clin. Immunol. Rev.* 2:1, 1983.

Normark, B. H. and Normark, S. Evolution and spread of antibiotic resistance. *J. Intern. Med.* 252:91–106, 2002.

Stockley, I.H. (ed.). *Stockley's Drug Interactions* (6th ed.). London: Pharmaceutical Press, 2002.

13   Drug Toxicity

Desired effect and *toxic effect*, when used to describe the end results of the interaction of a drug and a biologic system, are relative terms. They take on real
meaning only within the context of the circumstances under which the chemical-
biologic reaction occurs. Certainly, *desired effect* indicates that the purpose for
which a drug is being used has been achieved. And *toxic effect* always means
that a harmful effect has been produced on some biologic mechanism. Yet the
two terms are occasionally synonymous, as for example when the action of a
pesticide like malathion saves a farmer's crop by eliminating a plant-destroying
insect. This same effect would be considered very undesirable from another
standpoint were the farmer accidentally exposed to quantities sufficient to make
him ill or cause his death.

Drug safety and drug toxicity are also relative concepts. The penicillin antibiotics are relatively safe and nontoxic because they can effectively eliminate the
bacteria responsible for certain diseases without harming most human or animal
hosts. Phenobarbital and other barbiturates were once considered relatively safe
drugs because the dose producing the desired effect in most individuals is appreciably lower than that producing toxicity in even a small percentage of the same
population (cf. Fig. 9-14). But malathion has never been regarded as safe
despite the fact that it is a useful insecticide. For even though, on the basis of
dose per unit of body weight, it is much less toxic to humans, other mammals
and birds than it is to many insects (cf. Chapter 8), its administration to these
higher animals produces no salutary effects. Its usefulness as an insecticide pre-
supposes that it can be administered by mechanical means in a manner and in
amounts that will harm only the uneconomic or undesirable species.

We can also evaluate the relative safety and toxicity of a drug by comparing
it with other drugs having similar actions and used for similar purposes. These
comparisons can be made on the basis of the relative margins of safety (the difference between the dose producing a lethal effect and that producing the
desired effect) or the relative severity or incidence of any undesirable effects.
Penicillin, for example, elicits a much higher incidence of allergic responses than

does the antibacterial agent neomycin. Yet in nonallergic individuals, penicillin is the safer drug by far since it is virtually nontoxic to host tissues and cells. The barbiturates are no longer considered relatively safe because of the discovery of the benzodiazepine class of drugs. The benzodiazepines have similar efficacy to the barbiturates but much greater margins of safety and have therefore replaced the barbiturates for many therapeutic indications.

What do these examples tell us about drug safety and harmfulness as relative phenomena? First, they tell us that the relative safety of a drug is judged in terms of its effects on a species considered desirable or economic[1]; relative drug toxicity can be evaluated in terms of both the economic and the uneconomic species. Second, when the sites of action for the desired and toxic effects occur within the same organism, the *dose* is the single factor that determines the degree of harmfulness of the compound (except when the harmful effect is the result of an immune response or a drug interaction). But when an economic species uses a chemical to eliminate an undesirable species, it is the degree of *species specificity* or *selective toxicity* that determines the margin of safety for the species which it is desirable to maintain.

When a drug is intended for use in an economic species, it is implicitly understood that dosage can be regulated to produce the desired effect in most individuals without causing significant harmful effects to them. This is true whether the purpose of administering the drug is to effect a change in the physiologic function of the economic species itself or to eliminate an uneconomic species. In contrast, if a chemical is not intended for use in an economic species there is no dose that can be introduced into the species that will be both effective and noninjurious. If the dose is sufficiently small there may be no effects, untoward or otherwise; but a dose large enough to produce an effect will produce only an undesirable effect. A substance that acts in a noxious manner and by physicochemical means to cause harmful or lethal effects when introduced into a biologic system is, by definition, a *poison*. Thus a chemical is considered a poison when it exerts an injurious action in the majority of cases in which it reacts with a living organism. There is no sharp line of demarcation, however, between a poison and a drug intended for introduction into an economic species; in large enough doses, *any* chemical agent, even food and water, can cause harmful effects. As Paracelsus recognized so long ago, 'All things are poisons, for there is nothing without poisonous properties. It is only the dose which makes a thing a poison.'

The study of the harmful actions of chemicals on living organisms is the particular province of that branch of pharmacology known as toxicology. Since any chemical agent has the potential to cause injurious effects in some biologic mechanism, the subject matter of toxicology is, understandably, vast. We need formulate no new principles, however, to understand the essentials of toxicol-

---

[1]What constitutes an 'economic' species is also relative; it may be interpreted very differently by the public health official, the marine biologist, the agriculturalist, the ecologist and others concerned with the adverse effects of chemical compounds on biologic systems.

ogy; the principles of pharmacology are applicable to the study of both the beneficial and the toxic effects of chemicals that interact with living organisms. Thus the magnitude of the toxic response, like the intensity of any response (except an allergic one), is a function of the concentration of the chemical at the site(s) of action. And this in turn depends on many factors we have already discussed: (1) the physicochemical properties of the agent; (2) the route and rate of its introduction into the organism; (3) the rate of its absorption, distribution, biotransformation and excretion; and (4) the many other variables influencing the response of a biologic system. A separate discussion of the adverse effects of chemicals is warranted nevertheless, since toxicity has become a crucial aspect of the use of therapeutic agents and a major societal problem in the form of exposure to chemicals contaminating the atmosphere, food or water.

We shall limit our discussion to considerations of the types of toxic reactions and the means by which they occur, the incidence of untoward effects of chemicals, and the general principles underlying the treatment of drug toxicity. We shall simplify our task by dividing the many biologically reactive chemicals into two distinct categories based on whether or not they are intended for use in humans. All the drugs used in the treatment, cure, prevention, or diagnosis of disease; for population control; as food additives (sweeteners, flavoring agents and preservatives); or as cosmetics will fall into one category. For convenience, we shall refer to this category as *therapeutic* agents or *medicinals*, even though the purpose of administering food additives and cosmetics is not to produce biologic effects. The second category comprises those chemicals that are not intended for introduction into humans, but which are potentially capable of producing biologic effects upon incidental, accidental, or (maliciously) intentional exposure. This group includes agents produced for use by humans, such as cleaning and polishing agents, paints, petroleum products, and pesticides, as well as industrial waste materials, noxious gases, and nonfood plants. We shall refer to chemicals in this second category as *poisons*.

CLASSIFICATIONS OF TOXIC REACTIONS

In textbooks of toxicology, toxic agents are usually grouped by chemical classes, e.g. heavy metals, oxidizing agents, acids. The various chemicals may also be grouped according to the locale of exposure to the source of toxicity – household poisons, industrial poisons and so forth. From the standpoint of pharmacology, classification based on the types of toxic effects produced or the sites in the body where they occur is more appropriate.

Types of Toxic Effects Produced

Toxic reactions may be classified as *acute, subacute,* or *chronic* on the basis of the rate of onset of symptoms and the rate and duration of exposure to the offending agent. Toxicity is said to be acute when symptoms that imperil the individual develop shortly after introduction of the drug into the body. Acute skin or in the respiratory tract. A topical agent that causes destruction of tissues at the site of application is termed a *caustic* or *corrosive* agent. These caustic chemicals are called *primary irritants*; their action is nonselective and occurs in all cells in direct proportion to the concentration in contact with the tissue. Strong acids such as hydrochloric, sulfuric or nitric, and strong alkalis like sodium, potassium or ammonium hydroxide, are examples of agents that produce severe structural damage to tissues. A primary irritant effect may also be produced by gases that are converted to acids or bases when they react with water. High concentrations of ammonia gas, for example, can produce local injury to tissues when inhaled and converted to ammonium hydroxide on contact with the moist pulmonary surfaces. Gases such as sulfur dioxide and nitrogen dioxide, which are encountered as atmospheric pollutants (especially under smog conditions), also owe their toxic effects to conversion to acids within the lungs.

Primary irritants that are therapeutic agents are used topically for their **antiseptic** or **germicidal** properties (see Appendix 3, V). Many such agents are available in a variety of proprietary preparations, e.g. various derivatives of phenol (hexylresorcinol; hexachlorophene) or cresol (Lysol); inorganic compounds, such as iodine and silver nitrate; and acids, such as boric acid. When these agents are employed topically and for legitimate therapeutic purposes, they have some beneficial and few toxic effects. When one of these agents is taken into the body, its corrosive action is exerted on any tissue with which it comes in contact.

Systemic Actions

A chemical acts systemically only after absorption into the circulation and distribution by the blood to the cells and tissues capable of responding to it. Therapeutic agents administered for systemic effects are usually introduced into the body by the oral route or by subcutaneous, intramuscular or intravenous injections. The lungs, the alimentary canal and the skin represent the most important sites of absorption of chemicals not intended for use in human beings.

NONSELECTIVE TOXICITY. The systemic action of some chemicals, like the local action of primary irritants, may be nonselective in that the drugs may act by altering functions vital to cells in general. Thus a drug that modifies an enzymic reaction essential for energy production, growth or reproduction will affect this enzyme in any cell in the body to which the drug can gain access. Drugs with such actions are called *cytotoxic poisons*. The term cytotoxic implies a lethal effect on the cell and distinguishes the effect from a reversible side-effect. Many mechanisms may result in a cytotoxic effect with death of the cell occurring by either necrosis or apoptosis. These two forms of cell death differ in the structural and functional changes that occur in response to the toxic chemical. We have already noted that the toxic effect of cyanide in oxygen-dependent animals is mediated through its ability to inhibit cellular utilization of oxygen. Many heavy metals, such as arsenic and mercury, although markedly different in their physical and chemical characteristics, share the property of inhibiting various enzyme systems essential to normal cellular metabolism. As a result, the symptoms of poisoning by these heavy metals are referable to many tissues, organs and systems. The tissues and cells most easily disrupted are those with the greatest metabolic requirements or the lowest reserve capacity to carry on their overall function. Thus, rapidly proliferating tissues like the gastrointestinal mucosa and the blood-cell-forming elements of bone marrow, and the cells of the renal tubules and nervous system, show early signs of toxicity.

It is noteworthy that the cytotoxic action of each of the agents cited is a *specific* action of the particular agent. The *nonselectivity* of the action of any one of these agents arises from the fact that it can exert its cytotoxic effect on many tissues and organs. When such drugs possess selectivity as well as specificity, the toxicity will be manifested in certain cells but not in others. The rationale for the use of cytotoxic agents in the treatment of cancer, for example, is based on the fact that these agents selectively attack rapidly proliferating cells. This selectivity is limited, however, since the anticancer drugs do not always discriminate between malignant and normal cells; thus they may also be toxic to the rapidly multiplying cells of the bone marrow and gastrointestinal mucosa.

SELECTIVE TOXICITY OF THERAPEUTIC AGENTS. In contrast to the nonselective activity and toxicity of cytotoxic poisons, most therapeutic agents have a relatively high degree of selectivity or specificity of action, or both. As we have seen, selectivity and specificity are the most important characteristics of a drug in determining its therapeutic usefulness (cf. Chapter 9). The greater the selectivity and specificity, the less likelihood of toxic effects occurring when therapeutic agents are used in recommended dosage. Toxic effects unrelated to idiosyncrasy, allergy, concurrent drug therapy, or pathology are unlikely in the majority of individuals given normal doses of drugs that have highly selective and specific sites and mechanisms of action. Excessive doses will produce toxic effects in all individuals. And obviously, except for the immune response or a drug interaction, whenever a therapeutic agent produces a harmful effect, regardless of circumstantial or predisposing factors, the dose administered must be considered an overdose. The type of toxicity observed may be the result of a continuation of the therapeutic effect (e.g. the occurrence of hemorrhage following overdosage with an anticoagulant), or the toxicity may be produced by mechanisms unrelated to those responsible for the desired or intended effect of the drug (e.g. the necrotic damage to the liver following overdosage with acetaminophen).

The frequency of unwanted effects associated with therapeutic agents depends on the circumstances of their use. However, even when we exclude accidental or voluntary overdosage and consider only the adverse effects of the correct drugs used in recommended dosage for the right indications, we find the incidence of untoward effects not insignificant. Although the true incidence is unknown for the general population, it is estimated that 15% of hospital admissions are due to adverse drug reactions and between 5 and 10% of hospitalized patients experience some unwanted effects of drug therapy. Between 20 and

25% of these are allergic manifestations. The remainder, in order of frequency, are referable to effects on the central nervous system, the gastrointestinal tract, and the cardiovascular system. The most common effects include drowsiness, dizziness, nervousness, headache, insomnia, nausea, heartburn, abdominal distention, vomiting, and diarrhea. Many of the effects that occur most often are not harmful and do not necessarily require withdrawal of the offending drug. Yet nonspecific changes in general well-being can be life-threatening when, for example, a drug induces suicidal tendencies. Excessive vomiting or diarrhea merits consideration as being serious in every instance.

The more serious aspects of the toxicity induced by therapeutic agents are those relating to pathologic changes in specific organs. The frequency with which these changes occur may be low (e.g. only a few tenths of 1% of those using the drug) or even rare (e.g. less than 2 in 50,000 patients). Nevertheless, they represent the most hazardous and unpredictable complications of drug therapy. The sites most frequently affected are the liver, kidney, and blood-forming elements of bone marrow. For example, drugs like acetaminophen, ethanol, and androgenic steroids may produce hepatotoxicity; renal tubular damage is a severe toxic effect of some antibiotics like tetracycline and the aminoglycosides; and drugs like the antipsychotic agent clozapine may produce disorders of the blood. The liver and kidney are particularly vulnerable, because many drugs attain high concentrations in these organs. Some of the effects on the liver, kidney, and bone marrow may be manifestations of drug allergy.

Chemicals that induce abnormal fetal development when administered to the pregnant animal are called *chemical teratogens*. That this type of toxic phenomenon could be induced by an ordinary, and supposedly harmless, therapeutic agent was dramatically and tragically demonstrated by what has since become known as the 'thalidomide disaster of 1960–1962.' In the aftermath of this tragedy, a wide range of medicinals, both old and new, have been tested and shown to have teratogenic effects in animals. The potential teratogenicity of most of these agents in humans is unknown since only a very few have met the criteria essential for proof of human teratogenicity (Table 13-1). But these investigations and the retrospective analysis of the effects of thalidomide indicate that there is a specific critical period during fetal development when malformations can be induced. The embryo is most susceptible to teratogenic effects during the period corresponding to organogenesis. In the human, this extends from about the twentieth day of gestation to the end of the first trimester. This means that part of the period of greatest vulnerability occurs in many instances before pregnancy is recognized or diagnosed. The uncertainty of the risk to the human embryo of drugs known to be teratogenic in animals obviously dictates their cautious use in any woman of child-bearing age. And until a drug is known to be reasonably safe by virtue of thorough investigation or long usage, it should be avoided altogether in women known to be pregnant. For example, although conclusions about the human teratogenicity of caffeine cannot be drawn at this time, the Food and Drug Administration has asked

Table 13-1. *Examples of chemicals producing teratogenicity in humans[1]*

Anticancer drugs
  Cyclophosphamide
  Busulfan
Anti-epileptics
  Phenytoin
  Valproic acid
Antithyroid drugs
  Propylthiouracil
Coumarin anticoagulants
Diethylstilbestrol (an estrogen)
Ethanol
Lithium
Tetracyclines
Thalidomide
Vitamin A (high doses)
  13-*cis*-Retinoic acid (ISOTRETINOIN, ACCUTANE)

[1]The criteria essential for proof of human teratogenicity are:
a. Documented exposure to agent during critical period of fetal development.
b. Careful delineation of the defect or syndrome.
c. Consistent findings in at least two nonbiased, controlled epidemiologic studies.

practitioners to counsel patients who are or may become pregnant to avoid or limit consumption of foods and drugs containing caffeine.

Whereas the potential teratogenicity of some drugs has been recognized only recently, the tendency of some chemicals to produce cancer in animals and humans has been known for about half a century. Legally, except for one group of therapeutic agents, no chemical may be designated for use in humans which has been found to be capable of producing cancer in laboratory animals (cf. Chapter 16). The exception is the group of chemicals used to treat cancers in humans; many of these agents have been shown to be carcinogenic for laboratory animals. The unknown etiology of most spontaneous cancers, the long latent period involved in the chemical production of tumors and the low predictive power of animal tests for carcinogenicity make it impossible, however, to say that a compound will not be carcinogenic in humans.

SELECTIVE TOXICITY OF POISONS. *Selectivity* has somewhat different connotations when used in connection with the actions of poisons and when used to refer to the actions of therapeutic agents. Chemicals not intended for introduction into humans have selectivity only with regard to the types of toxic effects they may produce; they are not selectively capable of producing effects which are not harmful to humans. The selectivity of action of poisons may be manifested as an immediate harmful effect on a particular function or organ or as a delayed pathologic change in one or more specific organs. Many chemicals are capable of producing both immediate and delayed effects; the particular toxic symptoms that develop are determined by the conditions of exposure. For example, the initial effects of the ingestion of methyl alcohol (methanol or wood alcohol) are referable to the central nervous system and resemble those of intoxication with ethyl alcohol. The most serious toxic effect of methanol is the selective injury to retinal cells, which results from the products of methanol biotransformation (formaldehyde, formic acid; cf. p. 171). As little as half an ounce (15 ml) of methanol has caused blindness. The immediate effects of carbon tetrachloride (CCl_4), following either ingestion or inhalation of quantities sufficient to cause toxicity, are also initially on the central nervous system and consist of dizziness, headache, stupor, convulsions, and coma. The delayed toxic effects of CCl_4 are on hepatic or renal tubular cells, or both. These delayed effects may either follow recovery from acute poisoning or occur as a result of chronic exposure in the absence of any marked effects on the central nervous system. The extent of tissue damage is a dose-related phenomenon, and the reversibility of the damage depends on the efficiency of the mechanisms of tissue repair. In chronic exposure to any chemical that produces tissue damage, the tissue will be able to perform its functions only as long as the rate of repair keeps pace with the rate of injury.

That constant exposure to certain chemicals can induce cancer in humans was recognized as early as 1775, when soot was implicated as a causative factor in the high incidence of scrotal cancer among chimney sweeps. Many other examples of cancer as an occupational hazard came to light in the second half of the nineteenth century. These indicated that cancer-producing substances are also present in coal tar, crude paraffins, pitch, mineral oils and certain dyestuffs. But it was not until the early part of the twentieth century that cancer was produced by chemical means in experimental animals. Then the earlier clinical observations made in humans were confirmed by laboratory demonstrations of the carcinogenic activity of the suspect chemicals. The responsible agents were subsequently isolated and identified and found to be polycyclic hydrocarbons, such as benzopyrene, and aromatic amines like naphthylamine. There are at present stringent laws to safeguard workers in those occupations in which a high incidence of cancer has been associated with particular chemicals.

A great variety of compounds besides the polycyclic hydrocarbons and aromatic amines are now known to be capable of producing cancer in animals. Many mechanisms have been elucidated that explain the carcinogenic potential of some chemicals. In some cases the compounds are genotoxic, meaning they damage DNA or impair DNA-repair mechanisms. As a result, mutations arise that either 1) activate genes that cause transformation of the cell into a neoplastic form ('oncogenes') or 2) inhibit genes that act to suppress tumor formation ('tumor suppressor genes'). Many of these chemicals occur in the environment and are derived from various sources, and some have been clearly incriminated in the production of cancer in humans. Since large segments of the population undoubtedly have contact with these agents, it becomes essential to determine how much of a hazard they constitute. However, establishing tolerance levels for potential environmental carcinogens and formulating measures to protect the general public pose serious practical problems that are as yet unresolved.

EVALUATION OF DRUG TOXICITY

The introduction of any new chemical into medicine, industry or everyday living carries with it certain potential hazards that must be assessed prior to its use. This potential toxicity is evaluated initially by measurements using *in vitro* systems and experimental animals. The nature of the tests carried out is dictated by the intended use of the new chemical.

Chemicals Intended for Use in Humans

If the chemical is a potential therapeutic agent, toxicity studies are conducted with a dual purpose in mind. First, since no active medicinal agent is without undesirable effects, it is essential to delineate the conditions under which these effects occur and to define the type(s) of toxicity that may be encountered. Second, the expected beneficial effects must be weighed against any possible harmful aspects of the agent's use, so that its margin of safety may be determined (cf. Chapter 9). These tests are carried out as *in vitro* studies and as acute, subacute, and chronic studies in several species of laboratory animals in accordance with the guidelines established by regulatory agencies (cf. Chapter 16). In the United States this agency is the Food and Drug Administration. The rationale of these preclinical studies is based on the assumption that toxicity determinations in animals have predictive value for the harmful effects likely to occur in humans. This assumption is often valid, particularly when the toxic effect involves a physiologic function equally important to all species concerned, or when it is a continuum of the therapeutically desired effect. Sometimes, however, a newly introduced drug thought to be free of undue toxicity turns out to have serious toxic effects in humans of a nature unforeseen from the animal tests. In general, preclinical tests in animals fail to provide clues about human toxicity when the toxicity is a rare event or the toxic effect is detectable only in humans.

The number of animals feasible to use in toxicity tests is very small compared with the large number of patients who will receive the drug once it is in widespread use. Therefore, a toxic effect with a low incidence is unlikely to be detected in preclinical animal testing; effects with an incidence of less than 1% are unlikely to be disclosed in most animal studies. Some drugs cause toxic effects such as the blood disorders in less than 0.1% of patients, but it may take widespread clinical use for several years before the toxicity is attributed to the drug itself.

Several toxic effects occur in humans that appear to have no counterpart in animals. The most serious among these are allergic reactions, skin lesions, some blood disorders and many central nervous system effects. Nausea, headache, dizziness, amnesia, and mild depression are examples of minor effects not readily observable in animals which, nevertheless, frequently limit the use of a drug. But even when we exclude from consideration the effects that cannot be demonstrated in animals, toxicity tests in various species do not necessarily predict the kinds of effects that will be observed in humans. The magnitude of the problem of extrapolating data from animal experiments to humans is

Act of 1947 as amended in 1972, 1975, 1978, 1980 and 1988 are administered by the Pesticide Registration Division of the EPA. The purpose of this act is to ensure that quality products are available to the public and that when properly used these products will provide consumers with effective pest control without causing unreasonable risk to health or adverse effects upon the environment. Under the law as amended, all pesticides must be registered prior to distribution, sale or use. This regulation applies to newly developed pesticides and to those marketed prior to changes in the law. Since registration is effective for a period of only 5 years from the time of registration, products are required to be reregistered.

Before a registration can be obtained, however, the manufacturer must submit data to the Registration Division of the EPA showing that the product, when used as directed, (1) will not present an unreasonable risk to humans, animals or crops; (2) will not cause unreasonable adverse effects to the environment; and (3) will not result in residues on food or feed greater than the established 'safe' residue level. Increasing attention has been directed at assessing risk in potentially vulnerable populations such as pregnant women and children.

The development of a pesticide includes preliminary studies conducted in the laboratory, greenhouse and small field plots in order to determine its inherent effectiveness against specific pests. Once this is established, additional evidence of its safety and usefulness is obtained through advanced large-scale laboratory and field testing procedures that more closely approach anticipated use conditions and that employ commercial application equipment. All tests consider factors of degree and duration of pest control and crop yield and quality.

The pesticide hazard to humans and domestic animals is assessed following administration by mouth, by application to the skin and eyes and, in some cases, by inhalation. Acute toxicity by the oral route is determined in mammalian species, preferably the rat, whereas the rabbit is the animal of choice for dermal LD_{50} studies. When the physical and chemical nature of the pesticide under conditions of use is likely to result in a respirable product, acute toxicity by the inhalation route is also evaluated. Subacute and chronic toxicity studies are designed to determine the adverse effects of multiple or continuous exposure for various periods; these may include assessment of carcinogenic, mutagenic, teratogenic, reproductive, and metabolic effects. If the pesticide is intended for outdoor use, data on acute and subacute toxicity to avian species and acute toxicity to fish are obtained. And if the pesticide may be expected to move readily from the application site by means of drift, volatilization or leaching in soil, then studies on toxic effects to susceptible nontarget plants are also undertaken.

The regulations governing research and development of a pesticide – a chemical that is intended to be used by, but not in humans – are now as stringent as are those for drugs that are intended for use in humans (cf. Chapter. 16). No pesticide is registered by the EPA unless it has been shown to be safe when used as directed. To promote effective and safe use of pesticides, the law also requires that products be properly labeled. The label on each package of pesticide must include: name and address of the producer; intended product use; composition by percentages for both active and inactive ingredients; directions for use; pests to be controlled; crops, animals or sites to be treated; dosage, time and method of application; and warnings to protect user, consumer of treated foods and beneficial plants and animals. Antidotes and first-aid instructions are required only on products that have been judged 'highly toxic'; the labels on such products must also bear the word DANGER. If the product is considered highly toxic on the basis of its oral, inhalation or dermal toxicity (as distinct from local effect on skin and eye), the label must also bear the skull and crossbones and the word POISON in red on a contrasting background (Table 13-3). The signal words on the label, such as *Danger*, *Warning* and *Caution*, are set by law and reflect the degree of toxicity of the pesticide as determined in studies involving five areas (indicators) of toxicity. The more toxic products are also classified on a use-by-use basis as 'Restricted Use' after it has been determined that the incremental risks of unrestricted use outweigh the incremental benefits of use. Pesticides classified for restricted use are described on the labeling, and their use is permitted only by appropriate applicators or by persons acting under their direct supervision.

Toxic Substances Encountered in the Workplace

There are at least 3,000,000 known chemicals! Although no one is certain exactly how many are in use today, this extraordinary number includes the more than 100,000 different industrial chemicals that are incorporated into more than 300,000 consumer products marketed in the United States. Since every chemical has an inherent potential for producing toxicity, the average individual is exposed to an enormous number and variety of chemical hazards as an integral part of our industrial society. It is the workers who manufacture or handle these chemicals, however, who are the population at greatest risk. In 1970 alone the estimated new cases of occupational disease in the United States totaled 300,000, many of which were due to exposure to toxic substances in the workplace. In consideration of annual figures such as this, Congress passed the Occupational Safety and Health Act of 1970 'to assure so far as possible every working man and woman in the nation safe and healthful working conditions and to preserve our human resources.' Under the provisions of the act, the Occupational Safety and Health Administration (OSHA) was created within the Department of Labor to (1) encourage employers and employees to reduce hazards in the workplace and to implement new or improve existing safety and health programs and (2) develop mandatory job safety and health standards and enforce them effectively. Since its formation OSHA has established standards that stipulate allowable exposure levels to more than 400 chemicals in occupational settings. Many of these standards were originally derived from the guidelines of the American Conference of Governmental Industrial Hygienists (ACGIH) for good industry practice and once adopted by OSHA became mandatory and enforceable by law.

Some common environmental contaminants and their permissible limits are listed in Table 13-4. The values are estimations based on human experience, measurable physiologic responses and toxicologic data derived from animal studies; they represent levels of contamination to which it is believed nearly all humans may be repeatedly exposed day after day without adverse effects. (These are, of course, subject to change whenever they are found to be inadequate.) The standards are expressed as parts of gas or vapor per million parts of air (ppm), or approximate milligrams of particulate per cubic meter of air (mg/m^3). Two exposure standards are usually set. One, which is referred to as the threshold limit value of the time-weighted average (TLV-TWA), is the average concentration for an 8-hour shift of a 40-hour work week. The second stipulates the maximum short-term exposure level (usually 15 minutes) and is referred to as the TLV-STEL. Sometimes a ceiling level (TLV-C) is provided, which indicates the maximum concentration on brief exposure.

The current convention of expressing the toxicity of airborne chemicals in terms of parts per million parts of air, or milligrams per cubic meter, and of chemicals given or taken by other routes in terms of LD_{50} values has little meaning for the average individual. Even though dangerous or lethal doses of toxic agents are only tentatively established for humans, there is a need to express the relative toxicity of different chemicals in simple, understandable language. The American Industrial Hygiene Association has suggested the six categories given in Table 13-5 as a way of translating oral toxicity data obtained in animals into terms that are more meaningful to the general population.

Despite the great strides made in reducing gross occupational hazards and making both employers and employees more aware of the dangers associated with exposure to injurious chemicals in the workplace, occupational toxicity continues to present major problems. One of these, quantifying the effect on reproduction of exposure to chemicals in the workplace, remains difficult at best because of the lack of parameters to measure reproductive function. Even the teratogenic potential of these chemicals is largely unknown since of the roughly 55,000 chemicals in common use in the United States, only 3000 have been tested for their ability to cause birth defects. About one-third of those tested proved to be animal teratogens on the basis of the high doses called for in animal teratogen test protocols, but very few have met the criteria to be

Table 13–5. *Interpreting animal toxicity data*

LD_{50} of single oral dose in animals (dose/kg)	Degree of toxicity	Probable lethal dose for 70-kg man
0.1 mg	Extremely toxic	A taste
1–50 mg	Highly toxic	A teaspoonful
50–500 mg	Moderately toxic	An ounce
0.5–5.0 g	Slightly toxic	A pint
5–15 g	Practically nontoxic	A quart
15 g	Relatively harmless	More than a quart

Source: From H.C. Hodge and J.H. Sterner, *Am. Ind. Hyg. Assoc. Q.* 10:93, 1949.

designated as human teratogens. Among the environmentally encountered chemicals that can be added to the list of teratogens in humans (cf. Table 13-1) are the chlorobiphenyls, lead, and organic mercurials.

The most serious problem of occupational toxicity is cancer (Table 13-6). To what degree occupational exposure to chemical carcinogens contributes to the cancer incidence rates in the United States is not known. The National Institute for Occupational Safety and Health (NIOSH), which recommends standards for OSHA's adoption, has obtained evidence to indicate that more than 10% of the thousands of substances on its Toxic Substance List may be carcinogenic. The first new health standard under the 1970 Occupational Safety and Health Act drastically curtailed workers' exposure to asbestos, a known carcinogen. And all of the 16 health standards OSHA set between 1970 and 1988 involved cancer-causing substances. One of these is vinyl chloride, the basic ingredient in making polyvinyl chloride (PVC), which is used in plastic products. OSHA acted swiftly in response to the discovery that vinyl chloride causes a rare form of cancer and is a potent killer. Within 3 months of the first reports of cancer an emergency temporary standard of 50 ppm was set. Six months later, a permanent standard of 1 ppm was promulgated when animal studies indicated that the temporary limit was too high. The fact that vinyl chloride was once considered so free of hazard that it was used as a general anesthetic agent illustrates the difficulties encountered in assessing the real carcinogenic potential of a chemical.

The latent period between first exposure and the development of cancer is much longer for most carcinogens than it is for vinyl chloride – usually 10–50 years. Since the annual rate at which new chemicals enter the workplace is about 7%, how can workers be protected from potential but unknown occupational carcinogens? The only answer can be to treat all chemicals as potential hazards until proved otherwise and to regulate exposures through enforcement of universal standards.

Environmental Toxicity

The hazards associated with the many chemical substances that are constantly being developed, produced and used in industry can reach well beyond the workplace, endangering the residents of a particular community or even the population as a whole. Poisoning of water, air, land, and food, and the cost of clean-up of environmental contamination has been the steep price society pays for technologic advance. The year 1970 marked the beginning of the comprehensive program and concerted effort to deal with the problems of widespread pollution of the biosphere when Congress established the United States Environmental Protection Agency (EPA). The creation of the EPA ended the piecemeal approach to the nation's environmental problems and filled the need for a single, strong agency to mount an integrated, coordinated attack on pollution.

The EPA is, first and foremost, a regulatory agency, having responsibilities for establishing and enforcing environmental standards. The process of setting

Table 13-6. *Carcinogens encountered in the workplace*

Agent	Organ affected	Occupation
Wood	Nasal cavity and sinuses	Woodworkers
Leather	Nasal cavity and sinuses, urinary bladder	Leather and shoe workers
Iron oxide	Lung, larynx	Iron ore miners; metal grinders and polishers; silver finishers; iron foundry workers
Nickel	Nasal sinuses, lung	Nickel smelters, mixers and roasters; electrolysis workers
Arsenic	Skin, lung, liver	Miners; smelters; insecticide makers and sprayers; tanners; chemical workers; oil refiners; vintners
Chromium	Nasal cavity and sinuses, lung, larynx	Chromium producers, processors and users; acetylene and aniline workers; bleachers; glass, pottery and linoleum workers; battery makers
Asbestos	Lung (pleural and peritoneal mesothelioma)	Miners; textile, insulation and shipyard workers
Petroleum, petroleum coke, wax, creosote, anthracene, paraffin, shale and mineral oils	Nasal cavity, larynx, lung, skin, scrotum	Contact with lubricating, cooling, paraffin, wax, fuel oils or coke; rubber fillers; retort workers; textile weavers; diesel jet testers
Vinyl chloride	Liver, brain	Plastic workers
Coal soot, coal tar and other products of coal combustion	Lung, larynx, skin, scrotum, urinary bladder	Gashouse workers, stokers and producers; asphalt, coal tar and pitch workers; coke oven workers; miners
Benzene	Bone marrow	Explosives, benzene or rubber cement workers; distillers; dye users; painters; shoemakers
Benzidine	Urinary bladder	Dyestuffs manufacturers and users; rubber workers; textile dyers; paint manufacturers

standards, however, begins with a scientific research and monitoring program, since the hazard of pollutants and exposure assessment must be known before the environment can be treated. The EPA, therefore, carries out a diversified research program at the laboratories of its Office of Research and Development and also gathers information from scientific and technical advisory committees, from industry and from the scientific community as a whole. The aim is to obtain the basic knowledge needed to safeguard public health and to balance the benefits of a specific product against the hazards it might pose for the environment. Thus studies are designed to determine not only what a specific level of a specific pollutant does to human beings, but also what it does to crops and other vegetation; to domestic animals and wildlife; to marine plant and animal life; to concrete, steel and other building materials; to painted surfaces; and to fabrics.

Whereas research constitutes the essential scientific foundation for action to improve environmental quality, the EPA's authority to enforce the standards established subsequent to research is derived from the various laws passed by Congress since 1970. These include (1) the Clean Air Act; (2) the Federal Water Pollution Control Act; (3) the Marine Protection, Research and Sanctuaries Act, known as the 'Ocean Dumping Act'; (4) the Safe Drinking Water Act; (5) the Federal Insecticide, Fungicide and Rodenticide Act; (6) the Toxic Substances Control Act (TSCA); (7) the Comprehensive Environmental Response, Compensation and Liability Act of 1980, known as 'Superfund', and (8) the Pollution Prevention Act of 1990. The TSCA is intended to provide additional regulatory authorities to deal with all hazardous chemicals that might lead to health and environmental damage. The TSCA mandates the EPA to obtain *from industry* data on the production, use and health effects of chemicals and to require testing of chemicals suspected of being harmful. If a new or existing chemical is determined to pose significant environmental or health hazards, its use may be banned or otherwise regulated by the EPA. Many cancer authorities believe that the TSCA will be a major step in controlling occupational cancer.

In the years since enactment of the laws creating the EPA and giving it the authority to implement and enforce regulations and standards, there have been significant areas of improvement in the quality of our environment. For example, in 1971 ambient (outside) air quality standards for five major air pollutants were set by EPA under the Clean Air Act[2]. As a result of this action, the national emission levels of four of the five major air pollutants declined between the years 1970 and 1975: total suspended particulates were reduced 33%; sulfur dioxide, 4%; hydrocarbons, 9%; and carbon monoxide, 15% from the 1970 level. In 1978 the ambient standard for lead was promulgated and set at 1.5 mg/m^3 averaged over 3 months. According to EPA reports, the trend toward cleaner air continues. The biggest improvement is in lead emissions, down 87%

---

[2]A sixth air quality standard, that for photochemical oxidants (ozone), was also set, but data for this pollutant have been recorded for too short a time to be able to assess the effects of the regulations.

in the years since the standard for lead was promulgated and tighter restrictions were placed on lead additives in gasoline. Since 1977 there has been a 37% reduction in sulfur dioxide, 32% in carbon monoxide, 14% in nitrogen dioxide and 21% in ambient ozone. There has also been marked success from the voluntary program dubbed '33/50' under which chemical companies signed on to reduce the 1988 emission levels of 17 of the most critical air pollutants by 33% by 1992 and by 50% by 1995.

The changes in air quality, which resulted from emission control plans, indicate that fewer Americans are being exposed to unhealthy levels of air pollution. But since these are annual averages of air quality nationwide, the encouraging downward trends do not reflect conditions in a local area or short-term changes in degree of air pollution. The EPA estimates, for example, that, although there has been a remarkable decrease in ambient ozone nationwide, ozone remains the major ambient air problem, affecting about 75 million people living in large urban areas that violate the ozone standard. The continuous monitoring and reporting of levels of air pollution by regional or local control stations are designed, however, to advise their respective communities of any possible adverse health effects resulting from extant air pollution. The Pollutants Standards Index (PSI) was developed by the Council on Environmental Quality and the EPA to achieve consistent and reliable reporting of the daily health effects associated with the quality of the air we breathe. The PSI values for five major pollutants are shown in Table 13-7. The establishment of descriptive categories (GOOD through HAZARDOUS) for varying degrees of air pollution are based on air quality criteria documents. These documents, which provide the scientific basis for standards, are required by the Clean Air Act to reflect accurately the latest scientific knowledge useful in indicating the kind and extent of all identifiable effects on public health or welfare from pollutants in the ambient air. The PSI values can be used to report the daily status of air pollution in a local area in much the same way as the 'burning index' is used to report the danger of forest fires. The guidelines for using the PSI advise reporting any index value that exceeds 100 in order to 'alert' the public that the standard has been exceeded. For example, the air quality index for a particular day might be reported in a typical news broadcast as: 'The PSI for today is 150, which falls into the unhealthful category. The pollutant causing this condition is sulfur dioxide. Persons with existing heart or respiratory ailments should reduce physical exertion and outdoor activities.'

INCIDENCE OF POISONING

Awareness has been growing throughout the world of the increasing incidence of acute poisoning. It is estimated that in the United States alone the number of nonfatal poisonings exceeds four million a year, although only about one-half of this figure is actually reported and tabulated at present. Several sources provide data to track the incidence of poisoning in the United States. One source is the National Center for Health Statistics of the Center for Disease Control, which reports fatal poison based on death certificates. A second source is the Toxic Exposure Surveillance System (TESS) of the American Association of Poison Control Centers (AAPCC). This data collection method was started in 1983 with 16 poison control centers. Since its inception, the number of participating centers has increased dramatically; in 2002 there were 64 centers serving a population of 291.6 million, more than 90% of the population of the United States. The data are collected by the AAPCC and summarized in annual reports published each September in the *American Journal of Emergency Medicine*. As the number of centers participating and reporting grew year to year, so did the reported incidence of human poison exposures, from 5.8 exposures per thousand in 1983 to 8.2 per thousand in 2002 (see Table 13-11). This increase probably reflects in part greater public awareness of the services available through poison centers rather than a true increase in poisoning. It is hard to believe that almost 1 out of every 100 people in the United States is exposed to a substance that precipitated a poison center contact. Of course, it is not known how many cases of poisoning occur that are not reported, or whether the unreported cases have the same characteristics as the cases reported to the centers. Nevertheless, poison control case reports provide useful information on the relative frequency and trends of exposure and poisoning from various substances, their relative harmfulness, and victim demographics.

The TESS data reveal that more than 90% of exposure incidents take place in the home, and about the same percentage of all reported cases are accidental or unintentional rather than intentional. Of these unintentional exposures nearly 10% involve therapeutic errors; the most common is inadvertently taking a medication twice, 'double-dosing'. Fortunately the vast majority of these accidental poisonings have a favorable outcome, yet the mortality rates of unintentional poisonings have shown a disturbing increase since 1984 (Table 13-8). The annual number of deaths caused by accidental exposure to carbon monoxide and other noxious gases and vapors has declined throughout the 1990s (Table 13–8). But the death toll due to ingestion of solids and liquids has continued to rise. This increase is attributable primarily to fatalities from poisoning by medicinals, including those used for both medical and nonmedical purposes. Medicinals account for almost 90% of all accidental poisoning fatalities (Table 13-8). The number of deaths due to accidental poisoning by therapeutic agents is not surprising, however, since pharmaceuticals represent about 50% of the types of exposures currently reported to Poison Control Centers.

Until the mid 1970s, one group of drugs – the barbiturates – accounted for more than one-third of all the fatalities caused by medicinal agents. Since then the number of fatal poisonings with barbiturates has declined dramatically (1% of the total reported to Poison Control Centers in 2002). This outcome results from the marked decline in the use of these drugs and has been offset by a continuing increase in poisoning by other types of agents including analgesics, other sedative/hypnotic/psychotic drugs such as the benzodiazepines, antidepressants, stimulants, and street drugs such as cocaine (Tables 13-9 and 13-10).

One of the most distressing sets of statistics on accidental poisoning is that

Table 13-7. *Pollutants Standards Index for reporting possible adverse health effects resulting from air pollution*

Index value	Air Quality Level and health effect descriptor	Pollutant levels ($\mu g/m^3$)					General health effects	Cautionary statements
		Suspended particulates (24-hour)	Sulfur dioxide (24-hour)	Carbon monoxide (8-hour) (mg/m^3)	Oxidants (1-hour)	Nitrogen dioxide (1-hour)		
500	Significant harm HAZARDOUS	1000	2620	57.5	1200	3750	Premature death of ill and elderly; healthy people will experience adverse symptoms that affect their normal activity and avoid traffic	All persons should remain indoors, keeping windows and doors closed All persons should minimize physical exertion
400	Emergency HAZARDOUS	875	2100	46.0	1000	3000	Premature onset of certain diseases in addition to significant aggravation of symptoms and decreased exercise tolerance in healthy persons	The elderly and persons with existing diseases should stay indoors and avoid physical exertion General population should avoid outdoor activity
300	Warning VERY	625	1600	34.0	800	2260	Significant aggravation of symptoms and	The elderly and persons with existing heart or

UNHEALTHFUL	200	375	800	17.0	400	1130	decreased exercise tolerance in persons with heart or lung disease with widespread symptoms in the healthy population	lung disease should stay indoors and reduce physical activity
Alert								
UNHEALTHFUL								
National Ambient Air Quality Standards	100	150	365	10.0	240	100	Mild aggravation of symptoms in susceptible persons with irritation symptoms in the healthy population	Persons with existing heart or respiratory ailments should reduce physical exertion and outdoor activity
MODERATE								
50% of National Ambient Air Quality Standards	50	50	80	5.0	120			
GOOD								

Table 13-8. *Number of deaths due to accidental poisoning by type of substance, 1980–1997*

Type of substance	Year				
	1980	*1986*	*1990*	*1994*	*1997*
All solids and liquids	3089	4731	5055	8309	9587
Medicinals	(2492)	(4187)	(4506)	(7828)	(9099)
Nonmedicinals[1]	(597)	(544)	(549)	(481)	(488)
Gases and vapors	1242	1009	748	685	576
Total	4331	5740	5803	8974	10163

Data from National Center for Health Statistics, Center for Disease Control, United States.
[1]Includes alcohol.

Table 13-9. *Deaths due to exposures in all age groups, 2002*

Type of substance	Deaths
Analgesics	659
Sedative/hypnotics/psychotics	364
Antidepressants	318
Stimulants and street drugs	242
Cardiovascular drugs	181
Alcohols	139
Antihistamines	71
Anticonvulsansts	65
Total	1153

Source: 2002 Annual Report of the American Association of Poison Control Centers.

Table 13-10. *Pharmaceuticals most frequently involved in human exposures in 2002*

Substance	Number of exposures	
	Under 6 years	*Total all ages*
Analgesics	90,295	256,843
Cough and cold preparations	62,107	100,612
Antimicrobials	33,764	63,372
Sedatives, hypnotics, antipsychotics	10,254	111,001
Antidepressants	13,836	99,860
Vitamins	45,239	57,313

Source: 2002 Annual Report of the American Association of Poison Control Centers.

Table 13-11. *Report of accidental exposures to poisons in children under 6 years of age and total exposures for all ages, 1965–2002*

Year	Under 6 years Number	Percentage of total cases	Total cases all ages	Exposures/thousand population[1]
1965	66,352	88.4	75,059	—
1974	109,614	68.3	160,533	—
1983	160,090	63.7	251,012	5.8
1991	1,097,485	59.7	1,837,939	9.2
1997	1,149,599	52.4	2,192,088	8.8
2002	1,227,381	51.6	2,380,028	8.2

Source: For years 1965–1974 the figures are from individual case reports submitted to the National Clearinghouse for Poison Control Centers. For later years, figures are from annual reports of the American Association of Poison Control Centers.
[1]Based on total population served by participating centers.

for children under 6 years of age (Table 13-11). In 1965, accidental ingestion of potentially harmful chemicals by children in this age group accounted for 88% of all the *reported* cases. Fortunately, the mortality was proportionately much lower, since the 379 children under age 6 who died by poisoning that year represented only 18% of the total deaths from poisons. Whereas there was a steady decrease in the percentage of both fatal and nonfatal poisonings in children under 6 years age in the years that followed, unintentional poisoning in this age group still accounts for about one-half of all reported cases. Since the number of reported cases has risen dramatically over the years, poisoning in children under 6 years of age remains a major public health problem. What is more noteworthy and reassuring is that this increased incidence of childhood poisoning has not been paralleled by an increase in mortality. On the contrary, there has been a decline in both the death rate and the actual number of deaths due to accidental poisoning of the very young. By 1986, the mortality within this age group from all accidental poisonings (due to drugs, nondrug solids, and liquids, and gases and vapors) dropped to 69. Based on the 2002 TESS data this number had decreased further to 23, which represented 2% of all the fatalities reported to Poison Control Centers and only 0.01% of the cases of exposure in that age group. These numbers document a remarkable decrease in mortality within this age group, while the number of fatal poisonings for the entire population was increasing. However, it is difficult to draw any conclusions concerning trends in accidental poisoning deaths in adults, since many of them are likely to be misclassified. Most forensic scientists believe that truly accidental poisoning deaths in adults are rare events and that most drug deaths are suicides. That opinion is supported by data from the cases reported to Poison Control Centers in 2002; 81% of adult fatalities and 89% of adolescent deaths resulted from intentional exposures.

The promising downward trend in deaths from accidental poisoning among children under 6 years of age can be accounted in part by the sharp decline in the number of fatalities due to ingestion of medicines. This decline in deaths attributable to medicinals is associated with a dramatic drop in the number of fatal poisonings due to aspirin – the drug that had been the number one killer and poisoner in the very young. From 1965 to 1978 there was a decrease in fatal poisoning of 78% for all medicines and 91% for aspirin and its congeners; in 1987 and again in 2002, no fatalities due to aspirin were recorded in this age group. The decrease in mortality due to poisoning by aspirin is a reflection of the lowered incidence of its ingestion among children under 6 years of age. The credit for this successful reduction in the ingestion of aspirin by children can be shared by (1) the pharmaceutical industry, which voluntarily set a limit of 36 baby aspirin tablets to a bottle; (2) the governmental and private organizations that campaigned intensively to make the public aware of the problem; and (3) the firms that instituted safety packaging on their own accord during 1970. Safety packaging for aspirin as well as other medicines became law in 1970 with the passage of the Poison Prevention Packaging Act, but the first safety packaging regulations only became effective in the latter part of 1972. That these packaging precautions are a powerful deterrent to poisoning by medicinals among children under 6 years of age is clearly evidenced by the mortality data for 1972 and 1974. Between 1972 and 1974 there was a 38% drop in the number of deaths from accidental poisoning by all medicinals and an even more dramatic decline of 57% for those attributable to aspirin. The incidence of nonfatal poisoning also shows a steady decline, and aspirin alone or in combination with other analgesics in 2002 accounted for only about 1% of all childhood cases of poisoning by pharmaceuticals (Table 13-12).

The steady decline in the number of fatal poisonings in very young children certainly must also be partly related to the widespread growth of poison control centers and the consequent increased accessibility of information about poisons. Each poison control center is provided with an index, filed for rapid retrieval, which contains information on composition, toxicity, symptoms of poisoning and recommended treatment for most of the products sold and distributed within the United States. In addition to therapeutic agents for human and veterinary use, the file contains references to household products, toiletries, cosmetics, pesticides, industrial chemicals, plants and fungi. Commercial firms whose products are included have cooperated willingly in providing the necessary data, despite the fact that trade secrets have had to be divulged. The centers are open to telephone inquiries 24 hours a day and provide information to anyone seeking help.

A clearinghouse for the exchange of pesticide information has also been established by the EPA in conjunction with Texas Technical University School of Medicine. The service provides free general, technical and emergency information on pesticides and maintains up-to-date information on each pesticide as well as names of experts to be contacted at various geographic locations. The service is designed to educate the public on pesticides and their effects on human health and the environment.

Table 13-12. *Poisoning exposure cases in 1979 and 2002 by type of substance among children under 6 years of age and in all ages*

Type of substance	1979		2002	
	Under 6 Years	Total all ages	Under 6 years	Total all ages
Pharmaceuticals[1]	34,710	65,791	543,764	1,281,336
Household cleaning and polishing agents	12,692	17,701	121,841	212,660
Plants	10,754	13,793	62,306	84,578
Cosmetics and personal care products	9563	10,782	162,946	219,877
Pesticides	4359	7683	50,415	96,112
Paints and stripping agents	3520	5727	13,049	24,727
Hydrocarbons	2468	5117	21,738	59,132

[1]Includes internal, external and combination medicines.
Source: Individual case reports submitted to the National Clearinghouse for Poison Control Centers in 1979; Annual Report of the American Association of Poison Control Centers, 2002.

TREATMENT OF TOXICITY

Treatment of poisoning by either specific or nonspecific means is referred to as *antidotal therapy*. Any chemical agent used to counteract the action of the poison is termed an *antidote*. Only when the mechanism of action of a poison has been elucidated is it possible to develop effective measures to antagonize specifically the action of the offending agent. This has been achieved for only a minority of the known poisons; a specific antidote is available in less than 2% of all cases of poisoning. For the most part, treatment consists in applying basic pharmacologic principles to deal with the signs and symptoms of poisoning as they arise.

The General Principles of Antidotal Treatment

It is axiomatic that prevention of poisoning is preferable to treatment and cure. But once poisoning has occurred, all antidotal treatment, both specific and non-specific, is aimed at lessening the magnitude of the effect(s) produced by the chemical-biologic interaction. The intensity of any drug effect, whether toxic or salutary, is a function of the concentration of drug at the site where the action-effects sequence is initiated. And the concentration of drug at a site of action is a function both of dose – the quantity administered – and of time – the time involved in getting a drug to and from its site of action. Provided that the effect is reversible, it will be produced only when and as long as there is an effective concentration of drug at the site. It follows that treatment of poisoning must be directed toward reducing the effective concentration at the site where the chem-

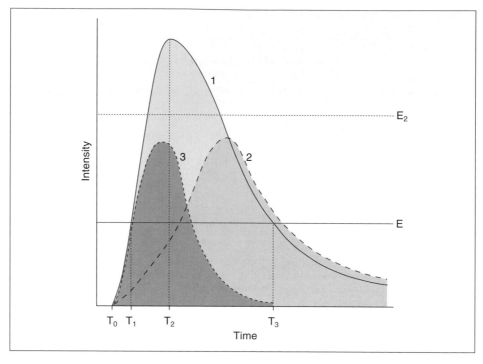

Figure 13-2. *Intensity of toxicity as a function of time. Exposure to drug at time 0 (T_0). T_0 to T_1 = time for onset of toxic effect; T_0 to T_2 = time to peak toxic effect; E = minimal level of measurable toxic response; T_1 to T_3 = duration of action; curve 1 = time course of toxicity; curve 2 = time course of toxicity when antidotal treatment decreases rate of absorption of toxic agent; curve 3 = time course of toxicity when antidotal treatment increases rate of elimination of toxic agent; E_2 = minimal level of measurable toxic response when antidotal treatment raises threshold of toxicity.*

ical interaction occurs. Thus to formulate the general principles of antidotal treatment, we need only apply what we already know about the relationship between time and drug effect.

Let us consider the case of a poison introduced into the body by the oral route at a dose sufficient to produce toxic but not lethal effects. The solid curve in Figure 13-2 represents the time course of action of such a poison. This curve is identical to that of Figure 10-2, except that we now consider E the minimum level of measurable toxic effect. The duration of the toxic effect extends from T_1 to T_3, and the intensity of the effect at any point in time is measured by the height of the curve above E. The faster the rate of absorption and distribution, the sooner the onset of toxic effects. The faster the rate of absorption relative to elimination, the sooner the maximum drug concentration is attained at a site of action and the greater is the intensity of effect. Or, from the standpoint of elimination, the slower the rate of elimination relative to absorption, the higher the maximum drug concentration (and the intensity of effect) and the longer the duration of action. Since the aim of antidotal treatment is to reduce the intensity and duration of the toxic effect (to decrease the area under the curve above E), there are two obvious ways in which this goal can be attained. Either the rate of access of the drug to its site of action can be slowed (curve 2), or its rate of removal from the body can be increased (curve 3). By either procedure, the rate of elimination becomes faster *relative* to absorption and distribution; the maximum level of drug in the body and the intensity of effect are reduced. In practice, a reduction in the rate of access of drug to an effector site is achieved by removing the unabsorbed portion of the poison from the site of entry into the body, preventing further absorption or preventing distribution of the absorbed poison to its site of action. The rate of elimination is enhanced by mechanically or chemically increasing the rate of excretion or by combining the poison with another chemical to form a less toxic, stable complex.

There is still a third procedure by which the aim of antidotal therapy can be achieved, and that is to elevate the minimal or threshold concentration at which the toxic effect occurs (E_2). This is accomplished either by administering a physiologic or pharmacologic antagonist or by employing mechanical procedures that compensate for the function(s) impaired by the poison. Now let us briefly examine the ways in which these principles are applied in both the nonspecific and the specific treatment of poisoning.

Nonspecific Therapy

The treatment of acute poisoning is always an emergency, but the judicious and rational use of therapeutic procedures is more effective than heroic measures, which may do more damage than the poison itself. More than 40 years ago the Committee on Toxicology of the American Medical Association published some excellent recommendations for first-aid measures to be used in poisoning emergencies, and these are presented in their entirety in Table 13-13 since they are still relevant.

The essentials of the nonspecific treatment of poisoning include (1) removal of the poison; (2) its identification; (3) administration of a suitable antidote; (4) promotion of elimination of the poison; and (5) supportive treatment of the patient. The order in which these actions are taken depends on the general condition of the victim, on the route of administration of the poison and on the poison itself.

The maintenance of respiration and circulation takes precedence over all other considerations. In essence, this is an application of the third procedure for accomplishing the goal of antidotal therapy. The maintenance of respiration by mechanical means and the administration of therapeutic agents to support the circulation are procedures for elevating the threshold to toxicity. The poison continues to exert its effect at its site of action, but the effect is overcome by measures that compensate for the physiologic functions impaired by the offending agent. There is also need to identify the poison as soon as possible so that

Table 13-13. *First aid measures for poisoning*

The following recommendations on first-aid measures for poisoning have been adopted by the Committee on Toxicology of the American Medical Association. These recommendations are made in response to numerous requests to the American Medical Association for general instructions for poisoning emergencies. They are intended for use in educating the public in what to do when poisoning occurs.

Emergency telephone numbers:

Physician _ _ _ _ _ _ _ _ _ _ _ _ _ _ _   Fire Dept. _ _ _ _ _ _ _ _

Hospital_ _ _ _ _ _ _ _ _ _ _ _ _ _ _ _ (resuscitator)

Pharmacist _ _ _ _ _ _ _ _ _ _ _ _ _   Police _ _ _ _ _ _ _ _ _

Rescue Squads _ _ _ _ _ _ _ _ _ _ _ _ _

The aim of first-aid measures is to help prevent absorption of the poison. SPEED is essential. First-aid measures must be started at once. If possible, one person should begin treatment while another calls a physician. When this is not possible, the nature of the poison will determine whether to call a physician first or begin first-aid measures and then notify a physician. Save a poison container and material itself if any remains. If the poison is not known, save a sample of the vomitus.

Measures to be Taken Before Arrival of Physician

I. SWALLOWED POISONS

Many products used in and around the home, although not labeled 'poison,' may be dangerous if taken internally. For example, some medications which are beneficial when used correctly may endanger life if used improperly or in excessive amounts.

In all cases, except those indicated below, REMOVE POISON FROM PATIENT'S STOMACH IMMEDIATELY by inducing vomiting. This cannot be overemphasized, for it is the essence of the treatment and is often a life-saving procedure. Prevent chilling by wrapping patient in blankets if necessary. Do not give alcohol in any form.

II. INHALED POISONS

1. Carry patient (do not let him walk) to fresh air immediately.
2. Open all doors and windows.
3. Loosen all tight clothing.
4. Apply artificial respiration if breathing has stopped or is irregular.
5. Prevent chilling (wrap patient in blankets).
6. Keep patient as quiet as possible.
7. If patient is convulsing, keep him in bed in a semidark room; avoid jarring or noise.
8. Do not give alcohol in any form.

III. SKIN CONTAMINATION

1. Drench skin with water (shower, hose, faucet).
2. Apply stream of water on skin while removing clothing.
3. Cleanse skin thoroughly with water; rapidity in washing is most important in reducing extent of injury.

IV. EYE CONTAMINATION

1. Hold eyelids open, wash eyes with gentle stream of running water immediately. Delay of a few seconds greatly increases extent of injury.
2. Continue washing until physician arrives.
3. Do not use chemicals; they may increase extent of injury.

A. Do not induce vomiting if:

1. Patient is in coma or unconscious.

2. Patient is in convulsions.

3. Patient has swallowed petroleum products (kerosene, gasoline, lighter fluid).

4. Patient has swallowed a corrosive poison (symptoms: severe pain, burning sensation in mouth and throat, vomiting). CALL PHYSICIAN IMMEDIATELY.

(a) Acid and acid-like corrosives: sodium acid sulfate (toilet bowl cleaners), acetic acid (glacial), sulfuric acid, nitric acid, oxalic acid, hydrofluoric acid (rust removers), iodine, silver nitrate (styptic pencil).

(b) Alkali corrosives: sodium hydroxide (lye, drain cleaners), sodium carbonate (washing soda), ammonia water, sodium hypochlorite (household bleach)

If the patient can swallow after ingesting a corrosive poison, the following substances (and amounts) may be given:

For acids: milk, water, or milk of magnesia (1 tablespoon to 1 cup of water). For alkalis: milk, water, any fruit juice, or vinegar.

For patient 1–5 years old: 1 to 2 cups.

For patient 5 years or older: up to 1 quart.

B. Induce vomiting when noncorrosive substances have been swallowed:

1. Give milk or water (for patient 1–5 years old, 1 to 2 cups; for patient over 5 years, up to 1 quart).

2. Induce vomiting by placing the blunt end of a spoon or your finger at the back of the patient's throat, or by use of this emetic: 2 tablespoons of salt in a glass of warm water.

When retching and vomiting begin, place patient face down with head lower than hips. This prevents vomitus from entering the lungs and causing further damage

V. INJECTED POISONS

(scorpion and snake bites)

1. Make patient lie down as soon as possible.

2. Do not give alcohol in any form.

3. Apply tourniquet above injection site (e.g. between arm or leg and heart). The pulse in vessels below the tourniquet should not disappear, nor should the tourniquet produce a throbbing sensation. Tourniquet should be loosened for 1 minute every 15 minutes.

4. Apply ice-pack to the site of the bite.

5. Carry patient to physician or hospital; DO NOT LET THEM WALK.

VI. CHEMICAL BURNS

1. Wash with large quantities of running water (except those burns caused by phosphorus).

2. Immediately cover with loosely applied clean cloth.

3. Avoid use of ointments, greases, powders and other drugs in first-aid treatment of burns.

4. Treat shock by keeping patient flat, keeping him warm, and reassuring him until arrival of physician.

Measures to Prevent Poisoning Accidents

A. Keep all drugs, poisonous substances and household chemicals out of the reach of children.

B. Do not store nonedible products on shelves used for storing food.

C. Keep all poisonous substances in their original containers; do not transfer to unlabeled containers.

D. When medicines are discarded, destroy them. Do not throw them where they might be reached by children or pets.

E. When giving flavored and/or brightly colored medicine to children, always refer to it as medicine – never as candy.

F. Do not take or give medicine in the dark.

G. READ LABELS before using chemical products.

Source: From Council on Drugs, *JAMA* 165:686. 1957.

rational and specific treatment may be instituted promptly. The immediate measures taken to prevent or retard absorption into the circulation depend on the route of drug entry into the body and on the general class of agent involved in the poisoning (Table 13-13). Copious washing with water is appropriate for the removal of any poison from the external surface of the body. But the procedures employed to remove unabsorbed poison from the gastrointestinal tract are dictated by the patient's condition and the type of poison ingested.

Vomiting is never induced as a means of removing ingested poisons in an unconscious patient or in the conscious patient when the toxic agent is a petroleum product or a corrosive substance. There is too much danger of inhaling the poison into the lungs or of perforating a corroded esophagus or stomach. Gastric lavage may be used in the comatose patient, however, to remove a noncorrosive agent when appropriate precautions are taken to avoid the possibility of asphyxiation by inhalation of the stomach contents.

In the conscious patient, both gastric lavage and emetics can be employed to remove ingested poisons. Vomiting can be induced by the parenteral injection of apomorphine, which acts on the vomiting center in the brain, or by oral administration of syrup of ipecac, which acts on receptors in the gastric mucosa. Apomorphine, however, has side-effects and ipecac is relatively ineffective unless used rapidly after the ingestion. These agents are now used infrequently. The preferred approach for reducing absorption of poisons from the gastrointestinal tract is administration of large quantities of activated charcoal. If given within an hour of ingestion of a poison, it will effectively absorb a variety of agents, such as aspirin, chlorpheniramine (an antihistaminic agent), pentobarbital, propoxyphene (DARVON), strychnine, morphine, atropine, mercury, and arsenic. Laxatives may also be used at times to hasten transit of poorly absorbed poison through the bowel, thus decreasing the opportunity for absorption of any material not removed by emesis.

In nonspecific antidotal therapy, an increase in the rate of drug elimination is usually the result of increasing the rate of urinary excretion of the poison. This can be achieved by administering large amounts of water and a suitable diuretic agent in order to produce a copious flow of urine. The larger quantities of fluid entering the renal tubules may provide a less favorable concentration gradient for reabsorption of the poison and, in turn, the lower drug concentration may protect the renal tissue from damage by the poison. When the poison is known to be a weak organic electrolyte, the urinary pH may be appropriately adjusted to favor ionization of the drug and, thereby, further inhibit reabsorption from the tubular urine (cf. Chapter 7). Alkalinization of the urine by the administration of agents such as sodium bicarbonate, for example, may be indicated in cases of poisoning by salicylates.

Other approaches to remove poisons from the body include methods that filter the blood to extract the poison such as hemodialysis and hemoperfusion. Hemodialysis has the advantage of also correcting pH and electrolyte abnormalities such as those that occur in salicylate poisoning. Hemoperfusion, which filters blood over an adsorbent material, may be especially effective in extracting high molecular weight compounds with low aqueous solubility. Peritoneal dialysis is a less efficient method than hemodialysis, but it involves a much simpler procedure – normally, only the irrigation of the peritoneal cavity with an isotonic fluid.

Specific Therapy

Specific therapy for poisoning differs from nonspecific treatment only with regard to the availability of a specific antidote to counteract the toxic effect of a particular agent or group of agents. All the other measures used in the non-specific treatment may still be required, even though a specific antidote is available. A specific antidote opposes the toxic effect(s) of another agent by acting as a chemical, pharmacologic, or biochemical antagonist.

Prevention of Absorption or Distribution to Site of Action

The antidotes used to prevent further absorption of a toxic agent act locally as chemical antagonists (Table 13-14). They neutralize the offending agent either by a chemical reaction that leads to the formation of a new, harmless or nonab-sorbable compound or by complexing or binding the toxic agent. The use of weak bases, such as magnesium oxide or milk of magnesia, to neutralize ingested acids or of weak acids, such as vinegar or lemon juice, to neutralize alkalis are examples of such chemical reactions. Detoxification by the mechanism of complex formation is exemplified by the use of deferoxamine in poisoning by therapeutic preparations of iron. This is an all-too-frequent occurrence in children. In 1997, in the United States, 2810 children under 6 years of age were poi-soned following the ingestion of ferrous sulfate and other iron-containing tablets intended for adults being treated for iron-deficiency anemias. The oral administration of an antidotal agent, such as deferoxamine, can prevent the absorption of iron by the formation of a nonabsorbable complex that is eventu-ally excreted in the feces.

The antidotal treatment of cyanide poisoning is an example of how chemical antagonism when carried out quickly can prevent a poison from gaining access to its site of action and also can increase its rate of removal from its site of action and from the body. Thus, therapy is directed toward removing the cyanide *before* it can reach cells and, if cyanide has combined with intracellular respiratory enzymes, toward removing it from the enzyme protein. The combi-nation of cyanide with methemoglobin to form a nontoxic complex achieves this end. However, there is usually insufficient preformed methemoglobin in normal individuals to bind much cyanide. So to make sufficient amounts available for this reaction, sodium nitrite is administered to quickly oxidize hemoglobin to methemoglobin. Methemoglobinemia itself does not present serious problems until more than half the available hemoglobin is converted to the non-oxygen-carrying form. Yet conversion of about 50% of hemoglobin yields enough methemoglobin to combine with more than a fatal dose of cyanide. Cyanide may also be converted to the harmless thiocyanate ion by an enzyme that occurs

Table 13-14. *Toxic agents, specific antidotes and mechanisms of antidotal action*

	Specific antidote	Mechanism of action
Prevention of absorption		
Iron	Sodium bicarbonate	Formation of relatively insoluble ferrous carbonate
Iron	Deferoxamine	Formation of nonabsorbable complex
Silver nitrate	Sodium chloride	Formation of insoluble silver chloride
Fluoride ion	Calcium salt (milk, calcium lactate)	Formation of insoluble calcium fluoride
Prevention of distribution to site of action		
Heparin	Protamine	Formation of complex that is removed by urinary excretion
Methanol	Ethanol, fomepizole	Prevents formation of poisonous metabolite
Enhancement of rate of elimination		
Acetaminophen	Acetylcysteine	Restores glutathione that inactivates toxic metabolite
Lithium	Sodium chloride	Accelerates excretion in urine
Lead, nickel, cobalt and copper	Calcium disodium edetate (EDTA)	Removes metals from tissue binding sites by complex formation
Mercury, arsenic, gold and antimony	Dimercaprol (BAL)	
Copper	Penicillamine	
Botulinus toxin and other toxins	Botulinus antitoxin and other antitoxins	Forms complex with toxin
Organic phosphate insecticides (Parathion)	Pralidoxime	Removes poison from enzyme cholinesterase
Elevation of threshold of toxicity		
Opioid analgesics	Naloxone and related antagonists	
Benzodiazepines	Flumazenil	
Carbon monoxide	Oxygen	Pharmacologic antagonism at site where toxic action is produced
Warfarin	Vitamin K	
Organic phosphate insecticides	Atropine	

normally in mammals. The reaction requires sulfate ion, however, and this is usually in short supply. When sulfate is supplied by the administration of thiosulfate, cyanide is rapidly biotransformed to the innocuous sulfur derivative. Thus the treatment of cyanide poisoning involves two mechanisms: (1) complexing with methemoglobin, whose formation is induced by sodium nitrite, and (2) acceleration by thiosulfate of the rate of cyanide's biotransformation to the nontoxic thiocyanate, which is readily excreted in urine.

In contrast to cyanide poisoning, in which part of the treatment depends on the acceleration of its biotransformation, the specific antidotal treatment for methanol poisoning involves the inhibition of its biotransformation by alcohol dehydrogenase. Methyl alcohol is converted to formaldehyde and formic acid (cf. Chapter 8), both of which severely inhibit essential metabolic processes. The actions of these metabolites are potentially more toxic than the central nervous system depressant activity of the parent compound. The same enzyme that oxidizes methanol is responsible for the metabolism of ethanol, but conversion of the latter gives rise to harmless metabolites and proceeds at a rate five times faster than the corresponding reaction with methanol. This difference provides the basis for the treatment of methanol intoxication. The administration of ethanol slows the rate of methanol biotransformation by competing for the oxidative enzyme, thereby slowing the rate of accumulation of the toxic metabolites of methanol. This antidotal strategy has been improved by the development of a selective inhibitor of alcohol dehydrogenase, the drug fomepizole, which unlike ethanol, does not have effects on the brain.

Enhancement of Rate of Elimination

The treatment of intoxication due to acetaminophen overdosage provides another example of the use of antidotes that accelerate the rate of elimination, in this case by increasing the rate of biotransformation of normal but potentially toxic metabolites. The hepatotoxic effects of acetaminophen, associated with doses above 10 g, occur as a result of saturation of normal conjugation reactions. The major pathway for elimination of acetaminophen is by conjugation of a reactive metabolite with glucuronide or sulfate. The reactive metabolite formed by microsomal oxidation is toxic, but it is normally inactivated by conjugation with glutathione to a nontoxic compound. Cytotoxicity only occurs when glutathione is depleted and the toxic metabolites accumulate. Glutathione synthesis depends on the availability of cysteine, but the supply of this amino acid may in itself be limited. Therefore antidotal treatment of acetaminophen overdosage involves the administration of acetylcysteine to replenish glutathione stores by increasing its synthesis.

As already described for cyanide poisoning, the removal of a toxic agent from its site of action through complex formation can be a very effective mechanism of detoxification. The action of the poison is terminated even before it is removed from the body. The agents dimercaprol (BAL, or British antilewisite) and calcium disodium edetate (EDTA) used in the treatment of poisoning by heavy metals are examples of specific antidotal complexing agents. Additional examples are given in Table 13-14. The great value of compounds like BAL and EDTA lies in their ability to form tightly bound, nondissociable complexes with metal ions. This binding effectively removes the metal ions from circulation and promotes the continuing dissociation and removal of any metal that is reversibly bound to enzymes and other tissue components. The metal complexes are water-soluble and are readily excreted in the urine. Thus, the complexing agent not only terminates the action of the poison but also serves to eliminate it from the body. For example, following the administration of EDTA to victims of lead poisoning, the urinary excretion of lead as the EDTA-lead complex may be as much as 50 times greater than in the untreated state.

Elevation of the Threshold of Toxicity

When the ability of an agonist to combine with its receptor is altered by the presence of a second drug that interacts with the same receptor, the phenomenon is known as pharmacologic antagonism. In the presence of a pharmacologic antagonist, the agonist acts as though it has become a less potent drug; much more agonist is required to produce responses equal in magnitude to those elicited before the addition of the antagonist. Thus, in the presence of a pharmacologic antagonist, there is an increase in the minimal concentration of agonist required to produce a demonstrable effect; the dose-effect curve of the agonist is shifted to the right (cf. Chapter 9).

All the specific antidotes acting to elevate the threshold to toxicity are pharmacologic antagonists (Table 13-14). They decrease the response to a given dose of a toxic agent by preventing the latter from exerting its full effect at the site where the toxic action is produced. For example, oxygen is a specific antidote for carbon monoxide poisoning, since oxygen competes with the noxious gas for hemoglobin and displaces the carbon monoxide bound to the protein. This is very different from the use of oxygen as a physiological antagonist in the treatment of barbiturate or opioid poisoning, in which respiration is depressed by direct action of the poison on the respiratory center of the brain. The use of atropine in the treatment of poisoning by organic phosphate insecticides is another example of antidotal therapy utilizing the mechanism of pharmacologic antagonism. The toxicity of these insecticides is mediated through their inhibition of the enzyme cholinesterase. In the presence of the enzyme inhibitors, acetylcholine is not metabolized and accumulates to excessive amounts. Atropine, as an antagonist at muscarinic acetylcholine receptors (cf. Chapter 9), diminishes some of the adverse effects produced by the inhibition of cholinesterase activity. The agent pralidoxime is another specific antidote used in the treatment of poisoning by organic phosphate insecticides (Table 13-14). However, pralidoxime acts as a complexing agent and removes the offending drugs from combination with cholinesterase, thereby restoring the activity of the enzyme. The difference in the mechanisms by which atropine and pralidoxime act as specific antidotes in poisoning resulting from cholinesterase inhibition is an important distinction. In the presence of a pharmacologic antagonist, the toxic action of an offending chemical may be reduced, but the toxic agent is neither detoxified nor removed from the body by the specific antidote. This is in sharp contrast to the fate of a toxic agent in the presence of a complexing agent. Therefore, when pharmacologic antagonists are employed, the toxic effect of a poison may reappear if the rate of elimination of the antagonist is more rapid than that of the toxic agent. And it must always be borne in mind that the use of any chemical agent, even an antidote, carries its own potential for producing unwanted and toxic effects.

SYNOPSIS

A drug, in the broadest sense, is any chemical substance (except food) that affects a living organism. Even when we limit consideration of these chemical-biologic reactions to the species *Homo sapiens*, the number of substances that this broad definition embraces remains extraordinarily high. And since any chemical agent, whether intended for use in humans or not, has some dose at which it will produce a harmful effect, the potential for chemicals to affect the human organism adversely is enormous.

The toxicity of agents intended for use in humans has become the most critical aspect of modern therapeutics. The introduction of more effective and more potent agents for therapeutic use has brought with it drug-induced adverse effects that are now called 'diseases of medical progress.' This is all the more reason for therapeutic agents to be used carefully and wisely, so that the expected benefits to be derived will outweigh the possible risks involved.

Whereas drug-induced diseases may be part of the price that has to be paid for more effective and better therapeutic agents, the toxicity associated with the nontherapeutic use of these chemicals can only be deplored. Poisoning by chemicals not intended for use in humans is also a major health problem. However, from the published morbidity and mortality statistics, it is apparent that the major incidence of poisoning is due to accidental rather than intentional use of therapeutic agents. And the vast majority of these accidental poisonings occur in children under 6 years of age. Increasing concern has led to many constructive measures to correct and reduce the hazards involved in the everyday exposure to potentially harmful chemicals of all types. But since exposure to many of these chemicals is unavoidable, more effort must be aimed at preventing the occurrence of toxicologic problems.

The best treatment for drug toxicity is prevention. But when poisoning occurs, nonspecific treatment is aimed first at supporting the vital physiologic functions, such as respiration and circulation, and at limiting further exposure to the offending agent. Removing the poison from the patient (or the patient from the toxic agent in the case of a contaminated atmosphere) and continuing adequate supportive measures as needed to antagonize and control the toxic effects may be all that is necessary. Given a little time, the normal mechanisms of drug elimination can be depended on to terminate the action of the offending agents.

Safe and effective specific antidotes are known for only a relatively few drugs. Yet because there are such specific agents, a positive identification of the cause of poisoning often facilitates therapy. Specific antidotes that prevent an agent from exerting its effects or that permanently remove it from its site of action are the most effective. Outstanding examples are sodium nitrite and thiosulfate used to treat cyanide poisoning, or the complexing agents used to treat heavy metal poisoning. The use of antidotal chemicals is not without hazard, however, and should be restricted to those situations in which irreparable damage or death may occur in the absence of their use. The objective of antidotal therapy, as with all therapy, is to achieve salutary effects without harm to the patient.

GUIDES FOR STUDY AND REVIEW

When is a chemical considered a poison? When does a chemical intended for use in humans become a poison? What is the single most important factor in determining the margin of safety of a chemical when the sites of action for the desired and toxic effects occur within the same organism? when an economic species uses a chemical to eliminate an undesirable species?

How do acute, subacute and chronic toxicities differ from each other?

What do we mean by nonselective toxicity? selective toxicity?

What is the approximate incidence of adverse effects of therapeutic agents when these agents are correctly used in recommended dosage for the right indication? What kind of untoward effect is most common? What other untoward effects are commonly encountered? What effects represent the most hazardous and unpredictable complication of drug therapy? What is the one group of therapeutic agents that can be legally designated for use in humans even though they may have been found capable of producing cancers in laboratory animals?

In general, how is the toxicity of a chemical intended for use in humans evaluated? What regulatory agency in the United States set the guidelines for this evaluation?

What types of toxic reactions are unlikely to be discovered in laboratory animal testing? What kinds of problems are encountered in extrapolating data from animal experiments to humans?

In general, how are chemicals that are used by humans to eliminate pests evaluated for their safety? for their efficacy? Is such assessment required by law? In layman's terms, when would a chemical be considered 'extremely toxic'? 'relatively harmless'? What information is required by law to appear on the label of a package of pesticide? How is the degree of toxicity of the product indicated on the label?

According to the published morbidity and mortality statistics, is the major incidence of poisoning (either accidental or intentional) due to use of therapeutic agents or nontherapeutic chemicals? What kinds of therapeutic agents are most responsible for fatal poisoning? What factors in recent years are responsible for the decline in the number of fatal poisonings in young children? Do you know how to get professional help in a case of suspected poisoning?

What do we mean by antidotal therapy? What is an antidote?

What is the aim of all antidotal treatment? What are the three general procedures by which this aim can be achieved? What general procedures can be used to slow the rate of access of the drug to its site of action? What general procedures can be used to increase the rate of drug excretion? What procedures can be used to elevate the threshold concentration of drug needed to produce the toxic effect?

What are the essentials of the nonspecific treatment of poisoning? What measures take precedence over all other measures? Why is the maintenance of respiration or the administration of agents to support the circulation an example of procedures used to elevate the threshold of toxicity?

What first-aid measures should be taken if poisoning is by inhalation? by skin contamination? by injection? by ingestion?

What first-aid measures should be taken in the case of chemical burns?

What measures should be taken to prevent poisoning accidents?

What do we mean by specific therapy of poisoning? What is a specific antidote for poisoning by therapeutic iron preparations that acts by preventing absorption of the drug from the gastrointestinal tract? What is the specific antidote for poisoning by methanol, and how does it act? What is the specific antidote for the treatment of lead poisoning, and how does it act? What are the specific antidotes for the treatment of poisoning by morphine and other opioid analgesics, and how do they act to elevate the threshold of toxicity? What is the specific antidote for the treatment of poisoning by cyanide? by carbon monoxide?

SUGGESTED READING

Albert, A. *Selective Toxicity* (7th ed.). London: Methuen, 1985.

Gosselin, R.E., Smith, R.P. and Hodge, H.C. *Clinical Toxicology of Commercial Products* (5th ed.). Baltimore: Williams & Wilkins, 1984.

Hayes, A.W. (ed.). *Principles and Methods in Toxicology* (4th ed.). Philadelphia: Taylor & Francis, 2001.

Kales, S.N. and Christiani, D.C. Acute chemical emergencies. *N. Engl. J. Med.* 350:800–808, 2003.

Klaassen, C.D. (ed.) *Casarett and Doull's Toxicology: The Basic Science of Poisons* (6th ed.). New York: McGraw-Hill, 2001.

Watson, W.A., Litovitz, T. L., Rodgers, G.C., Klein-Schwartz, W., Youniss, J., Rutherfoord Rose, S., Borys, D. and May, M.E. 2002 Annual Report of the American Association of Poison Control Centers Toxic Exposure Surveillance System. *Am. J. Emerg. Med*. 21:353–421, 2003.

Loomis, T.A. *Essentials of Toxicology*. Philadelphia: Lea & Febiger, 1970.

Reed, D. J. Glutathione toxicological implications. *Annu. Rev. Pharmacol. Toxicol*. 30:603, 1990.

14   How Drugs Alter Physiologic Function

As described earlier (Chapter 1), evaluation of the effects of drugs on physiologic function provides a critical tool for understanding biological mechanisms. As Claude Bernard pointed out more than a century ago, the drug 'becomes an instrument that dissects and analyzes the most delicate phenomena of the living machine.' His studies led to understanding the unique properties of the neuromuscular junction and its inhibition by the poison curare. Commonly, these investigations lead to important new therapeutics, such as the development of tubocurarine, used as a skeletal muscle relaxant in surgery. In this chapter we will consider the properties of the peripheral nervous system, especially the autonomic component, with respect to the target sites of drugs. Using the cardiovascular system as an example, we will examine how drugs can interact with several different targets to reduce elevated blood pressure or hypertension.

DRUG ACTIONS INFLUENCING THE AUTONOMIC NERVOUS SYSTEM

Traditionally the nervous system is divided into the *central nervous system* (CNS) consisting of the brain and spinal cord (cf. Chapter 15), and the *peripheral nervous system* comprising the cranial, spinal and peripheral nerves with their motor and sensory endings. The peripheral nervous system, in turn, is subdivided into the *somatic nervous system* and the *autonomic nervous system* (ANS). The somatic nervous system innervates those parts of the body that are under voluntary control; it is concerned with consciously influenced functions such as movement of the muscles of locomotion and posture. In contrast, the ANS supplies all structures of the body except the skeletal muscles; it is concerned with the maintenance of homeostasis, does not require conscious activation and is largely automatic in its operation. Indeed, many of the organs innervated by the ANS can continue to carry out some of their functions when their nervous connections to the CNS are severed; intestinal segments can contract and the heart can beat and pump fluid even when completely removed from the body. However, only an intact ANS can provide the tight control of cardiac function, blood flow, digestion and other **visceral** or internal functions of the body essential for maintaining the internal environment within the limits compatible with life.

The classic division of the nervous system into central and peripheral and somatic and autonomic, although descriptively convenient, implies separations that really do not exist either anatomically or functionally. Skeletal muscles, for example, are supplied by **motor** nerve fibers that are axons of cells entirely within the CNS. And the normal functioning of the ANS is dependent on centers of integration within the brain such as those in the hypothalamus that regulate body temperature, water balance, fat and carbohydrate metabolism and other visceral functions (cf. Chapter 15). Whereas there are distinct differences between autonomic and somatic efferent neurons (Fig. 14-1, Table 14-1),

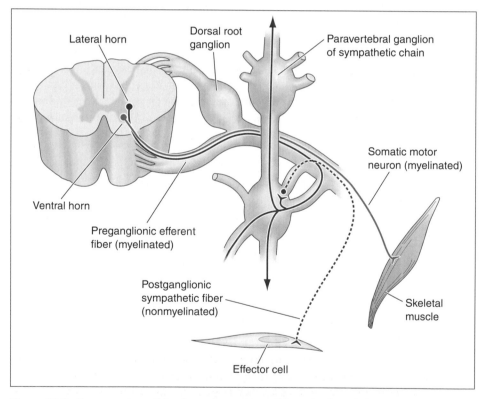

Figure 14-1. *Cross-section of the thoracic segment of the spinal cord showing general arrangement of somatic and autonomic efferent neurons. The somatic neuron (solid line) has its cell body in the anterior horn and its axon terminal in skeletal muscle. The preganglionic fiber of the sympathetic autonomic nervous system has its cell body in the lateral horn and synapses in the ganglion outside the spinal cord with the postganglionic fiber (dashed line) to the effector cell.*

Table 14-1. *Differences between autonomic and somatic motor nerves*

	Autonomic	Somatic
Structures innervated	All structures of the body except skeletal muscles	Skeletal muscles
Neuron in functional contact with effector:		
Cell body	Completely outside CNS	Within CNS
Axon	Generally nonmyelinated	Myelinated
Effect of interruption of cerebrospinal nerve	Some automatic activity independent of innervation	Complete paralysis of skeletal muscle innervated

the **afferent** components of these two systems are identical, and in the CNS there is extensive overlay between autonomic and somatic centers of integration. Somatic responses are always accompanied by visceral responses, and visceral activity modifies somatic reactions. For instance, the sight and smell of a steak cooking over a charcoal fire stimulates the flow of saliva and gastric juices in preparation for ingestion and digestion; during digestion the increased blood flow through the gastrointestinal tract tends to decrease the capacity of skeletal muscle to do work. Thus the activities of the somatic and autonomic nervous systems are coordinated and interdependent.

Although the sensory components and the CNS control centers of the ANS are essential to its normal functioning, we shall focus our discussion on its efferent pathways and **effector** organs. Knowledge of structure, physiologic function and biochemical processes in the peripheral ANS is sufficiently detailed to explain the mechanism of action of drugs that affect the system. To facilitate understanding of these mechanisms, we shall briefly describe the most relevant aspects of the anatomy and physiology of the efferent autonomic system and discuss the biochemical reactions underlying transmission of information within the system.

General Aspects of the Anatomy and Function of the Peripheral Autonomic Nervous System

On the motor side, the ANS is separated into two main divisions, the *sympathetic* and the *parasympathetic*. The motor pathways of both systems consist of two types of neurons; the first, the *preganglionic* fiber, has its origin within the brain or spinal cord but synapses with the second, the *postganglionic* fiber, outside the CNS. Most viscera are supplied with postganglionic fibers of both divisions. However, even though most viscera are functionally innervated by both the sympathetic and parasympathetic nerves, the actions of these two systems are frequently physiologically antagonistic (see Table 14-3). Although the efferents of both divisions are similar in origin and number of neurons, their respective preganglionic fibers issue from entirely different segments of the CNS and synapse differently in relation to the viscera innervated. These and the other differences between the two divisions (noted below and summarized in Table 14-2) clearly establish that differentiation of the efferent ANS into two major divisions has both structural and functional significance.

Another nervous system that is sometimes considered part of the ANS is the *enteric nervous system*, which regulates and coordinates the motor activity and secretory functions of the gastrointestinal tract. Efferent nerves from both main divisions of the ANS connect with enteric neurons, but the enteric nervous system can act on its own even in the absence of sympathetic and parasympathetic innervation. The function of the latter two systems is to modulate rather than control the motor and secretory activities of gastrointestinal tissues.

Anatomic Considerations

SYMPATHETIC NERVOUS SYSTEM. The sympathetic division of the ANS is also called the *thoracicolumbar division* since the cells that give rise to its preganglionic fibers are located primarily in the thoracic and upper lumbar segments of the spinal cord (Fig. 14-2). The myelinated axons from these cells leave the spinal cord in the anterior nerve roots and form synapses with postganglionic sympathetic nerves lying in ganglia outside the CNS. These synapses reside either in the ganglia of the paravertebral sympathetic chains that lie on each side of the spinal column throughout its length or in special collateral ganglia such as the superior mesenteric ganglia. The paravertebral ganglia are

Table 14-2. *Characteristic differences between the sympathetic and parasympathetic nervous systems*

	Sympathetic	Parasympathetic
Origin of preganglionic fibers	Thoracic and upper lumbar segments of spinal cord	Brainstem and sacral segment of spinal cord
Ganglia	Near CNS	Near effector cell
Length of fibers:		
Preganglionic	Short	Long
Postganglionic	Long	Short
Ratio of pre- to postganglionic fibers	High, may be 1:20 or more	Usually low – 1:1 or 1:2
Response to stimulation	Diffuse	Discrete
Preganglionic transmitter	Acetylcholine (ACh)	ACh
Postganglionic transmitter	Norepinephrine (most cases); ACh for sweat glands and blood vessels of skeletal muscles	ACh

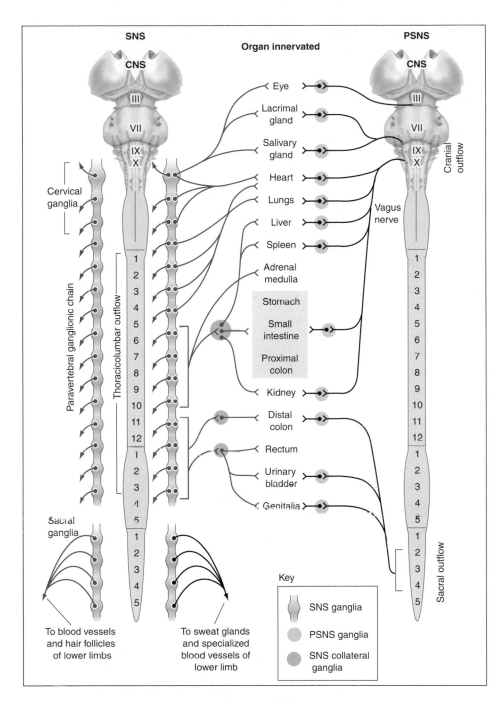

Figure 14-2. *Schematic diagram of the divisions of the autonomic nervous system. The diagram on the left shows the origin of the sympathetic nerves and the organs they innervate; that on the right shows the parasympathetic system and the organs it innervates.*

connected to each other by nerve trunks; preganglionic fibers issuing from one level may pass up or down the chain before forming synapses with more than one sympathetic ganglion en route. Thus a single preganglionic fiber may make contact with a large number of postganglionic fibers, and one ganglion may be innervated by several preganglionic nerves. These ramifications of preganglionic and postganglionic fibers account in large part for the diffuse response that usually follows stimulation of the sympathetic division of the ANS.

PARASYMPATHETIC NERVOUS SYSTEM. The preganglionic fibers that issue from the midbrain, the medulla oblongata and the sacral part of the

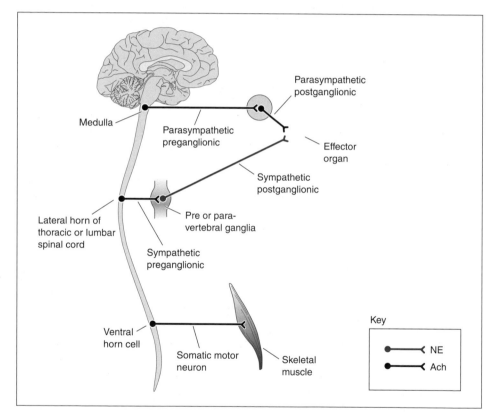

Figure 14-3. *Schematic diagram of differences between sympathetic and parasympathetic neurons. The relatively short preganglionic fiber of the sympathetic division originating in the thoracic segment of the cord forms a synapse in the ganglion outside the central nervous system (CNS); a relatively long postganglionic fiber of the sympathetic division terminates in an effector cell and releases norepinephrine on stimulation. The relatively long preganglionic neuron of the parasympathetic division originating in the medulla terminates in the effector organ with the relatively short postganglionic fiber. The somatic axon originating in the lower segment of the cord goes directly to skeletal muscle. Acetylcholine is released by preganglionic fibers of both sympathetic and parasympathetic nerves, by postganglionic parasympathetic fibers and by somatic neurons.*

spinal cord constitute the parasympathetic or craniosacral division of the ANS (see Fig. 14-2). The ganglia in which these fibers form synapses are in, on or near the organs innervated and, consequently, the postganglionic fibers of the parasympathetic division are very short (Fig. 14-3). This anatomic arrangement of motor neurons largely accounts for the limited and discrete response that is characteristically evoked by stimulation of parasympathetic fibers.

ENTERIC NERVOUS SYSTEM. The enteric nervous system is contained within the wall of the gastrointestinal tract and consists of a tremendous number of neurons, whose cell bodies form intramural plexuses. The plexuses are interconnected, receive preganglionic parasympathetic and postganglionic sympathetic fibers and have afferent neurons that respond to chemical and mechanical stimuli providing local control of function without input from the ANS.

Functional Considerations

As stated above, the ANS is an important part of the complex machinery by which the body keeps its internal environment constant. It maintains body temperature, fluid balance and the ionic composition of the blood; it regulates, in whole or in part, respiration, circulation, digestion, metabolism, the secretion of various **exocrine** glands and, in general, all those bodily activities that are not under voluntary control and that ordinarily function below the level of consciousness. The fine and rapid adjustment to ever-changing internal and external environments, the coordinated response to emergencies or vigorous muscular activity and the conservation and restoration of energy are made possible because the component parts of the ANS, the sympathetic and parasympathetic divisions, have distinct and usually contrasting functions (Table 14-3).

The sympathetic nervous system is normally active at all times. As a dynamic system, it not only is involved in the moment-to-moment control of homeostatic needs during ordinary activity but is also capable of responding rapidly to emergencies and stressful situations. Anatomically the sympathetic division is geared to influence several organs simultaneously or to discharge as a unit and affect all the sympathetically innervated structures of the body. For example, in a situation that provokes fear or rage there is an increase in heart rate, a rise in blood pressure, an increase in blood flow to skeletal muscles, a rise in the blood sugar concentration, a dilation of the bronchioles and increase in respiratory rate, a curtailment of gastrointestinal activity and dilation of the pupils of the eyes – all measures designed for 'fight or flight'. Many of these effects of massive discharge of the sympathetic system are reinforced by the epinephrine simultaneously released into the blood by the adrenal medulla.

Although the sympathetic division is capable of profoundly affecting the functional activity of the organism, this system and its associated adrenal medulla are not essential to life. In the sheltered confines of the laboratory, the sympathectomized animal can continue a fairly normal existence. In the absence of sympathoadrenal functions, however, such an animal is much less resistant to

Table 14-3. *Basic effects on some major organ systems produced by stimulation of autonomic nervous system*

Effector	Sympathetic	Parasympathetic
Eye		
Pupil	Dilated	Constricted
Ciliary muscle	Relaxed for far vision	Contracted for near vision
Heart		
Rate (direct effect)	Increased	Decreased
Contractility	Increased	Slightly decreased or no effect
Bronchiolar smooth muscle	Relaxed	Contracted
Gastrointestinal tract		
Motility	Decreased	Increased
Sphincters	Constricted	Relaxed
Secretory activity	May be decreased	Increased
Salivary glands		
Secretory activity	Increased; thick mucus	Increased; watery, dilute saliva

environmental changes and is seriously deficient in protecting itself under stressful conditions.

The parasympathetic nervous system is concerned primarily with conserving and restoring energy. It slows the heart, lowers the blood pressure, constricts the pupil of the eye (protecting the retina from excessive light), contracts the urinary bladder and the rectum for emptying of these organs and aids in the digestion and absorption of nutrients by stimulating gastrointestinal movements and secretions. In general, the parasympathetic division controls functions essential for life. It is anatomically organized for discrete and localized actions on individual organs or regions; no useful purpose would be served were the parasympathetic system to participate in the massive discharge characteristic of the sympathetic division.

As we stated earlier, in many of the **smooth muscles** and visceral organs that are innervated by both divisions of the ANS, the effects of the two systems are reciprocal. This is certainly the case, for example, in the heart, the bronchi, the gastrointestinal tract and the bladder (see Table 14-3). In other organs such as the salivary glands and pancreas, however, the influence of the two divisions is in the same direction – both stimulate secretion. And sometimes what appears functionally to be opposing actions may be the result of similar actions of the two divisions on opposing structures of the same organ. The involuntary adjustment of the eyes to changing light conditions is a case in point. The pupil of the eye dilates in response to sympathetic stimulation and constricts in response to increased parasympathetic activity. However, the nerve impulses of both divisions cause a muscle of the iris to contract; contraction of the radially oriented muscle innervated by sympathetic fibers produces dilation, and contraction of the circular muscle innervated by parasympathetic neurons produces constriction. Finally, it is important to point out that some organs are functionally innervated by only one division of the ANS: the adrenal medulla, spleen, sweat glands and probably the blood vessels of the viscera, skin and skeletal muscle are supplied only by the sympathetic division; focusing of the lens of the eye and lacrimation are controlled almost exclusively by the parasympathetic system.

The integrative neuronal network of the enteric nervous system is, obviously, involved only with control of the functions of the gastrointestinal tract which, from a pharmacologic point of view, are gastric secretion and motility of the bowel.

Biochemical Aspects of Autonomic Nervous System Activity

The ability of the ANS to elicit the appropriate diffuse or discrete response to change in the internal or external environment depends upon the transmittal of information from sensors to effectors. The operation of this information system is partly electrical and partly chemical. Electrical phenomena account for the rapid transfer of information along the neuron; this passage of impulses along the nerve fiber to the nerve terminal is called *conduction. Transmission,* the process of passing information across a synapse from one neuron to another, or across a neuro-effector junction from nerve terminals to the cells innervated, is a chemical rather than an electrical process.

Transmission is mediated by specific chemical agents known as *neurotransmitters,* which are synthesized in the neuron and stored in small vesicles at the axonal terminals. The sequence of events involved in neurohumoral transmission is as follows: (1) the arrival of the nerve impulse at the axonal terminals; (2) the release of the neurotransmitter elicited by the nerve impulse; (3) diffusion of the transmitter across the synaptic space or neuroeffector junction; (4) combination of the transmitter with postjunctional receptors; (5) initiation of electrical or chemical activity in the postjunctional neuron or effector cell; and (6) destruction or removal of the neurotransmitter from the site of action.

The concept that nerves transmit their messages across junctions by means of specific chemical agents is the foundation of the theory of neurohumoral transmission. This theory, which was first postulated in the early 1900s[1] and which received direct experimental confirmation in the 1930s[2], is now universally

[1]T.R. Elliott, while a graduate student at Cambridge, England, postulated that sympathetic nerve impulses released an epinephrine-like substance and that this substance was the chemical step in junctional transmission. He published this hypothesis in *J. Physiol.* (London) 32:401–467, 1905.

[2]Otto Loewi, who won the Nobel Prize in 1936 for work begun in 1921, established the first real proof of the chemical transmission of nerve impulses. The story of his brilliant research can be read in the words of Dr Loewi, published a year before his death as 'An Autobiographic Sketch' in *Perspect. Biol. Med.* 4:325, 1960.

accepted. Initially, only two agents were firmly established as neurotransmitters. These two were acetylcholine and norepinephrine. The extensive data that were collected concerning the details of chemical transmission in the peripheral nervous system (PNS) clearly showed that acetylcholine and norepinephrine each fulfilled all the criteria of a putative neurotransmitter. (1) Acetylcholine and norephinephrine were shown to be present at the axonal terminals of appropriate motor nerves. So too were the enzymes necessary for their synthesis and the structures required for their storage – two factors essential for ensuring that sufficient material would be available for release upon arrival of the propagated nerve impulse. (2) In experiments using isolated preparations, stimulation of appropriately innervated structures led to the corresponding release of either acetylcholine or norepinephrine. The amounts of each compound recovered during periods of nerve stimulation were found to be in excess of those recoverable in the absence of stimulation. (3) The pharmacologic effects produced by the appropriate local administration of either acetylcholine or norepinephrine were demonstrated to be identical with those elicited by stimulation of nerves containing the respective compound. (4) The responses elicited by stimulation of appropriate nerves or by the corresponding local administration of either acetylcholine or norepinephrine were also shown to be affected by the same drugs and in like manner. (5) Finally, mechanisms were identified for the rapid removal of acetylcholine and norepinephrine from the immediate vicinity of their respective receptor sites. This termination of the action of the transmitters is essential if they are to be effective under dynamic conditions.

The requirements for chemically mediated transfer of information – the processes involved in synthesis, storage, release and inactivation – have now been shown to be satisfied, wholly or in part, by many endogenous chemicals, in addition to acetylcholine and norepinephrine. Among these substances are dopamine, serotonin (5-HT), gamma-aminobutyric acid (GABA), adenosine triphosphate (ATP), nitric oxide (NO), and substance P and a number of other peptides. Some of these, such as 5-HT, GABA and dopamine are also neurotransmitters in the CNS and others like histamine and the amino acids, glutamic and aspartic acids, are neurotransmitters only in the CNS (cf. Chapter 15).

From the brief discussion above it is evident that the ANS is more complex than its simple representations in Figures 14-2 and 14-3 would lead us to believe. These descriptions of the ANS, while oversimplified, aptly serve as a basis for discussion of how drugs act to produce their effects on the PNS. Therefore, let us now examine in a more detail the individual steps in transmission as they apply specifically to acetylcholine and to norepinephrine. We will then be ready to turn our attention to how the actions of **autonomic drugs** can be related to the individual events in neurohumoral transmission.

Acetylcholine

Acetylcholine is the chemical mediator at the axonal terminals of (1) all preganglionic fibers of both divisions of the ANS and preganglionic nerves to the adrenal medulla; (2) all postganglionic fibers of the parasympathetic nervous system; and (3) some postganglionic fibers of the sympathetic nervous system such as those that innervate the sweat glands. Acetylcholine has also been clearly established as the chemical transmitter in all motor nerves of the somatic nervous system. Nerves that contain acetylcholine as the neurotransmitter are, by definition, *cholinergic nerves.*

The synthesis of acetylcholine is an example of the conjugation of a naturally occurring compound (see Table 8-1). Acetylcholine is the end product of the acetylation of choline, a normal dietary constituent as well as a compound that can be synthesized in the body from the amino acid serine. This conjugation reaction takes place in the axonal terminals of cholinergic nerves and is catalyzed by *choline acetyltransferase (choline acetylase),* an enzyme that is also synthesized by the neuron.

The acetylcholine that is synthesized in the cytoplasm is stored in vesicles ('synaptic vesicles') in highly concentrated ionic form; it has been estimated that a single nerve terminal may contain 300,000 or more vesicles and that each vesicle may store from 1000 to 50,000 molecules of acetylcholine.

When an impulse arrives at the nerve terminal, 100 or more of these vesicles synchronously discharge their content of acetylcholine, which then diffuses across the junctional cleft and combines with the specialized receptor of the postjunctional membrane. Binding of acetylcholine to its receptor activates the opening of a channel within the receptor to permit the inflow of Na^+. This event depolarizes the post-synaptic cell and leads to generation of an impulse in a postganglionic neuron (or contraction of skeletal muscle innervated by somatic nerves).

Destruction of the acetylcholine released in the process of cholinergic stimulation is accomplished by the enzyme acetylcholinesterase, which hydrolyzes the mediator to choline and acetic acid. So rapid is this hydrolysis at some sites, that within milliseconds the action of acetylcholine can be terminated and the postjunctional membrane can again be made responsive to nerve impulses. It is the strategic localization of acetylcholinesterase at the surface of postjunctional membranes that accounts for this rapid inactivation of the transmitter.

Norepinephrine

The role of norepinephrine as a neurotransmitter is confined to postganglionic fibers of the sympathetic nervous system. Even within this system there are exceptions since, as noted above, the fibers to sweat glands and some vasodilator fibers (found primarily in skeletal muscle) are cholinergic fibers. Nerves that release norepinephrine upon stimulation are called *adrenergic nerves.*

SYNTHESIS. The amino acids phenylalanine or tyrosine, both of which are present in body fluids, are the starting points for the synthesis of norepinephrine by the body, but the total synthesis is more complicated than that for acetylcholine (Fig. 14-4). First of all, not all of the enzymes involved have the same locus of action: step 1, the hydroxylation of phenylalanine takes place outside

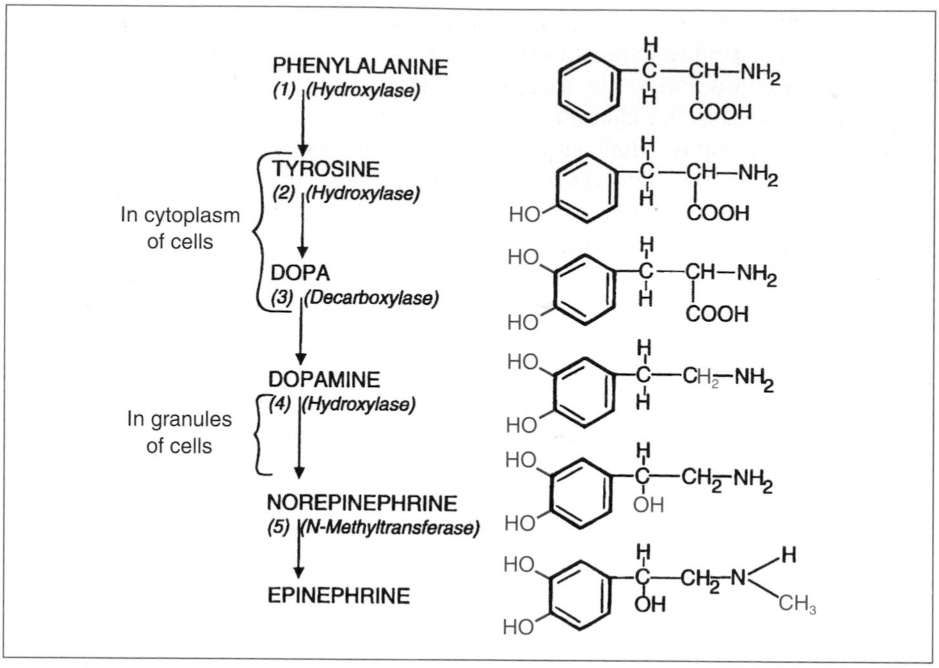

Figure 14-4. *Synthesis of norepinephrine and epinephrine.*

the nerve terminals and then the tyrosine formed or that already present is actively transported into the nerve ending; steps 2 and 3 take place within the cytoplasm of the nerve ending; and step 4, the final step, within the vesicle. Second, none of the enzymes in the sequence is specific for norepinephrine; the enzymes involved can catalyze similar reactions using other endogenous compounds and some drugs as substrates. For example, methyldopa, a drug formerly used in the treatment of hypertension, not only inhibits the metabolism of dopa to dopamine (step 3) but can itself participate in steps 3 and 4 and be converted to α-methylnorepinephrine. We shall see later the pharmacologic significance of these interactions and how they can be used to explain mechanisms of drug action.

STORAGE AND RELEASE. The processes involved in the storage and release of the adrenergic transmitter are also more complicated than those for the cholinergic transmitter – some of the norepinephrine content of the nerve terminal exists as a dissociable complex within the synaptic vesicle. This form of the transmitter is in equilibrium with an unbound form of norepinephrine which in turn is in equilibrium with the norepinephrine outside the storage granules, the cytoplasmic pool. The intravesicular pools containing the more recently synthesized transmitter account for the norepinephrine that is released from adrenergic fibers in response to nerve stimulation. An active transport system helps to maintain a high concentration gradient within the vesicle.

DEPOSITION OF RELEASED NOREPINEPHRINE. Although there are two major enzymes, *catechol-O-methyltransferase* and *monoamine oxidase,* that can inactivate released norepinephrine (cf. pp. 163, 169), neither plays an important role in terminating the action of the adrenergic transmitter. Some small portion of the released norepinephrine diffuses away from the extracellular region and is metabolized, but the mechanism primarily responsible for the removal of norepinephrine from its receptor sites is the active reuptake by the axonal terminals. Obviously, this reentry into the nerve also conserves the transmitter and provides a source other than synthesis for maintaining adequate supplies in readiness for its functioning as a neurotransmitter. Whereas diffusion along concentration gradients can account for the movement of released norepinephrine out of the axonal terminal, active transport processes are required for its reuptake: one transport system for reentry into the cytoplasmic pool and a second for active transport across the membrane of the synaptic vesicle. These transporters are the sites of actions for some drugs.

Pharmacologic Considerations

Elucidation of basic cellular function and better understanding of drug action usually proceed in parallel. Thus, the validation of the role of acetylcholine and norepinephrine in neurotransmission and the clarification of the sequence of events involved in the process at peripheral cholinergic and adrenergic terminals are of fundamental importance to pharmacology; the action of most drugs affecting the PNS as well as the CNS can be interpreted in terms of how they modify the synthesis, release, storage or disposition of a neurotransmitter or stimulate or inhibit its interactions at receptor sites. Table 14-4 lists the individual steps in transmission at both cholinergic and adrenergic terminals and some representative agents that act at each point.

Drug Actions Influencing Transmitter Synthesis, Storage and Release

There are, of course, more ways in which drugs alter adrenergic transmission than cholinergic transmission, simply because the processes involved in the synthesis, storage and release of norepinephrine are more complex than those for acetylcholine. Let us, for example, consider the modes of action of hemi-cholinium, α-methyltyrosine (α-MT) and methyldopa, each of which interferes with neurotransmitter synthesis, thereby limiting the store of chemical mediator available for release. Hemicholinium blocks the synthesis of acetylcholine by inhibiting the active transport of choline from extracellular fluid into the cytoplasm of axonal terminals where the final step of synthesis occurs. α-Methyltyrosine blocks the synthesis of norepinephrine by inhibiting the enzyme responsible for the conversion of tyrosine to dopa (step 2 in Fig. 14-4). Methyldopa, on the other hand, is an inhibitor of norepinephrine synthesis because it effectively competes with dopa, the precursor of the normal transmitter, for the enzyme that catalyzes step 3 (Fig. 14-4). Since the enzymes involved in the

Table 14-4. *Mechanisms of drug action in relation to the steps involved in neurohumoral transmission at cholinergic and adrenergic neuro-effector junctions*

Mechanism of drug action and effect produced	Neurotransmitter involved	
	Acetylcholine	*Norepinephrine*
Inhibition of synthesis of transmitter leading to its depletion	Hemicholinium	α-Methyltyrosine[1]
Biotransformation via same synthetic pathway as that of transmitter, leading to displacement of normal neurotransmitter by 'false transmitter'	...	Methyldopa[2]
Inhibition of active reuptake across membrane of vesicular storage, leading to depletion of transmitter	Vesamicol[1]	Reserpine[2]
Inhibition of active reuptake across membrane of nerve terminal, leading to accumulation and potentiation of activity of transmitter at receptor sites	...	Cocaine, imipramine
Rapid release of transmitter from axonal terminal, leading to initiation of activity at effector sites		Tyramine[1], ephedrine, amphetamine
Inhibition of release of transmitter, leading to inhibition of activity at effector sites	Botulinus toxin	Bretylium
Inhibition of enzymic destruction of neurotransmitter leading to accumulation and potentiation of activity of transmitter at receptor sites	Anticholinesterase agents (e.g. physostigmine, diisopropyl phosphofluoridate [DFP])	Monoamine oxidase inhibitors (pargyline, tranylcypromine) (see text for discussion)
Combination with postjunctional receptor sites, leading to qualitatively same effects as produced by transmitter	Methacholine[2], pilocarpine	Epinephrine, phenylephrine, isoproterenol
Blockade of endogenous transmitter at postjunctional receptor sites, leading to inhibition of activity at effector sites	Atropine, scopolamine, pirenzapine	Metoprolol, prazosin

[1] Used only as an experimental tool.
[2] Largely supplanted in therapy by newer agents; still used as experimental tool.

synthesis of norepinephrine are relatively nonspecific, methyldopa can be decarboxylated and hydroxylated (steps 3 and 4, Fig. 14-4) to form α-methylnorepinephrine; the latter can be stored in granules and released by nerve stimulation and, in general, act as a 'false transmitter' at adrenergic receptor sites. It is a false transmitter only in the sense that it replaces the normal neurotransmitter. However, α-methylnorepinephrine has activity at neuroeffector junctions qualitatively identical to that of norepinephrine, but quantitatively different at various sites of action.

There appear to be no drugs that interfere with the storage of acetylcholine in vesicles at the axonal terminal once it has been synthesized. And since little or none of the transmitter reenters the nerve terminal after its release, the available acetylcholine store is solely dependent on its synthesis. There are drugs that act, however, by preventing the release of acetylcholine upon nerve stimulation. The extremely poor prognosis following poisoning by botulinus toxin and β-bungarotoxin, two of the most potent poisons known, is attributable to their action in blocking the release of acetylcholine from cholinergic terminals throughout the nervous system; death, when it occurs, results from peripheral respiratory paralysis (cf. p. 90, and Table 13-14).

In the case of adrenergic transmission, the rather complicated pattern of norepinephrine's storage and release provides a number of potential points for drug attack. For example, bretylium acts in a fashion analogous to that of botulinus toxin since the **adrenergic blocking agent** prevents the release of norepinephrine from intravesicular pools in response to nerve stimulation. In contrast, the activity of the adrenergic neuron blocking agent, guanethidine, is due to impaired release of the neurotransmitter. Guanethidine initially mimics nerve stimulation but, by promoting a slow and prolonged release of the transmitter, leads to depletion of norepinephrine since the transmitter is deactivated before it can be recaptured. Reserpine also leads to depletion of the transmitter, but it does this by blocking the active transport of norepinephrine from the cytoplasm into the intravesicular pools; the adequate supply of transmitter within storage granules is dependent both on *de novo* synthesis and on recapture of norepinephrine previously released from the nerve terminal. The norepinephrine prevented by the action of reserpine from reentering the vesicle is largely destroyed by the monoamine oxidase present in the cytoplasm; the norepinephrine released from the vesicles by the action of guanethidine undergoes a similar fate. Thus, the long-lasting effects produced by both reserpine and guanethidine are more like those of adrenergic receptor blocking agent (e.g. prazosin) rather than those following release of the adrenergic transmitter. On the other hand, agents such as tyramine, ephedrine and amphetamine promote a rapid release of the transmitter and trigger action at the receptor site, that is, produce a **sympathomimetic** effect.

Drug Actions Influencing Transmitter Receptor Activity and Disposition of Transmitter

Drugs that act extracellularly can also produce their effects by a number of different mechanisms. In both the cholinergic and adrenergic systems there are a variety of agents that can combine with the receptors and mimic or antagonize the effects produced by the normal transmitter (see Table 14-4). At cholinergic nerve endings, the action of the acetylcholine released can be potentiated by anticholinesterase agents – drugs that inhibit its enzymic destruction. In the adrenergic system, however, drugs that inhibit the neuronal enzyme catechol-O-methyl transferase or the intracellular monoamine oxidase, the two enzymes primarily responsible for the metabolism of norepinephrine, apparently produce little enhancement of the effects of norepinephrine. But, as noted before, drugs that inhibit monoamine oxidase can lead to accumulation of tyramine, and this can have serious consequences when certain foods augment the normal body content of this sympathomimetic agent (cf. p. 316). Drugs such as the psychostimulant cocaine and the antidepressant imipramine act extracellularly, however, to potentiate the action of norepinephrine at its postjunctional receptor sites; these agents inhibit the active reuptake of the transmitter from the extracellular fluid, the major process responsible for the termination of the effects of adrenergic stimulation.

Postganglionic Receptor Sites

Up to this point we have explored the ways in which cells in the peripheral nervous system communicate with each other in terms of the steps involved in transmission but said little about reception. However, characterizing the nature of the recognition sites to which drugs bind – the receptor – is fundamental to our understanding of how this binding leads to a physiologic response. Application of gene technology to the study of the molecular organization of receptor proteins combined with measurements of ligand-receptor binding, pharmacologic studies and other experimental approaches has provided the basis for the classification of ANS receptors. Such information has already been helpful in explaining the action of important drugs and been of great significance for the development of new therapeutic agents with more selective activity than those already available.

ACETYLCHOLINE RECEPTORS. Studies of the actions of acetylcholine carried out by Dale in 1914 clearly showed that its pharmacologic activities could be divided into two categories, which he termed *muscarinic* and *nicotinic*[3]. This division corresponded closely to the principal physiologic functions of acetylcholine and laid the basis for classifying cholinergic receptors as either muscarinic or nicotinic. Nicotinic receptors occur in the periphery at neuromuscular junctions

---

[3]The muscarinic actions of acetylcholine are those that can be elicited by an injection of muscarine. The nicotinic actions of acetylcholine closely resemble those of nicotine and are elicited by large doses of acetylcholine after its muscarinic actions are blocked by atropine.

of the somatic nervous system and at ganglionic synapses of the ANS. These receptors belong to the family of ionotropic, ligand-gated ion channels. Muscarinic receptors are located at parasympathetic postganglionic neuroeffector junctions and are metabotropic, G-protein-coupled receptors (Fig. 14-5).

Studies of function and molecular structure showed that there are further divisions of both the nicotinic and muscarinic receptors. Differences in the structure of nicotinic receptors explain the selectivity of antagonists such as tubocurare for the neuromuscular junction and hexamethonium for the ganglia. In the case of muscarinic receptors, five different subtypes have been identified from their specific amino acid sequences and four have been characterized functionally. The first one so characterized was the M_1 receptor subtype, which was identified as the result of the development of a selective antagonist, pirenzepine, an inhibitor of gastric acid secretion (cf. Appendix 1). M_1 receptors are found on peripheral neuronal structures and gastric parietal cells. M_2 receptors are present in the heart and exert inhibitory effects when activated; M_3 receptors are present in smooth muscle and exocrine glands, and produce mainly excitatory effects such as stimulation of salivary secretion and smooth muscle contraction; and M_4 receptors are found in lungs where they play a role in bronchiolar constriction.

ADRENERGIC RECEPTORS. That several subclasses of the adrenergic

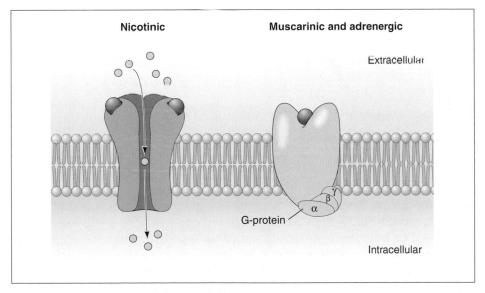

Figure 14-5. *Model of the structures of cholinergic and adrenergic receptors. Nicotinic cholinergic receptors are ligand-gated ion channels, allowing Na⁺ to enter upon binding by acetylcholine. Acetylcholine activates muscarinic receptors and norepinephrine activates adrenergic receptors coupled to G-proteins, which mediate a series of signaling events leading to changes in membrane ion permeability (via ion channels) or transcriptional activity.*

receptor exist in the body was clearly demonstrated as early as 1948 by Ahlquist. He postulated that sympathetically innervated organs had two different types of receptors, α and β, which he differentiated on the basis of responses to norepinephrine, epinephrine and the synthetic agent isoproterenol. Later the use of various selective antagonists confirmed Ahlquist's original classification and demonstrated that the α and β receptors could be further subdivided into several subtypes of each receptor, including α_1, α_2, β_1, β_2. These subtypes differ in their tissue distribution and in the response to their activation. They share similarity in structure and signaling mechanism, since they are all G-protein-coupled receptors (GPCRs) (see Chapter 3). Receptor activation releases the G-protein αβγ complex (Fig. 14-5), which causes a downstream event such as enzyme activation. The physiologic response to subtype activation depends upon the G-protein to which the receptor is coupled (e.g. Gs and Gi). Because the response results from the effects of the G-protein, activation of receptors from other families can produce the same effect as that of an adrenergic receptor subtype, if it is expressed in the same tissue and coupled to the same G-protein.

The identification of the various subtypes of adrenergic receptors led to the development of agents that are more selective and have fewer side-effects. For example, agonists were discovered that selectively target β_2 receptors, which are located in smooth muscle of the airways. Activation of these receptors relaxes the muscles, opens the airways (bronchodilation), and makes breathing easier. These drugs (e.g. albuterol) are important agents in the treatment of asthma. The selectivity for the one adrenergic subtype (as well as their administration by inhalation rather than by ingestion) minimizes the risk of side-effects from activation of other adrenergic receptors such as those in the heart. We will explore the importance of receptor-subtype selective agents in the context of drugs that target the cardiovascular system.

Autonomic Control of Cardiovascular Function: A Target for Antihypertensive Drugs

The cardiovascular system comprises the heart, vessels, and blood, and it serves the critical role of delivering oxygen, glucose, and other nutrients to tissues, and removing carbon dioxide and other waste products. The physiological activity of the cardiovascular system is tightly regulated by the autonomic nervous system and influenced by the actions of hormones and peptides (Fig. 14-6). The heart is innervated by both the sympathetic and parasympathetic branches of the autonomic nervous system. Norepinephrine, released from the adrenergic nerve endings, as well as epinephrine released from the adrenal medulla, activates β_1 receptors in the sinus node, to increase heart rate, and those in the cardiac muscle, to increase the force of contraction. Acetylcholine, released from the vagus nerve, activates muscarinic receptors in the sinus node and slows the heart rate. Blood vessels are innervated by the sympathetic nervous system, primarily through neurons that release norepinephrine. (Fibers to some vessels such as those in skeletal muscle release acetylcholine.) Norepinephrine activates

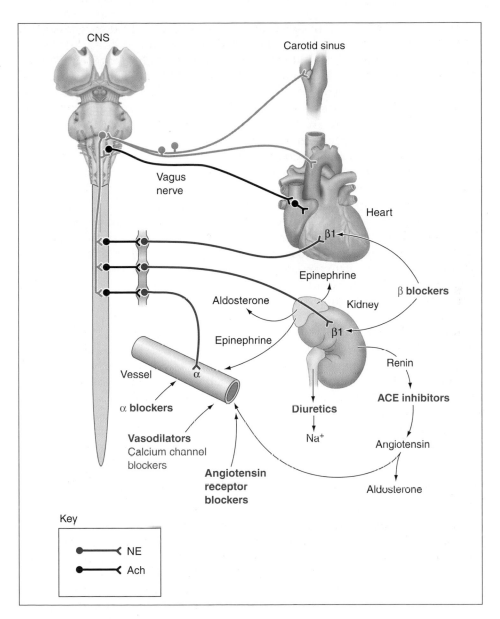

Figure 14-6. *Innervation of the heart and blood vessels by the sympathetic and parasympathetic nervous system and sites of action of drugs used to treat hypertension. The peripheral neurons in black release acetylcholine (Ach); those in blue release norepinephrine (NE).*

the α_1 receptor subtype on the post-synaptic membrane and causes constriction of the blood vessel.

The pressure in the heart and vessels is critical to the flow of blood throughout the body. Pressure is determined by the output of blood from the heart, the diameter of the blood vessels, and the volume of the blood. Reflexes play a role in modulating these factors to maintain the pressure within an appropriate range. For example, there are pressure sensors in the aorta and in the carotid vessels to the brain. They send signals to the brainstem that increase firing of the sympathetic nerves and inhibit the vagus, if the pressure is too high, and the converse if the pressure is too low (see Fig. 14-6). This mechanism, called the baroreceptor reflex, is critical to maintaining pressure on shifts of body position, such as occur when standing from a recumbent position.

Other mechanisms regulate the volume of the blood. Sympathetic nerve fibers innervate a structure within the kidney that releases a small protein, angiotensin. This peptide is converted by an enzyme (angiotensin converting enzyme, ACE) to an active moiety, which constricts blood vessels and causes release of aldosterone from the adrenal cortex. Aldosterone acts in the renal distal tubules and collecting ducts to cause the retention of sodium and water and therefore the expansion of the blood volume (see Chapter 7).

Understanding the regulatory mechanisms of the autonomic nervous system has been critical to the discovery and development of drugs for treating hypertension, the chronic elevation of blood pressure. Hypertension, which affects about 50 million individuals in the US population, is a risk factor for vascular disease, leading to heart attacks, heart failure, strokes, blindness, and kidney failure. The first generation of drugs used to reduce blood pressure dampened the hypertensive effect of the sympathetic nervous system. Among the drugs acting by this mechanism were reserpine and guanethidine, which depleted norepinephrine from its nerve endings. Initially, other drugs like α-methyldopa were thought to affect norepinephrine storage and release, but subsequently were found to act in the brainstem to reduce the activity of the sympathetic nervous system. Another approach to inhibit the sympathetic input to the heart and vessels was the use of drugs (e.g. hexamethonium) acting at sympathetic ganglia to block the nicotinic receptor. The norepinephrine depletors and ganglionic blockers proved to be nonselective in their effect, as could be predicted from the mechanism of action, and caused many side-effects.

Later, adrenergic receptor antagonists were developed to antagonize selectively either the α receptor on blood vessels or the β receptor on the heart. The α receptor antagonists effectively dilate blood vessels and reduce blood pressure. But due to activation of the baroreceptor reflex as pressure drops, they typically cause an increase in heart rate, problematic in a patient with hypertension. The choice of drugs in this class was improved when drugs such as prazosin were discovered with selectivity for the α_1 receptor, relative to the α_2 receptor. This change slightly reduced the degree of adverse effect on heart rate. Drugs with β receptor blocking activity decrease the rate and force of contraction of the heart, and therefore they also lower blood pressure. Like the α-blockers, the initial drugs in this class such as propranolol did not distinguish among the adrenergic subtypes. As a result, these nonselective β-blockers antagonized the β_2 receptor subtype, which is important in relaxing smooth muscle of the airways. The nonselective β-blockers were most problematic with respect to their ability to aggravate symptoms in asthmatic patients. Their use in the treatment of hypertension has been supplanted by the more selective β_1 receptor antagonists such as metoprolol.

As indicated in Fig. 14-6, other classes of antihypertensive agents act on targets other than receptors of the autonomic nervous system. Diuretics such as chlorothiazide act on a Na, Cl transporter in the kidney to increase sodium loss and decrease extracellular fluid volume. ACE inhibitors act on the enzyme that converts angiotensin to its active form. Angiotensin receptor blockers bind to the receptor and prevent interaction with the active peptide. These effects reduce the vasoconstrictive activity of the peptide and decrease its stimulation of aldosterone release from the adrenal cortex. Other agents such as calcium channel blockers act within the smooth muscle of blood vessels to inhibit the influx of calcium, a critical mediator of contractile signaling, and cause vasodilation. The variety of targets involved in regulation of blood pressure, including receptors, enzymes, and transporters, has led to development of many classes of agents, sometimes used in combination in patients with hypertension. More target discoveries are likely with the prospect of new drug classes with ever improving selectivity.

GUIDES FOR STUDY AND REVIEW

What are the traditional subdivisions of the nervous system? of the peripheral nervous system? Do these divisions have anatomic significance? functional significance?

How does the somatic nervous system differ from the autonomic nervous system? In what ways are these two systems similar?

What are the two major divisions of the autonomic nervous system? What are the major structural differences in these two systems? functional differences?

What factors account for the diffuse response of the sympathetic nervous system to stimulation? What factors account for the discrete and localized actions of the parasympathetic nervous system? What is the functional significance of this difference in the general type of response of the two systems?

How are the terms *conduction* and *transmission* distinguished from one another with respect to nervous activity? What is the sequence of events involved in neurohumoral transmission? What are the criteria that must be fulfilled for an endogenous material to be a neurotransmitter?

At what axonal terminals is acetylcholine the neurotransmitter? What is the name given to nerves that release acetylcholine?

How and where is acetylcholine synthesized? stored? released? metabolized? What factors are responsible for the termination of the action of acetylcholine?

At what axonal terminals is norepinephrine the neurotransmitter? What is the name given to neurons that release norepinephrine?

In general terms, how and where is norepinephrine synthesized? Does the entire synthetic process occur in one or more loci? Are the enzymes involved in the synthesis of norepinephrine specific or relatively nonspecific?

How and where is norepinephrine stored? released? metabolized? What factors are responsible for the termination of the action of norepinephrine?

In general, how may drugs that affect the autonomic nervous system produce their effects? How may drugs interfere with the synthesis of acetylcholine? norepinephrine? What are the consequences of such interference?

How may drugs interfere with the storage of norepinephrine? with its release? Are there drugs known to interfere with the storage or release of acetylcholine?

How may drugs influence transmitter receptor activity and the disposition of transmitter? How does the disposition of acetylcholine differ from that of norepinephrine? What is the significance of this difference? How do drugs that inhibit the metabolism of acetylcholine affect activity at receptor sites? How do drugs that inhibit the enzymic inactivation of norepinephrine affect activity at receptor sites?

What structural types of receptors mediate the effects of acetylcholine? of norepinephrine? What is the significance of the existence of subtypes of these receptors with respect to the selectivity of drug action?

What are the major regulatory effects of the autonomic nervous system on the heart and blood vessels? What target sites in the cardiovascular system explain the therapeutic effects of drugs used to treat hypertension?

SUGGESTED READING

Amara, S.G. and Kuhar, M.J. Neurotransmitter transporters: recent progress. *Annu. Rev. Neurosci.* 16:73, 1993.

Appenzeller, O. *The Autonomic Nervous System*. Amsterdam: Elsevier, 1982.

Bell, C. Dopamine precursor or transmitter in sympathetically innervated tissues? *Blood Vessels* 24:234, 1987.

Bredt, D.S. and Snyder, S.H. Nitric oxide: a novel neuronal messenger. *Neuron* 8:3, 1992.

Burnstock, G. The changing face of autonomic transmission. *Acta Physiol. Scand.* 126:67, 1986.

Doyle, A.E. Comparison of beta-adrenoceptor blockers and calcium antagonists in hypertension. *Hypertension* 5:II103, 1983.

von Euler, U.S. Historical perspective: growth and impact of the concept of chemical neurotransmission. In: L. Stjune, P. Hedquist, H. Lagercrantz and A. Wennmalm (eds). *Chemical Neurotransmission – 75 Years*. London: Academic, 1981:3.

Furness, J.B. and Costa, M. *The Enteric Nervous System*. Edinburgh: Churchill Livingstone, 1987.

Hokfelt, T. Neuropeptides in perspective: the last ten years. *Neuron* 7:867, 1991.

Kelly, R.B. Storage and release of neurotransmitters. *Cell/Neuron* 72 (Suppl. 43): 1993.

Levine, R.R. and Birdsall, N.J.M. (eds). Proceedings of the Sixth Symposium on Subtypes of Muscarinic Receptors. *Life Sci.* 5:1, 1995.

Parsons, S.M., Prior, C. and Marshall, I.G. Acetylcholine transport, storage and release. *Int. Rev. Neurobiol.* 35:279, 1993.

Summers, R.J. and McMartin, L.R. Adrenoceptors and their second messenger systems. *J. Neurochem.* 60:10, 1993.

15   The Pharmacologic Aspects of Drug Abuse

The earliest records of the search by humans for means to cope with the demands of the environment attest to a remarkable ingenuity in finding drugs that allay anxiety, elevate mood and, in general, furnish pleasure and satisfaction. Certainly, most ethnic groups had independently found methods of producing alcohol during a primitive stage in their development. Opium, the source of morphine, and solanaceous plants, the source of atropine and scopolamine, as well as the sources of hashish, nicotine, cocaine, caffeine and similar drugs, were also discoveries of primitive peoples. Among these agents known and used since antiquity are some that remain part of our modern therapeutic armamentarium. But these and many other ancient drugs are also among those that pose serious problems in our contemporary culture through their use for nonmedical purposes. Whether the ancients also recognized the social ills attendant on the use of drugs that provide the user with an escape from reality is clearly documented only in the case of alcohol. It was not until the late 1600s that descriptions of abuse appeared in the annals of medicine for other drugs (even opium, so widely used in ancient times for its soporific and analgesic properties). But surely there must have been individuals among ancient civilizations who used these drugs in a manner at odds with the society of their times. And in this context, drug abuse and drug dependence are as old as some of the drugs associated with these phenomena.

The term *drug abuse* refers to the excessive and persistent use, usually by self-administration, of any drug without due regard for accepted medical practice. The vast majority of drugs of abuse are agents that act on the central nervous system (CNS) to produce profound effects on mood, feeling and behavior. This broad definition of drug abuse also includes the habitual use by laymen of drugs like laxatives, headache remedies, antacids and vitamins. However, inclusion of the word *persistent* excludes from classification as abusive the occasional nonmedical or inappropriate medical use of a drug, such as the indiscriminate use of antibiotics to treat the common cold. This use of drugs for purposes or conditions for which they are unsuited (or even their appropriate use but in improper dosage) is better termed *drug misuse.*

The abuse of some drugs that act in the CNS often leads to *dependence* and *addiction.* Both *dependence* and *addiction* are often preceded by some degree of tolerance (see Chapter 12). *Dependence* is a condition in which the body functions normally only in the presence of the drug[1]. If the drug is removed, the person suffers from several physiologic changes that are unpleasant at the least, or even fatal at most. *Addiction* is a condition in which a person feels compelled to use a drug, despite negative health and social consequences. The person has lost control over this compulsive use, and if the drug is not available, the addict suffers intense craving that usually leads to renewed drug-seeking behavior or relapse.

We shall be concerned in this chapter only with the neurobiological aspects of drug dependence and addiction and not with the social, economic, psychologic, moral, or legal issues that also enter into the complex phenomenon of drug abuse. Since drugs of abuse produce their psychoactive effects by acting on the CNS, we shall begin with an abbreviated account of the functional anatomy of the CNS.

THE FUNCTIONAL ORGANIZATION OF THE CENTRAL NERVOUS SYSTEM: A BRIEF REVIEW

The billions of cells of the body, each a unit in its own right, are transformed into interdependent and cooperatively functioning parts of a single entity – a human being – largely through the activities of the nervous system. The endocrine system and other chemical mechanisms also play important roles in the control and integration of the body functions. But it is the CNS that is the principal coordinator and director of all the activities of the tissues and organs of the body. By virtue of its capacity for rapid response, the CNS also provides the most effective mechanism by which the human can adjust to changes in the external environment. And it is the high degree of specialization of the brain that sets the human apart from all other animals in the ability to correlate and integrate information, to reason abstractly and to think creatively.

The CNS, enclosed by the vertebrae and the skull, is made up of the spinal cord, and the brain, both of which contain billions of nerve cells. The *nerve cell* or *neuron,* the impulse-conducting unit, characteristically consists of a nucleated *cell body* (or soma), *dendrites* and a long process known as the *axon* or nerve fiber (Fig. 15-1). The dendrites, of which there may be many, receive impulses from the neurons and conduct them to the cell body. The axon, a single

---

[1]The term 'dependence' used here is not the same as that described by the American Psychiatric Association DSM-IV for the diagnosis of substance dependence. According to the DSM-IV, substance dependence is a maladaptive pattern of substance use leading to significant impairment, and requires at least three manifestations during a 12-month period, such as tolerance, withdrawal, increasing dosage over time, unsuccessful control of use, drug-seeking behavior, loss of social/recreational/occupational activities, and continued drug use despite negative consequences. Physiological dependence requires evidence of tolerance or withdrawal.

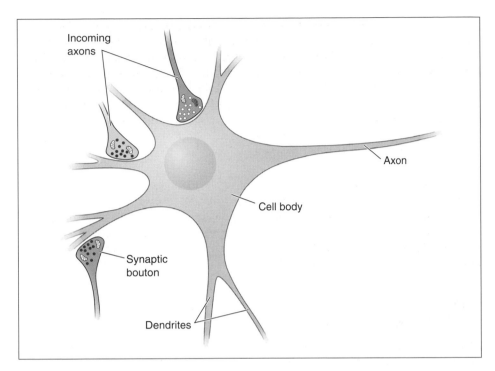

Figure 15-1. *Nerve cell. A neuron may have many dendrites but has only one axon, which carries impulses away from the cell body. Nerve impulses from other nerve cells are transmitted from terminals (synaptic boutons) of incoming axons to dendrites or directly to the nerve cell body. A single neuron may receive impulses from many other neurons.*

cytoplasmic extension of the cell body, conducts impulses away from the soma and stimulates other cells; there is usually only one axon, but this may have numerous branches or *collaterals*. Neurons vary widely in shape and size and in the number, length and degree of branching of their processes. Their structure may be specific to a certain function. For example, with respect to the peripheral nervous system, neurons can be divided into two main categories: *afferent* or *sensory* and *efferent* or *motor* neurons. Neurons that conduct impulses toward the CNS from the sense organs (e.g. eye or ear), or from receptors in tissues that respond to different stimuli, are afferent neurons. Efferent neurons carry impulses outward from the CNS to the muscles, glands, or other tissues and organs.

Neurons do not occur singly in vertebrates; the nerves that are visible on dissection are composed of bundles of both efferent and afferent nerve fibers. Outside the CNS these bundles are called *nerve trunks*; within the CNS they are usually referred to as a tract, or a column. A cluster of cell bodies is known as a *ganglion,* but within the CNS the terms *nucleus, body,* or *corpus* are also used to designate a group of associated nerve cell bodies.

The junction between two neurons at which impulses are transmitted from one to another is called a *synapse*. (The junction between an efferent fiber and a muscle or other tissue or organ which it innervates is known as a neuro-effector junction.) Transmission at the synapse is unidirectional, the impulse being conveyed from the axon of one neuron (the presynaptic cell) to the soma or dendrite, or both (or in some cases, the axon), of another neuron (the postsynaptic cell). The terminal branches of a single axon may impinge on a number of different cells, so that one axon may transmit impulses to hundreds of other neurons. Conversely, any one neuron may receive impulses from many different axons.

Transmission of impulses at the synapse is brought about chemically, not electrically as in the case of impulse **conduction** along the axon. At synapses the collaterals of the axon end in synaptic boutons, or terminal buttons, which contain numerous small vesicles. Nerve impulses arriving at the terminal cause these vesicles to liberate their contents into the synaptic space, and the discharged chemical, rather than an electric current, affects the adjacent neuron. Outside the CNS, the chemical transmitters released upon nerve stimulation have been identified as acetylcholine at all synapses and between nerves and skeletal muscles, and as acetylcholine or norepinephrine at most other neuroeffector junctions (see Chapter 14). Within the CNS, the transmitters at specific synapses are also known. For example, in the spinal cord, acetylcholine is known to be the transmitter at the synapse between the Renshaw cell and the motor neuron; in the cerebellum, norepinephrine is a neurotransmitter that modulates the firing of Purkinje cells. And in the hippocampus, a structure important in learning and memory, glutamate is the transmitter between pyramidal cells. In addition acetylcholine, histamine, serotonin (5-hydroxytryptamine; 5-HT), dopamine, gamma-aminobutyric acid (GABA) and glycine function as neurotransmitters within the CNS; a modulatory role of other amino acids or peptides is common throughout the CNS. The identities of the transmitters and their receptors at different loci in the CNS help to establish the precise mechanisms of action of many drugs that act on the CNS. Outside the CNS, many drugs are known to produce their effects either by mimicking, potentiating or inhibiting the actions of acetylcholine and norepinephrine or by altering the synthesis, storage, release or catabolism of these neurotransmitters (see Chapter 14). The drugs acting on the CNS may also produce their characteristic effects directly or indirectly by altering the ability of neurons to transmit information to one another.

The *spinal cord* consists mainly of nerve fibers segregated into special functional groups, some transmitting sensory nerve impulses upward (the ascending tracts), others conveying efferent impulses downward to peripheral nerves and muscles (the descending tracts). The spinal nerves, 31 pairs in all, enter and emerge from each side of the spinal cord through spaces between the vertebrae (see Fig. 14-2). Each spinal nerve consists of a posterior (dorsal) root and an anterior (ventral) root. The posterior root contains the small bundles of afferent fibers that have united at each segment before entering the spinal cord, and the anterior root carries the efferent fibers that will divide after leaving the cord. Drugs may produce some of their effects by actions directly on the nerves within the spinal cord. Amphetamine, for example, enhances excitatory activities of some simple reflexes, such as the knee jerk elicited in response to a tap below the kneecap. This reflex involves only a single synapse between the afferent fibers carrying the sensory impulses and the efferent fibers to the leg muscles.

The *medulla oblongata* is a direct extension of the spinal cord (Fig. 15-2). This region of the brain contains the vital centers that regulate respiration, blood pressure (vasomotor center), heart rate and contractile force (cardiac center). The groups of synapses concerned with the reflex control of swallowing, coughing and vomiting also lie within the medulla. There are many drugs that produce their effects by stimulating or depressing one or another of these medullary centers. For example, respiration is depressed by alcohol, the barbiturates and opioid analgesics through their actions on the respiratory center. Some drugs owe their therapeutic usefulness to their ability to affect a specific medullary center at doses usually below those which produce effects at other sites, e.g. cough suppression by codeine or the induction of vomiting by apomorphine.

The *pons* and *midbrain* along with the medulla constitute the *brainstem,* the part of the brain below the cerebrum. Ascending and descending tracts of fibers course through the pons, some of the descending fibers forming synapses with neurons which enter the cerebellum. The midbrain also serves as a relay station for messages to and from the higher regions of the brain as well as for impulses concerned with vision and hearing.

The *cerebellum* lies close to and somewhat above the medulla and is connected to the brainstem by large tracts of fibers. Its primary functions are the modulation and control of equilibrium, posture and movements. Through feedback mechanisms to the periphery of the body and to other parts of the brain, the cerebellum coordinates and refines muscular activity and movement. Drugs such as alcohol and benzodiazepines, which produce motor incoordination or ataxia, affect neurotransmission within the cerebellum.

The *hypothalamus,* the area underlying the thalamus, is one of the central elements of systems concerned with control of the emotional state, of wakefulness and sleep and of alertness and excitement. The hypothalamus, as the principal locus of integration of the entire autonomic nervous system (see Chapter 14), is also involved in the subconscious control of many of the body's internal activities, including regulation of arterial blood pressure, respiration, body temperature, body fluid volume, gastrointestinal activity and fat and carbohydrate metabolism. The hormonal secretions of the endocrine glands, particularly those of the pituitary, are also influenced by the activities of the hypothalamus. Through its links with the thalamus and cerebrum, with various other regions of the brain and with organs involved in the basic life functions, the hypothalamus is in a most strategic position. It is not surprising that drugs that influence hypothalamic activity, either directly or indirectly, produce marked changes in an individual's behavior or in the ability to adapt to changes in the internal and external environments. For example, amphetamines have multiple actions, many of which result from effects on the hypothalamus. Amphetamines disrupt temperature regulation, causing hyperthermia, and they inhibit areas of the hypothalamus that regulate hunger, accounting for the anorectic effects.

The *limbic system,* intimately connected with the hypothalamus, is a collection of structurally and functionally interrelated brain centers lying deep inside the cerebral hemispheres and surrounding the thalamus and hypothalamus. The *amygdala* and *hippocampus* are two of the better-studied components of the system. The limbic system is concerned with the complex emotions and instincts for survival – fear, feeding and mating. Thus it is involved with the integration of the emotional state with somatic and autonomic activities (cf. Chapter 14). Drugs such as the morphine-like opioids and antipsychotic agents that affect behavior may do so, in part, by altering the activity of the limbic system.

The *thalamus,* lying atop and to the right and left of the midbrain, is concerned primarily with sensory transmission and perception. All sensory impulses entering the spinal cord or brainstem arrive in the thalamus and are coordinated and interpreted before being relayed to the cerebral cortex. However, thalamic perception and interpretation of sensations of heat, cold, pain, touch or other types of sensory phenomena are rather gross and nondiscriminatory; the more refined, advanced sensations contributing to consciousness are interpreted through the cerebrum. Drugs that act on the thalamus, such as morphine, may interfere with the orderly transmittal of sensory impulses such as pain, and this interference may be partially responsible for the action of opioid analgesics.

The *cerebrum,* by far the largest part of the human brain, is incompletely separated into right and left *hemispheres* by a median longitudinal fissure. At the base of this cleft, a band of fibers known as the *corpus callosum* connects the two cerebral hemispheres. The *cerebral cortex* is the outer layer covering each hemisphere and the four large areas, or lobes, into which each half of the brain is divided (Fig. 15-3). The *frontal lobe* contains areas concerned with the control of muscular movements and speech as well as centers involved in coordinating muscular activity with the functions of the vital organs. The *parietal lobe* is responsible for the interpretation of sensations of heat, cold, touch and pressure with a specificity and fine discrimination not realized in the thalamus. The *occipital lobe* is the area for the perception and interpretation of visual stimuli, and a large part of the *temporal lobe* is involved with the process of hearing.

In lower mammals, almost the whole surface of the cortex is concerned with specific sensory or motor activities. In contrast, in humans the greatest bulk of the cerebral cortex is given over to associational fibers which form complex interconnections among all the impulses received in this region of the brain. These *association areas* make up almost all of the frontal and parietal lobes and much of the temporal and occipital lobes, and it is the size and degree of devel-

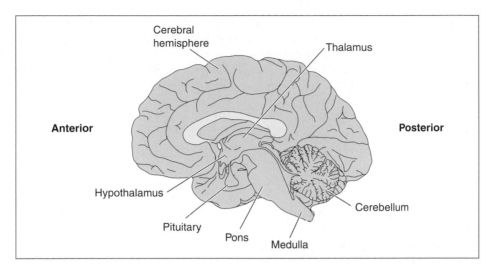

Figure 15-2. *Structural and functional relationships of various parts of the CNS. The medulla contains control centers for respiration, blood pressure, heart rate and vomiting. The cerebellum is primarily concerned with the modulation and control of equilibrium, posture and movement. The hypothalamus is involved in the control and regulation of blood pressure, respiration, body temperature, body fluid volume, gastrointestinal activity and metabolism. Hypothalamic pathways also influence the emotional state, sleep and wakefulness. The thalamus is concerned primarily with sensory transmission and perception. The cerebrum is concerned with learning, memory, intelligence, reasoning, creative thought and imagination as well as with specific sensory and motor activities. The reticular formation, extending between the medulla and the thalamus, influences the overall degree of activity of the CNS and is responsible for normal wakefulness and alertness.*

opment of these association areas which place humans above other mammals. Learning and memory, intelligence and reasoning and those ideational processes unique to humans – creative thought and imagination – appear to be functions of the association areas.

Cortical activity may be depressed by drugs such as alcohol, phenobarbital, or benzodiazepines, or stimulated by agents such as amphetamine and caffeine. The depressant activity may be manifested as a decrease in the acuity of sensory perception or as a decrease in muscular activity. Stimulation may be expressed as reduced fatigue, wakefulness, elation or increased mental or muscular activity. However, the basic actions of the drugs that produce either depression or stimulation are exerted on portions of the brain not directly concerned with motor activity.

Although it is possible to identify specific regions of the brain with particular functions, such as control of respiration, muscular activity, sensory perception and so forth, no one area of the CNS operates independently. Even though each part may have its own responsibilities, the various sections of the brain and spinal cord are interconnected and are constantly interacting with each other.

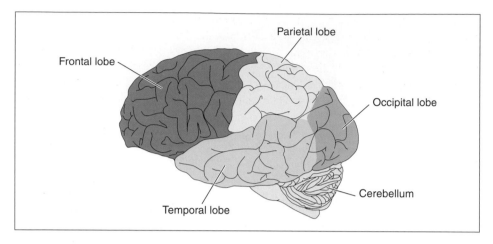

Figure 15-3. *Lateral view of left cerebral hemisphere of the human brain, illustrating position of the four lobes.*

This is perhaps best illustrated by considering how the *reticular formation* influences the overall degree of activity of the CNS.

The reticular formation, a complex network of cell bodies and interlacing fibers, begins in the medulla and extends upward through the midbrain to the thalamus (see Fig. 15-2). From the thalamus, fibers fan out to virtually all areas of the cerebral cortex. These upward projections of the reticular formation and thalamus are called the *ascending reticular activating system* (RAS). This system functions to control the overall degree of CNS activity and is basically responsible for normal wakefulness and alertness. The RAS has little intrinsic activity of its own, and in the absence of sensory impulses it is quiescent and the individual is relaxed, drowsy or asleep. Yet this system is instantly responsive to almost any type of sensory impulse, and stimulation of the RAS produces an arousal reaction and a state of wakefulness. By means of descending fibers the cortex is also able to increase the degree of activity of the RAS. Thus, once the RAS is stimulated, a 'feedback' system from the excited cortex helps to maintain increased activity in the RAS.

The RAS also has an important descending component that can lead to increased or decreased activity of the peripheral muscles. When muscular activity is increased, this in turn feeds back to the RAS and promotes continued excitation. Many of the vital functions of the body are stimulated by the RAS, and this type of increased activity provides another feedback loop. Thus, once an individual has been awakened by the activation of the RAS, the feedback impulses from both the cerebral cortex and the periphery function to keep the individual awake. The neurons of the RAS are not capable of maintaining activity indefinitely, however, and after prolonged wakefulness they become fatigued or less excitable. The cycle then reverses itself, and the lessened activity of the RAS produces less and less activity in the feedback loops until most of the components of this complex system become inactivated and a state of sleep ensues. Drugs such as the barbiturates, which inhibit the RAS, can depress brain activity, induce sleep and, if the dose is large enough, may lead to unconsciousness and coma. Despite the discontinuation of barbiturates for use as sedative/hypnotic drugs because of their toxicity, these drugs are still abused. Many other drugs, such as the general anesthetics and other sedatives/hypnotics, also decrease the activity of the RAS.

During the wakeful state, the RAS also controls the general level of attentiveness to external surroundings. But through its links with the thalamus, the RAS can excite or inhibit *specific* areas of the cortex. The latter may be one of the mechanisms whereby an individual can direct attention to certain aspects of the conscious mind while ignoring others. It would appear that the RAS plays a role in selecting the appropriate response to a given stimulus or condition and, in general, provides for integration of the activity of various parts of the CNS. Some of the effects of low doses of alcohol are the consequences of a depression of this integrating activity of the RAS (cf. General Depressants of the Central Nervous System; p. 404).

GENERAL CHARACTERISTICS OF DRUG DEPENDENCE AND ADDICTION

Drug dependence is sometimes referred to as physical or psychological. *Physical dependence* is an altered or adaptive physiologic state produced in an individual by the repeated administration of a drug. That physical dependence has been induced during the prolonged use of a drug is revealed only when the drug is abruptly discontinued or when its actions are diminished by the administration of a specific antagonist. Physical dependence manifests itself as intense physiologic disturbances called the *withdrawal* or *abstinence syndrome*. Often these 'withdrawal symptoms' are opposite to the physiological effects of the drug itself. For example, a person can become dependent on the anti-anxiety drug, alprazolam (XANAX), and if he/she stops taking alprazolam abruptly, intense anxiety or even seizures can ensue. The degree of physical dependence can be measured only by the severity of the withdrawal symptoms. For drugs like alcohol, the benzodiazepines, and the opioid analgesics, the withdrawal syndromes are so unpleasant and sometimes life-threatening that they are important factors motivating drug-seeking behavior and continued drug use to prevent their appearance. The term *drug dependence* carries no connotation of the degree of serious harm to the drug user or to society. In fact, it is possible to be dependent on a drug, without misusing or abusing that drug. Cancer patients may be treated chronically with opioid compounds for pain and they may be dependent (and tolerant as well), but these patients are not abusing drugs and they are not addicted.

Psychologic dependence is a term that has been used historically to denote a condition characterized by an emotional or mental drive to continue taking a drug whose effects the user feels are necessary to maintain a sense of optimal well-being. Although the definition does not include somatic 'withdrawal' symptoms upon drug cessation, newer brain imaging techniques demonstrate that changes do take place in the brain, even in response to a cue. Thus, the term *psychologic dependence* is no longer used in the pharmacologic arena (although it is used still in the psychiatry or psychological arenas). Instead, psychopharmacologists prefer to use the term, *craving*, to describe this intense desire for the drug, especially when it is not available. Addiction is characterized by the compulsion to use drugs despite negative health and social consequences. Smokers who are trying to abstain can experience intense craving for a cigarette; alcoholics can experience an overpowering obsession to obtain alcohol by knowingly drinking unusual or poisonous mixtures. Addiction represents the major problem of drug abuse, since it indicates that the user has lost control over the drug.

Addiction is usually accompanied by physical dependence – this is common with drugs such as alcohol, barbiturates, and the opioids. Moreover, physical dependence is a powerful factor in reinforcing the compulsion to continue taking the drug. In some cases, addiction develops to drugs that do not induce significant physical dependence and which, therefore, do not give rise to grossly observable abstinence syndrome after discontinuance of drug use. For example, addiction to nicotine or cocaine can be very strong, yet only mild withdrawal symptoms are evident when these drugs are abruptly discontinued. However, craving for the drug is considerable, and it is the craving that drives the user back to taking the drug. Other drugs that are abused may produce only mild addiction or even none at all. For many years it was thought that marihuana did not produce addiction (or dependence, for that matter). However, today we find a considerable number of compulsive users of marihuana, leading physicians and psychologists to conclude that marihuana can be addictive in some individuals. On the other hand, hallucinogens such as lysergic acid diethylamide (LSD) are not usually used compulsively, and therefore are not considered to be addicting. One exception is phencyclidine (PCP), which can produce addiction and has actions within the brain reward system (see below).

The fact that some individuals do not develop addiction to a drug that can induce this phenomenon in others points to the presence of predisposing factors in the person. One explanation that is widely accepted is that many personality factors, life history, and the existence of underlying psychiatric disease contribute to drug abuse. What we do not know, unfortunately, is why some individuals can occasionally use drugs like alcohol or experience other drugs of abuse and not be compelled to use the agents repeatedly, whereas others become drug abusers.

Many of the drugs that induce dependence also have the capacity to produce tolerance, the adaptive state characterized by diminished response to the same dose of a drug (cf. pp. 300–305). Yet tolerance and drug dependence are separate phenomena and may develop independently of each other. Tolerance may be produced by many agents, such as beta-adrenergic antagonists used for asthma, which have no potential for abuse (see Chapter 12). On the other hand, drug dependence and addiction may occur in the absence of the development of any demonstrable tolerance. For example, no apparent tolerance develops to cocaine despite the fact that it produces strong addiction. Moreover, tolerance developed to drugs that are subject to abuse is not necessarily accompanied by physical dependence. The abuse of LSD is a case in point; marked tolerance develops to LSD, but withdrawal symptoms are not seen upon abrupt discontinuance of drug use. However, tolerance is almost invariably associated to some degree with the use of agents that do induce physical dependence, and at times euphoria.

DRUG-SEEKING BEHAVIOR AND THE REWARD PATHWAY

Almost all of the drugs of abuse mentioned in this chapter, with the exception of the hallucinogens, interact with a brain pathway important in reward and positive reinforcement (i.e. drug-seeking behavior). This pathway, the 'reward pathway' (see Fig. 15-4), includes a *mesolimbic* projection of neurons arising in an area of the brainstem called the ventral tegmental area (VTA), to a forebrain structure, the nucleus accumbens. Also important is a *mesocortical* projection of neurons from the VTA to areas of the prefrontal cortex. Additional components of this pathway are shown in Fig. 15-4 and discussed in more detail below. Details about this pathway emerged from studies using animal models for drug addiction; rats and monkeys will self-administer intravenously or

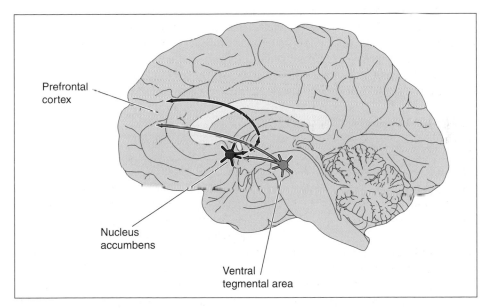

Prefrontal cortex

Nucleus accumbens

Ventral tegmental area

Figure 15-4. *Major pathways involved in rewarding properties of abused drugs are shown. Neurons arising in the brainstem area, the ventral tegmental area (VTA) project to the nucleus accumbens (NA) and to areas of the prefrontal cortex. Nucleus accumbens neurons project to the prefrontal cortex and back to the VTA. Each of these projections contains the neurotransmitter dopamine. Drugs that have rewarding properties increase the release of dopamine in the NA either directly or indirectly by acting on other neurons that connect with this pathway.*

directly into the reward pathway those drugs that are positively-reinforcing and addictive in humans (Table 15-1). This model for 'compulsive use' in animals is a fairly reliable predictor for the addictive potential of a drug. For example, animals do not self-administer drugs that do not produce addiction in humans, such as LSD and other hallucinogens, or antidepressants.

The reward pathway is believed to be important in the ability of natural reinforcers, such as food, water, and sex, to ensure survival of our species. The major neurotransmitter released at the synapses in the nucleus accumbens and the prefrontal cortex is dopamine, and most drugs that cause addiction also cause the release of dopamine, either directly or indirectly, within this circuit. Drugs that increase the release of dopamine indirectly work through other neurotransmitter systems, including opioid, GABAergic, and glutamatergic. Both the rewarding or pleasurable effects of abused drugs and the craving when the drugs are not available are mediated via the reward pathway.

GENERAL CHARACTERISTICS OF ABUSED DRUGS

The drugs that are subject to abuse may be classified on the basis of their characteristic pharmacologic effect on the CNS, i.e. general depressants, opioid analgesics, stimulants, and hallucinogens. Each of these classes of drugs interacts with a major neurotransmitter system to produce the characteristic pharmacologic effects. The CNS depressants act at GABA synapses, the opioid analgesics act at endogenous opioid (i.e. enkephalin, endorphin) synapses, stimulants act at dopamine and norepinephrine synapses, and hallucinogens act at serotonin synapses. The pharmacologic characteristics of these classes of drugs are discussed below in the context of their abuse. A summary is presented in Table 15-2.

Table 15-1. *Self-administered drugs in animals may be addictive in humans*

Drugs self-administered	Drugs not self-administered
Alcohol	Fluoxetine (PROZAC)
Amphetamines	LSD
Barbiturates	Mescaline
Caffeine*	Psilocybin
Cocaine	
Diazepam*	
Gamma-hydroxybutyrate (GHB)	
Heroin	
MDMA (Ecstasy)	
Morphine	
Nicotine	
Phencyclidine	
Δ^9-THC	

*Although we do not associate these drugs with addiction, they are positively reinforcing and are associated with compulsive use in some individuals.

Table 15-2. *Characteristics of tolerance, dependence, and addiction in users of psychoactive drugs*

Agents	Tolerance	Physical dependence	Withdrawal syndrome	Addiction
General depressants				
Alcohol	Irregular and incomplete; little tolerance to adverse effects of high doses; cross-tolerance among members of group	Develops slowly but to marked degree	Varies in intensity with duration and amount of drug intake; potentially severe and most dangerous; characterized by convulsions; deaths not uncommon	Strong with alcohol and barbiturates; rare with benzodiazepines
Sedative-hypnotics				
Barbiturates				
Benzodiazepines				
Anti-anxiety drugs				
Meprobamate				
Benzodiazepines				
Opioid analgesics				
Natural opiates	Striking degree of tolerance to all, but effects on pupil and gastrointestinal tract; cross-tolerance with other opioids	Early development which increases in intensity paralleling increase in dosage	Severe symptoms, but not life-threatening; may be precipitated by administration of narcotic antagonist	Strong with all opioids
Synthetic derivatives of opiates				
Synthetic opioids				
Stimulants				
Amphetamines	Marked, but incomplete; cross-tolerance with amphetamine-like agents but not with cocaine	? (see text)	? (see text)	Strong with most CNS stimulants; exception, MDMA
Cocaine		? (see text)	? (see text)	Intense craving
Nicotine		Develops slowly, but to marked degree	Varies in intensity, but not life-threatening	Intense craving
Hallucinogens				
LSD	Marked	None	None	None
Other drugs with hallucinogenic properties				
Marihuana	Low degree developed to high doses	None	None	Strong in some people
Phencyclidine	Low degree to both behavioral and toxic effects	Mild (but still questionable)	Mild but prolonged (still questionable)	Strong

GENERAL DEPRESSANTS OF THE CENTRAL NERVOUS SYSTEM

A variety of agents widely used for subjective purposes have in common the ability to produce a nonspecific but generalized depression of the CNS. Included in this category are ethyl alcohol; the sedative-hypnotics, including the barbiturates and the benzodiazepines; the anxiolytics; and anesthetic agents (Table 15-3). While all of these drugs act at GABA receptors and increase the ability of GABA to inhibit neuronal firing, they differ markedly in their physicochemical properties and in some of their pharmacologic actions; these differences account for their classification and therapeutic usefulness specifically as sedatives, hypnotics, anxiolytics or anesthetics (cf. Appendix 5, Alcohol and General Anesthetic Agents, and Appendix 6). But despite the differences that exist among the individual agents within the group, the pattern of dependence developed to the entire group is remarkably consistent.

All the general depressants of the CNS are abused to one degree or another for similar reasons: the drugs act to allay anxiety, decrease tension, and produce sedation. All the agents in this group produce the same dose-related signs and symptoms characteristic of increasing depression of the CNS. The agents also resemble one another with respect to the pattern and the degree of tolerance acquired with continued use. Physical dependence develops to all these agents, and the discontinuance of the use of any of them produces similar symptomatology. The drugs are essentially additive and interchangeable; they show *cross-dependence,* the ability of one drug to suppress the manifestations of physical dependence induced by another and to substitute for the other in maintaining the physically dependent state. Alcohol and the barbiturates, at all doses, produce a primary and continuous depression of the CNS. At low doses the effects are principally the result of depression of the reticular system, the more primitive part of the brain concerned with the maintenance of consciousness and the control of responsible behavior. Since the impulses ascending from the

Table 15-3. *General depressants of the CNS used for nonmedical purposes*

Ethyl alcohol	Anxiolytics
Sedative-hypnotics	Diazepam (VALIUM)
Barbiturates	Alprazolam (XANAX)
Secobarbital (SECONAL)	General anesthetics
Pentobarbital (NEMBUTAL)	Ether
Amobarbital (AMYTAL)	Nitrous oxide (laughing gas)
Methaqualone	Inhalants
Gamma-hydroxybutyrate (GHB)	Glue
Benzodiazepines	Paint thinners
Flurazepam (DALMANE)	Lacquer thinners
Triazolam (HALCION)	Gasoline
Diazepam (VALIUM)	
Flunitrazepam (ROHYPNOL)	

reticular activating system to the cortex can be either excitatory or inhibitory, the behavioral responses that are observed will depend on which pathway is initially depressed. Thus the effects of low doses of alcohol and barbiturates are contingent on the degree of excitability of the CNS at the time of drug administration. This, in turn, depends on the environmental setting of drug use and on the personality of the user. In a quiet, nonsocial environment, the ascending excitatory influence may be impaired, and the sedation and drowsiness produced by the drugs are then readily equated with depression of the CNS. In a social setting, where there is a great deal of sensory input, the cortex may be freed from its integrating control by depression of the ascending reticular system. Under these circumstances the effects of low doses of drug are perceived as stimulation, whereas in fact they are the result of release from inhibition secondary to depression of those pathways of the reticular activating system that inhibit specific areas of the cortex. The paradoxical excitement – the talkativeness, the heightened vivacity, the increased self-confidence and the general loss of self-restraint – may be likened to the situation of an automobile parked on an incline being suddenly set in motion by releasing the brake. There is also loss of mental acuity and judgment and impaired motor coordination. As the dose is increased, and during chronic intoxication, these agents produce more of the same effects. There may be slurred speech; staggering; loss of balance and falling; loss of emotional control; stupor from which arousal is difficult; severe respiratory depression; and finally, coma and death. Although low doses of alcohol and barbiturates impair mental and motor function to one degree or another, it is the untoward effects of high doses that can produce the greatest harm to the individual and to society.

In the abuse of alcohol there may be overt pathologic changes in tissues and organs, e.g. the liver, a factor not associated with chronic use of other drugs of abuse. Alcohol, unlike other drugs, can be utilized by the body as a source of energy. This supply of calories often suppresses appetite, leading to dietary deficiencies which may be responsible in part for the pathologic conditions seen in chronic alcoholism

Drug abuse and drug dependence occur in all degrees with alcohol and other CNS depressants. Abuse ranges from occasional sprees of gross intoxication to prolonged, daily use and chronic intoxication. Ethyl alcohol is the agent most widely used and abused, and indeed, in Western cultures, alcoholism is still the most prevalent type of drug abuse. Ethyl alcohol is also the only potent pharmacologic agent used for nonmedical purposes that is socially and culturally acceptable. However, daily use of these drugs is not necessarily abuse or indicative of a state of dependence. For example, since drinking alcoholic beverages is socially acceptable, daily consumption is considered a normal part of the culture of many countries. Problems begin when the evening cocktail or the wine at dinner is escalated to several drinks. Development of tolerance to alcohol develops easily and this leads to an increase in the amount of alcohol that one might drink to provide the desired effect. The onset of tolerance to alcohol sets the stage for the development of dependence. At first, this is insidious, since the dependent state frequently goes unrecognized in its mild form; it becomes apparent only when daily consumption exceeds accepted norms and deviates from established cultural patterns. Similarly, the taking of medically prescribed benzodiazepines daily for anxiety or sleep disorders is not considered abusive drug use. However, dependence can develop to therapeutic doses of benzodiazepines that are used for extended periods. Although this can vary greatly from individual to individual, dependence may be more likely to develop with short versus long half-life benzodiazepines. In fact, withdrawal symptoms develop more rapidly and are more intense after abrupt cessation of short-acting benzodiazepines (alprazolam, triazolam) compared to long-acting benzodiazepines (diazepam).

Thus, mild degrees of dependence may develop to the CNS depressant drugs when they are used in low or therapeutically recommended dosage. Although this pattern of intake may lead to their continued use, drug administration may be stopped without serious subjective disturbances. When there is need for increased drug consumption because of incomplete relief of anxiety and tension, then the development of tolerance enhances the need for more drug, and the development of physical dependence reinforces compulsive use to avoid withdrawal symptoms.

The tolerance that develops to the CNS depressants is erratic and incomplete and never reaches the degree observed with the opioids. Drug-dependent individuals appear less intoxicated and less impaired in performance at a given blood level of drug than do nontolerant individuals. However, the lethal dose of any of these agents is not much greater in the drug-dependent individual than in the nontolerant subject.

The most distinguishing feature of the dependence on CNS depressants is the abstinence syndrome that appears upon abrupt cessation of prolonged administration of high doses. The withdrawal symptoms are usually far more dangerous than those resulting from withdrawal of the opioids or other agents of abuse to which physical dependence may be developed. However, the severity of symptoms depends on the length of drug abuse and the degree of intoxication. In the typical course of alcohol withdrawal, symptoms begin within the first 24 hours after discontinuance of the drug, reach their peak intensity within 2–3 days but are self-limiting and usually disappear within 1–2 weeks. During the first days of alcohol withdrawal there may be headaches, anxiety, involuntary twitching of muscles, tremor of hands, weakness, insomnia and nausea. During the next 48 hours the symptoms become progressively more intense: there may be a precipitous fall in blood pressure; fever; delirium characterized by disorientation, delusions and vivid visual hallucinations; and convulsions similar to those exhibited in grand mal epilepsy. The fever, delirium and convulsions are the most serious symptoms and may lead to fatality.

OPIOID ANALGESICS

The **opioid** analgesics were originally referred to as the 'narcotic analgesics'. In legal parlance the term **narcotic** includes drugs with morphine-like activity, as well as marihuana and cocaine; the last two drugs are pharmacologically unrelated to morphine and induce entirely different states of dependence. In medicine, *narcotic* applies only to drugs having both analgesic and sedative action; the term essentially embraces only those drugs, either natural or synthetic, that have morphine-like pharmacologic activity. Often, the term *narcotic analgesic,* is used interchangeably with *opiate* or *opioid*. Opiates are the active chemicals found in the opium poppy. Any compound that acts like an opiate is termed an opioid. The term opioid is now used to avoid the confusion inherent in the legal classification and is therefore better terminology to designate the morphine-like drugs.

The drugs classified as opioids, for which morphine is the standard of reference, include the natural opiates, their partially synthetic derivatives, and wholly synthetic morphine-like drugs. Heroin, a semisynthetic form of morphine, is the most common street opioid. A listing of the commonly used opioids includes:

Natural opiates obtained from opium
    Morphine
    Codeine

Semisynthetic opioids
    Buprenorphine (SUBUTEX)
    Dihydromorphinone (DILAUDID)
    Heroin
    Oxycodone (OXYCONTIN)

Synthetic opioids
    Fentanyl (SUBLIMAZE)
    Meperidine (DEMEROL)
    Diphenoxylate (with atropine as LOMOTIL)
    Methadone (DOLOPHINE)
    Propoxyphene (DARVON)

Opioid antagonists
    Naloxone (NARCAN)
    Naltrexone (TREXAN)

Although the opioids differ in chemical structure, in their analgesic potency and in their potential to become drugs of abuse, they have basically similar pharmacologic profiles (cf. Appendix 5, Analgesics, II). Even some opioids that have antagonistic properties, when used alone, have pharmacologic actions like those of morphine; these agents are referred to as **mixed agonists/antagonists**. Only the antagonists naloxone and naltrexone differ in this respect from the other opioid antagonists. The opioids are also alike in their ability to induce and maintain some degree of physical dependence and to develop tolerance. With the exception of the opioid antagonists, these agents may be substituted for one another to prevent the appearance of the withdrawal syndrome. And when this syndrome does occur, the signs and symptoms of abstinence are the same for all the opioids.

Dependence on opioids is extraordinary in that the *first* dose of an opioid may set in motion the mechanisms leading to physical dependence and to the development of tolerance. Dependence can be initiated with small doses well within the therapeutic range; the intensity and rapidity with which dependence and tolerance develop vary with the agent but parallel the increase in dosage. This is very different from the dependence on the CNS depressants that develops gradually and then only when the daily dose is increased appreciably above therapeutic levels.

In contrast to alcohol and other general CNS depressants, the opioids are *selective* depressants of the CNS. For example, doses of 5–10 mg of morphine may produce relief of pain without producing any change in the perception of other sensory stimuli (touch, light, sound and so forth); analgesia may occur before and often without sleep. Typically, however, analgesia is accompanied by drowsiness, mood alteration, mental clouding, and some respiratory depression. An essential feature of the analgesic action of morphine is its ability to alter the *reaction* to pain, rather than merely to decrease the perception of the painful stimulus itself. The opioid analgesics also relieve anxiety, tension and fear, the reactions evoked by the specific sensation of pain. Thus the patient, freed from suffering or distress, feels more comfortable, and is able to tolerate the pain even when the patient knows it is still present.

The relief from worry, tension, and fatigue, and the mental fogginess or 'other-worldly' sensation produced by the opioids are interpreted by some subjects as pleasurable (euphoric). These effects account in large measure for the abuse potential of the opioid analgesics. To the opioid abuser everything 'looks rosy' and is 'as it should be'. However, the naive subject may find the effects of morphine quite unpleasant, with nausea, vomiting, itching, and sweating as the predominant effects. In the compulsive drug user there is a state of drive satiation; the drug reduces hunger and diminishes the sexual drive. And, unlike alcohol, the opioids also suppress aggressive behavior. Violence is often characteristic of the compulsive opioid user only when the drug is not available and the addict must resort to criminal activity to satisfy the craving. The rapid development of tolerance and physical dependence upon repeated administration reinforces the emotional need to continue taking the drug and to obtain it by any means.

The rate at which tolerance develops to the opioid analgesics depends on the rate of administration, and it is significant only when administration continues on a more or less daily basis. However, the degree of tolerance may reach phenomenal proportions; some habitual users have been known to take as much as 5 g of morphine per day (500 times the usual analgesic dose). Tolerance develops to all the effects which the chronic user considers desirable: analgesia, sedation and euphoria. Tolerance also develops to the respiratory depression produced by all the opioids. Since respiratory failure is the cause of death in opioid poisoning, this tolerance makes it possible for the compulsive user to satisfy a need with doses that would otherwise be lethal. Tolerance does not develop, however, to the initial 'rush' experienced with i.v. opioids, the constricting effect on the pupil of the eye (cf. p. 34), or the constipating effect on the gastrointestinal tract.

The severity of the abstinence syndrome upon discontinuance of opioid administration is determined by the degree of dependence. Although the symptoms of withdrawal are not nearly as serious as those seen upon withdrawal from alcohol, the morphine abstinence syndrome is nevertheless characterized by changes in most major organs and systems. Symptoms appear shortly before the time for the next scheduled dose, intensify over the next several days and then gradually subside and disappear within 7–10 days. The signs and symptoms include anxiety; restlessness; irritability; lacrimation; generalized body aches; insomnia; perspiration; dilated pupils; gooseflesh ('cold turkey'); hot flushes; nausea; vomiting; diarrhea; fever; increased heart rate and blood pressure; and abdominal and other muscle cramps. The vomiting and diarrhea, combined with the inability to retain water and food, lead to dehydration and loss of weight. All these symptoms, excepting dehydration and weight loss, can be suppressed by administering the drug of dependence or another opioid analgesic. However, the abstinence syndrome does not necessarily require suppression, because it is self-limiting. When the abstinence syndrome is precipitated by the administration of one of the opioid antagonists, the symptoms are the same but the first signs appear within minutes, reach their peak within a half hour and are much more severe.

For opioid-dependent individuals, the harm to the individual and society does not result from the direct pharmacologic effects of the drugs as it does in alcohol-dependent individuals. Rather, ill health, personal neglect, social irresponsibility, economic loss and crime are the indirect consequences of the user's need to procure the drug at all costs. When the opioid-dependent individual is able to obtain the drug by legitimate means, or has adequate funds, and is also able to control the dosage, the user can work productively, discharge social obligations and remain healthy. The capacity of the opioid analgesics to induce *compulsive drug-seeking behavior* is their most malignant property; it is more pernicious than for alcohol with respect to the rapidity with which such behavior can be initiated in susceptible individuals by the repeated administration of small doses.

Over the past several years, there has been considerable progress toward the disclosure of the mechanisms underlying the actions of opioids and opioid addiction. The actions of opiods are mediated by their binding to specific receptors on neuronal membranes. There are multiple opioid receptors in the brain and other organs; in the CNS there is now solid evidence for three major types of receptors in the G-protein-coupled family (termed mu, kappa, and delta).

Why should there be highly stereospecific receptors in mammalian brain that interact with chemicals of *exogenous* origin – with chemicals like the opioids that are entirely foreign to the body? The logical answer is that such receptors were not developed to bind opioids but are receptors for normal components of the body, for either *endogenous* molecules whose functional role is still undefined or endogenous substances as yet undiscovered. Investigations using the latter conceptual approach proved highly successful. Less than 5 years after the disclosure of the existence of specific binding sites for opiate drugs, endogenous substances capable of binding and interacting as agonists at opioid binding sites were discovered and characterized. These 'endogenous opioids' are called *endorphins* or *enkephalins*. The endorphins and enkephalins have been extracted from the brain and pituitary gland of various animal species and from the human pituitary gland, cerebrospinal fluid, and various other areas of the CNS as well as from some peripheral organs and tissues; all have been identified as **peptides** containing 5–30 amino acid residues. Although the physiologic role of the opioid peptides has not been fully elucidated as yet, they are important modulators of neuronal activity associated with pain perception, endocrine function, gastrointestinal function, respiration, and feelings of pleasure.

The euphoria and pleasurable feelings associated with opioid abuse are mediated by actions within the reward pathway. Researchers have identified the ventral tegmental area (VTA) as a key target for opioid-mediated reward and drug-taking behavior (see Figure 15–4). Within the VTA, there are small neurons containing endogenous opioids. The opioids released from these 'interneurons' bind to opioid receptors on interneurons containing the neurotransmitter, GABA. Since activation of both opioid and GABA receptors decreases the firing rate of neurons, the actions of opioids indirectly cause the VTA neurons to increase their firing rate, releasing dopamine in the nucleus accumbens.

STIMULANTS OF THE CENTRAL NERVOUS SYSTEM

Drugs may produce increased activity of the central nervous system either by blocking pathways that normally inhibit activity or by directly enhancing excitation. The drugs used for abusive purposes and classified as CNS stimulants activate specific pathways in the brain to produce behavioral stimulation. In humans the cortical stimulation is seen as garrulousness, restlessness, increased motor activity and excitement. These stimulants also produce a lessened sense of fatigue, so that physical performance and work may be improved and prolonged when they have been impaired by fatigue or lack of sleep (see Appendix 8). Prolonged use or use of large doses is nearly always followed by lethargy and mental depression.

The amphetamines, cocaine, and nicotine are the principal agents of abuse among the stimulants of the CNS (Table 15-4). CNS stimulants such as amphetamines and cocaine differ significantly in many of their pharmacologic actions but are remarkably similar in their subjective effects, toxic symptoms, and present-day patterns of abuse. We shall therefore use amphetamine as the standard of reference for the group and indicate the ways in which dependence on cocaine differs from that on amphetamines. Nicotine will be considered separately.

Table 15-4. *Commonly abused CNS stimulants*

Amphetamines
  Dextroamphetamine (DEXEDRINE)
  Amphetamine (BENZEDRINE)
  Methamphetamine (METHEDRINE, DESOXYN)
  3,4-Methylenedioxymethamphetamine (MDMA)
Cocaine
Methylphenidate (RITALIN)
Mephentermine (WYAMINE)
Nicotine

The ability of the amphetamines to elevate mood, combat fatigue, reduce appetite and induce a general state of well-being accounts for their widespread use as stimulants and appetite suppressants. These effects are typical and occur even in those using the drugs for the first time. This is in contrast to the effects of the opioids, which many first-time users find unpleasant. These typical responses to the amphetamines also form the basis for their abuse potential. Many normal individuals take amphetamines in the course of treatment for obesity and experience the drug-induced mood elevation, yet do not become compulsive drug users. With prolonged and continuous administration, tolerance develops, and the user feels the need to increase both the quantity and the frequency of administration in order to obtain the desired mood elevation. This phenomenon is similar to the development of tolerance to alcohol. The same pattern of abuse may be followed by long-distance drivers or students who use amphetamines to ward off sleep. However, the great majority of persons who abuse the amphetamines and other stimulants do so specifically for their euphoric effects. And this type of abuse commonly involves the intravenous rather than the oral route of administration.

Tolerance develops to many effects of the amphetamines, particularly to those which are most desired by the compulsive user. Although the tolerance develops slowly, it reaches such magnitudes that in order to obtain a state of elation, the habitual user may require doses several hundred-fold greater than the usual therapeutic dose. There have been reports of the use of more than 10 g of methamphetamine intravenously over a 24-hour period. (The therapeutic dose of methamphetamine is about 10 mg.) Such parenteral use of large doses can be particularly hazardous; intracranial hemorrhage associated with severe hypertension has occurred frequently.

Tolerance does not develop evenly to all the CNS effects, and the user may show increased nervousness and persistent insomnia as the dose of amphetamine is increased. After weeks or months of continued use, a toxic psychosis resembling schizophrenia may develop which is characterized by delusions and hallucinations, both auditory and visual. These psychologic disturbances may also appear within a day or two after ingestion of a single large dose or after 2–4 days of chronic use; this psychosis is usually self-limiting and disappears within a week of discontinuing drug use.

The patterns of cocaine use are similar to those of amphetamine with some notable exceptions. The use of cocaine as a stimulant has its roots in antiquity, and the centuries-old custom of chewing coca leaves is still prevalent among the Peruvian Indians of the high Andes Mountains. The leaves of *Erythroxylon coca,* a shrub growing at 1000–3000 meters above sea level, are rich in cocaine and are chewed or sucked by highland inhabitants for the sense of well-being the stimulant provides. Although coca is freely available for the Indians, it is used most often for religious rituals and only occasionally for individual enjoyment. Cases of chronic toxicity or the development of a psychosis are practically unknown, and Andeans have no difficulty in discontinuing their use of coca leaves when they move to lower altitudes. In contrast, drug toxicity, drug dependence, and drug-seeking behavior are closely associated with the smoking of coca paste (60–80% cocaine) by urban-dwelling Peruvians. The problems of addiction to cocaine in the United States and Europe can also be linked directly to the change in its route of self-administration – from the almost nonexistent drug addiction associated with the oral route of slow absorption and distribution to the near-epidemic proportion of addiction coupled to use by routes that provide almost instant delivery of cocaine to centers in the CNS responsible for its euphoric effects (Fig. 15-5). This became alarmingly apparent in 1985 with the widespread availability of a preparation of cocaine that could be smoked. Cocaine hydrochloride, the crystalline powder that is snuffed ('snorted') or injected intravenously, decomposes when heated, but cocaine free base ('crack') melts at 93°C, a temperature low enough to be vaporized by heating in a pipe. The fact that inhaling cocaine vapor gets the drug to the brain as fast as injecting it into a vein adds extra dimension to the problems of cocaine abuse: first, the faster the drug reaches the brain and then leaves the brain, the more likely the user will 'binge' and become addicted; second, inhaling cocaine vapor avoids the additional hazards of intravenous administration and circumvents some individuals' fears and reluctance to use needles.

As in the case of the opioids, even brief use of injected or smoked cocaine by some individuals can initiate a cycle in which they cannot control their drug use. However, unlike the opioid-dependent individual, but like the amphetamine abuser, the typical cocaine addict is a binge user, not a daily user. Thus cocaine, like amphetamine, is employed in huge quantities during these binges – as much as 10 g per day. This excessive dosage is not indicative of the development of tolerance, since cocaine is so rapidly biotransformed that the effect of each administration may last only minutes. The use of large doses of cocaine is associated, however, with toxic psychoses similar to those seen with the amphetamines. Moreover, death from acute intoxication is no longer unusual, yet no one can predict which users are at risk of cardiac arrest, lethal convulsions or respiratory failure. Seizures and fatal cardiac arrhythmias represent toxicities more common with cocaine than amphetamine. These toxic actions may result from the local anesthetic properties of cocaine, which amphetamine lacks.

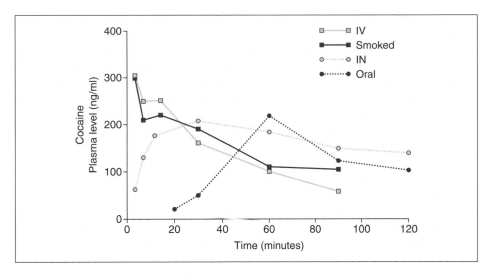

Figure 15-5. *Plasma concentrations of cocaine following administration of the hydrochloride salt by the oral, intranasal (IN) or intravenous (IV) route, or of cocaine base by inhalation. (Redrawn from M.W. Fischman,* J. Clin. Psychiatry *49:2 (Suppl.), 1988.)*

Abrupt discontinuance of the use of amphetamines does not lead to a physiologically disruptive state, and withdrawal of the drugs is never life-threatening. Upon abrupt withdrawal there is a period of prolonged sleep, lethargy and often a precipitous depressive reaction. This state of depression, as well as anhedonia (the inability to feel pleasure), and the intense craving that ensues, probably motivate continuation of drug use. There is a growing consensus that these symptoms, which appear regularly when the amphetamine-like drugs are discontinued, constitute a mild form of abstinence syndrome. Similar symptoms appear when the use of cocaine is abruptly terminated. The harm to the individual and to society of the compulsive use of CNS stimulants can arise during the toxic episodes induced by large doses. The compulsive user of the stimulant drugs has enhanced drives, in contrast to the decreased drives of the opioid user. The hyperactivity, the feeling of great muscular strength, the paranoid delusions and the auditory and visual hallucinations often combine to make the user a dangerous individual capable of committing serious antisocial acts. Chronic users of amphetamines are also prone to accidents, since they are unaware of their fatigue until it overcomes them at an inopportune time.

Another CNS stimulant related to amphetamine is 3,4-methylene-dioxymethamphetamine (MDMA), the active ingredient in Ecstasy. MDMA not only has CNS stimulant properties, but it also has hallucinogenic properties similar to mescaline (see below). Because abuse of MDMA is a relatively recent phenomenon and it is used intermittently, for example, at 'raves', clear evidence for dependence and addiction is still lacking. However, individuals typically feel depressed, irritable, and hungry after using MDMA repeatedly, which may indicate some form of withdrawal. Moreover, monkeys will self-administer MDMA, and the drug increases dopamine release within the reward pathway. MDMA also increases serotonin levels, which explains its hallucinogenic actions and ability to alter perception. As abuse of this drug increases within the population, its ability to produce addiction will become more clear.

A socially accepted form of stimulant abuse is nicotine, the active ingredient in cigarettes. Cigarette smoking itself is rather unpleasant at first; the user may choke and experience nausea due to the nicotine. However, tolerance develops to the nausea rather quickly, and the user may continue to smoke to attain the same pharmacologic actions that are produced by amphetamines and cocaine: increased alertness, elevated mood, and appetite suppression. As smoking becomes a chronic activity, physiologic dependence to nicotine ensues. In this case, the abstinence syndrome is rather mild; it includes restlessness, irritability, and hunger when the user stops smoking. Smokers typically smoke to keep the blood levels of nicotine high enough throughout the day to avoid these symptoms. When smokers try to quit, the craving for cigarettes is intense, and along with stress, it accounts for the high relapse rate.

All of the CNS stimulants interact with the reward pathway to increase dopamine release within the nucleus accumbens (see Fig. 15-4). Amphetamines (including MDMA) increase the release of dopamine directly at the terminals of the VTA neurons in the nucleus accumbens; cocaine prevents the reuptake of dopamine at the same terminals. Nicotine has two actions – it increases the firing rate of VTA neurons (by activating nicotinic receptors on the VTA neurons) and it increases the release of dopamine at the terminals of VTA neurons in the nucleus accumbens. The actions of these CNS stimulants within the reward pathway underlie their ability to produce feelings of pleasure, euphoria, and drug-seeking behavior. The pathway also plays an important role in the craving that ensues when the user tries to stop taking these drugs.

HALLUCINOGENS

The term *hallucinogen* designates a drug that acts on the CNS to produce a state of perception of objects with no reality or of sensations with no external cause. Among the commonly abused drugs included in this category are lysergic acid diethylamide (LSD); psilocybin and psilocin (from the Aztec mushroom); and mescaline (from the peyote cactus plant). (Diethyltryptamine (DET), dimethyltryptamine (DMT) and a number of other synthetic agents are also classified as hallucinogens.) The hallucinogens are also referred to as *psychotomimetics*. The word *psychotomimetic* suggests that the effects produced by the hallucinogens mimic the naturally occurring psychoses. However, most hallucinogenic drugs do not model natural schizophrenia, which is characterized by predominantly auditory hallucinations. Other classes of abused drugs have hallucinogenic properties as well. These include the dissociative anesthetics phencyclidine (PCP) and ketamine; cannabinoids – the active ingredients in marihuana; and MDMA.

Even drugs such as the amphetamines and cocaine can induce illusions and delusions.

The pharmacologic characteristics and patterns of abuse of the various hallucinogenic agents are not sufficiently alike to permit them to be described as a single type. We shall discuss LSD as a prototype hallucinogen, and include some discussion of marihuana and PCP.

LSD-type Hallucinogens

The hallucinogenic properties of LSD are also characteristic of those produced by its related derivatives and by mescaline, psilocybin and psilocin. These agents, which bind to different subtypes of serotonin receptors, differ in potency and duration of action. The action of LSD as a partial agonist at a subtype of serotonin receptors, 5HT-2A, in the noradrenergic *locus coeruleus* and in the cerebral cortex appears to underlie its ability to cause distortions in cognition, perception, and affect.

Very small amounts of LSD (microgram range) may produce effects in susceptible individuals, and these may last from 8–12 hours. The nature of the hallucinogenic state is not predictable in advance and is influenced by the setting of drug use as well as by the mood and expectations of the user. However, certain physical, psychological and perceptual effects are included in most descriptions of the drug experience ('trip'), and these are summarized in Table 15-5. The perceptual changes are the most notable.

The patterns of abuse in the LSD group of drugs are different from that in most other drugs of abuse. The most common pattern is an occasional use at weekly or monthly intervals. Regular use of LSD following initial exposure is now the exception rather than the rule. Even among chronic users the drugs are rarely taken more than twice a week.

Although marked tolerance develops rapidly to the behavioral effects of LSD, it also disappears quickly. Since no physical dependence develops, the user has little compulsion to increase dose or to continue use to avoid the discomfort of its absence. Likewise, there is no evidence that LSD and related

Table 15-5. *The major effects produced by the LSD group of drugs*

Physical: Dizziness; increased heart rate; pupillary dilation; muscular weakness; numbness; tremors; dry mouth; nausea, vomiting; decreased appetite

Psychologic: Altered moods; inner tension relieved by laughing or crying; euphoria (sometimes dysphoria); sense of retardation of time; decreased ability to concentrate; difficulty in expressing thoughts and feelings; depersonalization; introspection; dream-like state; poor memory; rapid thoughts; impaired judgment; great anxiety and tension

Perceptual: Blurred vision; altered shapes and colors; great heightening of color intensity; increased acuity of hearing; colors are heard, sounds may be seen; perceptual distortion of space; organized visual illusions and hallucinations

---

compounds interact with the brain's reward pathway. The real and potential hazards of the hallucinogenic drugs lie in the unpredictability and unreliability of the effects which they may produce and in the frequency of unpleasant or disastrous experiences ('bad trips'). The syndromes produced by these hallucinogens are psychologically harmful to the individual and may be manifested as either acute, recurrent, or prolonged reactions.

The acute reactions, estimated to occur in about 10% of those who experiment with LSD or related drugs, are of short duration and are usually treatable by reassurance or by sedative/hypnotic or antipsychotic drugs. The acute psychotoxic reactions may be characterized by uncontrollable excitement, confusion, acute paranoia, or all of these. The acute panic reactions appear as secondary responses to drug-induced effects. The sensory distortions and powerful emotions elicited by the drug produce in some individuals an overwhelming tension and anxiety, a fear of losing one's mind and an abject sense of helplessness. In the grip of such reactions individuals may expose themselves to dangerous situations or engage in behavior that threatens their life. Deaths attributable to the direct actions of the drugs are unknown, but deaths by drowning, falling out of windows and walking into the path of automobiles have occurred.

In the heavy LSD user, recurrent reactions may appear up to a year after the last use of drug and without further exposure to the hallucinogen. They usually involve the spontaneous return of perceptual distortions and a reliving of the earlier traumatic experiences. These 'flashbacks' may vary in length from a few seconds to a half hour, but occur unpredictably.

The prolonged reactions may be exhibited as chronic anxiety states or chronic psychoses. The former are a relatively common occurrence and are accompanied by time and space distortion, difficulty in functioning and depression stemming from the morbid or terrifying feelings or thoughts experienced during drug use. It is not certain whether the small number of individuals who develop prolonged psychotic reactions would have developed these same conditions in the absence of the use of psychedelic drugs.

The use of the LSD group of drugs was at an all time high during the 1960s. In the 1970s usage declined perhaps as a consequence of the recognition of the real hazards attendant on their use. But current use of LSD and other psychedelic drugs among 18- to 25-year-olds is about 1–2%, about twice that among older individuals, and is rising.

Marihuana: Cannabinoids

The hemp plant *Cannabis sativa* is the source of the ancient drug cannabis and its products, variously referred to as *hashish, charas, bhang, ganja, dagga,* and *marihuana.* Active ingredients are found in all parts of both male and female plants, with the highest concentration occurring in the flowers. The most potent natural supply of cannabis is the resinous exudate obtained from the flower clusters; in the Middle East and North Africa the resin is called *hashish.* In the

United States, the term *marihuana* is used to refer to any part of the plant or its extracts. The drug is most commonly used in Western countries as a mixture of leaves and flowers incorporated into cigarettes.

The active ingredients in cannabis are tetrahydrocannabinols (THC); the particular isomer believed to be responsible for most of the psychologic effects characteristic of marihuana is delta-9-tetrahydrocannabinol (Δ^9-THC). This active ingredient has been synthesized, and studies with the pure compound have indicated that one of the metabolic products of Δ^9-THC is capable of producing CNS effects similar to those of its parent compound. Specific receptors for Δ^9-THC (cannabinoid receptors) have been identified in various parts of the CNS. They are particularly abundant in the hippocampus, an area important in learning and memory. The binding of Δ^9-THC to cannabinoid receptors decreases neuronal firing rate—accounting for disruption of short-term memory caused by smoking marihuana. Soon after the discovery of cannabinoid receptors, an endogenous compound, anandamide, was isolated from the brain. More recently, a series of endogenous cannabinoids (endocannabinoids) have been identified. Although these compounds bind cannabinoid receptors in the CNS, their physiologic roles have not been established fully. Recent studies indicate that the endocannabinoids may be involved in analgesia, memory disruption, and immunosuppression.

As with LSD, the subjective effects produced by marihuana are influenced by the state of mind, mood and expectations of the user and by the specific circumstances in which the drug is used. Alone and in a quiet setting, the user usually feels drowsy; in company, the user is inclined to be talkative and hilarious. Experience also plays a role in the effects produced. Naive subjects appear to experience fewer of the subjective effects for which marihuana is used and more impairment of motor and intellectual ability than experienced smokers.

The content of active ingredients contained in materials available for smoking varies rather widely because of normal variation in the plant itself and methods of preparing the cigarettes. However, the experienced smoker usually requires only one to two cigarettes to produce the desired effects. These are generally described as a sleepy, happy, dreamy state of altered consciousness, associated with uncontrollable and freely flowing ideas and changes in the perception of time, space, objects and sounds. Delta^9-THC can produce subjective effects that are remarkably like those elicited by low doses of LSD (Table 15-6), while those induced by marihuana are usually milder and more predictable. Also, a much lower degree of tolerance is developed to the effects of marihuana than to those of LSD. But despite the similarity in their subjective effects, the two drugs show no cross-tolerance, a fact indicative of different mechanisms of action. Moreover, there are dissimilarities in the physiologic effects produced by the two drugs. Unlike LSD, marihuana has a sedative action, does not dilate pupils, and does not significantly alter blood pressure.

Marihuana and alcohol are also frequently compared with each other, since the patterns of their social group use are similar. First, the recreational use of either drug in low or moderate doses does not necessarily lead to a state of drug

Table 15-6. *The major effects produced by tetrahydrocannabinol*

Physical: Dizziness; increased heart rate; reddening of the conjunctivae ('red eyes'); dry mouth; nausea; vomiting; drowsiness; increased appetite

Psychologic: Altered mood; euphoria; elation; uncontrollable laughter; sense of retardation of time; decreased ability to concentrate; difficulty in expressing thoughts and feelings; depersonalization; introspection; dream-like state; poor memory (later good); rapid thoughts; impairment of judgment

Perceptual: Blurred vision; altered shapes and colors; heightening of color intensity; increased acuity of hearing; colors are heard, sounds may be seen; perceptual distortion of space; vivid hallucinations

dependence. Second, although low doses of both drugs tend to produce sedation in nonsocial use, in the group environment they induce a loquacious euphoria and increased sociability, often accompanied by hilarity. These effects are characteristic of a depression of inhibitory control mechanisms. As a consequence, judgment is impaired and motor skills affected, which make the user of low doses of either marihuana or alcohol a potential hazard behind the wheel of an automobile; these hazards are increased when there is concurrent use of both drugs, since marihuana and alcohol produce additive impairment of performance of some motor tasks. In the use of marihuana, alterations in the perception of time and space may also contribute to decreased driving skills. Marihuana intoxication also interferes with immediate memory and with a wide range of intellectual tasks and consequently may impair classroom learning. However, the individual who is 'high' on marihuana, unlike the user of alcohol, does not show ataxia, or motor incoordination, and thus does not alert those around him to his inability to function responsibly.

There are still other dissimilarities between the effects of low or moderate doses of marihuana and alcohol which may be of even more significance in their use. Marihuana, even when used in the group setting, tends to make the user introspective, whereas persons under the influence of alcohol behave like extroverts. Such differences in the behavioral response to the two drugs may account for the fact that the individual under the influence of marihuana is unlikely to be aggressive and violent and less likely to commit crime than is the person intoxicated with alcohol. Nor does the development of addiction drive the marihuana user to commit crime to appease his drug hunger. On the other hand, the smoking of only a few marihuana cigarettes can produce a temporary state of paranoia in some individuals, a side-effect rarely associated with the use of low doses of alcohol. Studies with synthetic tetrahydrocannabinol show that these psychotic reactions may also occur in some subjects who receive small doses of the pure chemical.

Unlike alcohol, chronic use of marihuana does not lead to appreciable tolerance and physical dependence. There is no characteristic abstinence syndrome when the use of marihuana is discontinued and little compulsion to continue its use to avoid discomfort. However, many individuals using marihuana chronically display marked lethargy, inertia, and self-neglect; they may be subject to severe psychologic reactions, and resort to compulsive use. This latter phenomenon suggests that addiction can and does develop to marihuana use, depending on the user. In fact, there are cannabinoid receptors located in the reward pathway; their activation produces an increase in dopamine release similar to other drugs that produce addiction. Moderate social use of marihuana does not appear to be seriously deleterious, although it markedly impairs short-term memory. Recent studies indicate that cognitive impairment can exist even after stopping marihuana use. The effects of long-term, chronic use in addition to those discussed above, include impairment of lung function, to a greater extent than tobacco cigarettes, and immunosuppression, which renders the user more susceptible to respiratory infections.

It is well-established that in some societies the continued abuse of potent preparations, particularly hashish, has been associated with social degradation; it is not clear, however, which is the cause and which is the effect. More knowledge of the physical, personal, and social consequences of the use and abuse of marihuana is required before definitive judgments can be made. But it must be borne in mind that alcohol, the drug most widely used for social purposes, is also the drug most frequently abused in Western society. Although millions of people use alcohol for a temporary escape from reality and are able to control their drug use, other millions lose control over their intake and become drug-dependent. It is also interesting to note that alcoholism, known since biblical times, became a serious sociologic problem only after the invention of distillation and the introduction of alcoholic beverages more potent than the previously used wine or beer. The problems of opioid and cocaine abuse were also magnified by technologic advances: the isolation of the pure drugs from their plant origin and the invention of the syringe. Now, not only have the active ingredients of *Cannabis sativa* been isolated in pure form, but Δ^9-THC has also been synthesized. Thus, until more factual knowledge is available, there is some justification for viewing the sequelae of the continued abuse of marihuana from the perspective of past experience with other drugs of abuse. It is noteworthy that the *Cannabis sativa* plants contain more Δ^9-THC today than in the 1960s and 1970s (when compulsive use was not very apparent). While use of marihuana appeared to have leveled off in the mid 1980s, it is now on the rise.

Currently, efforts to gain a better understanding of the long-term consequences of the abuse of marihuana are continuing. At the same time, researchers are studying the potential value of cannabinoids as therapeutic agents. There appears to be little hazard associated with the moderate, controlled use of marihuana, and numerous studies have shown that Δ^9-THC has a wide margin of safety. This has led to an FDA-approved form of Δ^9-THC (MARINOL) for the treatment of glaucoma and as an anti-emetic drug. Some states have also authorized marihuana use by physicians for the treatment of patients undergoing cancer chemotherapy (although superior drugs do exist for these conditions). It is unlikely that the FDA will ever approve the sale of marihuana cigarettes as a prescription drug due to the harmful effects of smoking. Any potential pharmacotherapy for cannabinoids will require safer delivery systems.

Phencyclidine

Phencyclidine (PCP), or 'angel dust' as it is better known to drug abusers, was developed in the 1950s as a general anesthetic for use in animals and humans. Its therapeutic use in humans was short-lived because patients experienced severe postoperative thought disturbances and agitation. Because of the occurrence of psychotic-like symptoms and other adverse reactions, PCP acquired a bad street reputation and was only abused sporadically in the 1960s. However, in the mid 1970s, after its mode of use changed from oral ingestion to smoking or snorting, PCP became a serious problem as a widely abused drug. The popularity of PCP was short-lived, since its use declined sharply in the 1980s. More recently, ketamine, a dissociative anesthetic like PCP has become a popular drug of abuse. This drug is used clinically to obtain dissociative anesthesia, such as during the changing of dressings on burn victims, yet it does not produce the degree of psychosis observed with PCP.

Phencyclidine and its chemically similar analogs, although often classed as hallucinogens, are different from LSD in terms of their actions in humans and animal models. For example, unlike LSD, PCP manifests its hallucinogenic activity primarily by body image and proprioceptive disturbances, often accompanied by thought disorders. Unlike other hallucinogens, PCP is self-administered by monkeys and produces addiction in humans. Phencyclidine has an unusual pharmacologic profile with CNS stimulant, CNS depressant, hallucinogenic, analgesic and local anesthetic activities. This wide range of effects results from the interaction of PCP with several neurotransmitter systems, including dopaminergic, cholinergic, and glutamatergic systems. In fact, PCP is a classic example of a drug that lacks specificity. PCP binds to several different targets, including glutamate, GABA, and acetylcholine receptors. Its interaction with a glutamate receptor subtype, the N-methyl-d-aspartate (NMDA) receptor, may account for many of the behavioral and psychological actions.

The wide range of physical and psychologic effects produced by PCP is illustrated in Table 15-7. These dose-related symptoms are likely to be encountered when its use requires treatment at a hospital emergency room. At low doses, in addition to the physical symptoms associated with intoxication, the patient may also exhibit hostile and bizarre and even criminal behavior. The toxic psychosis induced by low doses is characterized by overt symptoms of schizophrenia, not by hallucinations. Persistent problems with speech and memory, and difficulty with thinking may follow long periods of regular drug use. Chronic users also report insomnia, decreased appetite, constipation, and urinary hesitancy. The deaths associated with the use of PCP in low doses appear to be secondary to the behavioral toxicity produced, whereas the cause of death with high doses of PCP is primary respiratory depression.

Table 15-7. *The major effects produced by phencyclidine (PCP) and its chemically related analogs*

Low doses (up to 5 mg): Agitation and excitement; gross incoordination; blank stare; slurred speech; nystagmus; catatonic muscular rigidity; sweating; numbness of extremities; changes in body image; disorganization of thought; drowsiness; apathy

Moderate doses (5–10 mg): Coma or stupor (eyes remain open); vomiting; hypersalivation; muscle rigidity on stimulation; repetitive movements; fever; decreased peripheral sensation; heart rate and blood pressure increased

High doses (over 10 mg): Prolonged coma (eyes closed); muscular rigidity; convulsions; absent peripheral sensation; decreased or absent gag and corneal reflexes

In view of the widely noted and acknowledged negative aspects of the PCP experience, one wonders why the use of PCP persists, although it is apparently declining. The answer will be forthcoming only when we have a better understanding of the underlying personality problems that lead to abuse of drugs like PCP.

DRUGS USED TO TREAT DRUG DEPENDENCE

The development and identification of compounds to treat drug dependence and addiction has become a priority of the National Institute of Drug Abuse, part of the NIH. Considerable progress has been made in the treatment of opioid dependence and addiction. Three types of compounds are now in use, including, opioid agonists, partial agonists, and antagonists. These compounds are useful because they reduce the addict's drug-seeking behavior and associated criminal activities and the risk of HIV infection from use of contaminated needles. Methadone is among the first of the compounds used for treating opioid dependence under the supervision of the medical establishment. This opioid agonist suppresses withdrawal and reduces craving. It still produces dependence, although not as strong as that produced by morphine or heroin. Because of its pharmacokinetic profile, patients must make frequent visits to a clinic to obtain their oral doses. This problem has been addressed with a newly approved opioid partial agonist, buprenorphine (SUPENEX), which has a longer half-life and requires less frequent dosing. This property increases the likelihood that the patient will adhere to the treatment. As a partial agonist, buprenorphine causes little euphoria or dependence. Moreover, it suppresses the euphoria produced by morphine or heroin. Naltrexone, the opioid antagonist, is also used to treat opioid addicts, but since it produces no euphoria, only the most committed patients are likely to benefit from this strategy. Interestingly, naltrexone has been used to treat alcohol and cocaine addicts after withdrawal to prevent relapse, with limited success. Since the reward pathway contains an opioid component, the idea of using an opioid antagonist to reduce craving and relapse during withdrawal from other positively reinforcing drugs is a clever strategy.

Treatment of nicotine addiction during smoking cessation has had limited success with the advent of nicotine gum, lozenges, and the skin patch. The antidepressant bupropion (WELLBUTRIN, ZYBAN) has also been used to reduce nicotine craving and facilitate smoking cessation. Whether this drug's ability to increase dopamine release is the basis for its limited success is not clear.

SYNOPSIS

The drugs most likely to be used, if not compulsively abused, for nonmedical purposes are those which affect the CNS; they alter mood and behavior in ways that satisfy the emotional needs of certain individuals. Some agents have legitimate therapeutic uses but are abused because of their ability to produce pleasurable feelings. These include the sedative-hypnotics like the benzodiazepines and the opioid analgesics. Other drugs once had some therapeutic use, including the amphetamines and cocaine. The agents without proved therapeutic usefulness that are most widely abused are LSD, marihuana, and phencyclidine. However, all these compounds represent only a fraction of the agents of both synthetic and plant origin that are involved in contemporary drug abuse.

All the psychoactive agents used for nonmedical purposes have one property in common: they are capable of eliciting in certain individuals a state of mind in which the user feels that the effects produced by the drug are necessary for well-being. These psychologic effects may range from a persistent desire for the drug to an undeniable compulsion to obtain and take the drug at any cost. Addiction develops in some, but not all, persons who use a drug repeatedly. Personality disturbances antecedent to drug use, and the environment may contribute to abuse in susceptible individuals.

The periodic or continuous administration of psychoactive drugs leads to an altered physiologic state. This condition of physical dependence is revealed only when the body is forced to do without the drug or, in the case of opioids, when a specific antagonist is administered. Tolerance, the need for increased dosage to produce the desired effect, is also induced by many of the drugs that cause physical dependence. Physical dependence and tolerance are powerful factors in reinforcing drug-seeking behavior.

Physical dependence, accompanied by marked tolerance, occurs with continuous use of general depressants of the CNS and with the opioids. Alcohol is the most commonly abused depressant. This group also includes sedative-hypnotics such as barbiturates and benzodiazepines. Dependence occurs with all types of opioid agonists, regardless of whether they are natural or synthetic. The nature of dependence to CNS depressants like alcohol differs from opioid dependence with respect to (1) the symptoms exhibited during drug use; (2) the course of development of dependence; (3) the withdrawal syndrome precipitated by discontinuance of drug administration; and (4) the limits of tolerance developed.

During chronic intoxication with alcohol, the user is accident-prone through incomplete development of tolerance to the sedative action and to the effects of the drugs on motor coordination. There is also impairment of mental acuity, confusion and increased emotional instability. Aggressiveness, violence and crime are associated with the use of general depressants, not only in the user's efforts to procure the drug but also during the time the user is under the influence of the drug. In contrast, the opioid user can function with reasonable efficiency both occupationally and socially as long as there is an adequate supply of drug. With opioid dependence, violence and crime are primarily related to the user's need to procure the drug.

Physical dependence and tolerance develop only after continued use of doses above the socially acceptable levels of alcohol. On the other hand, opioid dependence is created by doses within the therapeutic range and may be set in motion in the very first dose. The symptoms of withdrawal from alcohol and from the opioids are extremely unpleasant and severe. But abrupt withdrawal from the general depressant drugs is much more dangerous than that from the opioids and may be life-threatening. The tolerance developed to alcohol is incomplete; there is considerable persistence of behavioral disturbances and little increase in the dose levels that produce toxic symptoms or death in nontolerant individuals. In contrast, marked tolerance develops to all the effects of the morphine-like drugs with the exception of their effects on the pupil and gastrointestinal tract.

The development of physical dependence is also produced by CNS stimulants. However, the degree of physical dependence developed to the CNS stimulant drugs is mild and is revealed upon withdrawal as a state of mental and physical depression. While tolerance develops to amphetamines, it is not characteristic of cocaine use. Other abused drugs such as the hallucinogens (e.g. LSD), marihuana, and MDMA do not produce physical dependence and, consequently, there is no characteristic abstinence syndrome. While tolerance does not develop readily to marihuana and MDMA, marked tolerance does develop with the persistent use of LSD.

The addiction that develops to the amphetamines or cocaine can lead to a profound and dangerous type of drug abuse. Unlike the opioid addict, the amphetamine or cocaine addict is hyperactive and may respond by violence and criminal activity to the paranoid delusions associated with the toxicity induced by high doses. Hallucinogens do not produce addiction, as compulsive use is not characteristic of these compounds. There is still some question as to whether the long-term use of marihuana can produce addiction. In some instances, the chronic abuse of marihuana, as opposed to its periodic use, may be a symptom of emotional disturbance or mental instability. If marihuana use becomes compulsive, as it has in some individuals, we can conclude that users risk possible addiction to yet another drug with psychoactive properties.

A common pathway for the rewarding or reinforcing properties of drugs that cause drug-seeking behavior is known as the reward pathway. Although the pharmacodynamic actions of abused drugs such as heroin, cocaine, or alcohol differ substantially, these drugs all interact with the reward pathway to increase dopaminergic transmission. In dependent individuals, craving is a major factor in relapse after withdrawal, and therefore, efforts to treat drug dependence and addiction in abstinent users have focused on strategies to suppress withdrawal and reduce craving. These pharmacological strategies are targeted to modify the function of the reward pathway, without eliciting dependence on yet another compound.

GUIDES FOR STUDY AND REVIEW

What is the basic cell unit of the nervous system? What is an afferent or sensory neuron? an efferent or motor neuron? What is a synapse? How is information transmitted from one unit of the nervous system to another? What are neurotransmitters and what is their function? What are the two most important chemicals identified as neurotransmitters outside the CNS?

The hypothalamus is concerned with the control and regulation of what important bodily functions? What is the functional role of the cerebral cortex in humans? the limbic system? What is the functional role of the reticular activating system (the RAS)? In general how do various types of drugs influence the activity of the RAS and what is the result of such interaction? How can the effect of low doses of alcohol be explained in terms of their influence on the RAS?

What does the term *drug abuse* mean? What kinds of therapeutic agents and nonmedicinal chemicals are commonly drugs of abuse? What do we mean by the term *drug misuse?*

What does the term *drug dependence* mean? What does the term *addiction* mean? Can physical dependence develop to some drugs that are not drugs of abuse? Can physical dependence develop to some drugs of abuse under conditions which do not lead to addiction? What is the most characteristic feature of the state of physical dependence?

What is the relationship between the phenomena of drug tolerance and drug dependence? Can tolerance be developed to drugs that have little potential for abusive use? Does tolerance develop to all drugs that are drugs of abuse? With what types of drugs of abuse is the phenomenon of tolerance almost invariably associated?

What drugs are included in the category of 'general depressants of the CNS'? Does physical dependence develop to all these agents? What are the characteristic symptoms of withdrawal of these agents? How does the severity of the withdrawal syndrome associated with alcohol differ from that of morphine?

How do the limits of tolerance developed to the general depressants of the CNS differ from those developed to the opioid analgesics?

What drugs are included in the category of opioid analgesics? What are the characteristics of the drug-dependent state that develops to this category of drugs? How does the course of development of dependence to the opioid analgesics differ from that to the general depressants of the CNS? What is the outstanding difference between the morphine and alcohol types of drug dependence with respect to harm to the drug abuser and society when the drug may be obtained by legitimate means?

What are some of the commonly abused drugs classified as CNS stimulants? How does the drug-dependent state developed to amphetamine differ from that to cocaine, particularly with respect to physical dependence and tolerance? Why is the compulsive use of CNS stimulants a serious threat to the life of the drug abuser and to society?

How is the term *hallucinogen* defined? Does abuse of hallucinogens produce dependence and addiction characteristic of other psychoactive agents? Tolerance development? How do the chronic effects of marihuana use differ from those of alcohol? Do dependence and addiction develop to marihuana use?

Why do humans (and animals) have a reward pathway? What is the major neurotransmitter system in the reward pathway? Which psychoactive drugs are most likely to interact with the reward pathway? How do these drugs interact with the reward pathway?

What is the rationale for treating abstinent alcoholics or cocaine addicts with an opioid antagonist?

SUGGESTED READING

Abood, M.E. and Martin, B.R. Neurobiology of marihuana abuse. *Trends Pharmacol. Sci.* 13:201, 1992.

Aghajanian, G.K. and Marek, G.J. Serotonin and hallucinogens. *Neuropsychopharmacology* 21:16S, 1999.

American Psychiatric Association. *Diagnostic and Statistical Manual of Mental Disorders* (4th ed.). Washington, DC, American Psychiatric Association, 1994.

Bloom, F.E. and Kupfer, D.J. (eds). *Psychopharmacology: The Fourth Generation of Progress*. New York: Raven Press, 1995.

Brownstein, M.J. A brief history of opiates, opioid peptides and opioid receptors. *Proc. Natl Acad. Sci.* U.S.A. 90:5391, 1993.

Kornetsky C. Action of opioid drugs on the brain-reward system. *NIDA Res. Monogr.* 147:33, 1995.

Devane, W.A. New dawn of cannabinoid pharmacology. *Trends Pharmacol. Sci.* 15:40, 1994.

Di Chiara, G. and North, R.A. Neurobiology of opiate abuse. *Trends Pharmacol. Sci.* 13:185, 1992.

Gardner, E.L. Addictive potential of cannabinoids: the underlying neurobiology. *Chem. Phys. Lipids* 121:267, 2002.

Goldstein, A. *Addiction, From Biology to Drug Policy*. New York: W.H. Freeman & Co., 1994.

Green, A.R., Mechan, A.O., Elliott, J.M., O'Shea, E. and Colado, M.I. The pharmacology and clinical pharmacology of 3,4-methylenedioxymethamphetamine (MDMA, 'ecstasy'). *Pharmacol. Rev.* 55:463, 2003.

Hammer, R.P. (ed.). *The Neurobiology of Opiates*. Boca Raton: CRC Press, 1992.

Hyman S.E. and Malenka R.C. Addiction and the brain: the neurobiology of compulsion and its persistence. *Nat. Rev. Neurosci.* 2:695, 2001.

Koob, G.F. Drugs of abuse: anatomy, pharmacology and function of reward pathways. *Trends Pharmacol. Sci.* 13:177, 1992.

Koob, G.F., Ahmed, S.H., Boutrel B., Chen, S.A., Kenny, P.J., Markou, A., O'Dell, L.E., Parsons, L.H. and Sanna, P.P. Neurobiological mechanisms in the transition from drug use to drug dependence. *Neurosci. Biobehav. Rev.* 27:739, 2004.

Nestler, E.J. From neurobiology to treatment: progress against addiction. *Nature Neurosci.* 5 Suppl:1076, 2002.

Robinson, S.E. Buprenorphine: an analgesic with an expanding role in the treatment of opioid addiction. *CNS Drug Rev.* 8:377, 2002

Samson, H.H. and Harris, R.A. Neurobiology of alcohol abuse. *Trends Pharmacol. Sci.* 13:206, 1992.

Snyder, S.H. *Drugs and the Brain*. New York, Scientific American Library. W.H. Freeman & Co., 1986.

Various authors. Mini-reviews on addiction. *J. Neurosci.* 22:3303, 2002.

Watson, R.R. *Alcohol and Neurobiology: Receptors, Membranes, and Channels*. Boca Raton: CRC Press, 1992.

Woolverton, W.L. and Johnson, K.M. Neurobiology of cocaine abuse. *Trends Pharmacol. Sci.* 13:193, 1992.

16   The Development and Evaluation of New Drugs

Until the early part of the nineteenth century, the only drugs available were crude preparations of plant, animal or mineral origin. The modern era of pharmacology was ushered in with advances in chemistry and the development of fundamental and essential methods of physiologic experimentation. The former permitted the isolation, purification, and identification of active components of older preparations as well as the synthesis of new agents. And the development of experimental methods made it possible not only to distinguish worthless remedies from those that were useful, but also to determine how drugs produce their effects in the living organism.

Once given the necessary tools and techniques, pharmacology grew at an accelerating pace, paralleling the rapid advances in related disciplines and spurred on by the extensive research and development within the pharmaceutical industry itself. The proliferation of new drugs, the increased number of diseases beneficially affected by drugs, and the progress in understanding basic mechanisms of drug action are the tangible effects of this evolution. This growth reached its peak in the decade following World War II with the almost explosive expansion of basic research in the biomedical sciences. The rate of development, at least of new drugs, then declined and leveled off, until advances in molecular biology spurred another growth phase in drug discovery. Advances are continually being made, and new agents are constantly being added to the therapeutic armamentarium. In this chapter we shall trace the development of a new drug from its genesis in the chemist's laboratory to its final acceptance as a safe and useful therapeutic agent.

DEVELOPMENT AND EVALUATION IN THE LABORATORY

The First Step – Discovering a Drug

Serendipity coupled with astute observations by alert investigators has played a role in the development of some very important drugs. The classic example is the discovery of penicillin by Fleming, which heralded the beginning of anti-biotic therapy[1]. Such chance observations occur rarely, so that almost all the new drugs available today are the original products of the research and develop-ment efforts primarily of the large pharmaceutical firms, but with academic and governmental research playing significant roles. Leads for therapeutic discover-ies have been and are being provided by both empiric and rational approaches: by the large-scale testing of natural or synthetic products and by the deliberate exploitation of side-effects of older agents, of unexpected clinical findings during the use of known drugs, or of newly discovered causes of disease.

Natural Products

During the first half of the twentieth century, natural products received only modest attention as potential sources of new drugs. However, interest in the study of plants was intensified in 1952 when reserpine was isolated from *Rau-wolfia serpentina* and shown to be useful in the treatment of hypertension and in treating psychotic patients. Since preparations of *Rauwolfia* had been used in India for centuries for various therapeutic purposes, the discovery of its active principle stimulated the re-examination of folklore medicinals. While much of this folk medicine has provided only false clues to the pharmacologic value of plant remedies, some useful compounds have been discovered. For example, a study of the periwinkle plant *(Vinca rosea)*, reputed to be beneficial in diabetes, did not disclose any compounds with antidiabetic activity, but did yield drugs effective against some types of cancer.

The investigation of natural products for potentially useful agents is ordinar-ily carried out by a relatively simplified procedure of extracting a sample of the material and testing the extract in a biologic system. Such a process is usually referred to as screening. This empiric approach is time-consuming since large numbers of compounds or random samples are tested to determine whether or not they possess exploitable pharmacologic activity. For example, thousands of samples of soil may be tested in the search for a new antibiotic. This seemingly inefficient approach is nonetheless valuable, since many chemical substances produced by soil microbes have been isolated and found to be therapeutically useful as antimicrobial agents. The discovery of Mexican yams as an inexpensive source of starting materials for the synthesis of steroid hormones such as corti-sone and progesterone is another example of how large-scale screening of natural products can lead to desirable end products. A more recent example of a natural product that has been the source of novel drugs is paclitaxel (TAXOL) isolated from the bark of the Pacific yew tree and effective in the treatment of refractory ovarian cancer and advanced breast cancer. In this respect, it is note-worthy that the US National Cancer Institute has contracted with various insti-

---

[1]In 1928, Fleming noticed that a stray mold (genus *Penicillium*) on a plate culture of staphylococci had inhibited the growth of the bacteria.

tutions, world-renowned for their botanical expertise, to provide authenticated, plant-derived materials for evaluation as potential pharmaceutical agents.

Once a useful pharmaceutical has been identified from a natural product, the ultimate goal is to synthesize it in the medicinal chemist's laboratory. Natural products, however, remain the primary source of supply of many of our drugs of ancient heritage, for even though compounds like morphine have been synthesized in the laboratory, it is more economical to obtain them from their natural sources. Unlike the older preparations, however, these modern drugs of plant or animal origin are isolated and purified compounds. And drugs of natural origin like morphine and the digitalis derivatives, or the newer ones like antibiotics and hormones, continue to represent a large fraction of the total annual volume of drug sales. However, in cases where the natural product is required, attempts are being made to increase yields by exploiting plant and marine cell culture technologies.

New technologies have also provided very powerful methodologies for separation, structure elucidation, and bioassay, which contribute to the rapid characterization of natural products as innovative leads for pharmaceutical development. As a result of these advances in technology and the current popularity and use of natural products for self-medication and as dietary supplements, there has been a renaissance of interest within the pharmaceutical industry for exploitation of plant-derived products to serve as discovery leads to new prototypes.

The increased popularity and widespread availability of natural products has challenged the Food and Drug Administration (FDA) to seek additional ways to protect the public. Under the Dietary Supplement Health and Education Act of 1994, products such as herbal medicines and dietary supplements need not be evaluated for safety and efficacy. The law requires only that these products be explicitly labeled as dietary supplements and not make any therapeutic claims. Calcium to prevent bone loss and folic acid to prevent certain birth defects (in pregnant women) are the only two dietary supplements that have FDA-approved therapeutic claims. With the increasing use of these products there are newly raised concerns about the lack of standardization of the contents, the presence of contaminants, and the risk of side-effects, including drug interactions.

Synthetic Chemicals

The products of the synthetic chemist's laboratory are the source of the greatest number of new drugs; their potential pharmacologic activity is also discovered by screening processes. In the empiric approach, the screening process may involve a battery of experimental procedures to determine the total pharmacologic profile of a new chemical. Alternatively, groups of chemically related compounds may be put through a limited number of tests designed to reveal a specific type of activity, such as effect on blood pressure or kidney function, or interaction with a specific isolated receptor. This so-called partially empiric approach, based on the concept of a relationship between structure and activity, has been utilized in several different ways, each of which has led to the synthesis of many valuable drugs.

One approach has been to modify systematically the molecular structure of an established drug in order to develop a congener that has more desirable properties than the original compound. The aim may be to improve the margin of safety, to eliminate a particular type of side-effect, to prolong or shorten the duration of action or to improve absorption from the gastrointestinal tract (Table 16-1). The success that may be achieved by such structural manipulation is dramatically illustrated by the development of the oral contraceptive agents. The synthetically modified estrogenic and progestational hormones have the same pharmacologic activity as the natural hormones. However, the partially synthetic derivatives, unlike the natural products, are effective when administered orally. The natural hormones are metabolically degraded in the intestine or liver, or both, before they reach the systemic circulation. Thus the introduction of synthetically modified hormones that retain their activity when taken by mouth revolutionized gynecologic and contraceptive therapy.

It happens all too often that structural modifications of an existing drug yield congeners with pharmacologic profiles insignificantly different from that of the parent compound. Although these new agents offer little advantage over the drug already available, they are marketed for competitive reasons and become 'me-too' drugs. The practice is sometimes difficult to justify unless the 'me-too' drug is less expensive to manufacture. On the other hand, a multiplicity of drugs with similar pharmacologic activity may represent therapeutic insurance for patients who are either unresponsive or allergic to other drugs within the group. In addition, when resistance develops to a particular drug, as for example in parasitic infections, the availability of 'backstop' drugs – drugs of pharmacologic equivalence – may be exceedingly important. This has proved to be the case for one of a group of compounds that was studied during World War II and found to have antimalarial activity. Halofantrine was not developed at the time as a 'me-too' drug, however, when chloroquine was found to be most effective. When plasmodia developed resistance to chloroquine, pyrimethamine, and quinine, there was a real need for additional chemotherapeutic agents that would be active against *P. falciparum*. Such an agent is halofantrine, which was marketed in 1992.

At the same time, systematic modifications of the structure of an existing drug have led frequently to the synthesis of agents with therapeutic applications or pharmacologic properties markedly different from those anticipated. Meprobamate, the forerunner of today's anti-anxiety agents, for example, was originally synthesized as a potential muscle relaxant. It was one of more than 1200 derivatives investigated in a search for a long-acting successor to mephenesin, a muscle relaxant of short duration of action and unreliable absorption. Meprobamate was found to be effective orally, to have a satisfactory duration of action and to possess the looked-for muscle-relaxant activity. But it was also noted during the screening tests that meprobamate had the ability to allay

Table 16-1. *Development of new drugs by modification of older or established drugs*

Established drug	New drug	Advantage of newer over older drug
Procaine	Lidocaine	Effective when applied to body surfaces; little potential for allergic reactions; more stable to biotransformation at site of injection, hence longer acting
Procaine	Tetracaine	Much more potent, but relative therapeutic ratio with respect to lethal toxicity is only slightly increased
Codeine	Dextromethorphan	Much greater selectivity of action as a cough suppressant; no analgesic properties and no abuse potential
Atropine	Atropine methyl nitrate (quaternary ammonium compound)	Fewer side-effects relative to the central nervous system because of decreased ability to penetrate into brain
Pentobarbital	Thiopental	Much faster penetration into brain due to increased lipid solubility, therefore useful as an intravenous anesthetic agent
Penicillin G	Phenoxymethyl penicillin	More completely absorbed from the gastrointestinal tract; more stable in acid medium
Penicillin G	Oxacillin	More completely absorbed from the gastrointestinal tract; not degraded by penicillinase, therefore useful against penicillin-resistant organisms
Morphine	Methadone	Less costly to produce; longer duration of action; effective by oral route
Terfenadine	Fexofenadine	Effective antihistamine (H_1 receptor antagonist) but without cardiotoxic effect of its precursor

anxiety without producing too much drowsiness. These latter pharmacologic properties account for its early exploitation as a sedative to reduce tension and worry and for the later development of more effective anti-anxiety agents.

The ability of meprobamate to produce sedation might well be regarded as a side-effect of the drug if one were looking merely for muscle-relaxant activity. Such a side-effect occurring during a large-scale screening program might easily escape notice in the absence of a competent and alert investigator. But when careful observation is coupled with recognition of the potential usefulness of a side-effect, new drugs may be discovered or new uses found for older agents.

There are many significant advances in therapy that had their origin in the clues provided by the observed side-effects of existing drugs. For example, when sulfanilamide was first introduced as an antibacterial agent, careful clinical observation indicated that it produces a slight increase in both the volume and pH of urine. Subsequently, the drug was found to inhibit the enzyme carbonic anhydrase, which in turn was found to prevent the normal acidification of the urine (cf. Appendix 2, I.C). Structural manipulations led to the development of more potent carbonic anhydrase inhibitors, such as acetazolamide. Although the carbonic anhydrase inhibitors have limited usefulness as diuretic agents, they played a significant role in the elucidation of normal kidney function. Moreover, further modification of the acetazolamide molecule produced the therapeutically important thiazide diuretics, of which chlorothiazide is the prototype (cf. Appendix 2, I.D.). A useful class of orally effective antidiabetic drugs also evolved from the antibacterial sulfonamides. The impetus for the development of these hypoglycemic agents was the clinical finding of a lowered blood sugar as a side-effect of the treatment of typhoid fever with a sulfonamide. It is noteworthy that these different structural modifications of sulfonamides eliminated their antibacterial activity and yielded diuretics with limited hypoglycemic activity or antidiabetic drugs without diuretic activity.

Probenecid is a good example of a drug developed for one purpose that later found a new and more important use. When penicillin was first introduced, its rapid elimination in the urine was of practical concern, since the antibiotic was both expensive and scarce. A systematic study was undertaken to find an organic acid that would compete with penicillin for the renal tubular secretory process and thereby inhibit penicillin's rapid loss from the body (cf. p. 246). Probenecid was the answer. It was also found that large doses of probenecid enhance the excretion of uric acid by inhibiting its reabsorption from the tubular urine. This uricosuric action of probenecid was usefully applied in the treatment of gout, a disease characterized by high levels of uric acid in the body (cf. Appendix 4, Analgesics, I.E). The deliberate approach to achieve a specific pharmacologic objective has led to the development of a number of useful agents like probenecid that act by competitively antagonizing the actions of other drugs or of functionally important endogenous substances.

In some cases discovery of an alternative indication for a class of compounds occurs during the drug development process. For example, a compound with activity as an inhibitor of the enzyme phosphodiesterase was predicted to be effective for cardiovascular indications. However, early investigations revealed efficacy in prolonging erection in men. This observation led to the development of a new class of agents for treatment of male erectile dysfunction. The first marketed drug in this class, sildenafil (VIAGRA), was soon followed by a number of others that differ in their duration of action.

The search for new types of drugs may also be guided by rational concepts when the biochemical or physiologic abnormality underlying a disease state is revealed. The treatment of parkinsonism, for example, was dramatically changed with the disclosure that the major defect in the disease is a decreased content of dopamine in certain areas of the brain. Dopamine itself cannot be used effectively to correct the biochemical defect, since it does not readily pass the blood-brain barrier. But the drug levodopa does gain access to the brain, where it is metabolically converted to dopamine. Levodopa is an example of a prodrug – an agent that is administered as the precursor of a drug and is converted in the body to the active therapeutic agent. The development and use of prodrugs to achieve appropriate distribution and clinical effectiveness have become an important approach in drug development.

The synthesis of effective drugs tailored to fit predetermined specifications occurs all too infrequently. However, the unquestioned success of levodopa as an approach to the treatment of parkinsonism gives substance to the hope that more and more drugs will be developed from such sound theoretical considerations. In this respect, the use of computers to simulate the drug target and to design chemical structures that might interact with the drug receptor has become exceedingly useful in the development of new drugs.

Structure-based drug design is a modern version of Ehrlich's famous 'lock and key' analogy (cf. Chapter 3) using computer-generated three-dimensional structures to speed discovery and refinement of lead compounds. The target is usually a structure obtained from crystallography or by nuclear magnetic resonance (NMR) techniques and may be a critical enzyme, a hormone, a pharmacological receptor, or a nucleic acid. The actual discovery step is computationally intensive, but the computer attacks the problem much the same way we solve jigsaw puzzles. Through trial and error the computer finds the 'pieces' – the compounds – that best fit the target and then these are further examined and selected for testing. Structure-based drug design has been successful, for example, in the discovery of drugs now used successfully in the treatment of HIV infection and acquired immune deficiency syndrome (AIDS).

An alternative and different approach to drug discovery is high throughput screening (HTS). HTS, along with related robotic systems, a diversity of chemical compounds, and sophisticated database management systems, has revolutionized the way in which the search for new drugs is carried out. In HTS, large numbers of compounds are evaluated in specific assays with the goal of identifying an active compound more by random chance than by design. The success of HTS depends on having a large number of automated, well-substantiated, biological assays and good test compounds of chemical diversity. Technological developments in automation have provided the kind of cost effective assays needed – those with high levels of sensitivity to relevant compounds but with resistance to irrelevant chemicals. The large number and diversity of test samples are provided by the in-house libraries of chemical compounds in many pharmaceutical and chemical companies, by natural products, and by the new technology available to medicinal chemists. It is now feasible to evaluate up to 15,000 compounds a month in 10–20 assays. Examples of drugs that have already been uncovered by HTS are lovastatin, a cholesterol-lowering drug; rapamycin, an immunosuppressive agent derived from a soil microorganism; and ivermectin, an anthelmintic.

The technological advance in chemistry that has revolutionized drug discovery is called *combinatorial chemistry*. Medicinal chemists are exploiting this new synthetic strategy to make huge numbers of molecules available for screening as drug leads. Combinatorial chemistry is a way of turning out candidate compounds quickly and affordably and increasing the range of molecular diversity available by harnessing randomness in the synthesis of molecules. The success of this new technology for speeding up the early phases of drug discovery depends on its integration with traditional and structure-based drug discovery approaches in concert with the development of novel, rapid and cost-effective assays for potential biologic activity.

New technologies developed by biotechnology companies are also providing the pharmaceutical industry with a wealth of novel drugs and **drug discovery targets**. These newer targets are frequently proteins that function as ligands or as receptors in a pathway that contributes to a disease process. New technologies such as microarray gene chips allow for the detection of changes in the expression of genes in disease. From these studies, the protein products are analyzed and evaluated as drug targets. Studies of this type that characterize the production and function of proteins based on new technologies are referred to as proteomics. These techniques have driven the pharmaceutical industry increasingly to focus its efforts on the development of innovative therapeutics for previously intractable or poorly treated diseases. Numerous protein drugs are now used in therapeutics, e.g. growth hormone, insulin, erythropoietin, DNAse, TNFα antagonists, and the α- and β-interferons. The usefulness of protein drugs is somewhat limited because of their molecular size and chemical reactivity, precluding noninvasive forms of administration. However, technological advances in protein formulation have made it possible to deliver drugs via the pulmonary route (e.g. DNAse) and modify the chemical structures to achieve longer half-lives in the blood. The production of therapeutic proteins by recombinant technologies, using the human genetic sequence to code for all or part of the molecule, has substantially reduced the risk of hypersensitivity reactions for those drugs previously derived from an animal source, such as insulin and growth hormone.

Studies in Animals or Laboratory Models

The Initial Evaluation of Potential Usefulness

The first tests a compound undergoes in animals are part of the initial screening to determine whether the agent has any biologic activity of potential pharmacologic interest. As already indicated, this may involve either a general, or profile, screen or a specific screen for a definite type of pharmacologic activity. In the general screen a small number of mice or rats are given several doses of the compound under consideration and are then observed for several hours or days. Careful observation at this stage may disclose unusual activity and provide leads to the kinds of pharmacologic action that might be worth pursuing. Frequently, these profile screens are standardized to yield reliable data at minimum cost and labor.

Screening for specific types of pharmacologic activity may follow the clues provided by the profile screen or may be used at the outset when the compound to be tested has been fashioned for a particular purpose. The screen may be either organ-oriented or disease-oriented. In either case, the potential drug is used in experimental animal preparations designed to reveal changes in certain physiologic states or functions. For example, in the search for an agent useful in treating hypertension, animals are prepared so that changes in blood pressure may be monitored in response to drug administration. Or, if a potential anti-malarial agent is being tested, the drug is administered to birds infected with the malarial parasite. *In vitro* screening procedures using isolated tissue or organ preparation (cf. Fig. 9-2), receptor-binding systems or specific enzyme systems may also serve to demonstrate an effect on some physiologic or biochemical function. The difficulty generally associated with any testing procedure, particularly with the disease-oriented test, is finding or producing in animals a relevant counterpart of the physiologic state or disease seen in humans. Although there is no absolute assurance that the drug's effect in the animal model will be duplicated in humans, these tests have predictive value and have been successfully employed to find new agents of benefit to humans. Normally, hundreds of compounds are screened before a potentially active drug is found.

Once a drug survives the initial qualitative assessment of its potential usefulness, it must be subjected to quantitative determinations of its potency and toxicity. The quantitative procedure used to determine the relationship between the dose administered and the magnitude of response is called a *bioassay*. A bioassay to determine the potency of a new agent compared with that of an established drug may have been part of the initial screening procedure. But now the purpose of the bioassay is mainly to determine the relationship between the doses producing a desired effect and those eliciting an undesirable or toxic effect. At this stage of the evaluation, many drugs are found to be unsatisfactory for further trial, since their therapeutic indices indicate a small margin of safety between doses that yield desirable and undesirable effects.

The bioassay is also an essential feature of the standardization of impure drugs of natural origin, such as digitalis, heparin or hormones. The tests are carried out in strict conformity with the rigorous regulations set by appropriate public agencies. The Center for Biologics Evaluation and Research of the FDA, for example, sets the standards for vaccines, serums and other so-called biologics; standards for hormones are set by the *United States Pharmacopeia*.

The Preclinical Evaluation of Safety and Efficacy

When a compound has been found in the profile or specific screening test and in confirmatory testing to produce an effect that suggests it is a potentially useful drug, it is selected for step-by-step, detailed and exhaustive *in vivo* (in animals) and *in vitro* studies. The aim of these preclinical studies is to obtain data on the drug's safety and efficacy sufficient to demonstrate that there will be no unreasonable hazard in initiating trials in human beings.

Regardless of the precise sequence, studies are carried out to determine the effectiveness of the drug in several species of animals. While these studies are directed to the compound's major pharmacologic activity (e.g. analgesia), other

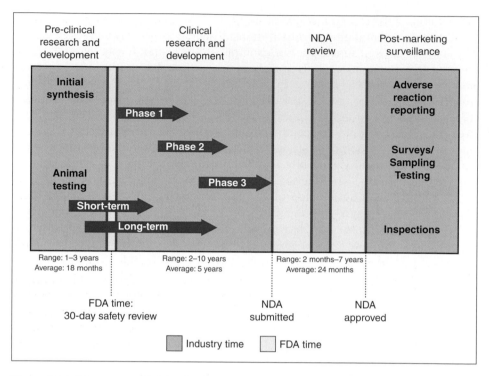

Figure 16-1. *Time course for the development of a new drug.*

experiments are conducted to determine its effect on various organ systems such as heart, lungs, kidneys, intestine, brain and muscle. A serious adverse effect on any of these organs can and may preclude further consideration of the compound as a therapeutic agent. The total process of gathering efficacy and safety data can take several years, and the drug may be discarded at any stage of the evaluation because of inadequate effectiveness or signs of toxicity (Fig. 16-1).

Regulatory agencies have set stringent requirements for the kinds of data that must be submitted in order to obtain permission for trials in human subjects. In the United States, the regulatory authority is the FDA; similar agencies exist in most other countries. In recent years the International Conference on Harmonization has worked to standardize the drug approval promise in the United States, Japan, and Europe in order to decrease regulatory review times and drug development costs. Guidelines issued by the FDA for studies of new drugs specify the number and types of animals to be used in tests of toxicity and efficacy. These guidelines are flexible and change from time to time as experience indicates the utility of newer or better approaches.

The preclinical studies are directed initially toward defining the safety of the drug. To this end, its acute, subacute and chronic toxicities are determined in several animal species (cf. pp. 277–279). The common measure of acute toxicity is the median lethal dose (LD_{50}). It is usually determined, as previously described, by giving groups of animals single doses, some of which are lethal (cf. pp. 205–207). The toxic symptoms developed by the animals and the time at which they appear are also noted. Such observations may provide clues about the mechanisms of toxicity. For example, delayed death may be due to the toxicity of a metabolite rather than of the parent drug. At least three species of animals, one not a rodent, are used, and the acute toxicity is usually determined by more than one route of administration. These initial evaluations of toxicity give some indication of the species differences that may be anticipated, the harmful effects that may be expected and the dosage at which they may be evoked. They have little predictive value, however, unless accompanied by longer-term studies using measures of toxicity other than death.

The subacute toxicity studies must be conducted in at least two animal species. The duration of treatment usually lasts from 4–13 weeks. In each species at least three dose levels are employed, varying from near-therapeutic doses to a level sufficiently high to produce clear-cut toxicity. The drug is administered one or more times daily by the route(s) to be used in the human trials. Routine laboratory examinations, such as hematologic studies and tests of liver and kidney function, are carried out during the period of observation. At the termination of the study, the animals are sacrificed and thorough pathologic examinations are made of organs and tissues.

Chronic toxicity studies must be carried out in at least two species, one of which is usually a rodent. These studies last from a minimum of 6 months to 2 years or longer, depending on the intended duration of drug use in humans. Three dose levels are commonly employed, varying from a nontoxic but greater-than-therapeutic dose to a level high enough to produce a toxic response upon repeated administration. These chronic studies permit many correlated observations to be made which are not practical during the short-term studies. For example, the effect of the drug on food consumption, body weight and growth may be assessed. Again, routine laboratory tests are made at intervals during the long period of drug administration in order to evaluate the possibility of deleterious effects on various bodily functions. Some animals are sacrificed periodically for gross and histologic postmortem examinations. Potential carcinogenic activity is also assessed in specially designed experiments. Extensive reproduction experiments are carried out in rats and rabbits to detect any alterations in the reproductive cycle or any harmful effects on the unborn. Tests for potential teratogenic effects became a routine part of drug toxicity studies only after the thalidomide catastrophe of 1961 focused attention on the need for evaluation of the special effects of drugs upon the fetus (cf. p. 332). These special animal tests and the longer chronic toxicity studies may be conducted concurrently with the initial studies in human subjects. This is particularly true when the drug is intended only for short-term use in humans.

Emphasis in the preclinical phase of investigation is placed on toxicity studies, since adequate scientific evidence must be secured to demonstrate that the drug is safe for human trial under the conditions proposed for its use. The efficacy of the drug does not have to be proved before permission is granted to initiate human studies. But, even though it is recognized that a drug's effect on animals is only predictive of benefit in human disease, the rationale for its proposed use in humans must be documented by animal experimentation. Thus, preclinical tests are also carried out to define more explicitly the drug's full spectrum of pharmacologic properties, and its absorption, distribution, biotransformation and excretion.

The rate and extent of absorption and excretion are usually determined during the course of the subacute toxicity studies by following the changes in plasma concentration of the drug after oral and parenteral administration. Measurements of plasma concentration following intravenous administration provide some information on the extent of tissue distribution as well. And the temporal relationship between plasma concentrations of the drug and its pharmacologic actions may suggest the way in which the drug produces its effect. For example, a lack of relationship may indicate that the drug acts through a metabolite. Measurements of the change in plasma concentration of drug (or metabolites) during the chronic toxicity studies may help to determine whether drug accumulation or enzyme induction occurs upon repeated administration. Additionally, organs and tissues may have to be analyzed directly for their content of drug or metabolites. In order for any of these biochemical studies to be conducted, it is obvious that a sensitive and specific method must be available or developed for the determination of the drug and its metabolite(s) in animal tissues or model systems.

At this stage of drug development, the studies of absorption and elimination performed in animals are only preparatory to carrying out similar studies in humans when human trials are authorized. Detailed investigation of how the body affects the drug is not warranted at this point, since it has limited value in incipient clinical studies. Additional animal studies are usually conducted concurrently with clinical studies. However, preliminary data on the fate of a drug in animals may provide an opportunity to determine which species more closely resembles the human and, thus, which species may provide toxicity data more directly related to humans.

The Formulation of the Drug Product

Before proceeding to a discussion of clinical studies, mention must be made of the formulation of the drug product to be used in treating patients. Drugs are formulated as liquids, capsules, tablets, injectable solutions, or special drug delivery systems. The formulation contains an excipient such as lactose if it is a capsule or tablet, a solvent of some sort for liquids or injectables, a preservative, coloring agent, and so forth. The formulated product provides greater ease in administering the correct dosage, and proper formulation can enhance absorption, whereas improper formulation can retard absorption even to the point of decreasing drug efficacy. The appropriate drug formulation can give the drug product stability so that it does not deteriorate with age as rapidly as it otherwise might and the use of drug delivery technologies can improve its bioavailability and safety.

Formulation studies usually begin early in the investigation of a promising compound, and data are obtained by administration of the drug product to animals and by *in vitro* studies. The final formulation may have to be adjusted after clinical trials are started.

CLINICAL STUDIES

When a compound passes pharmacologic, toxicologic and biochemical tests in animals, the crucial question arises, 'What does it do in humans?' Many adverse effects produced by drugs simply cannot be discerned in animals. For example, symptoms such as nausea, dizziness, headache, ringing in the ears, heartburn and depression would not be recognized in animal studies. In fact it has been estimated that at least half the undesirable effects seen most frequently in the widespread use of drugs can be ascertained *only* during human trial. Moreover, for many human diseases and illnesses there are no reliable animal models. This is particularly true for noninfectious diseases such as arthritis. Thus, no matter how extensive the studies in animals may be, they can only complement, not take the place of, trials in human subjects. Species variation, which may be manifested as qualitative or quantitative differences in the pharmacodynamics or pharmacokinetics of drug action, or both, necessitates the use of human subjects to obtain evidence of the clinical safety and efficacy of a drug.

The initial trials in humans of a potentially useful agent must, obviously, be carried out with extreme caution by qualified investigators in carefully planned studies. Yet only in the last half century has federal legislation been enacted to regulate the manner in which drugs are introduced for human use. The first law, enacted in 1906 as the Federal Food, Drug and Cosmetic Act, was concerned only with standards of purity for drugs already on the market. It designated *The Pharmacopeia of the United States* and *The National Formulary* as the compendia of official standards and empowered the federal government to enforce these standards and require that a drug possess the purity and strength claimed for it. However, it was not until 1939 that new drugs had to be judged safe for their intended use before they could be sold. The Federal Food, Drug and Cosmetic Act of 1938 required, for the first time, that manufacturers submit a new drug application to the FDA for review and approval of studies undertaken to demonstrate the safety of the newly proposed therapeutic agent. It took the death of more than 100 people in the 'elixir of sulfanilamide' disaster of 1937 to gain passage of the law. The so-called elixir of sulfanilamide contained diethylene glycol as a liquid vehicle in the absence of any investigation of the toxicity of this solvent. Diethylene glycol produces severe kidney and liver damage; death results from kidney failure or respiratory failure due to pulmonary edema. Today, an accepted remedy, even one used for years, is considered to be a 'new drug' if manufactured in a new form, and it requires evaluation by the FDA.

The Kefauver-Harris Drug Amendment of 1962 changed the 1938 act to include a requirement that the manufacturer provide 'substantial evidence' that a new drug is not only safe but also effective. The law defines substantial evidence as 'adequate and well-controlled investigations, including clinical investigations, by experts qualified by scientific training and experience to evaluate the effectiveness of the drug involved.' The efficacy provisions were also made retroactive to include products marketed between 1938 and 1962. Agents marketed under the 1938 act constitute a large percentage of the drugs sold today – about 4000 preparations[2]. But the 1962 law and subsequent amendments to the 1938 act did more than require a demonstration of the substantial efficacy of a drug before it could be marketed. These laws also increased governmental regulatory authority (1) to ensure that adequate preclinical studies are completed before human studies are initiated and (2) to provide greater control and surveillance over the distribution and clinical testing of investigational drugs.

Before starting tests of a new drug in humans, the sponsor (usually a pharmaceutical firm, sometimes an individual physician or a research institute) must supply the Center for Drug Evaluation and Research of the FDA with the information specified by the Federal Food, Drug and Cosmetic Act. This application is the Investigational New Drug application, usually referred to as the 'IND'. A new drug is defined as (1) any chemical or substance not previously used in humans for the treatment of disease; (2) combinations of approved drugs or of old drugs, even though the individual components are not new drugs; (3) an approved drug employed for uses other than those approved[3]; (4) a new dosage form of an approved drug; and (5) even a drug used *in vitro* as a diagnostic agent when its use will influence the diagnosis or treatment of disease in a human patient.

The IND submitted to the FDA contains the results of all the preclinical investigations carried out in animals, including complete toxicity data, the full pharmacologic spectrum of the drug and any studies of absorption, distribution, biotransformation and excretion. In addition, the IND must provide the following information:

1. Complete composition of the drug, its source and manufacturing data with details of all quality control measures employed to ensure exact reproducibility of manufacture and identification of all ingredients.
2. Specifications of the dosage forms to be given to humans.
3. A description of the investigations to be undertaken, including the doses to

---

[2]The review of these drugs was carried out under the auspices of the National Academy of Sciences – National Research Council. Thirty panels of experts, each responsible for particular categories of disease, carried out surveys of the effectiveness of the 1938–1962 drugs based on information submitted by the drug manufacturers.

[3]In accordance with the **FDA Modernization Act of 1997**, the FDA issued a proposed rule to permit manufacturers to distribute written information of both efficacy and safety on new and unapproved uses of approved drugs, biologics and devices.

be administered, the route and duration of drug administration and the specific clinical observations and laboratory examinations to be performed.

4 The names and qualifications of, and the facilities available to, each investigator who will participate in the initial studies (phase 1).

5. Copies of all informational material supplied to each investigator (the data sheets supplied to the investigator incorporate the data submitted in the IND itself).

6. An agreement from the sponsor to notify the FDA and all investigators if any adverse effects arise during either the continuing animal studies or human tests.

7. Agreement to submit annual progress reports.

8. Certification that 'informed consent' will be obtained from the subjects or patients to whom the drug will be given.

Investigations in humans may begin as soon as the FDA has indicated its approval, or 30 days from submission of the IND if no formal notice has been received. The clinical studies are divided into three phases, the first two of which are described as clinical pharmacology (Table 16-2).

Conditions Essential to the Proper Execution of Clinical Studies

Before any investigational drug is used in human beings, the law requires that the physician 'obtain the consent of such human beings or their representatives except when it is not possible or when in his professional judgment it is contrary to the best interest of such human beings.' The basic elements of informed

Table 16-2. *Time course for the development of a new drug*

	Number of patients	*Length*	*Purpose*	*Percentage of drugs successfully completing[1]*
Phase 1	20–100	Several months	Mainly safety	70%
Phase 2	Up to several hundred	Several months to 2 years	Some short-term safety, but mainly effectiveness	33%
Phase 3	Several hundred up to five thousand	1–4 years	Safety, effectiveness, dosage	25–30%

[1]For example, of 100 drugs for which investigational new drug applications are submitted to FDA, about 70 will successfully complete phase 1 trials and go on to phase 2; about 33 will complete phase 2 and go to phase 3; and 25 to 30 will clear phase 3 (and, on average, about 20 of the original 100 will ultimately be approved for marketing).

consent include (1) a fair explanation of the procedures to be followed, including an identification of those which are experimental; (2) a description of the attendant discomforts and risks; (3) a description of the benefits anticipated; (4) a disclosure of appropriate alternative procedures that would be advantageous for the subject; (5) an offer to answer any inquiries concerning the procedures; and (6) an instruction that the subject is free to withdraw consent and to discontinue participation in the project at any time. In the early phases of trials in human subjects there can be no exceptions to the rule of obtaining consent, since the drug is being administered primarily for the accumulation of scientific data. Only in later stages of testing, where patients are given a new drug for treatment, may exceptional circumstances warrant drug administration without informed consent. The law defines these exceptions as situations 'where as a matter of professional judgment exercised in the best interest of a particular patient under the investigator's care it would be contrary to the patient's welfare to obtain his consent.' Thus, although large numbers of subjects participate in clinical studies, almost every patient involved is fully informed of the actions of the drug, the purpose of the study and the benefits to be derived from it.

Additional procedures for safeguarding the rights and welfare of human subjects participating in clinical trials of drugs have been established by many institutions where such studies are being performed. These procedures are a direct outgrowth of the policies of the Department of Health and Human Services (HHS). The HHS stipulates that 'no grant or contract for an activity involving human subjects shall be made unless the application for such support has been reviewed and approved by an appropriate institutional committee.' Subsequent to the formation of such committees, many institutions decided that it was their responsibility to safeguard the welfare of all human subjects, not just those involved in activities supported by HHS funds. As a result, most clinical studies in the United States are initiated only after an Institutional Review Board (IRB) has carefully examined applications, protocols or descriptions for the proposed studies and arrived at an independent determination of possible risks. Favorable recommendation is given when this review determines that (1) the rights and welfare of the subjects involved are adequately protected; (2) the risks to an individual are outweighed by the potential benefits to him or by the importance of the knowledge to be gained; and (3) that informed consent has been obtained by methods that are appropriate and adequate.

Women with child-bearing potential are never subjects for clinical trials unless the appropriate teratologic studies in animals have been completed. Such studies must show that administration of 10–20 times the therapeutic dose produces no teratogenic or toxic effects on the embryo or fetus and no adverse effects on the mother. Also, with the obvious exception of trials of new contraceptive drugs, no women are used as subjects when pregnant or if they plan to become pregnant either during or immediately after the clinical study.

Children have rarely been the subjects of clinical trials despite the use of drugs in this age group. A new regulation of the FDA, the Pediatric Research

Equity Act of 2003, is designed to correct this problem. A challenge to the appropriate implementation of this act is the issue of informed consent of minors, which usually must be provided by parental guardians. It is expected that guidelines for IRBs and clinical investigators will be expanded to improve understanding of pediatric risks and education of parents about the components of clinical trials.

In any experiment, the aim is to establish the reliability of and confidence in the outcome of the study by ruling out error and providing a standard of comparison. Thus clinical studies are usually conducted as *controlled* experiments. Whereas what constitutes an adequately controlled study of a new drug in humans varies, by necessity, with the nature of the drug and drug effect being evaluated, there are certain indispensable requirements for all clinical studies. An adequate number of subjects must be used, and the drug effect(s) must be evaluated by appropriate and sensitive methods. The new drug must be concurrently compared with a reference drug over a range of doses. The data must be collected without bias and subjected to valid statistical analysis.

The efficacy of a new drug can be evaluated, with rare exception, only by comparison with one or more accepted agents as standards of reference. The rare exception occurs, for example, when a new drug produces cure of a previously fatal disease, as when the mortality of miliary-meningeal tuberculosis was reduced from 100% to 5% by streptomycin. In most instances, however, the patients are randomly assigned to two or more experimental groups; each group is then treated with a different drug, either the new drug or the older agent(s) available for the specific illness.

To minimize the bias of the patient or investigator, or both, many of the clinical trials are conducted as *single-blind* or *double-blind* studies. A single-blind study is one in which the patient is unaware of the nature of the medication. This does not mean, however, that the new drug is administered without informed consent. The patient is informed that the drug can be properly tested only in a controlled fashion and that, on a randomly selected basis, some patients will receive the new drug while others receive different treatments, including a placebo (see below). In a double-blind study, both the patients and the investigators who supervise the patients and evaluate the data are unaware of which medication has been assigned to a particular individual. The medication each patient received is revealed only after all evaluations of drug effects have been completed. Then the comparisons between the new drug and the standard preparation(s) can be made on the basis of unbiased observations. Properly designed studies using sufficiently large numbers of patients and appropriate statistical analysis of the differences between treatment groups can reveal whether the new agent is inferior, superior or equal to the established treatment. Studies under blind conditions are particularly important in evaluating the efficacy of drugs that produce subjective effects, such as relief of pain.

A new drug is also compared with a placebo (cf. p. 283) as an aid in distinguishing pharmacologic effects from those which are temporally correlated with the mere administration of the drug. However, the use of placebo controls is necessary and appropriate only under certain circumstances. Placebos have a rightful place in studies carried out on normal, healthy volunteers in which the active drug is of no direct therapeutic benefit to the subject. This is also a particularly helpful design when the subjective effects of a drug are under study. Placebos are equally appropriate, if not essential, in studies of wholly new drugs for which there are no existing counterparts. For example, the efficacy of an entirely new vaccine in preventing an infectious disease could hardly be assessed in the absence of a placebo group to determine the normal concurrent incidence of the infection. Placebo controls are not permissible, however, when to give them means withholding a drug from a group of patients who would benefit from its use. Therefore placebos have no place in studies of a new drug in patients suffering from conditions for which an effective drug is already available. The new drug should properly be compared with the existing drug.

Studies in Normal Individuals: Phase 1 of the FDA Regulations

In phase 1 the studies are conducted under carefully controlled conditions in a comparatively small number of subjects, mainly healthy volunteers. The investigator, usually a trained clinical pharmacologist, must be able to evaluate human toxicologic and pharmacologic data. The primary objective of this necessarily cautious phase of the investigation is to determine a safe and tolerated dosage in humans. However, observations of pharmacologic activity, toxicity (if it occurs), absorption, metabolism and excretion may also be made during phase 1. Measurements of blood and urinary levels of the new drug are particularly important at this stage if the drug appears to be ineffective in humans. Only with such data can the investigator decide whether the deficiency is in drug action rather than in a lack of absorption or too rapid elimination.

Although the goal of the phase 1 study remains the same, tests of certain classes of drugs such as the anticancer agents are carried out only in patients. Higher levels of toxicity are accepted for these drugs and the patients are informed that there is no therapeutic intent.

Limited Studies in Patients: Phase 2 of the FDA Regulations

When encouraging results are obtained in phase 1, the studies designated as phase 2 may be started. Most phase 2 studies are randomized controlled trials. Additional pharmacologic studies in animals may also be necessary to indicate the safety of entering this second phase of clinical investigation. Phase 2 consists of initial trials of the value of the drug in the treatment or prevention of the disease for which it is intended. The drug is administered to a limited number of patients under careful supervision to determine its safety and effectiveness. Here the clinician needs to be familiar with the conditions to be treated, the drugs used in these conditions and the methods of their evaluation.

These are, perhaps, the most crucial tests in the development and evaluation of a new drug. The decision to proceed with extensive trials in large populations must be made on the basis of the data obtained in a relatively small number of patients. It is at this point that additional studies of the rates of absorption, metabolism and excretion in individual patients may facilitate further investigations. Evidence of the drug's safety or efficacy may depend on the ability to demonstrate that some patients metabolize or excrete the drug so slowly that high plasma levels lead to toxicity or, conversely, that some patients eliminate the drug so rapidly that effective plasma levels cannot be attained. However, the need or utility of carrying out more or less extensive metabolic studies is guided by the characteristics of the drug under study. For example, when the pharmacologic effect can be measured by following changes in prothrombin time, blood sugar, blood uric acid, and so forth, the need for determining plasma concentrations of the drug may be less critical. Thus, flexibility in the design of additional studies is most desirable at this stage of investigation. Trained and capable investigators can then carry out the kinds of studies that will do the most to ensure safe and effective drug use. However, any changes in the original protocol require the submission of amendments to the IND and may require review by institutional review committees.

In 1987, the FDA made some revisions in the regulations on IND applications, which are noteworthy. The first of these revisions encourages problem-solving meetings with the FDA, sets deadlines for reporting any adverse effects that may occur during the clinical trials, and increases sponsor control over the design of initial tests in humans, provided that subjects face no unreasonable, significant risks. The most important revision, however, concerns the treatment use of investigational new drugs, which can bring promising and important – but still experimental – drugs to desperately ill patients years earlier than was formerly the case. The new regulation allows thousands of patients access to promising new drugs that are still in the experimental stage of development. Patients with immediately life-threatening diseases, such as acquired immune deficiency syndrome (AIDS) and deadly cancers may now get treatment with experimental drugs provided that no other satisfactory approved therapy exists. This regulation applies only to drugs already being studied in controlled clinical trials (phase 2) that show reasonable evidence of potential benefit without unreasonable risk. FDA approval of zidovudine (AZT) illustrates this policy; AZT was made available to 4000 AIDS patients just 1 week after phase 2 studies were terminated (Table 16-3). Another example involves the use of a relatively toxic cancer therapy for patients with advanced melanoma or advanced kidney cancer. Despite the treatment's toxicity, the National Cancer Institute, which requested the approval from the FDA, believed expanded use was warranted because these advanced cancers are almost always fatal and some patients had complete disappearance of tumors in response to treatment. The FDA on the recommendation of its Oncologic Drugs Advisory Committee[4] approved the use

---

[4]The Oncologic Drugs Advisory Committee is one of many committees that advise the FDA about the safety and effectiveness of drugs and biologic products. These committees comprise nine to 15 outside experts as appointed members.

Table 16-3. *Time course for development of zidovudine, the first antiviral drug approved for the treatment of acquired immune deficiency syndrome (AIDS)*

1964	Azidothymidine (AZT, now known as zidovudine) developed as potential cancer treatment. Shelved because of ineffectiveness
October 1984	Preclinical tests begin for use as antiviral to treat acquired immune deficiency syndrome (AIDS)
May 1985	Investigational new drug exemption (IND) submitted
July 1985	Phase 1 tests begin
February 1986	Phase 2 tests begin
September 1986	Trials terminated; phase 3 not conducted[1]
October 1986	Treatment IND approved[2]
December 1986	New drug application (NDA) submitted
March 1987	NDA approved.

[1]The study was stopped because patients on the drug clearly were living longer than those given a placebo. It was deemed unethical to continue to withhold treatment from the control group.
[2]Treatment protocol that allows access to the new drug before approval for marketing for patients who meet the medical criteria of the study protocol.

of interleukin-2 combined with lymphokine-activated killer cells within 1 month of the initial approach by the National Cancer Institute.

The new regulation applies also to investigational new drugs that may effectively treat or improve treatment for the serious but not immediately life-threatening illness. Approval by the FDA for the expanded availability of PROTOPIN, a cloned form of human growth hormone, for use in the treatment of hormone-deficiency diseases is an example of the implementation of the new regulation; it is also an example of the approval of a drug developed through recombinant DNA technology – through genetic engineering.

The Expedited Drug Approval Act of 1992 increased the flexibility in these approval standards by permitting approval of drugs and biologicals for serious or life-threatening illnesses on the basis of surrogate endpoints that are 'reasonably likely' to predict clinical benefit. These newer regulations also included provisions for phase 4 studies, restrictions on distribution and use, premarket review of promotional materials and market withdrawal of the drug. Stavudine, for example, was cleared by the FDA in 1994 through the accelerated approval mechanisms for the treatment of adults with advanced human immunodeficiency virus (HIV) who are unable to take other anti-HIV drugs. The approval of stavudine was based on interim results from a phase 3 trial using as the surrogate marker counts of cells that determine the outcome of the infection.

Large-scale Controlled Studies: Phase 3 of the FDA Regulations

Studies on a limited number of normal subjects and patients are primarily aimed at ascertaining whether a new drug merits further investigation. The figures in Table 16-4 indicate that a large percentage of the INDs originally submitted to

Table 16-4. *Tabulation of the number of original INDs[1] submitted, INDs discontinued, original NDAs[2] submitted,[3] NDAs approved[4] and new chemical entities approved[5] by FDA for calendar years 1970–1998*

Year	Original INDs submitted	INDs discontinued by sponsor	Original NDAs submitted	NDAs approved	New chemical entities
1970	1127	. . .	87	53	18
1974	802	399	129	95	23
1977	925	802	124	63	21
1980	1087	626	162	114	12
1983	1798	913	269	94	14
1984	2112	742	217	142	22
1986	1596	1429	120	98	20
1987	1346	1831	142	69	21
1988	1337	961	126	67	20
1994	2156	. . .[6]	. . .[6]	62	22
1995	1924	. . .[6]	. . .[6]	82	28
1997	1996	. . .[6]	. . .[6]	121	39
1998	2419	. . .[6]	. . .[6]	90	30

[1]Applications submitted to FDA for permission to begin investigations in humans.
[2]NDA = New Drug Application.
[3]Applications submitted to FDA for permission to market a new drug.
[4]New drugs marketed as totally new entities or as revisions of older drugs.
[5]Newly discovered drugs.
[6]Figures not available from FDA.
Source: Food and Drug Administration, Public Health Service, Department of Health and Human Services.

the FDA are discontinued by the sponsor of the new drug or preparation. It is likely that many of these projects are terminated during initial studies and before extension of the clinical testing to phase 3. But when the data obtained in phases 1 and 2 provide reasonable assurance of the safety of the drug and a promise of clinical efficacy, proposals are made for the extensive trials of phase 3. It is at this point that representatives of the drug sponsor meet with FDA staff to discuss plans for phase 3. The studies in the final phase must yield data on which the sponsor and the FDA can base a decision that the drug is marketable as safe and effective for its intended use. Thus, in phase 3, controlled clinical trials are conducted by a sufficient number of qualified investigators on a large enough population of patients to obtain the necessary data to substantiate claims of safety and efficacy. As many as 150 clinicians may participate in these studies, and the patients under their supervision usually number over 1500 and may even exceed 3000. The clinical trial (phases 1–3) can, and usually does, take a long time to complete – from 2 to 10 years with an average of 5 years.

At the beginning of phase 3, the IND must be revised to reflect any modifications in the investigations to be undertaken. The FDA must also be informed of the qualifications of the new investigators who have agreed to study the drug under the conditions specified in the IND. In addition to experienced clinical pharmacologists, physicians who are not specialists may serve as investigators so that a broad background of experience may be secured in a large number of patients. The objective of phase 3 testing and of joint FDA–drug sponsor consultations is to develop data that will permit the drug to be marketed and used safely and effectively.

The value of carrying out extensive studies on the biotransformation of a new drug during phase 3 is largely dictated by the usefulness of such information in the evaluation of safety and efficacy. However, more detailed studies are usually carried out at this time to determine the drug's capacity to bind to plasma proteins, to induce or inhibit enzymes and to interact in various ways with other drugs.

It is at this point that pharmacogenomics can be a potentially useful tool to increase the probability of success of the candidate drug. Pharmacogenomic testing can identify those patients who are likely to show little or no response or a toxic response as a result of genetic differences in pharmacodynamics.

THE NEW DRUG APPLICATION (NDA)

The clinical studies of phase 3 are completed when, in the opinion of the sponsor, sufficient data have been collected to permit the judgment that the drug is safe and effective. There are no hard and fast rules on what constitutes 'safety' or 'efficacy'; these qualities must be judged in relation to the specific clinical conditions for which the drug is to be used. For example, a lesser degree of efficacy and a smaller margin of safety are acceptable for an agent to be used to treat cancer than for a drug to treat a self-limiting, nondebilitating and nonfatal disease. In the latter case, or when an effective drug of the same type is already available, efficacy in a high proportion of patients and a low incidence of adverse effects would have to be demonstrated. When the sponsor is convinced that the data obtained in phase 3 studies justify approval of the drug as safe and effective for the use(s) intended, a New Drug Application (NDA) is submitted. Usually at least 5 years or more will have elapsed between the time the drug was selected from the original pharmacologic screen and the date of completion and filing of its NDA.

The NDA contains all the chemical, pharmacologic, clinical and manufacturing data that have been collected since research on the drug was initiated. The FDA also requires samples of the drug, its labels and the *package insert* that will accompany the drug in all shipments to physicians and pharmacies to provide FDA-approved guidance on how to use the drug. In some cases, the NDA may also contain data of bioequivalence and bioavailability as defined and determined by the procedures included in the 1977 amendment to the Federal Food, Drug and Cosmetic Act. Traditionally, physical and chemical tests were used to demonstrate that a drug product met the appropriate standards of strength, quality and purity and had its purported identity. With the development of biopharmaceutics and pharmacokinetics, however, it became possible to characterize a drug product more fully by determining its biologic availability. Therefore, standards for certain drug products were amended to include bioequivalence and bioavailability requirements. Bioequivalence data are required whenever there is evidence that drug products containing the same active drug ingredient or therapeutic moiety and intended to be used interchangeably for the same therapeutic effect are not or might not be bioequivalent drug products (cf. p. 95). *In vivo* bioavailability data must be included in the NDA unless other information is sufficient to permit the FDA to waive this requirement. However, *in vivo* bioavailability data are always required for certain classes of drugs such as anticoagulants, anticonvulsants, antibacterials, cardiac glycosides, and anti-anxiety agents[5].

The Center for Drug Evaluation and Research (CDER) is responsible for receiving and evaluating the NDA and is required to act on the application within a relatively short period of time. The FDA's CDER usually insists that sponsoring companies file the results of two well-controlled phase 3 studies in order for their submission to be considered for approval. A review clock is started, by law, on the date the FDA receives an NDA, and the FDA has 180 days to review the application and either approve or reject it. Theoretically, if the NDA is 'complete', it will be promptly approved and then the new agent may be marketed (Table 16-3). What is more frequently the case, however, is that the application is considered 'incomplete'. The sponsor is informed of the specific data that are lacking and has the opportunity to resubmit the NDA with the additional required information or studies. The sponsor may also request a hearing when there is disagreement with the conclusions reached by the professional staff of the Bureau of Medicine. A negative ruling following a hearing

---

[5]'(a) Pharmaceutical equivalents: drug products that contain identical amounts of the identical active drug ingredient, i.e. the same salt or ester of the same therapeutic moiety, in identical dosage forms, but not necessarily containing the same inactive ingredients, and that meet the identical compendial or other applicable standard of identity, strength, quality, and purity, including potency and, where applicable, content uniformity, disintegration times and/or dissolution rates. (b) Pharmaceutical alternatives: drug products that contain the identical therapeutic moiety, or its precursor, but not necessarily in the same amount or dosage form or as the same salt or ester. Each such drug product individually meets either the identical or its own respective compendial or other applicable standard of identity, strength, quality, and purity, including potency and, where applicable, content uniformity, disintegration times and/or dissolution rates. (c) Bioequivalent drug products: pharmaceutical equivalents or pharmaceutical alternatives whose rate and extent of absorption do not show a significant difference when administered at the same molar dose of the therapeutic moiety under similar experimental conditions, either single dose or multiple dose. Some pharmaceutical equivalents or pharmaceutical alternatives may be equivalent in the extent of their absorption but not in their rate of absorption and yet may be considered bioequivalent because such differences in the rate of absorption are intentional and are reflected in the labeling, are not essential to the attainment of effective body drug concentrations on chronic use, or are considered medically insignificant for the particular drug product studied. (d) Bioavailability: the rate and extent to which the active drug ingredient or therapeutic moiety is absorbed from a drug product and becomes available at the site of drug action.' (From *Fed. Reg.* 42:1624, 1977.)

may be appealed to the courts. It is obvious from the figures in Table 16-4, however, that a sizable number of NDAs fails to gain FDA approval.

The data in Table 16-4 also clearly indicate that new molecular entities, i.e. active moieties not yet marketed in the United States by any drug manufacturer either as a single entity or as part of a combination product, represent, on the average, only 25–30% of all the new drugs approved for marketing. The majority of the NDAs approved is for either a new salt, new formulation, new indication for use, new combination of drugs previously marketed by the same or different sponsor, or for a drug that duplicates an already marketed drug product. Of the new chemical entities (NCEs) approved in the 18-year period from 1970 to 1988, only one-quarter were evaluated as offering 'important therapeutic gain' and one-third as offering 'modest therapeutic gain' by the FDA. In making this type of evaluation, the FDA considered only the degree of therapeutic gain deemed to have been offered by the drug at the time of its introduction in the light of available therapeutic alternatives, without reference to subsequent experience. The criteria used were (1) *important therapeutic gain* – the drug may provide effective therapy or diagnosis (by virtue of greatly increased efficacy or safety) for a disease not adequately treated or diagnosed by any marketed drug, or provide markedly improved treatment of a disease through improved efficacy or safety (including decreased abuse potential); (2) *modest therapeutic gain* – the drug has a modest, but real advantage over other available marketed drugs, e.g. somewhat greater effectiveness, decreased adverse reactions, or less frequent dosing in situations in which frequent dosage is a problem.

In view of its limited resources, the FDA has now established a classification system for the order in which NDAs are reviewed so that priority will be given to drugs with the greatest potential benefit. Thus, a drug that is a new molecular entity and represents an important therapeutic gain is designated '1P' for priority review; a drug that is substantially equivalent to existing therapies is rated '1S' for standard review, and the designation '4S' is given to a combination of a new agent and an already marketed compound that is substantially equivalent to existing therapies. Priority NDAs are earmarked for greater attention by reviewers and an expedited review process. For example, 36 of the NCEs approved by the FDA for marketing between 1990 and 1992 were designated 1P. The mean review time for the theoretically important priority drugs was 20.6 months, but drugs such as the anticancer agent paclitaxel, the antimalarial drug halofantrine, and levamisole, an anticancer as well as anthelmintic agent, took only 5.3, 6.5 and 7.5 months, respectively, to go through the review process. The 'standard' NCEs required 40.9 months on average for NDA approval – twice as long as the priority drugs. It is noteworthy, moreover, that new drugs are now being approved for use in the United States faster than ever before; 50% of NCE approvals now take less than 1 year and between 1995 and 1998, 145 NCEs were approved, more than in any similar period since 1962.

The Prescription Drug User Fee Act (PDUFA) of 1992, reauthorized in 1997 and 2002, has contributed to the reduction in NDA review times. The regulations require manufacturers to submit fees with the NDAs and in exchange the FDA increased its review personnel and agreed to adhere to goals for review time.

However, the total time for drug development has increased in the last several decades. For NCEs approved in 1990–1999, the preclinical phase, phases 1–3, and the approval phase averaged 3.8, 8.6, and 1.8 years for a total of 14.2 years. These figures vary according to therapeutic class. The average cost of the research and development of a newly approved drug, including the expense of drugs that fail, has been estimated as about $400 million (in 2000 dollars) in out-of-pocket expenditures and $800 million in capitalized costs, which include lost alternative investment opportunity.

In addition to the 1986–1987 regulations streamlining the process for getting new, safe, and effective drugs to market and making promising experimental drugs available to desperately ill patients, two new laws were enacted in the 1980s to encourage new drug development. The first of these, the Orphan Drug Act of 1983, was designed to foster the development of drugs that offer little or no profit to the manufacturer but do offer benefit to people with rare diseases. A rare disease is defined as one that affects less than 200,000 Americans, and there are an estimated 2000 such diseases. Although the drug industry had provided so-called *public service products* for some of them for many years using their own initiatives and resources, Congress recognized that the government had to assume more of the burden if patients suffering from many rare diseases were to be helped. The new law allows drug companies to take tax deductions for about two-thirds of the cost of their clinical studies and to have exclusive rights for 7 years for any orphan products that are approved. Also, the FDA can give high priority for review and can make grants in support of a sponsor's clinical research of an orphan drug. Eighteen of the 74 new chemical entities approved between 1990 and 1992 were given orphan drug status and required only 18.2 months on average for marketing approval.

The second law, the Drug Price Competition and Patent Term Restoration Act of 1984, expands the number of drugs suitable for an abbreviated new drug application (ANDA) Previously, manufacturers of a 'generic' drug (i.e. nonproprietary drug) had to carry out their own tests to prove that the active ingredient in their product was safe and effective. Since that had already been shown when the equivalent proprietary drug was first approved for marketing, that part of the NDA has been eliminated in the ANDA for a 'generic' drug. 'Generic' drugs must still go through scientific testing to show that they have the same bioavailability as the original proprietary drug. The new law makes it less costly and time-consuming for 'generic' drugs to reach the market. The second part of the law, Patent Term Restoration, referred to the 17 years of legal protection given a firm for each drug patent. The provisions of this part of the Act of 1984 have been replaced by provisions created by the General Agreement on Trade and Tariffs (GATT) of 1994. The biggest changes in the United States patent laws since 1952 went into effect in June, 1995 and include the following: (1) a 20-year patent term measured from the date of filing, and (2) a new type of filing – the provisional application. The 20 years from filing patent term replaces the previous 17 years from the patent's date of issue. The patent term for unexpired patents issued before June 8, 1995 will be the greater of 20 years from filing or 17 years from date of issue. A provisional application allows an applicant to file an incomplete application, which provides a priority benefit of the earlier filing date and a 12-month period to decide whether patent protection should be pursued in the United States or internationally.

Postmarketing Surveillance: Phase 4

The manufacturer's responsibilities do not end when a drug has finally been approved for marketing but continue well into the period of its general clinical use. Although there is no accepted definition of this phase of FDA regulations, the term *phase 4* is commonly applied to all aspects of investigation that follow the granting of an NDA and the general availability of a new drug in widespread clinical use. The sponsor's claims of drug efficacy and safety that are to appear in brochures or advertising are reviewed and approved by the FDA. Reports concerning current clinical studies must be sent to the FDA every 3 months during the first year, every 6 months in the second year and annually thereafter. These reports must also include information about the quantity of drug distributed and copies of mailing pieces, labeling and, for a prescription drug, advertising. Any unexpected side-effects, injury, toxic or allergic reactions or failure of the drug to exert its expected pharmacologic action that is made known to the manufacturer must, in turn, be transmitted to the FDA. Thus the FDA has responsibility not only for ensuring that drugs are safe and effective before being marketed, but also for continued surveillance of those drugs long after their introduction into general clinical use. The Office of Post-Marketing Drug Risk Assessment was established by the FDA in 1998 to enforce the reporting requirements of the FDA Modernization Act of 1997.

CONCLUDING REMARKS

There is little doubt that the steps taken to improve the standards of drug development and evaluation have provided increased protection to both the test subject and the consumer. That the FDA has fulfilled these responsibilities is evidenced by the fact that less than 3.5% of the new drugs introduced in the United States between 1979 and 1988 had to be discontinued for safety reasons; this figure dropped dramatically to less than 1.5% in the period between 1989 and 1998. But with all these safeguards, no new drug – or, for that matter, no established drug – is completely free of hazard. Nor can more and more regulatory control hope to achieve this end; indeed, the effects of greater restrictions in drug development and evaluation might serve to deny the public the benefits of improved drug therapy. Given the unique genetic makeup of each person and the pharmacologic individuality this confers, there will always be some people who respond to a drug in an unexpected manner. And the more widespread the use of a drug, the greater will be the number of incidents of drug ineffectiveness or drug toxicity. But the risks inherent in the use of any drug can be minimized if drug use, whether by physician or patient, is always based on current knowledge of the general principles and concepts of pharmacology.

> Knowledge is the root and practice is the bough and there is no bough without a root behind it, although roots may be found which can as yet boast no boughs.
>
> *Moses Maimonides*

GUIDES FOR STUDY AND REVIEW

How are new therapeutic agents discovered? What are the sources of therapeutic agents?

How are chemicals evaluated initially for their potential usefulness as therapeutic agents? What is a bioassay and how is it used to evaluate potential drug effectiveness and safety?

What kinds of information, in general, must be available about a potential therapeutic agent before clinical trials in humans can be initiated? What agency in the United States decides whether trials in humans can begin? When was this made law? What is an IND?

What do we mean by 'informed consent' with respect to the use of investigational drugs in humans? Are there any conditions under which informed consent for administration of an investigational drug is not needed? What regulations protect women with child-bearing potential?

How is the efficacy of a new drug evaluated? What kinds of drugs serve as a standard of reference? What is a single-blind study? a double-blind study?

When is the use of a placebo appropriate in the clinical trial of a new drug? When is its use inappropriate?

What subjects are generally used and how extensive are the clinical trials in phase 1 of the FDA regulations? in phase 2? in phase 3? What is the NDA and when is it submitted? Must efficacy as well as safety of a new drug be demonstrated? by law? When can a new agent be placed on the market? What responsibilities does the sponsor of the new drug have after it is placed on the market? How do the regulations for marketing new therapeutic agents resemble those for registering new economic poisons?

SUGGESTED READING

Berkowitz, B. and Sachs, G. Life cycle of a block buster: discovery and development of omeprazole (PRILOSEC). *Molecular Interventions* 2:6, 2002.

Borman, S. Combinatorial chemists focus on small molecules, molecular recognition, and automation. *Chem. Engineer. News* Feb. 12:28, 1996.

Day, S., Green, S. and Machin, D. (eds). *Textbook of Clinical Trials*. New York: John Wiley & Sons, 2004.

DeSmet, P.A.G.M. Herbal remedies. *N. Engl. J. Med*. 347:2046–2056, 2002.

DiMasi, J.A. New drug development in the United States from 1963 to 1999. *Clin. Pharmacol. Ther*. 69:286–296, 2001.

DiMasi, J.A. Risks in new drug development: approval success rates for investigational drugs. *Clin. Pharmacol. Ther*. 69:297, 2001.

DiMasi, J.A., Hansen, R.W. and Grabowski, H.G. The price of innovation: new estimates of drug development cost. *J. Health Economics* 22:151–185, 2003.

Drug Discovery. *Science* (Special Section) 303:1796–1822, 2004.

Flynn, J.T. Successes and shortcomings of the Food and Drug Modernization Act. *Am. J. Hypertens*. 16:889–891, 2003.

Friedman, L.M., Furberg, C.D. and DeMets, D.L. *Fundamentals of Clinical Trials* (3rd ed.). New York: Springer-Verlag, 1998.

Guarino, R.A. (ed.) *New Drug Approval Process: The Global Challenge* (3rd ed.). New York: Marcel Dekker, 2000.

Hampton, T. Pediatric drug studies required by law. *JAMA* 291:412–414, 2004.

Janzen, W.P. *High Throughput Screening: Methods and Protocols*. Totowa: Humana Press, 2002.

Lin, J. Sahakian, D.C., de Morais, S.M., Xu, J.J., Polzer, R.J. and Winter, S.M. The role of absorption, distribution, metabolism, excretion and toxicity in drug discovery. *Curr. Top. Med. Chem*. 3:1125–1154, 2003.

Nwaka, S. and Ridley, R.G. Virtual drug discovery and development for neglected diseases through public-private partnerships. *Nat. Rev. Drug Discovery* 2:919–928, 2003.

Paton, W.D.M. *Man and Mouse: Animals in Medical Research*. Oxford: Oxford University Press, 1995.

Schreiner, M.S. Paediatric clinical trials: redressing the imbalance. *Nat. Rev. Drug Discovery* 2:949–961, 2003.

Shulman, S.R., Hewitt, P. and Manocchia, M. Studies and inquiries into the FDA regulatory process: a historical review. *Drug Information J*. 29:385, 1993.

Stonier, P.D. *Discovering New Medicines: Careers in Pharmaceutical Research and Development*. New York: J. Wiley & Sons, 1995.

Glossary

acid   A molecule, ion or other entity that acts as a proton or hydrogen ion donor; a substance that ionizes in solution to form hydrogen ions; any substance that contains hydrogen capable of being replaced by basic radicals (cf. base).

additive effect   A term ordinarily used to describe the combined effects of two drugs, acting simultaneously, which elicit the same overt response by the same mechanism of action. As in summation (q.v.), the total effect is equal to that expected by simple addition. The magnitude of the combined effect must be within the capacity of the system to respond, e.g. the combined effect of aspirin and acetaminophen to relieve pain.

adrenergic blocking agent   An agent that selectively inhibits certain responses to adrenergic nerve stimulation and to epinephrine, norepinephrine, and other sympathomimetic drugs.

adrenergic nerve   A nerve that releases norepinephrine when it is stimulated, i.e. most postganglionic fibers of the sympathetic nervous system (cf. cholinergic nerve).

afferent nerve   *See* sensory nerve.

affinity   A measure of the effectiveness of the interaction between a receptor and a drug. The greater the affinity of a receptor for a given drug, the greater is the propensity of the receptor to bind that drug; a high affinity interaction means that a smaller concentration of drug is needed to produce the same intensity of response compared to a drug that interacts with a lesser affinity at the same receptor.

agonist   A drug that produces a response (it has intrinsic activity), typically by binding to a receptor or other protein target.

allergic response   An adverse response to a foreign chemical resulting from a previous exposure to that substance. It is manifested only after a second or subsequent exposure and then as a reaction different from the usual pharmacologic effect of the chemical. Since a minute amount of an otherwise safe drug may elicit the allergic response, the term *hypersensitivity* is frequently used to describe the sensitization reaction. *Hypersensitivity*, used to designate the allergic response, should not be confused with the extreme *sensitivity* displayed by certain individuals in whom very small doses of a drug elicit an intensity of pharmacologic effect primarily seen only at higher doses (cf. antibodies, antigen).

analgesic drug   An agent that relieves pain without producing a loss of consciousness. In the latter respect, an analgesic differs from an anesthetic drug (q.v.).

anesthetic drug   (Gk *an*, 'not', + *aisthesis*, 'feeling') An agent that causes reversible loss of feeling or sensation. General anesthesia affects the entire body, causing not only loss of sensation but also loss of consciousness. Local anesthetics cause loss of sensation only in the particular area where they are applied by blocking the transmission of nerve impulses from the affected area.

angina pectoris   A syndrome characterized by a transient interference with the flow of blood, oxygen and nutrients to heart muscle and associated with severe pain.

antagonist   (*See* drug antagonism) A drug that blocks the response of an agonist; it may lack the ability to produce a response in the absence of an agonist (no efficacy).

anthelmintics   Drugs used to rid the body of worms (helminths).

antibiotic   A chemical substance or metabolic product that is produced by microorganisms and that destroys or prevents the growth of other microorganisms or neoplastic cells.

antibodies   Substances in the tissues or fluids of an organism that act to antagonize specific foreign bodies. The first exposure of the body to a foreign antigen triggers certain cells to elaborate specific antibodies – large proteins identified as specific immunoglobulins. Subsequent exposure to the same (or a related) antigen leads to an immune response characterized by an increase in the amount of the induced antibody. The type of response to the antigen-antibody interaction differs radically for different antigens and in different hosts; it is independent of the pharmacologic effects produced by the eliciting drug but is determined by the mediators released by the antigen-antibody complex (cf. allergic response).

antidote   Any chemical agent used to overcome the action or the effects of a poison.

antigen   A substance which, when introduced into the body, is capable of inducing the formation of antibodies and subsequently of reacting in a recognizable fashion with the specific induced antibodies. All proteins foreign to the organism may be antigens; many purified polysaccharides and simpler chemical groups (such as drugs) also can become antigenic when coupled to proteins. The relatively simple compounds – haptens – that do not by themselves stimulate antibody formation may react specifically with the antibody after the latter is formed.

antirheumatic agent   A drug effective in the treatment of acute rheumatic fever.

antisense compounds   Short, synthetic pieces of nucleic acids (oligonucleotides) designed to block the action of specific genes by binding to their messenger RNA.

antiseptic   A chemical agent with bacteriostatic action that inhibits the growth of microorganisms but does not necessarily kill them.

ataxia   Lack of normal coordination of muscular movement, especially inability to coordinate voluntary muscular movements.

autonomic drug   Any agent that has its primary action on any part of the autonomic nervous system or on autonomic effector cells.

bactericide (disinfectant, germicide)   An agent that is capable of producing rapid death of microorganisms. *Disinfectant* and *germicide* are used more frequently for agents killing microorganisms on inanimate objects, but all three terms are synonymous (cf. antiseptic).

base   A molecule, ion or other entity that acts as an acceptor of protons or hydrogen ions; a substance that ionizes in solution to form hydroxyl ions; any substance that has the property of neutralizing acids to form salts; any substance that can replace the hydrogen of an acid (cf. acid).

bioassay   A procedure for determining the quantitative relationship between the dose of a drug and the intensity of the biologic response it evokes. Bioassays are used (1) to determine the potency of a drug relative to another drug or a standard of reference, or (2) to standardize preparations of impure drugs.

bioavailability   The rate and extent to which the active drug ingredient or therapeutic moiety is absorbed from a drug product and becomes available at the site of drug action (as defined by FDA regulations). Experimentally, bioavailability is assessed from measurements of the concentration of a drug in the plasma at various times after drug administration.

biochemical antagonism   *See* drug antagonism.

bioequivalent drug products   Pharmaceutical equivalents or pharmaceutical alternatives whose rate and extent of absorption do not show a significant difference when administered at the same molar dose of the therapeutic moiety under similar experimental conditions, either single dose or multiple dose (as defined by FDA regulations).

biopharmaceutics   The science and study of the ways in which the pharmaceutical formulation of administered agents can influence their pharmacodynamic and pharmacokinetic behavior.

biotransport   The translocation of a solute from one side of a biologic barrier to the other side, the transferred solute appearing in the same form on both sides of the biologic barrier.

blood-brain barrier   The circumferential tight junctions of the endothelial cells of the blood capillaries in the brain that account, in part, for the slow diffusion of water-soluble materials into brain tissue. The envelopment of the vessels by astrocytes (a type of glial cell) and the presence of efflux carrier proteins in the endothelial membrane contribute to the barrier.

certain safety factor (CSF)   A number that reflects the relative safety of a drug or of its selectivity of action. The CSF is derived from the extremes of the quantal dose-effect curves of the effects to be compared, e.g. LD_1/ED_{99}, the ratio of the lowest lethal and highest therapeutic levels of response (cf. standard safety margin, therapeutic index, selectivity).

chemical antagonism *See* drug antagonism.

chemical teratogens Chemicals that produce abnormalities of fetal development when administered to a pregnant animal.

chiral compound A molecule that has at least one pair of enantiomers (q.v.). Chiral molecules frequently differ in potency, pharmacological activity, biotransformation, urinary excretion kinetics and toxicity.

cholinergic nerve A nerve that releases acetylcholine when it is stimulated, i.e. all motor nerves of the somatic nervous system, all preganglionic fibers of the autonomic nervous system, all postganglionic fibers of the parasympathetic division and a few postganglionic fibers of the sympathetic division (cf. adrenergic nerve).

competitive antagonism *See* drug antagonism.

conduction The passage of an impulse along an axon or muscle fiber (cf. transmission).

congener A drug that belongs to a group of chemical compounds having the same parent compound.

Controlled Substances Act An act passed by the United States Congress under the title *Comprehensive Drug Abuse Prevention and Control Act of 1970* to replace the *Harrison Narcotic Act of 1914.* This act codifies the regulations covering drugs subject to abuse and divides narcotic and other drugs into five schedules according to legitimacy of medical use and potential for abuse. Schedule I contains those that have a high abuse and *no* currently accepted therapeutic use in the US, e.g. heroin, marihuana, MDMA, LSD, peyote, and mescaline. Drugs listed in schedule I may be obtained only for research or chemical analysis. Schedule II lists drugs that have a high abuse potential with strong physical dependence liability, e.g. opium, morphine, codeine, methadone, and other opioids; cocaine; amphetamines, methamphetamine, methylphenidate (RITALIN) and PCP; amobarbital, pentobarbital, and secobarbital; dronabinol. Schedule III contains drugs that have an abuse potential less than those in schedules I and II but may lead to moderate or mild physical dependence, e.g. anabolic steroids; nalorphine, buprenorphine; ketamine; barbiturates (except those listed in another schedule, compound mixtures containing limited quantities of morphine, codeine or other narcotic analgesics), Schedule IV contains drugs that have a low abuse potential and lead to only limited physical dependence compared to drugs in schedule III, e.g. phenobarbital; chloral hydrate; meprobamate; and benzodiazepines. Schedule V lists drugs with an abuse potential less than those in schedule IV, e.g. preparations of opioids mixed with nonopioid active medicinal ingredients.

convulsion An involuntary, generalized contraction of muscle, usually having its origin in disturbed function of the central nervous system. In clonic convulsions, the gross, rhythmic, coordinated movements of different parts of the body are characterized by alternating contraction and relaxation of opposing (reciprocally innervated) muscle groups. In tonic convulsions, an intense contraction is maintained in all muscle groups.

coordinate covalent bond   *See* covalent bond.

covalent bond   The chemical bond formed between two atoms when the atoms share a pair of electrons. A covalent bond can result from the sharing of electrons supplied by one atom only, the resulting bond being called a coordinate covalent bond. The covalent bond is about 20 times stronger than the ionic bond (q.v.).

cross-dependence   The ability of one drug to suppress the manifestations of physical dependence induced by another drug and to substitute for the other in maintaining the physically dependent state.

cross-sensitization   The phenomenon whereby the initial exposure to a drug may elicit an allergic response in an individual previously sensitized to a different but related drug or environmental chemical.

cytochrome P450s   A family of structurally similar oxidative enzymes located in the membranes of the smooth endoplasmic reticulum (the 'microsomal' fraction) of many cells, especially the liver. Important for the biotransformation of many drugs and other foreign chemicals.

demulcents   Substances of high molecular weight that form aqueous solutions capable of alleviating irritation particularly of mucous membranes and abraded surfaces, e.g. acacia (gum arabic), glycerin.

disintegration time   The time required for a tablet to break up into particles of smaller or specified size under carefully controlled experimental conditions. The degree of compression of the tablet and the type of binders used influence disintegration time. Rapid disintegration does not ensure rapid absorption, but the absorption of drugs that are rapidly transferred across a barrier may be rate-limited by a long disintegration time (cf. dissolution time).

dissolution time   The time required for a given quantity or fraction of drug to go into solution from a solid dosage form. Since solution of the drug is preliminary to absorption, slow dissolution may be rate-limiting for drugs that are rapidly absorbed.

diuretic   A drug that increases the volume of urine excreted.

dosage   The total quantity of drug to be administered over a period of time in order to produce a desired effect. Thus the usual oral dosage of penicillin is 500 mg to 2 g, given in individual doses of 125 to 500 mg four to six times a day. Loading dose refers to a large initial dose designed to produce the therapeutic effect; maintenance dose refers to the smaller dose taken repeatedly to continue the therapeutic effect.

dosage form   The physical state in which a drug is dispensed.

dose   The amount of drug needed at a given time to produce a particular biologic effect.

dose-effect curve (dose-response curve)   Graphic representation of the mathematical expression of the relationship between dose (the independent variable) and effect (the dependent variable). One of the most basic principles of pharmacology states that the intensity of response elicited by a drug is a function of the dose administered, i.e. a larger dose produces a greater effect than a smaller dose, up to the limit of the capacity of the biologic system to respond. The term *graded* is applied to the type of relationship in which the responding system is capable of showing a progressively increasing effect with increasing concentration of drug. The term *quantal* is applied to the type of relationship in which the number or proportion of individuals responding by a particular, stated (all-or-none) response increases as the dose increases.

drug   Any chemical agent that affects living organisms.

drug abuse   The excessive and persistent use, usually by self-administration, of any drug without due regard for accepted medical practice. The vast majority of drugs of abuse are agents that act on the central nervous system to produce profound effects on mood, feeling, and behavior.

drug addiction   The compulsive use of a drug, despite the negative consequences with respect to family and friends, job, and health.   The user loses complete control over the drug-taking behavior, and may become preoccupied with drug-taking and drug procurement.   Craving is a key feature of addiction when the drug is not available.

drug antagonism   Any interaction between two drugs in which the conjoint effect of the two agents is less than the sum of the effects of the drugs acting separately:

Pharmacologic antagonism is observed when a drug – the antagonist – reduces the effect of another drug – the agonist – by preventing the latter from combining with its receptor. Pharmacologic antagonism is competitive when the antagonist combines reversibly with the same binding sites as the agonist and can be displaced from these sites by an excess of the agonist. Pharmacologic antagonism is noncompetitive when the effects of the antagonist cannot be overcome by increasing concentration of the agonist.

Physiologic or functional antagonism is observed when two agonists, acting at different sites, counterbalance each other by producing opposite effects on the same physiologic function.

Biochemical antagonism is observed whenever one drug indirectly decreases the amount of a second drug that would otherwise be available to its site of action in the absence of the first drug (the antagonist). Biochemical antagonism is the converse of synergism (q.v.).

Chemical antagonism is simply the reaction between an agonist and an antagonist to form an inactive product. The agonist is inactivated in direct proportion to the extent of chemical interaction with the antagonist.

drug dependence   A condition in which the user requires the presence of the drug to function normally.   *Physical dependence* is an altered or adaptive physiologic state produced in an individual by the repeated administration of a drug. That physical dependence has been induced during the prolonged use of a drug is revealed only when the drug is abruptly discontinued or when its actions are diminished by the administration of a specific antagonist.   Physical dependence can occur in the absence of addiction (e.g. β-adrenergic agonists used for asthma).

drug discovery target   A substance or process identified or suspected of playing a role in causing a disease or sustaining its harmful effects. Targets include substances such as receptors and enzymes, and processes such as gene expression and signal transduction (q.v.).

drug misuse   The occasional nonmedical use (as opposed to the persistent non-medical use in drug abuse) or the inappropriate medical use of drugs for purposes or conditions for which they are unsuited, or their appropriate use in improper dosage.

drug resistance   A state of decreased response, or complete lack of response, to drugs that ordinarily inhibit cell growth or cause cell death. Drug resistance is therefore a phenomenon which, by definition, may be associated only with drugs used to eliminate (1) an uneconomic species, such as insects, bacteria or other parasites, or (2) rapidly growing cells, such as cancer cells in higher organisms.

drug tolerance   A condition of decreased responsiveness that is acquired after prior or repeated exposure to a given drug or one closely allied in pharmacologic activity. Tolerance is characterized by the necessity of increasing the size of successive doses in order to produce effects equal in magnitude or duration to those achieved initially. Alternatively, it is an inability of the subsequent administration of the same dose of a drug to be as effective as was the preceding dose.

The term *tachyphylaxis* is used to describe the acute development of tolerance to the rapid, repeated administration of a drug.

economic species   The desirable species, e.g. humans and domestic animals (cf. uneconomic species).

effector   Organ or cell that responds in a characteristic manner to a stimulus.

efferent nerve   *See* motor nerve.

elimination half-life   The time to reduce the amount of drug in the body or its plasma concentration by 50%. Dependent upon both the total plasma clearance and the volume of distribution of a drug.

emetic   A substance that induces vomiting.

emollients   Fats or oils used for their local, protective or softening action on the skin, e.g. olive oil, white petrolatum, lanolin.

enantiomers   Molecular structures that have the same chemical constituents and are related to each other as an object and its nonsuperimposable mirror image (cf. racemic mixture).

endocrine   Denoting an organ or structure whose function is to secrete into the blood or lymph a substance (hormone) that has a specific effect on another organ or part.

enteral   Pertains to administration of drugs into any part of the gastrointestinal tract, i.e. oral administration (swallowing of the drug), sublingual administration (under the tongue) and rectal administration (cf. parenteral).

enzyme   A protein catalyst, a product of living cells, which accelerates biochemical reactions but remains apparently unchanged by the process.

enzyme induction   The increase in synthesis and in activity of microsomal enzymes by prior administration of a variety of foreign agents to the intact animal.

equivalent   A term used in chemistry to connote equal combining power. The equivalent weight of an element is its atomic weight divided by its valence (q.v.) *in the particular reaction under consideration.* A gram-equivalent weight is the equivalent weight of an element (or formula weight of a radical) divided by its valence. A solution containing one gram-equivalent of a particular constituent of the solute in a liter of solution is called a normal solution.

excipient   An inert substance used to give a pharmaceutical preparation a suitable form or consistency.

exocrine   Denoting a gland that discharges its secretion through a duct opening on an internal or external surface of the body, e.g. lacrimal gland, salivary gland.

FDA Modernization Act of 1997   Provisions in this act cover pediatric market exclusivity (sponsors of new or marketed drugs with potential benefits for the pediatric population to receive market exclusivity); fast track designation requests; dissemination of off-label information and allowing companies to provide economic data to health care purchasers.

first-pass effect   After oral administration of a drug its biotransformation within the gastrointestinal tract or liver prior to its distribution into the systemic circulation.

first-order kinetics   Describes a   reaction with a velocity that is proportional to the concentration of a single substance. In an enzyme reaction there are two reactants: the substrate and the enzyme. However, in the intact organism it is the enzyme concentration that influences the kinetics of the reaction. Enzyme systems display first-order kinetics at concentrations of substrate that do not saturate the binding sites of the enzyme. Similarly, drug receptor interactions display first-order kinetics at drug concentrations which do not lead to 100% receptor occupancy. The rates of migration of substances across biologic barriers also display first-order kinetics when the mechanism of translocation is passive diffusion or when the mechanism is facilitated diffusion or active transport and the quantity of solute to be transferred does not saturate the carrier (cf. zero-order kinetics).

galenical   A medicinal prepared by extracting one or more active constituents of a plant.

genomics   The search for normal genes and gene variants, or alleles, related to disease; the term includes differential gene expression, differential protein expression and protein function and pathway analysis.

germicide   *See* bactericide.

hapten   A simple chemical capable of binding rather firmly with a protein conjugate to form a product that has antigenic properties (cf. antigen, antibodies, allergic response).

homeostasis   The maintenance of the constancy of the body's optimal internal environment with respect to the composition, pH and osmotic pressure of the body fluids.

hormone   (Gk hormaein, 'to stimulate') A specific chemical substance secreted by cells in one part of a living organism that in various ways influences the growth, development or behavior of other cells remote from the source of the hormone.

hydrogen bond   The chemical bond formed between a strongly electronegative atom and a hydrogen atom which is already bound by an ionic or covalent bond to another strongly electronegative atom such as oxygen, fluorine or nitrogen. The strength of the hydrogen bond is less than that of a true ionic bond.

hydrolysis   A chemical reaction in which a compound is cleaved by the addition of a molecule of water.

hydrostatic pressure   The pressure (force per unit area) exerted by water or an aqueous system normal to the surface on which it acts. In a moving fluid, the static pressure is measured at a right angle to the direction of flow.

hyperosmotic   *See* osmotic effect.

hypertonic   *See* isotonic.

hypnotic   A drug that produces a state clinically identical with sleep by means of an action on the central nervous system (cf. sedative, anesthetic drug).

hyposmotic   *See* osmotic effect.

hypotonic   *See* isotonic.

idiosyncratic response   A genetically determined abnormal response to a drug. The response may take the form of extreme sensitivity to low doses or extreme insensitivity to high doses of a drug the administration of which ordinarily produces qualitatively similar effects only at much higher or much lower doses, respectively. The drug reactions may also be qualitatively different from the usual effects observed in the majority of subjects. The discontinuity of a frequency-response curve is characteristic of the idiosyncratic response and distinguishes this type of reactivity from the normal resistance to high doses of a drug or sensitivity to low doses (cf. sensitivity).

interstitium   Structures such as cells and fibers lying between other structures and forming a supporting framework of tissue that binds together the organs that form the animal.

ionic bond   The chemical bond formed between two atoms by the outright transfer of one or more electrons from one atom to the other. The strength of this bond depends on the distance between the two ions and diminishes as the square of the distance between them.

isotonic   Pertaining to solutions that have the same osmotic pressure (are isosmotic) as the reference standards and that do not cause any volume change in cells. Solutions that induce a net loss of water from the cells are *hypertonic*; conversely, solutions that cause cells to take up water are *hypotonic* with respect to the cell contents.

law of mass action   When a chemical reaction reaches equilibrium at a constant temperature, the product of the active masses on one side of the chemical equation divided by the product of the active masses on the other side of the equation is a constant, regardless of the amount of each substance present at the beginning of the action. Thus for the ionization of an acid:

$$HA \leftrightharpoons [H^+] + [A^-]$$

$$\frac{[H^+] \times [A^-]}{[HA]} = \text{a constant}$$

ligand   An organic molecule that donates the necessary electrons to form coordinate covalent bonds with metallic ions. The term is also used to indicate any ion or molecule that reacts to form a complex with another molecule, frequently a macromolecule.

lipid   A broad term used to include all the ether-soluble, water-insoluble substances obtained from plant and animal sources. According to W.R. Bloor's definition: (1) Simple lipids are esters of fatty acids and various alcohols, classified as (a) fats and oils when they are esters of glycerol, a three-carbon, straight-chain alcohol with three hydroxyl groups, and (b) waxes when they are esters of alcohols other than glycerol. (2) Compound lipids are esters of fatty acids and alcohols containing additional groups: (a) phospholipids, containing a phosphoric acid group; (b) glycolipids, containing a carbohydrate and a nitrogen-containing compound but no phosphoric acid group; and (c) others, such as sulfolipids. (3) Derived lipids are compounds derived from the preceding groups and having the general properties of the lipids; the derived compounds include fatty acids, glycerol, sterols and long-chain alcohols.

margin of safety   The degree of separation between the doses of a drug producing a desirable or therapeutic effect and the doses at which undesirable or adverse effects are elicited; expressed as a therapeutic index (q.v.).

materia medica   The material or substances used in the composition of remedies for the treatment of disease. Also, the branch of medical science that deals with the sources, nature, properties and preparations of drugs.

maximum efficacy   The maximum intensity of a specific effect that can be produced by a given drug, regardless of how large a dose is administered. The maximum effect produced by a given drug may be less than the maximum response of which the reacting tissue is capable or less than the maximum effect that can be produced by another drug. Also referred to as the ceiling effect.

median effective dose   The smallest dose required to produce a stated effect in 50% of the population, usually designated by the abbreviation ED_{50}. When death is the response, the ED_{50} is termed the *median lethal dose,* or LD_{50}. Depending on the stated response, the median effective dose can also be designated AD_{50}, the median analgesic dose; CD_{50} the median convulsive dose, etc.

mEq   The abbreviation for milliequivalent, one thousandth of a gramequivalent weight (cf. equivalent).

mM   The abbreviation for millimolar, one thousandth of a mole in one liter of solution (q.v.).

mixed agonist/antagonist   A drug that has agonist properties at one subtype of a receptor and antagonist properties at another subtype of the same receptor – true for several opioid analgesics.

molarity   Pertaining to molecules, or to moles per unit volume; thus a molar solution is one containing one gram-molecular weight of solute per liter of solution.

mole   One gram-molecule of any substance, i.e. the expression in grams of the molecular weight of a substance; a gram-molecular weight (cf. molarity).

motor nerve or neuron   Pertains to nerves which carry impulses from the central nervous system to the muscles, glands or other tissues and organs (cf. sensory nerve or neuron).

narcotic   In medicine, the term *narcotic* applies only to drugs having both an analgesic and a sedative action. In legal parlance, the term includes drugs with morphine-like activity as well as marihuana and cocaine. The term *narcotic analgesic,* was once used interchangeably with *opiate* or *opioid* (q.v.); today the term opioid is preferred.

narcotic analgesic   *See* opioid.

neuro-effector junction   A junction between a neuron and an effector organ or cell such as a smooth muscle of the pupil of the eye, or a gland cell (cf. synapse).

neuromuscular junction   The junction between a somatic motor neuron and a skeletal muscle fiber; acetylcholine receptors are concentrated on the postsynaptic side of the junction.

noncompetitive antagonism   *See* drug antagonism.

nonpolar   A nonpolar compound is one in which the centers of positive and negative charge almost coincide, so that no permanent dipole moments are produced. Nonpolar compounds do not ionize or conduct electricity.

normal equivalent deviation (NED)   A multiple (1, 2, 3, etc.) of the standard deviation. The quantal log dose-response curve may be transformed to a straight line when the data are replotted on coordinates in which the ordinate is expressed as normal equivalent deviation. Each percentage responding is converted to an NED, i.e. to the corresponding multiple of the standard deviation:

NED	Percentage response	Probit
3	0.1	2
−2	2.3	3
−1	16	4
0	50	5
+1	84	6
+2	97.7	7
+3	99.9	8

A further refinement of the use of the NED as an expression of the percentage response in quantal dose-effect curves involves the elimination of the positive and negative signs by the expedient of adding 5 to each NED value. This new unit is called a *probit* (from a contraction of the term *probability unit).*

nucleic acids   A group of complex compounds of high molecular weight that occur in all plant and animal cells and in viruses. Nucleic acids are made up of long chains of nucleotides that are composed of four characteristic groups: (1) heterocyclic bases of the purine type; (2) heterocyclic bases of the pyrimidine type; (3) a carbohydrate, being either a ribose (five-carbon sugar) or a deoxyribose (ribose with one oxygen atom removed); and (4) phosphoric acid. Nucleic acids containing ribose are known as ribonucleic acids (RNA); the principal bases in RNA are the purines, adenine and guanine, and the pyrimidines, cytosine and uracil. Nucleic acids containing deoxyribose are called deoxyribonucleic acids (DNA); the principal purine bases are adenine and guanine and the pyrimidines are cytosine and thymine. The nucleic acids are intimately involved in the mechanisms of self-duplication that are basic to life and by which hereditary characteristics are transmitted from cell to cell.

opioid   A drug, either natural or synthetic, that has the same pharmacologic properties as opiates, obtained from the opium poppy (i.e. morphine). It has both an analgesic and a sedative action; the term essentially embraces only those drugs that have morphine-like pharmacologic activity.

osmotic effect   The effect produced on the net movement of water when two solutions of unequal concentration are separated by a semipermeable membrane that permits freer passage of water than of the dissolved substances. The direction of movement of water will be from the solution in which the water molecules are *more concentrated* (the more *dilute* solution, i.e. the solution containing fewer molecules of solute) to the solution in which the water molecules are *less concentrated* (the more *concentrated* solution, i.e. the solution containing more molecules of solute). The measure of the tendency of solvent to pass from the more dilute solution to the more concentrated solution is the *osmotic pressure;* osmotic pressure is the force or pressure required to prevent osmotic flow of water into a given solution.

Any two solutions that have the same osmotic pressure are *isosmotic.* Solutions that have a greater osmotic pressure than a given reference solution are *hyperosmotic;* solutions that have a smaller osmotic pressure than a given reference solution are *hyposmotic* (cf. isotonic).

oxidation   A chemical reaction in which oxygen is added to a compound or, by extension, the proportion of oxygen in a compound is increased by the removal of other groups (cf. reduction).

parenteral   Pertains to administration of drugs into any part of the body other than the gastrointestinal tract (cf. enteral), e.g. subcutaneous, intramuscular or intravenous injection; topical application to the skin or mucous membranes, inhalation through the lungs.

partition coefficient   The measure of the tendency of a solute to distribute itself between two phases, expressed as the ratio of the solute's concentration in one phase to its concentration in the second phase. An example is the lipid/water partition coefficient, the ratio of a solute's concentration in a lipid phase (oily-solvent) to its concentration in water after the system has come to equilibrium.

peptide   Any member of a class of compounds of low molecular weight that yield two or more amino acids on hydrolysis. Formed by the loss of water from the NH_2 and COOH groups of adjacent amino acids. Peptides form the constituent parts of proteins.

pH   (Fr. puissance d'hydrogen, 'power of hydrogen'). A chemical symbol used to express acidity and alkalinity in terms of the concentration of hydrogen ion. The pH equals the negative logarithm of the H^+ concentration in gram-atoms per liter, i.e. the logarithm of the reciprocal of the H^+ concentration. The concentration of H^+ in pure water at 25°C is taken as the point of neutrality, or pH = 7;   the concentration of H^+ is 10^{-7} M and the concentration of hydroxyl ion (OH^-) is also 10^{-7} M.   pH values may range from 0 to 14, numbers less than 7 indicating acidity and numbers greater than 7, alkalinity.

pharmaceutical alternatives   Drug products that contain the identical therapeutic moiety, or its precursor, but not necessarily in the same amount or dosage form or as the same salt or ester (as defined by FDA regulations).

pharmaceutical chemistry   The synthesis of new drugs either as a modification of an older or natural drug or as an entirely new chemical entity.

pharmaceutical equivalents   Drug products that contain identical amounts of the identical active drug ingredient, i.e. the same salt or ester of the same therapeutic moiety in identical dosage forms, but not necessarily containing the same inactive ingredients.

pharmacodynamics   The study of the actions and effects of chemicals at all levels of organization of living material and of the handling of chemicals by the organism.

General pharmacodynamics includes the fundamental principles or properties involved in the action of all drugs.

Special pharmacodynamics includes the additional factors necessary to understand the action of individual drugs or drugs of similar action.

pharmacogenetics   The scientific study of genetic factors that account for individual differences in the response to drugs.

pharmacogenomics   The study of the variability of response of patients to drugs as a result of genetic variability in pharmacodynamics.

pharmacognosy   The identification of the botanical source of drugs.

pharmacokinetics   The branch of pharmacology that deals with the study of the factors that influence the magnitude of drug effect by determining the concentration of drug at its various sites of action as a function of time after drug administration.

pharmacologic antagonism   *See* drug antagonism.

pharmacy   The preparing, compounding, and dispensing of chemical agents for therapeutic use.

phospholipids   Compound lipids that are esters of fatty acids and alcohols containing a phosphoric acid group (cf. lipid).

physiologic antagonism   *See* drug antagonism.

placebo   An inert substance, such as the sugar lactose, which is used as a sham drug. The placebo has no inherent pharmacologic activity but may produce a biologic response by virtue of the factor of suggestion attendant upon its administration.

poison A chemical not intended for introduction into humans, but is potentially capable of producing biologic effects upon incidental, accidental, or (maliciously) intentional exposure.

polar A polar compound is, in general, a compound that exhibits polarity, or local differences in electric properties, and has a dipole moment associated with one or more of its interatomic valence bonds. Polar compounds associate readily in most cases. In the most general use of the term, polar compounds include all electrolytes, most inorganic substances, and many organic ones.

polymer A compound formed by two or more molecules of a simpler compound, the relative amount of each element remaining the same. The meaning of this term has also been extended to denote any one of a number of compounds composed of the same elements or radicals and related in such a way that the molecular formulas are in the relation of whole-number multiples of each other.

population A collection of items defined by a common characteristic. In pharmacologic context, an example would be all individuals responding to the administration of atropine by an increase in the diameter of the pupil of the eye.

potency A comparative expression of drug activity measured in terms of the dose required to produce a particular effect of given intensity relative to a given or implied standard of reference. Potency, like affinity, varies inversely with the magnitude of the dose required to produce this effect. If two drugs are not both capable of producing an effect of equal magnitude, they cannot be compared with respect to potency; for example, the analgesic potency of aspirin cannot be compared with that of codeine, since no dose of aspirin can relieve pain of certain intensities which are effectively relieved by codeine (cf. ceiling effect).

prodrug A compound that is metabolized to the pharmacologically active agent after administration.

proteins Highly complex molecules that are universally present in all living matter. All proteins are built from the same subunits, the amino acids, which are joined together by primary bonds to form long chains. The bond, called a peptide bond, —CONH— is formed between the carboxylic acid group, —COOH, of one amino acid and the amino group, —NH_2, of another amino acid, with the splitting out of water. A single protein molecule may consist of a chain of 100 or more subunits made up of 20 different kinds of amino acids recurring many times along the length of the chain. The sequence in which the amino acids occur along the chain is characteristic for each protein. Some proteins, called conjugated proteins, contain other chemical groups in addition to amino acids. Nucleoproteins consist of proteins combined with nucleic acids; lipoproteins consist of proteins combined with lipids.

proteolipid A combination of a protein or peptide with a lipid, having the solubility characteristics of lipids.

proteomics   The study of protein production, protein function and pathways. Proteomics is considered a subset of genomics (q.v.).

racemic mixture   A 50:50 mixture of enantiomers (q.v.).

receptor   A macromolecular tissue constituent of functional significance at the site of drug action and to which endogenous substances and drugs bind.

receptor subtypes   Receptors in the same protein family with similar but not identical structures. Subtypes may respond identically to an endogenous agonist, but differ in their response to drugs.

reduction   A chemical reaction in which oxygen is removed from a compound or in which the alteration leads to a decrease in the proportion of oxygen in a compound (cf. oxidation).

renal plasma clearance   The volume of plasma needed to supply the amount of a specific substance excreted in the urine in 1 minute. The clearance of a substance that is completely filterable and neither reabsorbed nor secreted by the renal tubular cells measures the glomerular filtration rate (about 120 ml/min/70 kg). A substance that is so rapidly secreted by the renal tubular cells that it is almost completely cleared in one passage through the kidney can be used to measure the total amount of plasma flowing through the kidney (about 640 ml/min/kg).

sedative   An agent that can induce a state of drowsiness at a dose that does not produce sleep.

selectivity   The capacity of a drug to produce one particular effect in preference to other effects – to act in lower doses at one site than those required to produce effects at other sites. Selectivity can be measured by the same ratios used to assess drug safety. Selectivity should not be confused with potency. Potency is a comparative measure of the capacity of *several* drugs to produce an effect of equal intensity, whereas selectivity is a comparative measure of the propensity of a single drug to produce several effects (cf. specificity, certain safety factor, standard safety margin, therapeutic index).

sensitivity   The ability of a member of a population, relative to the abilities of other members of the same population, to respond in a qualitatively normal fashion to a particular dose of a drug. Sensitivity may be measured or described in terms of the normal distribution curve or the dose-effect curve in which a wide range of doses may separate the most sensitive from the least sensitive individuals. The individuals lying to the left of the median are the most sensitive; those to the right, the least sensitive. Any individual responding with a given preselected response to a dose of a drug is said to be sensitive to the drug. Individuals responding at the extremes of a normal distribution curve should not be confused with individuals showing an idiosyncratic response. The characteristic feature in the idiosyncratic response to low or high doses is a discontinuity from the normal distribution of dose sensitivities.

sensory nerve or neuron   Pertains to nerves that conduct impulses to the central nervous system from the sense organs (e.g. eye or ear), or from receptors in tissues that are adapted to respond to different stimuli (cf. motor nerve or neuron).

side-effect Any effect other than that for which a given drug is administered. The intensity of the side-effect is a function of the dose administered. A particular effect of a drug may be a side-effect under certain circumstances or the desired therapeutic effect under others; e.g. sedation and dry mouth are side-effects of scopolamine when the drug is being used to prevent motion sickness. When scopolamine is used during surgery, sedation and reduced salivation are the therapeutic effects.

signal transduction The chain of events that links the binding of the substance to its receptor and the ultimate physiological or biochemical response. The binding to the receptor is the 'signal' and this is changed or 'transduced' into the series of other intracellular events that lead to the final response.

smooth muscle The effector organ of much of the autonomic nervous system. *Multi-unit* smooth muscle such as that of the iris of the eye and probably vascular smooth muscle has innervation similar to that of skeletal muscle; the nerve supply is excitatory and the organ displays little or no spontaneous or rhythmic activity. *Visceral* smooth muscle contracts spontaneously and rhythmically, but this activity can be modified by autonomic nerves that either inhibit or enhance the intrinsic activity.

specificity The capacity of a drug to manifest its effects by a single mechanism of action. A drug is said to have specificity, even though it may produce a multiplicity of effects, if all the effects produced are due to a single mechanism of action. Scopolamine, for example, has great specificity of action since it antagonizes only the actions of acetylcholine (or other drugs closely resembling acetylcholine) at the acetylcholine receptor. The widespread distribution of the acetylcholine receptor accounts for the multiplicity of effects (or non-selectivity) of the action of scopolamine (cf. selectivity).

standard deviation A measure of variability about the mean value of a distribution. The standard deviation has no verbal definition and is defined only by its formula:

$$\text{SD, or } s = \sqrt{\frac{\Sigma(x-\bar{x})^2}{n}}$$

where
x = the arithmetic average
$(x-\bar{x})$ = the deviation, the difference between an individual number and the average
$\Sigma(x-\bar{x})^2$ = the sum of all the deviations squared
n = the number of observations

standard safety margin A number that is an assessment of the relative safety of a drug or of its selectivity of action. The standard safety margin is the percentage by which the dose effective in virtually all of a population (ED_{99}) has to be increased to produce a lethal effect in a minimum number of the population (the LD_1). Thus the standard safety margin is equal to:

$$\frac{(LD_1 - ED_{99})}{ED_{99}} \times 100$$

(cf. certain safety factor, therapeutic index, selectivity.)

stereoisomers   Two substances of the same composition and constitution that differ only in the relative spatial position of their constituent atoms and/or groups. The isomerism may be due to the relative spatial position of groups attached to atoms joined by a double bond (geometric isomerism), or it may be due to the presence of one or more asymmetric atoms, i.e. a quadrivalent atom of carbon, silicon, etc., to which four different atoms or radicals are attached, therefore possessing spatial geometric forms that cannot be superimposed, but are in fact mirror images.

summation   The algebraic sum of the individual effects of two drugs acting simultaneously that elicit the same overt response, regardless of the mechanism of action of each of the drugs, e.g. the combined effect of aspirin and codeine in relieving pain, in which the two drugs act by different mechanisms; or the combined effect of aspirin and acetaminophen in relieving pain, in which case the two drugs apparently act on the same receptors (cf. additive effect, synergism).

sympathomimetic   An adjective describing (1) an effect that resembles the response to stimulation of adrenergic nerves, or (2) an agent whose effects, in general, are similar to those elicited by adrenergic stimulation.

synapse   The junction between two neurons or between a neuron and muscle (cf. neuro-effector junction, neuromuscular junction).

syndrome   The complete picture of a disease, including all the signs and symptoms.

synergism   The situation in which the combined effect of two drugs acting simultaneously is greater than the algebraic sum of the individual effects of these drugs. The term is usually reserved for those cases in which two drugs act at different sites and one drug, the synergist, increases the effect of the second drug by altering its biotransformation, distribution or excretion. An example would be the exaggerated response to tyramine in individuals being treated with monoamine oxidase inhibitors (cf. summation, additive effect).

tachycardia   Excessive rapidity in the action of the heart; the term is usually applied to a heart rate above 100 beats per minute.

tachyphylaxis   *See* drug tolerance.

therapeutic index   A number that is an assessment of the relative safety of a drug or of its selectivity of action. A therapeutic index is ordinarily computed from the quantal dose-effect curves describing data obtained in experiments with animals. The term usually refers to the ratio LD_{50}/ED_{50} the ratio of the dose required to produce a lethal effect in 50% of the population to the dose required to produce the desired therapeutic effect in 50% of the population. The larger the ratio, the greater the relative safety of the drug. However, the LD_{50}/ED_{50} ratio is not sufficient for a true assessment of drug safety, since median doses tell nothing about the slopes of the dose-response curves being compared or the degree of overlap of the curves (cf. certain safety factor, standard safety margin, selectivity).

threshold dose The dose of a drug just sufficient to produce any preselected intensity of effect. If the preselected effect is the first detectable effect, the threshold dose is the smallest dose required to produce a detectable effect. The dose required to produce a 50% decrease in heart rate may be considered a threshold dose if the preselected effect is a 50% decrease in heart rate.

tinctures Alcoholic or hydroalcoholic solutions of the active principles of drugs, e.g. paregoric.

total plasma clearance The volume of plasma cleared of a drug by all routes and mechanisms per unit time. Includes renal clearance, clearance by biotransformation, and, for volatile substances and gases, clearance by exhalation.

toxic effect An effect of a drug on an organism that is deleterious to the well-being or life of the organism. A toxic effect may be a side-effect or undesired effect under some circumstances but under other circumstances may be the desired effect. A toxic effect is a side-effect when a drug is being used as a therapeutic agent in the prevention, treatment or diagnosis of disease. A toxic effect is the desired effect, and not a side-effect, when the drug is being used to eradicate microorganisms, pests or malignant cells and does so without harm to the user.

Toxic effects may be classified on the basis of rate of onset, duration of symptoms and rate of intake of the chemical. Acute toxicity is the type that occurs when absorption is rapid and when exposure is sudden and severe. Subacute toxicity results from frequent, repeated exposure over a period of several hours or days to a dose of drug that is insufficient to produce toxic effects when given as a single dose. Chronic toxicity is the type that usually occurs from repeated exposure over a long period to a substance which has a tendency to accumulate in the body.

transmission The passage of an impulse across a junction; the process by which a nerve ending activates the next structure in the pathway (cf. conduction).

uneconomic species Undesirable species; organisms that threaten human economic security, comfort or health, e.g. an insect or pathogenic bacterium (cf. economic species).

uricosuric agent A drug that increases the excretion of uric acid in the urine.

valence The property of an atom or radical to combine with other atoms or radicals in definite proportions. The valence of an atom or radical is designated by a number representing the proportion in which a given atom or radical combines. The standard of reference is hydrogen, which is assigned a valence of 1; and the valence of any given atom or radical is then the number of hydrogen atoms, or their equivalent, with which the given atom or radical combines. Many elements have more than one valence, and their compounds are classified and designated accordingly. The number of electrons in the outer shell of an atom determines the valence or valences of the atom. By gaining, losing or sharing these outer-shell electrons, atoms combine to form molecules.

Van der Waals forces   Weak attractive forces between any two neutral atoms or atomic groupings. The force of attraction is inversely proportional to the seventh power of the distance between the atoms.

viscera (pleural viscus)   The large interior organs in the three great cavities of the body (abdomen, pelvis, thorax), especially in the abdomen.

volume of distribution or **apparent volume of distribution**   The volume of body fluid in which a drug appears to be dissolved. In a normal, lean, 70-kg male, the whole body water comprises about 40 liters. The extracellular water is about one-third of the total, or about 12 liters, 3 liters of which is the volume of circulating plasma-water.

zero-order kinetics   The kinetics characteristic of a reaction that proceeds at a constant rate independent of the concentrations of reactants. Enzyme reactions display zero-order kinetics at levels of substrate that saturate the binding sites of the enzyme. In analogous fashion, drug-receptor interactions become zero order when the concentration of drug at the receptor produces complete receptor occupancy, and facilitated diffusion or active transport becomes zero order when the concentration of solute saturates the carrier mechanism (cf. first-order kinetics).

Appendixes

Appendix 1
Drugs for Treating
Gastrointestinal Tract Disorders

I. **Agents Used to Treat Peptic Ulcer**
   A. **General Considerations.** Peptic ulcer, occurring as lesions of either the gastric or duodenal mucosa, is the most common gastrointestinal disease and affects about 5–10% of the population. The major causes of peptic ulcers are now believed to be infection with *Helicobacter pylori* or use of substances such as nonsteroidal anti-inflammatory drugs (NSAIDs). Most patients with duodenal ulcer disease also show hypersecretion of gastric acid. Although the pathogenic role of gastric acid and pepsin in generating a lesion has not been clearly established, there is no doubt that both acid and pepsin prevent healing of the lesion and produce pain. Therefore, one goal of peptic ulcer therapy is to control gastric acidity and thereby reduce pepsin activity. The therapeutic objective is to raise gastric pH to about 3.5 from its normal range of 1–2 in order to relieve pain (the pain of peptic ulcer is reasonably well established to be the result of the action of the acid on the lesion). At pH 3.5, the decrease in the activity of pepsin may also contribute to the decreased corrosive action of gastric juice on the lesion.

   Gastric acidity may be reduced by either neutralization of the acid or inhibition of its secretion. Neutralization of the acid can be accomplished through the use of antacids (see below). The use of antacids provides relief from pain, but healing is promoted only if there is continuous neutralization of the gastric contents. This latter is difficult to achieve, particularly in view of the fact that neutralization of gastric contents, in itself, stimulates acid secretion. Antacids are most useful in the treatment of peptic ulcer when they are combined with the use of drugs that inhibit the physiologic stimuli acetylcholine, histamine and gastrin, or the enzyme that is the common mediator of acid secretion (cf. p. 479).

   A radical change in the treatment of peptic ulcer took place when *H. pylori,* a Gram-negative bacillus, was found to be present in mucus in 90% of duodenal ulcer patients and in 70% of gastric ulcer patients.

Although the role of the bacillus in the etiology of peptic ulcer is not understood, its eradication by antibiotics reduces the incidence of recurrence by about 90%. Treatment of peptic ulcer, therefore, now includes the use of antibiotics, in addition to agents that inhibit acid secretion, for those cases where *H. pylori* is known to be involved.

B. **Antimuscarinic Agents.** Whereas the older conventional antimuscarinic agents such as atropine show no real selectivity of action in reducing gastric acid secretion, agents have now been developed that act selectively at some muscarinic receptors and not at others. Pirenzepine is a muscarinic antagonist that selectively inhibits gastric acid secretion without appreciably affecting heart rate, salivary secretion or gastrointestinal smooth muscle. The discovery of pirenzepine as a selective antimuscarinic agent had far-reaching effects: it encouraged rethinking the concept of selectivity of drug action at muscarinic receptors and stimulated the search for additional selective muscarinic antagonists and agonists. As a consequence, a number of different muscarinic receptor subtypes have been identified and new drugs developed that act selectively at different muscarinic sites.

C. **Antagonists of Histamine; H_2 Antagonists**

1. **General Considerations.** It had long been recognized that histamine is a potent stimulus of gastric acid secretion. For a long time, however, there were no drugs that could block the effects of histamine on gastric secretion, and, therefore, conclusive evidence for the physiologic role of histamine in acid secretion was lacking. The discovery of agents capable of inhibiting the actions of histamine that are resistant to block by the original antihistaminic agents, the H_1 blockers (e.g. diphenhydramine and chlorpheniramine), provided incontrovertible evidence that endogenous histamine played a significant role in gastric secretion. These agents, called H_2-receptor blocking drugs, or simply H_2 blockers, also signaled a new and effective approach to the therapy of gastric hypersecretory states, particularly those involving peptic ulceration.

2. **Agents**
   a. Cimetidine (TAGAMET).
   b. Ranitidine (ZANTAC).
   c. Famotidine (PEPCID).
   d. Nizatidine (AXID).

3. **Effects**
   a. Reversible and potent inhibition of gastric secretion stimulated by not only histamine but also insulin and gastrin; also partial inhibition of acetylcholine-stimulated secretion.
   b. Relief of pain and promotion of healing of duodenal ulcers.
   c. Well-tolerated, and side-effects infrequent; sometimes cause confusion in elderly patients. The low incidence of side-effects is due, in part, to the limited distribution of H_2 receptors in the body.

      d. Cimetidine inhibits certain CYP450 enzymes and, therefore, can lead to adverse effects of concomitantly administered drugs that are biotransformed by these enzymes.

D. Proton-Pump Inhibitors

1. **General Considerations.** The H_2 blockers effectively inhibit the basal and histamine-induced acid secretion, but the strongest suppression of hydrochloric acid is achieved by the blockade of the final, common process in acid production. This kind of blockade is achieved by agents that inhibit H^+/K^+ ATPase (proton pump), a membrane pump that exchanges hydrogen ions for potassium ions. Thus the proton-pump inhibitors block the formation of acid, be it basal or stimulated by histamine, acetylcholine or gastrin.

2. **Agents:**
    a. Omeprazole (PRILOSEC).
    b. Esomeprazole (NEXIUM).

3. **Effects.** Proton pump inhibitors are prodrugs; the active metabolite of each drug combines irreversibly with the proton-pump. Regeneration of the ATPase is only possible by new synthesis. These drugs produce an especially rapid healing of peptic ulcers and are indicated for therapy in patients with acute gastric and duodenal ulcers or esophageal reflux disorders. Unwanted side-effects are not common but omeprazole can inhibit some CYP450 enzymes.

E. Gastric Antacids

1. **Definition.** Basic chemical substances that on ingestion react *locally* with the hydrochloric acid of the gastric contents to neutralize the acidity and raise the pH.

2. **General Considerations**
    a. **Effects**
        (1) Increase in gastric pH. The activity of an antacid is dependent upon the total acid-combining capacity of the compound and the length of time it remains in the stomach. The commonly used antacids do not make the gastric contents alkaline enough to damage gastrointestinal tissue.
        (2) Reduction of the protein-digestive action of pepsin at pH above 5. The reduction in pepsin activity is sufficient to decrease the corrosive action of gastric juice on an ulcerative lesion, but not to suppress completely the digestion of food proteins. Peptic activity is maximal at pH 2; at pH 7–8, pepsin becomes completely inactive.
        (3) Increase in rate of stomach emptying (except with aluminum hydroxide). The higher the pH is raised, the more rapidly the stomach empties. Antacids are expelled into the intestine with the rest of the stomach contents.
        (4) Mucosal-protecting actions. There is evidence to indicate that in low doses (lower than those that produce significant

changes in pH) antacids may: (1) enhance the synthesis of prostaglandin, a deficiency of which can contribute to ulcer formation, and (2) reduce the colonization of *Helicobacter pylori*, a strain of bacteria thought to influence ulcer pathogenesis.

b. Classification

(1) High bioavailability. Antacids that form compounds that are soluble in gastric and intestinal secretions. The products formed are readily absorbed.

(2) Low bioavailability. Agents that interact with HCl to form relatively insoluble compounds. The reaction products are not absorbed to any degree and therefore have little, if any, systemic effect.

c. Uses

(1) Therapeutic. In combination with inhibitors of acid secretion for the treatment of peptic ulcer and reflux esophagitis.

(2) Popular. For the treatment of indigestion (upset stomach; sour stomach; heartburn; acid indigestion). Antacids are one of the groups of widely advertised nostrums used most extensively, and sometimes inappropriately, by the general public.

d. High Bioavailability Antacids

(1) Agents

(a) Sodium bicarbonate.

(b) Sodium citrate. Common constituent of many proprietary preparations that 'fizz'. The preparations that contain sodium bicarbonate and citric acid react in solution to form sodium citrate and release carbon dioxide.

(2) Effects

(a) May increase gastric pH to 7 or greater and provoke rapid gastric emptying.

(b) Increases the concentration of sodium bicarbonate in blood and may produce systemic alkalosis and electrolyte disturbances that burden the kidney with electrolyte readjustments. Distortions in acid-base balance are usually clinically insignificant in persons with normal kidney function.

(c) Release of carbon dioxide from carbonate-containing antacids causes belching.

e. Low Bioavailability Antacids

(1) Agents

(a) Aluminum-containing antacids: aluminum hydroxide gel (AMPHOJEL), aluminum phosphate gel (PHOSPHALJEL).

(b) Magnesium-containing antacids: magnesium hydroxide (milk of magnesia).

        (c)   Calcium compounds: calcium carbonate (TUMS).

        (d)   Aluminum hydroxide and magnesium hydroxide. Most common combination; available as suspensions or tablets (MAALOX; GELUSIL; MYLANTA).

            Most preparations on the market are combinations of different chemicals in order to yield both fast and slow neutralization of hydrochloric acid and provide even and sustained action; or to offset the effect of one compound by that of another (e.g. constipation versus laxation).

    (2) Effects

        (a)   Gastrointestinal: some agents cause constipation (aluminum-containing antacids); some cause diarrhea (magnesium-containing antacids).

        (b)   Systemic: aluminum, magnesium and calcium are not well absorbed and are unlikely to cause systemic effects unless renal function is impaired.

F. Mucosal Protective Agents

    1.   **General Considerations.** Mucus-secreting cells are found throughout the surface of the gastric mucosa and the mucus secreted helps to protect the stomach wall from self-digestion by HCl and pepsin. Whereas the genesis of peptic ulcers is not resolved, it is known that mucosal-damaging mechanisms are increased in ulcer patients particularly when *H. pylori* is present in the gastric mucosa.

    2.   **Agents**

        a.   **Bismuth chelate (colloidal bismuth subsalicylate, PEPTO-BISMOL).** Has bacteriocidal activity and when used alone has been reported to eradicate *H. pylori* in 30% of ulcer patients. Its other mucosal-protecting actions include: coating the ulcer, adsorbing pepsin, enhancing prostaglandin synthesis and stimulating bicarbonate secretion. Short-term treatment is considered safe if renal function is normal. Unwanted effects include blackening of the tongue and feces.

        b.   **Sucralfate (CARAFATE).** A complex of aluminum hydroxide, sucrose and sulfate that complexes with proteins on the ulcer surface and thereby decreases the destructive action of pepsin and HCl. It also stimulates mucus and bicarbonate secretion, promoting rapid healing. Most common side-effect is constipation.

II. Agents Used to Promote Upper Gastrointestinal Motility

    A. General Considerations. Several agents are now used to increase gastrointestinal motility in a variety of situations. The most common is in patients with symptoms of 'heartburn' who suffer from acid reflux into the esophagus, a syndrome referred to as gastroesophageal reflux disorder. These drugs increase gastric emptying and thereby decrease esophageal reflux. These agents may act in part through cholinergic mechanisms, but probably by other pathways in the enteric nervous system as well, including dopaminergic and serotonergic. Their advantage is their greater selectivity compared to older cholinergic agonists such as bethanechol.

B. Agent: Metoclopramide (REGLAN).

III. Laxatives

A. Definition. Laxatives and cathartics are orally administered agents that promote intestinal evacuation. Although the two terms are frequently used interchangeably, they are more properly used to imply different intensities of effect. Laxative effect refers to the excretion of a soft, formed stool and may result from increased motor activity of the intestine or simply from changes in the water content of the stool. Cathartic effect implies a more fluid evacuation and is invariably the result of increased intestinal motor activity; cathartics may be administered in doses that produce only a laxative effect.

B. Uses and Contraindications

   1. Therapeutic Uses

     a. In cases of drug and food poisoning, to flush the offending substance from the intestinal tract (osmotic laxatives, such as sodium sulfate, are used for this purpose).

     b. To empty the gastrointestinal tract prior to radiologic examination of abdominal organs and prior to elective bowel surgery.

     c. To expel intestinal parasites and the drugs (anthelmintics) used to treat these parasitic infestations.

     d. To keep the stool soft and to prevent irritation and straining in patients with hernia (before and after surgery), cardiovascular disease or rectal disorders (emollient laxatives generally used).

     e. In the temporary treatment of chronic functional constipation when other measures are inadequate.

   2. Contraindications

     a. In all cases of constipation associated with organic disease.

     b. In all cases of gastrointestinal cramp, colic, nausea, vomiting or other symptoms of appendicitis or any undiagnosed abdominal pain.

C. Classification. Laxatives are generally classified on the basis of their general mechanism of action as stimulant, osmotic, bulk-forming and emollient laxatives.

D. Stimulant Laxatives

   1. Agents

     a. Castor oil.

     b. Cascara sagrada (NATURE'S REMEDY); senna (GENTLAX; SENOKOT)

     c. Bisacodyl (DULCOLAX).

   2. Site of Action. With the exception of castor oil, the effects of these agents are limited primarily to the large intestine and are produced only after a delay of 6 hours or more. Castor oil acts in the small intestine and, as a consequence, usually produces its cathartic effect within 3 hours.

3. **Mechanism of Action.** The increase in motor activity of the intestine is thought to result from local irritation of the intestinal mucosa or from a selective action upon the intestinal smooth muscle or nerve networks within the intestinal wall. These cathartics also reduce net absorption of water and electrolytes and increase the permeability of the mucosa.

Castor oil itself is nonirritant but, when acted upon by intestinal digestive enzymes (lipases), it is converted to glycerol and ricinoleic acid, and the latter agent produces the cathartic effect. Senna and bisacodyl preparations contain prodrugs that are converted in the large intestine to active agents by bacterial actions.

4. **Undesirable Effects**
   a. May cause griping, intestinal cramps, increased mucous secretion and excessive fluid evacuation.
   b. Prolonged use may cause dehydration, electrolyte disorders and damage to the colon.

E. Osmotic Laxatives (Saline Laxatives)
   1. **Agents**
      a. Magnesium salts: magnesium sulfate (epsom salt); milk of magnesia.
      b. Sodium salts: sodium sulfate (GLAUBER'S SALT); sodium phosphate (SAL HEPATICA).
      c. Lactulose (CONSTILAC, DUPHALAC).
      d. Polyethylene glycol (PEG).
   2. **Site of Action.** Throughout small and large intestine.
   3. **Mechanism of Action.** The osmotic laxatives are soluble salts or inert sugars that are only slightly and slowly absorbed from the digestive tract. Their presence in the intestinal lumen leads to a retention of water by osmotic forces that serves as a mechanical stimulus to increase intestinal motor activity. Lactulose, a semisynthetic disaccharide of fructose and galactose is converted in the colon by bacteria to yield acetic and lactic acids which function as osmotic laxatives; it takes 2–3 days to act.
   4. **Effects**
      a. Full doses of saline cathartics produce a semifluid or watery evacuation in 1–3 hours. Isotonic solutions of PEG and salts in formulations such as CO-LYTE are taken in large volume to clear the bowel prior to procedures such as colonoscopy.
      b. Some absorption of the saline cathartics does occur, but this causes little untoward effect if kidney function is adequate.

F. Bulk-forming Laxatives
   1. **Agents**
      a. Methylcellulose.

> **b.** Plantago or psyllium seed (METAMUCIL).
> **c.** Sodium carboxymethylcellulose (SCMC).

2. Site of Action. Throughout small and large intestine.

3. Mechanism of Action. The various natural and semisynthetic poly-saccharides and cellulose derivatives dissolve or swell in water, and the resulting increase in bulk of the intestinal contents acts as a mechanical stimulus. These agents also form an emollient gel or viscous solution that serves to keep the fecal material soft and hydrated.

4. Effects
  a. The laxative effect is usually apparent in 12–24 hours but full effect is not manifest until 2–3 days of medication.
  b. Essentially devoid of systemic effects because these laxatives are excreted almost quantitatively in the feces.
  c. If adequate fluids are not taken with the bulk-forming laxatives, they can cause fecal impaction and intestinal obstruction.

G. Emollient Laxatives (Stool Softeners)

1. Agents
  a. Docusate sodium (COLACE; DOXINATE).
  b. Glycerin suppositories.

2. Site of Action. Throughout small and large intestine.

3. Mechanism of Action. Promote defecation merely by softening the feces, without either direct or mechanical stimulation of intestinal motor activity.

IV. Antidiarrheal Agents

A. Definition. Drugs that slow the passage of unformed stool and decrease the frequency of unformed bowel movements.

B. General Considerations. Some compounds used to treat diarrhea are nonspecific, providing only relief of symptoms and not affecting the underlying cause of the diarrhea. The mechanisms of action by which prescription and nonprescription preparations of proved value exert their antidiarrheal effects on the gastrointestinal tract include alteration of intestinal motility with a decrease in transit rate of intestinal contents and increase in fluid and electrolyte absorption.

C. Drugs Altering Intestinal Motility

1. Naturally Occurring Opium Alkaloids (cf. Chapter 15)
  a. Agents
    (1) Codeine.
    (2) Paregoric (camphorated tincture of opium).
  b. Effects
    (1) Decrease diarrhea by increasing the nonpropulsive segmental contractions and markedly decreasing the propulsive contractions in both small and large intestine. These effects are produced at doses less than the analgesic dose, especially by oral route.

(2) See Appendix 5 for other effects.
   c. **Uses and Contraindications**
     (1) Most effective agents for treating diarrhea or causing consti-
pation. Especially valuable in treatment of exhausting diarrhea due to a variety of causes.
     (2) See Appendix 5 for contraindications.
  2. **Synthetic Opioids** (cf. Chapter 15)
   a. **Agents.** Synthetic opioids also produce a decrease in bowel
motility, but the following are used solely for treatment of diarrhea.
     (1) Diphenoxylate, used primarily in combination with atropine,
e.g. LOMOTIL (obtainable with prescription only).
     (2) Loperamide (IMODIUM). Relatively selective drug because of
efficient enterohepatic cycling, it is distributed primarily to
the intestine with limited access to the brain.
   b. **Effects**
     (1) Counteract diarrhea by slowing gastrointestinal motility.
     (2) In doses used to treat diarrhea, produce little or no opioid
subjective effects.
     (3) In high doses, diphenoxylate produces typical morphine-like
effects, e.g. euphoria, suppression of morphine abstinence
(see also Chapter 15 and Appendix 5). Low abuse potential
by parenteral routes because of poor aqueous solubility.
Atropine is present in combinations with diphenoxylate only
to prevent abuse, since undesired effects of atropine may
occur before morphine-like effects.
D. Other Agents: Bismuth subsalicylate, the active ingredient in commercial
preparations such as PEPTO-BISMOL. Has been shown to be effective in
decreasing various types of diarrhea. Mechanism of action is unknown,
but it is effective as a treatment of 'traveler's diarrhea'. It is not recommended to be taken prophylactically.
V. Agents Used for Inflammatory Bowel Disease
A. General Considerations. The pharmacologic therapy of the inflammatory
bowel diseases, ulcerative colitis and Crohn's disease, includes the use of
drugs that act by a variety of mechanisms to suppress the symptoms of
inflammation, including abdominal pain and diarrhea.
B. Agents
  1. **5-Aminosalicylic acid (5-ASA)-containing drugs:** 5-ASA, formulated
for release in the distal small intestine and colon, are believed to
act topically to suppress the inflammatory response, in part
through inhibiting activity of the proinflammatory transcription factor
NF-κB.
  2. **Glucocorticoids:** This class of steroids act by a variety of mechanisms
to inhibit the inflammatory response. A variety of glucocorticoid
preparations are available for treating inflammatory bowel disease.

Because glucocorticoids can produce many systemic side-effects, agents with low bioavailability are safer, such as the controlled-release formulation of budesonide (ENTOCORT), which undergoes substantial first-pass metabolism.

3. **TNFα Antagonist: Infliximab** (REMICADE) is a monoclonal antibody that binds specifically to the peptide TNFα. This prevents the interaction of TNFα with its receptor mediating the inflammatory effect.

Appendix 2
Drugs for Modifying Renal Function

I. **Diuretics**
   A. **Definition.** An agent that increases the volume flow of urine. Diuretics are primarily used clinically to remove excess water from extracellular spaces (edema), which occurs with certain diseases of the heart, liver, and kidney.
   B. **Osmotic Diuretics**
      1. **Agent: Mannitol** (administered by intravenous route)
      2. **Site of Diuretic Action.** In the proximal tubule where tubular urine remains isosmotic (cf. pp. 137–140) and in the loop of Henle with the latter being the primary site.
      3. **Mechanism of Action.** Increase in volume of tubular urine due to osmotic pressure exerted by the large amount of excess solute that is not absorbed. Increased volume causes decrease in Na$^+$ concentration in tubular urine, which makes active transport of Na$^+$ more difficult and less efficient   Na$^+$ has to be transported against a higher than usual concentration gradient. Rarely used except in prevention of acute renal failure and in acute cerebral edema.
      4. **Untoward Reactions.** Little if any when properly administered. May expand extracellular fluid space.
   C. **The Sulfonamide Derivatives – Carbonic Anhydrase Inhibitors**
      1. **Agent.** Acetazolamide (DIAMOX). No longer used as a diuretic but important because of its role in revealing fundamental renal physiology and pharmacology and in the development of effective diuretics.
      2. **Site of Action.** In the proximal tubule primarily, where H$^+$ from tubular cell is exchanged for Na$^+$ (cf. pp. 138–139).
      3. **Mechanism of Action.** Inhibition of carbonic anhydrase. Carbonic anhydrase accelerates the equilibrium reaction:

$$H_2O + CO_2 \rightleftharpoons H_2CO_3 \rightleftharpoons H^+ + HCO_3^-$$

Dissociation of H_2CO_3 in the tubular cell yields free H^+, which is necessary for reabsorption of HCO_3^- from tubular urine. When carbonic anhydrase is inhibited, H^+ is supplied in insufficient amounts and too slowly for the exchange reaction to occur at a normal rate. When the rate of exchange of Na^+ for H^+ is decreased, the reabsorption of HCO_3^- is inhibited. Net result: diuresis with increased HCO_3^- and Na^+ excretion. As HCO_3^- is eliminated, the amount of HCO_3^- delivered to the kidney decreases and the amount of H^+ available, even in the absence of carbonic anhydrase activity, is sufficient to exchange with Na^+, combine with the HCO_3^- , and account for reabsorption of all HCO_3^- filtered. Thus, the action of acetazolamide is limited; the duration of action is only about 24 hours.

4. **Fate in the Body.** Well absorbed when administered orally. Excreted by the kidney within 24 hours.

5. **Extrarenal Effects.** Inhibition of extrarenal carbonic anhydrase of the aqueous humor of the eye is clinically important and accounts for use in the treatment of glaucoma. Also used in treatment of altitude sickness.

6. **Untoward Reactions.** Few of serious nature.

D. **Sulfonamide Derivatives – Benzothiadiazine Derivatives**

1. **Agents.** Many, but the most commonly used are:
   a. Chlorothiazide (DIURIL);
   b. Hydrochlorothiazide.

   All benzothiadiazines have qualitatively the same properties but differ among themselves quantitatively. Synthesized as an outgrowth of studies on carbonic anhydrase inhibitors, but agents vary widely in their ability to inhibit carbonic anhydrase.

2. **Site of Diuretic Action.** Principal effect is close to the origin of the distal convoluted tubule.

3. **Mechanism of Diuretic Action.** All agents act primarily by binding to a Na/Cl cotransporter protein (TSC) and inhibiting its active cotransport of Na^+ and Cl^- , thus decreasing NaCl reabsorption by the kidney tubule.

   All potent diuretics which inhibit Na^+ reabsorption deliver more Na^+ to the site of exchange of Na^+ for K^+ and H^+ in the more distal portions of the nephron. As a consequence, more exchange of Na^+ for K^+ and H^+ takes place.

   The various derivatives of benzothiadiazine differ not only in potency (size of dose needed to produce a maximum effect) but also in the amount of NaCl excreted at the maximally effective dose.

4. **Pharmacologic Effects Other Than Diuresis**
   a. **Therapeutically useful effects**
   (1) **Hypotensive effect.** Used as hypotensive agents either alone or in association with other agents.
   (2) **Antidiuretic effect in diabetes insipidus.** Paradoxical effect;

mechanism unknown. Thiazides reduce volume of urine in patients with *diabetes insipidus* resulting from a failure of the renal tubule to respond to antidiuretic hormone (ADH) (cf. pp. 142–143).

   b. **Untoward reactions**

     (1) **Excessive loss of K^+.** The excessive loss of K^+ may lead to cardiac arrhythmias and is more likely in patients treated with digitalis glycosides, in patients with liver disease, and in patients receiving adrenocortical steroids.

     (2) **Hyperglycemia.** May aggravate established diabetes mellitus or bring to light latent diabetes. Symptoms provoked by thiazides are reversible on stopping the drugs.

     (3) **Uric acid retention.** Thiazides in therapeutic doses block uric acid secretion by the renal tubule. Use of thiazides may precipitate gout. Effect is quickly reversed on stopping the drugs.

     (4) **Other effects.** Hypersensitivity reactions such as skin rashes.

  5. **Route of Administration.** Oral.

  6. **Fate in the Body.** Chlorothiazide is incompletely absorbed from the gut, but other agents are well absorbed. All agents are excreted fairly rapidly by the kidneys, many by proximal tubular secretion, so that duration of action is about 12–24 hours.

E. Potassium-sparing Diuretics: Aldosterone Antagonists

  1. **Agent.** Spironolactone (ALDACTONE).

  2. **Site of Action.** In the kidney at sites where the hormone aldosterone has its activity – primarily in the distal and collecting tubules (cf. p. 142).

  3. **Mechanism of Action.** Spirolactones are structurally related to aldosterone, bind to the mineralocorticoid receptor and competitively block the interaction of aldosterone with this receptor; inhibition of receptor activation reduces sodium reabsorption and consequently decreases K^+ and H^+ secretion.

  4. **Route of Administration.** Spironolactone in the form first introduced was incompletely absorbed from the gut, but in the more recent, finely dispersed small-particle form, spironolactone is much better absorbed and is effective in about a quarter of the dose of the original material. This is an excellent example of how *pharmaceutical formulation* may greatly alter the activity of a drug.

  5. **Untoward Reactions.** Has other steroid effects including gynecomastia (swelling of breast tissue in men); a new analog (eplerenone) is less likely to produce these effects.

  6. **Therapeutic Uses.** Although spirolactones alone may produce a diuresis in some cases, delivery of a relatively large amount of Na^+ to the distal part of the nephron is essential for full effect, and this is achieved by the concomitant administration of another diuretic that increases Na$^+$ delivery to the distal tubule. The spirolactone ensures that Na$^+$ is not reabsorbed or exchanged for K$^+$ or H$^+$ under the influence of aldosterone. Therefore, the chief use of spirolactone is in combination with other diuretics to counteract the loss of K$^+$ and enhance the excretion of Na$^+$, especially in patients with hyperaldosteronism. Shown to decrease mortality in patients with heart failure when added to the usual drug regimen for this disease.

F. **Potassium-sparing Diuretics: Epithelial Na Channel Blockers**
1. **Agents**
   a. Triamterene (DYRENIUM).
   b. Amiloride (MIDAMOR).
2. **Site of Action.** In the last part of distal tubule and in the collecting duct.
3. **Mechanism of Action.** Increase the excretion of Na$^+$ but depress that of K$^+$ and H$^+$. These agents can produce this effect when aldosterone production is suppressed and in adrenalectomized patients. Effects are not due to aldosterone antagonism but to inhibition of Na$^+$ transport from the tubular lumen into cells via the epithelial sodium channel (ENaC); decreased Na$^+$ reabsorption leads to decreased K$^+$ and H$^+$ secretion from cell into urine. These agents are weak diuretics in comparison with the thiazide group of drugs.
4. **Untoward Reactions.** Serum potassium concentration may rise excessively during continuous treatment with these agents. Reduction in K$^+$ loss is one of the reasons for using them in combination with other diuretics that produce excess loss of K$^+$. However, there may be too much retention of K$^+$ on continuous therapy with the potassium-sparing diuretics.
5. **Therapeutic Use.** Main value is in combination with other diuretics when hypokalemia is a troublesome feature of treatment with other diuretics alone.

G. **Loop or High-ceiling Diuretics**
1. **Agents**
   a. Torsemide (DEMADEX).
   b. Furosemide (LASIX).
   c. Bumetanide (BUMEX).
2. **Site of Action.** Primarily on thick portion of ascending limb of loop of Henle.
3. **Mechanism of Diuretic Action.** Inhibit the reabsorption of Na$^+$ and Cl$^-$ by inhibiting the Na$^+$/K$^+$/Cl$^-$ carrier (co-transporter BSC1) in the luminal membrane of the ascending limb of loop of Henle.
4. **Routes of Administration.** Oral and intravenous.
5. **Fate in the Body**
   a. **Absorption.** Unlike the other agents furosemide has variable bioavailability after oral administration.
   b. **Excretion.** Excreted in urine and in feces via bile. Secreted by proximal tubular cells, a process essential for activity since the

loop diuretics act on luminal membrane of cells of thick part of ascending loop of Henle. The secretion is blocked by probenecid.

6. **Therapeutic Uses.** Loop diuretics are especially valuable if rapid and intensive diuresis is required. (As much as 25% of the glomerular filtrate may be excreted, compared with the normal 1% loss.) May be used prophylactically for acute renal failure or in patients with renal insufficiency.

7. **Side-effects.** Effects related to diuretic activity. Such potent diuretics that their use can lead to:
   a. Excessive loss of K^+ and/or Cl^-;
   b. Dehydration;
   c. Elevated blood uric acid, precipitation of gout;
   d. General fatigue and muscle cramps (reversed by K^+).

II. **Agents Used in Treatment of Gout.** Uric acid is the end product of purine metabolism in humans. Uric acid is freely filtered at the glomerulus but is mostly reabsorbed in the proximal tubule. A small amount is also secreted into the proximal tubule; the net result is urinary elimination of 8–12% of that originally filtered. The amount of uric acid in the body may be increased by overproduction, and/or impaired excretion. Because of the limited aqueous solubility of uric acid, in hyperuricemic conditions there is a tendency for urate crystals to precipitate in certain tissues (joints and kidneys) and to elicit inflammatory responses. The following drugs can prevent hyperuricemia or ameliorate its consequences.

A. **Uricosuric Agents**
   1. **Definition.** Agents that increase the renal excretion of uric acid.
   2. **Agents.** Probenecid; sulfinpyrazone (ANTURANE).
   3. **Site of Action.** Renal tubular cell, primarily in proximal tubule.
   4. **Mechanism of Action.** Inhibit the active reabsorption of uric acid by the renal tubular cells.
   5. **Route of Administration.** Oral.
   6. **Fate in the Body.** Well absorbed. Highly bound to plasma protein, but actively secreted into urine by tubular cells. Unless urine is markedly alkaline, probenecid is almost completely reabsorbed from tubular urine. Therefore, long duration of action.
   7. **Effects**
      a. Cause uric acid to be excreted at a rate sufficient to keep up with the rate of its formation in the body.
      b. Inhibit active tubular *secretion* of other organic acids such as para-aminohippuric acid (PAH), penicillin and loop diuretics by competing for same transport process via organic anionic transporter proteins.
   8. **Therapeutic Uses**
      a. In the treatment of chronic gout.
      b. As an adjunct in penicillin therapy in diseases that require very high doses of penicillin.

B. Agents Acting Extrarenally
1. **Allopurinol** (ZYLOPRIM).
    a. **Mechanism of Action.** Inhibition of xanthine oxidase, which catalyzes the final steps in the conversion of purines to uric acid.
    b. **Route of Administration.** Oral.
    c. **Fate in the Body.** Biotransformed by xanthine oxidase to active metabolites and the metabolites excreted in urine.
    d. **Effect.** Decreased formation of uric acid and consequent lower uric acid levels in blood; the deposition of urate crystals in tissues is reversed.
    e. Drug of choice in long-term treatment of gout; ineffective in an acute attack.
2. **Colchicine**
    a. **Mechanism of Action.** Suppression of inflammatory response to the deposition of urate crystals in joint tissues. Colchicine alters the functioning of microtubules. Microtubules are involved not only in cell division but also cell motility. It is believed that colchicine suppresses the motility of leukocytes by interacting with microtubules and preventing the infiltrative aspects of the inflammatory response. By so doing, the drug prevents a local decrease in pH that occurs as a result of leukocyte activity and, therefore, the further deposition of urate crystals.
    b. **Route of Administration.** Oral.
    c. **Fate in the Body.** Most of drug excreted in feces, remainder (10–20%) in urine.
    d. **Effect.** Largely effective as anti-inflammatory drug only against gouty arthritis. Provides dramatic relief of pain and swelling in acute attacks of gout and effective prophylactically against such attacks.
    e. **Untoward Effects.** Chronic administration may result in bone marrow suppression or damage to gastrointestinal tract. Side-effects reflect the action of the drug on rapidly proliferating cells.

Appendix 3
Drugs for Treating Infections and Cancer

I. **General Considerations**

Chemotherapy deals with the treatment of disease by chemical agents that can produce a toxic effect upon the disease-causing organism without producing undue harm to the host. Drugs used in the treatment of parasitic (microbial, viral, fungal, helmintic, etc.) and neoplastic diseases are termed *chemotherapeutic agents*. An *antibiotic* is a chemical substance produced by a microorganism that suppresses the growth of or directly kills another microorganism.

The goal of chemotherapy is to kill or to assist the body in the elimination of rapidly dividing, invading cells. This can be accomplished with minimal or no injury to the normal cells of the host by exploiting qualitative or quantitative differences between the biochemistry of invading cells and that of normal host cells. The more fundamental and the greater the difference between invading and host cells, the greater is the *selective toxicity* and the smaller is the likelihood of injury to the host (cf. pp. 280–281).

There are many different types of bacterial or other infections and of neoplastic diseases. These different types have differing sensitivities toward chemotherapeutic agents, so that each agent has its own spectrum of diseases against which it is effective.

Disease-causing cells have the capacity to become resistant to drugs that initially inhibited their growth (see pp. 287–293).

II. **Antimicrobial Agents**

A. **Drug-Parasite Interactions**

1. **Spectrum of Activity.** Refers to the range of specific microbes capable of being inhibited by a particular agent. The spectrum of activity of a drug is dependent to some degree on the dose administered. A *narrow*-spectrum antimicrobial agent is one that primarily affects a limited number of different microorganisms. Examples of narrow-spectrum antibiotics: penicillin, erythromycin.

A *broad*-spectrum drug is one capable of inhibiting a wide variety of microorganisms. Examples of broad-spectrum antibiotics: tetracyclines, streptomycin.

2. **Type of Activity.** Classification is based on the dosage used in therapeutics, not on the *in vitro* potential activity of an agent.
   a. **Bacteriostatic.** The ability of an agent to inhibit multiplication and growth of microorganisms. Examples of bacteriostatic agents: sulfonamides; tetracyclines; chloramphenicol.

      Prevention of bacterial growth suppresses the infection or total bacterial cell population thus enabling the normal defense mechanisms of the host (white blood cells, tissue phagocytes, and antibodies) to eradicate the disease.
   b. **Bactericidal.** The ability of a drug not only to inhibit growth but also to kill the parasite. Examples of bactericidal agents: penicillin, streptomycin, cephalosporins, bacitracin. Eradication of disease still depends to some degree on the activity of host defense mechanisms.

      In general, bactericidal activity is associated with those agents that act by disrupting the synthesis or function of the microbial cell wall.

3. **Activity Resulting from Combining Antimicrobial Agents**
   a. **Additive effect.** Usually obtained by combining two bacteriostatic agents or two bactericidal agents.
   b. **Antagonist effect.** May result from combination of a bacteriostatic agent with a bactericidal agent, since most bactericidal drugs act maximally on multiplying bacteria and bacteriostatic agents depress bacterial multiplication. However, results of combining bactericidal and bacteriostatic agents are unpredictable.
   c. **Delay in emergence of resistant organisms.** Combinations may delay the emergence of organisms resistant to either agent in the combination. Delay of emergence of resistant organisms is particularly important when long-term therapy is needed or in diseases caused by organisms that develop resistance rapidly. Example: the use of rifampin to delay resistance of tuberculous organisms to isoniazid or ethambutol when therapy may continue for many months.

4. **Mechanism of Antimicrobial Action**
   a. Inhibition of bacterial cell wall synthesis (penicillins, cephalosporins, bacitracin, vancomycin).
   b. Inhibition of bacterial protein synthesis (erythromycin, tetracyclines, chloramphenicol, streptomycin, clindamycin, linezolid).
   c. Inhibition of bacterial synthesis of the essential nonprotein metabolite tetrahydrofolic acid (sulfonamides, isoniazid).
   d. Alteration of permeability of cell membrane (polymyxin B).
   e. Inhibition of nucleic acid function (quinolones, rifampin).

B. Untoward Effects of Antimicrobial Therapy

1. Development of resistant organisms, a major public health problem that has necessitated the continued search for new antimicrobials and/or agents to prevent the development of resistance.

2. Development of *superinfection* as a result of changes in the normal microbial population of the intestinal, upper respiratory and genitourinary tracts. Superinfection is the appearance of a new infection by pathogenic microorganisms or fungi during antimicrobial therapy of a primary disease.

3. Interference with normal nutrition, e.g. reduction of intestinal microflora may decrease availability of vitamin K since considerable quantities of this essential nutrient are synthesized by intestinal bacteria.

4. Development of drug allergy from known or unknown exposure (see pp. 293–294).

5. Specific Drug Toxicities
   a. **Sulfonamides.** Decreased solubility of conjugated drug may lead to precipitation in urinary tract (see p. 162); blood disorders can occur in individuals with certain genetic enzyme deficiencies (see pp. 272, 273–275).
   b. **Penicillins.** Among the least toxic agents known, but can produce convulsion in very high doses or high incidence of allergic reactions even in extremely low doses.
   c. **Tetracyclines.** Since the tetracyclines can form complexes with calcium, they can be incorporated into tissues that are actively laying down calcium (teeth and bones) and can cause mottling and discoloration of teeth.
   d. **Streptomycin** (also neomycin, kanamycin, gentamicin). Can cause nerve damage leading to hearing loss and disturbances in the nonacoustic part of the inner ear (vestibular apparatus), which functions to orient the body during movement.
   e. **Chloramphenicol.** Can depress the blood-cell-forming tissues in bone marrow.

C. Host Factors Determining Response to Antimicrobial Agents

1. **Age.** Impaired ability of the very young or elderly patients to biotransform or excrete drugs (see pp. 261–265).

2. **Genetic Enzyme Deficiencies.** For example, in biotransformation of isoniazid (see p. 271); in enzymes of red blood cells producing idiosyncratic responses to sulfonamides (see pp. 274–275).

3. **Pregnancy.** Increased risk to both mother and fetus.

4. **Impaired Liver or Kidney Function.** Drug toxicity due to altered rate of drug elimination.

5. **Impaired Defense Mechanisms of Body**
   a. Due to disease: e.g. cancers of various types; HIV infections.
   b. Due to drugs: e.g. anticancer agents; corticosteroids.

D. Misuses and Causes of Failure of Antimicrobial Drug Therapy
1. Treatment of untreatable infections: e.g. 90% of viral infections of upper respiratory tract; measles; mumps.
2. Treatment of fever of undetermined origin or an undiagnosed condition.
3. Improper dosage: excessive amounts leading to drug toxicity; suboptimal doses; adequate doses but given for too short a period of time.
4. Self-medication with a drug that 'just happened to be around the house'. All antimicrobial agents, like any other therapeutic agents, may produce serious and even fatal reactions. *These drugs must never be taken without medical direction and supervision.*

III. Antifungal Agents
A. Treatment of Superficial Infections, e.g. tinea (ringworm) infections confined to the epidermis, hair and nails.
1. **Topically Administered Agents**
   a. Undecylenic acid (DESENEX; MYCODECYL; PEDZYL). Primarily fungistatic and has undoubted benefit in retarding growth of (but not eradicating) *tinea pedis* (athlete's foot).
   b. Tolnaftate (TINACTIN). Effective in a variety of fungal infections of the skin.
   c. Azoles, such as miconazole (MONISTAT). A variety of agents used to treat fungal infections of the skin and mucous membranes.
2. **Systemically Administered Agent.** Griseofulvin, an antibiotic, is a systemic agent available for treatment of superficial fungal infections of the scalp or nails. Griseofulvin acts by inhibiting fungal mitosis; it is fungistatic.

B. Treatment of Deep Infections, e.g. candidiasis (thrush); infection involving the mucous membranes, gastrointestinal tract and other visceral organs. In the last two decades the incidence of deadly fungal disease has increased exponentially. These infections are among the hardest to cure and are no longer confined to the tropics. The dramatic increase in these painful, debilitating, deadly diseases is due to several factors: (1) the widespread use of broad-spectrum antibiotics which affect nonpathogenic bacteria that normally compete with fungi; (2) the increased use of immunosuppressant and anticancer drugs, and (3) the AIDS epidemic and the number of individuals with compromised immune systems. These agents act by altering fungal cell permeability through interaction with fungal membrane sterols (ergosterol).
1. **Nystatin.** An antibiotic; fungistatic and fungicidal, depending on concentration. Useful treatment for candidiasis (thrush) infections that can be reached by topical application to mucous membranes of various body orifices. Not absorbed to any useful extent, but has local effect in bowel lumen. Not given parenterally.
2. **Amphotericin B.** An antibiotic, given parenterally (poorly absorbed orally) for systemic fungal infections. Adverse reactions occur in

almost all patients, and there is a high incidence of serious and toxic side-effects. However, before the availability of amphotericin B, certain fungal infections were 100% fatal. Therefore, a certain degree of toxicity in its use was acceptable.

3. **Azoles.** A number of azole antifungal agents, such as itraconazole (SPORANOX), are now available that are less toxic than amphotericin B. The azoles have the additional advantage of formulation for oral as well as intravenous administration. These drugs are effective in the treatment of many types of fungal infections. They act by inhibiting fungal CYP450 enzymes involved in synthesis of a component of the fungal cell wall.

IV. Antiviral Agents

Viruses are not cells and do not have a metabolism of their own; they can only proliferate in living host cells and have to use their host's metabolic processes. It is, therefore, difficult to find drugs that have *selective* toxicity for these pathogens. Most viral diseases cure themselves but some are life-threatening such as HIV-1 infection. The epidemic of this infection in the 1990s led to discoveries of a number of highly selective drugs that can prevent or cure viral diseases by interfering with one or more stages of the viral infection.

A. **Agent Preventing Effective Viral Penetration into Host Cells**. Enfuvirtide blocks interaction of the HIV virus with a host membrane receptor involved in viral penetration; rimantadine, effective against influenza A viruses, blocks release of viral RNA from the viral particle following uptake into invaginations of the host cell membrane.

B. **Agents Interfering with Viral Replication.** The replication cycle of the virus is so similar to that of the mammalian cell and, unlike most other infectious microorganisms, requires the participation of the intracellular processes of the host cell. Thus, agents capable of inhibiting or preventing viral replication are likely to be cytotoxic to the host cells as well. Major quantitative differences in intracellular enzyme activities between mammalian cells and viruses, however, have been exploited in the development of drugs that selectively inhibit viral replication.

1. **Pegylated interferon alpha-2b.** A long-acting interferon which acts by multiple mechanisms to inhibit replication of the hepatitis C virus in liver cells.

2. **Acyclovir and congeners.** Effective for treatment of herpes simplex virus and varicella zoster virus infections. Administered orally and topically for genital herpes; mitigates symptoms but does not prevent recurrence. Relatively selective antiviral activity through inhibitory effect on viral DNA polymerase.

3. **Reverse transcriptase inhibitors.** Nucleosides (NRTIs): zidovudine (AZT), didanosine (ddl), zalcitabine (ddC). Nonnucleosides (NNRTIS): nevirapine, efavirenz. Administered orally for treatment of acquired immune deficiency syndrome (AIDS) (cf. Chapter 16). These drugs inhibit the viral enzyme reverse transcriptase, which

makes a complementary DNA from the viral RNA. In HIV-1-infected individuals, these drugs delay the progression of the disease and reduce the incidence of opportunistic infections. AZT is used to reduce the risk of transmission of the virus from HIV-positive mothers to fetuses. Because of rapid development of viral resistance, these drugs are used in combination. The nucleoside and nonnucleoside inhibitors have different binding sites on the enzyme and therefore cross-resistance is not observed.

4. **Protease inhibitors (Indinavir, Saquinavir).** Agents that inhibit an HIV enzyme critical for the late stages of replication. These drugs are used only in combination with other drugs, in part to slow development of resistance.

V. Antiseptics and Disinfectants
A. Definitions
1. **Antiseptics** are substances that are applied to living tissue to kill or prevent the growth of microorganisms.
2. **Disinfectants** are bactericidal drugs that are applied to inanimate objects; they play a major role in public health sanitation and treatment of water supplies.
3. **Germicides** are agents that are toxic to microorganisms in general when applied to living tissue or inanimate objects; term is frequently used to cover both antiseptics and disinfectants.

B. Mechanisms of Action
1. Coagulation of protein.
2. Destruction of normal permeability characteristics of cell membrane.
3. Poisoning of enzyme systems of cell.

   In many cases, germicides destroy microorganisms in such a nonselective manner that normal host cells may also be injured (see p. 330).

C. Agents
1. Phenols
a. **Hexachlorophene.** Incorporated into soaps but evidence is lacking for the effectiveness and safety of use as an 'aid to personal hygiene'; 3% solutions used for reducing bacterial counts on surgeons' hands and forearms.

b. **Cresol.** Soapy emulsion (LYSOL) used as disinfectant and antiseptic.

2. Acids
a. **Benzoic acid.** Weak, tasteless, nontoxic, bacteriostatic agent used extensively as a preservative in food and drink at a concentration of 0.1%. Esters of hydroxybenzoic acid are used as preservatives in pharmaceutical and cosmetic preparations (eye-drops, ointments, etc.).

3. Surface-active agents
a. **Anionic agents.** Include common soaps; owe their action primarily to dislodging bacteria in the skin.

    b. **Cationic agents.** Benzalkonium (ZEPHIRAN); chlorhexidine glu-
conate. Commonly used for antisepsis of skin and disinfection of
instruments; included in various proprietary preparations such as
mouthwashes, etc.

  4. **Oxidizing Agents.** For example, hydrogen peroxide, widely used for
cleaning wounds.

  5. **Alcohols.** Ethyl and isopropyl are bactericidal and extensively used
as skin antiseptics.

  6. **Halogens**

    a. **Iodine.** Possesses high bactericidal, viricidal, fungicidal, sporici-
dal and protozoacidal activity.

    b. **Chlorine.** Chlorine-releasing compounds used principally to ster-
ilize water for sanitization.

VI. Antiprotozoal Agents

The infectious diseases of humans that are commonly caused by protozoa
include: malaria, amebiasis, trypanosomiasis (sleeping sickness) and trichomoniasis (a venereal disease). Malaria and amebiasis are the most
common protozoal diseases; they are worldwide diseases and afflict hundreds of millions of people.

A. Antimalarial Drugs. The malarial parasite is a protozoan of the genus
Plasmodium, four species of which are known to infect humans. The
insect vector is the female *Anopheles* mosquito. (The disease may also
be transmitted from one human to another through a transfusion of
blood containing malarial parasites or by syringes and needles contaminated with parasite-containing blood.) Each parasite of the four
species has a sexual cycle in the mosquito and an asexual cycle in the
tissues and blood of humans. The efficacy of drugs in the prevention and
treatment of malaria is related to the species of infecting parasite and to
its stage of development; there is no drug that is equally effective against
all stages.

Attempts to eradicate malaria with the use of insecticides and by
chemotherapy have not met with success primarily due to the increasing
resistance of mosquitos to the insecticides and of the malarial parasite to
drugs. Not only has there been an increase in malaria worldwide but the
development of drug resistance now poses a serious clinical problem with
P. falciparum, the most dangerous of the malarial parasites, accounting
for 85% of infections and much of the patient mortality. Intensive use of
chloroquine, previously the most effective and most widely used drug to
prevent and treat *P. falciparum,* has led to the development of strains of
the parasite that are relatively or absolutely resistant to its action.

The principal agents employed in therapy:

  1. Chloroquine

  2. Mefloquine

  3. Primaquine

  4. Quinine

5.   Pyrimethamine (usually used in combinations)
6.   Halofantrine
7.   Doxycycline.

The mechanism of action of chloroquine, mefloquine and primaquine, as well as the older agents, quinine and quinacrine (ATABRINE), is not known. Chloroquine is believed to cause its antimalarial effect by inhibiting enzymes involved in hemoglobin metabolism in the parasite. Whatever selective toxicity these drugs possess depends upon selective accumulation at the intracellular milieu of the parasite. These agents act rapidly, however, and sensitive strains develop resistance to them with relative difficulty. However, the incidence of resistant strains is increasing and results in part from increased removal of the drugs from sites of intracellular accumulation.

The mechanism of action of pyrimethamine is much more selective than that of the above group, but resistance to its action can be obtained more readily. Pyrimethamine inhibits the utilization of folic acid within the cell; it is effective against the plasmodial enzymes at doses lower than those that affect mammalian cells.

B. **Amebicides.** Amebiasis is caused by *Entamoeba histolytica.* There are two principal phases in its life cycle, the *cystic* and the *trophozoite.* Ingested cysts liberate the trophozoite in the intestine. The trophozoite is motile and can penetrate the intestine, eventually reaching the liver; it is the trophozoite that causes the intestinal and extraintestinal forms of amebiasis. While the parasite remains in its cystic form within the lumen of the bowel there may be little or no disturbance to the well-being of the host. However, it is the cyst excreted in the feces that is the potential source of infection to the host or to others.

The goal of therapy in amebiasis is to kill the trophozoite forms wherever they may exist. (1) In the bowel, cysts cease to be produced when all trophozoites are killed, thereby inhibiting the spread of the infection to other tissues or organs of the host as well as to other persons; (2) killing trophozoites at sites other than the intestine eradicates the extraintestinal forms of the disease.

The modern therapy of amebiasis also includes the treatment of persons who have intestinal amebiasis without acute symptoms. The asymptomatic passer of cysts is a potential source of infection to the patient and others, and is an extremely serious public health problem. Drugs poorly absorbed from the gastrointestinal tract are used to treat asymptomatic or mild intestinal infections, e.g. diloxanide, iodoquinol. Metronidazole is the mainstay of treatment for both extraintestinal and intestinal amebiasis. Because it is not effective against cysts, it is used with a luminal agent and is not used for asymptomatic disease. Metronidazole's success in all invasive stages of the disease has revolutionized the treatment of amebiasis. It is also effective in the treatment of trichomoniasis when given orally.

VII. Anthelmintic Drugs

A. General Considerations. Anthelmintics are drugs used to rid the body of parasitic worms (helminths); anthelmintics may act locally to expel the helminths from the gastrointestinal tract or to combat systemic infestations. Worm infections represent the most common parasitic disease in the world – they affect half of the world's population.

Worms parasitic for humans include: tapeworms (cestodes), roundworms (nematodes) and flukes (trematodes). The different species vary with respect to bodily structure, physiology, habitat in the human host and sensitivity to drugs.

Parasitic worms are harmful to the host for a number of reasons:

1. Worms may cause injury to the tissues and organs by blockade due to their size and number: e.g. roundworms may cause gut obstruction; filariae may block lymphatic channels and cause massive edema.

2. Heavy infestations may interfere with nutrition by robbing the host of food.

3. Toxic substances made by the parasite may be absorbed by the host.

4. They may make the host more susceptible to secondary infections by bacteria.

Intestinal worm infections in general are more easily treated than those in other locations in the body: the worms need not be killed by the drug, and the drug need not be absorbed when given orally. The treatment of worms in tissues or organs other than the intestine is more difficult because they must be killed or critically injured so that they may be destroyed and eliminated from the tissues and ultimately from the body. Since drugs used to treat extraintestinal infestations must reach the site of infestation, the drugs must either be given parenterally or be absorbed when given orally with consequent greater danger to the host if the drugs are toxic. In general, localization of worms in tissues makes them highly resistant to chemotherapeutic attack.

None of the anthelmintics used currently are effective against all worms. Each agent has its own spectrum of activity, and identification of the type of parasitic infection is essential before chemotherapy begins. Selective toxicity for the parasite is achieved either by exploiting quantitative biochemical differences between parasite and host or by limiting access of the drug to the host.

B. Mechanisms of Anthelmintic Activity

1. Paralysis of musculature of worms by blocking action of acetylcholine resulting in relaxation of the worms' hold on the intestinal mucosa and their subsequent expulsion by normal bowel evacuation or following use of cathartics. Agents having this mechanism of action: piperazine for roundworm infections and pyrantel for pinworm. Muscle paralysis

caused by praziquantal, an anti-tapeworm drug effective in schistosomiasis, probably occurs by another mechanism.

2. Inhibition of microtubule synthesis: e.g. mebendazole for roundworms and hookworm infections.

3. Paralysis of worm by potentiating GABA-mediated neural inhibition
(cf. Appendix 5, benzodiazepines), e.g. ivermectin used for thread-
worm infections.

4. Inhibition of ova production (probably by inhibiting DNA replication): e.g. oxamniquine for blood fluke infections (schistosomiasis).

VIII. Anticancer Agents

There are two outstanding differences between microbial infections and
neoplasms that account for the failure of cancer chemotherapy to achieve
the same dramatic success as microbial chemotherapy.

A. Use of drugs in the treatment of an infection allows the normal host
defense mechanisms to eliminate the infecting agent. In contrast, the
body appears to possess limited effective defenses against most neoplastic cells, so that successful treatment of the disease presumably depends
upon the destruction of every neoplastic cell. However, in several human
neoplasms, the detection of 'foreign' antigens suggests that immunologic
defenses of the host may play an important role in long-term remissions.

B. The many *qualitative* differences between microbial cells and those of the
host favor the development of selectively toxic drugs that inhibit growth
or kill infecting organisms with minimal or no injury to host cells. In contrast, only *quantitative* differences are known between neoplastic cells
and host cells; this allows for only a moderate degree of drug selectivity
and does not permit the inhibition of cancer cells without producing
harm to those host cells which also normally undergo rapid division.

Differences in rate of metabolism and reproduction are the
most important exploitable differences between neoplastic cells and host
cells. But those host cells that normally undergo rapid division are also
vulnerable to anticancer drugs; e.g. epithelial cells in the gastrointestinal
tract and skin, and the tissues involved in blood cell formation. Toxic
effects of anticancer drugs usually include, therefore, ulceration of the
gastrointestinal tract, skin rashes, loss of hair and decrease in the number
of circulating blood cells. Susceptibility to microbial infections usually
increases, since many antineoplastic agents also suppress the immune
response. Other consequences of the growth-inhibiting properties of
antineoplastic agents are fetal abnormalities, with resulting defects in
development, or fetal resorption. These adverse effects can be produced
by virtually all the drugs that have been specifically developed for the
treatment of cancer. Many drugs also produce specific untoward effects.

C. **Mechanism of Action.** The final pathway of all cancer growth is through
an aberrant nucleic acid sequence leading to more rapid cell growth.
Anticancer drugs produce their effects by interfering in one way or
another with DNA replication or nucleic acid synthesis. Thus the ability

to inhibit protein synthesis is the pharmacologic effect common to all anticancer drugs. The various drugs used to treat cancer may be classified according to the mechanism by which they produce this inhibition of protein synthesis.

1. **Alkylating Agents.** Highly reactive chemicals that inhibit cell division by binding to DNA and causing abnormal cross-linking of the DNA strands. This cross-linking makes DNA excessively stable and incapable of its usual reactivity and of carrying out its normal function.

   The original nitrogen mustards were highly reactive and had to be administered intravenously. The newer derivatives of nitrogen mustard (e.g. chlorambucil, melphalan, cyclophosphamide) have the advantage of being somewhat less reactive and therefore able to be given orally; they are also well absorbed from the gastrointestinal tract. However, the alkylating agent cisplatin is given intravenously.

2. **Antimetabolites.** Chemical substances that are specific antagonists of normal substrates in the metabolic reactions of living organisms. An antimetabolite exerts its effect by interacting with a particular enzyme in such a manner as to prevent the enzyme from catalyzing a specific biochemical reaction. All of the antimetabolites that are anticancer drugs selectively inhibit one or more enzymic steps which are critical for the synthesis of DNA.

   a. **Folic acid antagonists.** Interfere with nucleic acid synthesis by inhibiting the enzyme that converts folic acid to the form in which the folic acid participates as a coenzyme in the biosynthesis of nucleic acids. Methotrexate is the most commonly used agent.

   b. **Purine antagonists.** Structural analogs of the natural purines; do not act directly but are converted into ribonucleotides which then become the active inhibitors of a number of critical reactions involving nucleotide synthesis. This process is referred to as 'lethal synthesis'. 6-Mercaptopurine is the most important of the antipurine drugs.

   c. **Pyrimidine antagonists.** Agents that interfere with normal pathways of pyrimidine biosynthesis. The antipyrimidines are not active by themselves but are incorporated into nucleotides, and the fraudulent nucleotides inhibit the formation of DNA. 5-Fluorouracil and cytarabine are among the best-established agents in this group.

   d. **Antibiotics.** Dactinomycin (actinomycin D), doxorubicin and bleomycin form a complex with DNA and block DNA-dependent synthesis of mRNA.

3. **Arrest of Mitosis.** Several natural or semisynthetic products derived from plants have the ability to block mitosis and have proved useful in the treatment of ovarian and testicular cancer. These include the

vinca alkaloids, vinblastine and vincristine extracted from the periwinkle plant, and paclitaxel (TAXOL), a semisynthetic derivative of yew trees.

4. **Hormones and Hormone Antagonists.** These agents are not cytotoxic in the usual sense but are used for tumors whose growth is hormone-dependent, e.g. for prostate, uterine and breast cancer. Examples include tamoxifen, an estrogen antagonist, for breast cancer and flutamide, a testosterone antagonist, for prostate cancer.

5. **New Therapeutic Approaches**

   a. **Kinase inhibitors**. For some types of cancers a chromosomal translocation generates a new gene, called an oncogene because it codes for a protein that transforms a normal cell into a neoplastic one. An example is the Philadelphia chromosome observed in chronic myelogenous leukemia (CML). The chromosomal fusion results in an abnormal tyrosine kinase (BCR-ABL) that causes inhibition of growth control. The drug imatinib mesylate (GLEEVEC) was developed because of its selectivity for blocking the ATP binding site on this enzyme. It was found to cause apoptotic death of transformed cells and to prolong survival in patients with CML.

   b. **Angiogenesis inhibitors.** These agents, antiangiogenesis drugs, block the formation of blood vessels, and it has been shown that angiogenesis is fundamental to the growth of solid tumors. By blocking blood vessel formation, these agents prevent the tumor from receiving essential factors for growth and development and, as a result, tumors effectively starve to death. The first antiangiogenic agent bevacizumab (AVASTIN) was approved for clinical use in 2004. It is a monoclonal antibody that blocks the angiogenic effect of vascular endothelial growth factor (VEGF).

   c. **Antisense technology.** Antisense drugs are short, synthetic pieces of nucleic acid that inhibit the action of specific genes by binding to their messenger RNA. Antisense agents being designed for the treatment of various diseases are showing promise in stopping the spread of cancers such as ovarian cancer.

Appendix 4
Drugs for Treating Hypertension

I. **General Considerations.** Elevation of blood pressure, referred to as hypertension, is a common phenomenon, with an estimated 50 million afflicted individuals in the US population and 1 billion worldwide. Hypertension has been definitively established as a risk factor for a number of adverse outcomes, including heart failure, heart attacks (myocardial infarction), stroke, renal disease, peripheral vascular disease, and blindness. Based on epidemiologic evidence of the relationship between blood pressure and adverse outcomes, hypertension is now defined as blood pressure greater than 120 mm Hg systolic blood pressure or 80 mm Hg diastolic blood pressure. Hypertension is treatable with nonpharmacologic measures such as weight loss, physical activity, dietary modification including sodium reduction, and moderation of alcohol consumption. Often, however, pharmacologic treatment is required in order to achieve adequate blood pressure reduction. It is especially important for patients with other cardiovascular risk factors such as diabetes, hypercholesterolemia, family history, and older age. Blood pressure is determined by numerous factors, including the diameter of blood vessels (total peripheral resistance), the pumping action of the heart (cardiac output), and blood volume (see Chapter 14). These factors are influenced by the regulatory actions of nerves and hormones, as well as by pathophysiologic mediators. Many drug targets have been identified that have led to development of numerous classes of antihypertensive agents.

II. **Inhibitors of the Sympathetic Nervous System**

   A. **Alpha Blockers**

   1. **Agents.** Many alpha receptor antagonists ('blockers') have been developed for therapeutic use in hypertension. The prototype is **prazosin** (MINIPRESS). These agents exhibit selectivity for the α_1 as compared to the α_2 receptor subtype, which is an advantage because it reduces the risk of side-effects such as increased heart rate. Newer agents have longer half-lives and therefore only need to be taken once a day, which improves compliance.

2. **Site and Mechanism of Action.** Alpha blockers have affinity for α_1 receptors in the smooth muscle of blood vessels. Generally, they competitively block the interaction with this receptor of norepinephrine released from adrenergic nerve endings in vessels. Therefore, the primary effect is a reduction in the total peripheral resistance as a result of dilation of vessels, especially arterioles.

3. **Side-effects.** Alpha blockers may cause excessive hypotension upon rising from a supine or sitting position (postural hypotension), because they inhibit the action of norepinephrine that is released in response to a drop in blood pressure on rising (baroreceptor reflex). The decrease in blood pressure may also cause a reflex increase in heart rate (tachycardia), which may be problematic in patients with coronary heart disease.

B. Beta Blockers

1. **Agents.** As with the alpha blockers there are now many beta blockers for therapeutic use in hypertension. The first drug in this class, propranolol (INDERAL), is a nonselective beta blocker. Newer agents, such as **metoprolol** (LOPRESSOR), exhibit greater selectivity for the β_1 as compared to the β_2 receptor.

2. **Site and Mechanism of Action.** Beta blockers have affinity for β_1 receptors in the sinus node and muscle cells of the heart. They competitively block the interaction with this receptor of norepinephrine released from adrenergic innervation of the heart and of epinephrine released from the adrenal medulla. Therefore, the primary effect is a reduction in heart rate and force of contraction, which leads to a reduction in cardiac output. These agents also block the β_1 receptor-mediated release of renin from specialized cells in the kidney. This effect contributes to blood pressure reduction by both vasodilation and decreased salt and water retention. Despite the ability of beta blockers to reduce cardiac output, some of these drugs such as carvedilol (COREG) have been demonstrated in clinical trials to be effective in the treatment of heart failure.

3. **Side-effects.** Nonselective beta blockers may cause difficulty breathing, especially in patients with asthma or other types of lung disease. This side effect occurs because β_2 receptor activation dilates the airways; antagonism of β_2 receptors can lead to constriction of the airways. The reduction in cardiac output, and effects in the brain by some of these drugs, can lead to fatigue. Chronic use of beta blockers leads to increased sensitivity of cardiac beta receptors, which is observed if the drugs are inappropriately withdrawn abruptly.

C. Peripheral Sympatholytics

1. **Agents. Reserpine** and **guanethidine** were among the earliest drugs used to treat hypertension and have been replaced by the newer classes of agents that cause fewer side-effects.

2. **Site and Mechanism of Action.** These drugs block the actions of the

sympathetic nervous system in blood vessels and the heart by acting in the presynaptic nerve terminal to reduce the release of norepinephrine. Both agents, which affect the storage of norepinephrine in vesicles by different mechanisms, cause depletion of the neurotransmitter from nerve endings.

3. **Side-effects.** Reserpine acts in the brain to produce a number of effects including sedation and depression; guanethidine may cause postural hypotension and a number of drug interactions. Both agents cause diarrhea.

D. Central Sympatholytics

1. **Agents. Methyldopa** and **clonidine** are also older agents with undesirable side-effects.

2. **Site and Mechanism of Action.** These drugs act predominantly in a region of the brainstem that regulates the activity of the sympathetic nerves to the heart and blood vessels. Through selective activation of α_2 receptors in this region the activity of these nerves is inhibited. As a result both reduction in cardiac output and total peripheral resistance may contribute to the hypotensive effect.

3. **Side-effects.** Sedation, via an action in the brain, is the most prominent side-effect, limiting current use of these drugs.

III. Inhibitors of Angiotensin

A. Angiotensin Converting Enzyme (ACE) Inhibitors

1. **Agents. Captopril** (CAPOTEN), the first ACE inhibitor marketed for use in hypertension, was followed by many others, such as the prodrug **enalapril** (VASOTEC), which required only once-a-day dosing and did not cause as great a risk of hypersensitivity reactions.

2. **Site and Mechanism of Action.** These agents were designed to inhibit with high selectivity the angiotensin converting enzyme (ACE). This enzyme, present in the vascular endothelium, converts the peptide angiotensin I, generated in response to renal release of renin, to angiotensin II. Angiotensin II increases blood pressure by a variety of mechanisms, including constriction of blood vessels and sodium and water retention by the kidney. This latter effect results, in part, from angiotensin II-induced release from the adrenal cortex of aldosterone, a hormone that acts on the distal portion of the nephron. Angiotensin II also affects the structure of blood vessels and the heart, which contributes to pathological changes in certain cardiovascular diseases. ACE not only generates angiotensin II, it also inactivates the vasodilator peptide bradykinin. Inhibition of ACE decreases angiotensin II and increases bradykinin, which results in a reduction of total peripheral resistance and loss of sodium and water. ACE inhibitors do not cause reflex tachycardia, which contributes to their usefulness in treating heart failure and heart attacks. ACE inhibitors are also efficacious in preventing kidney damage in diabetic patients.

3. **Side-effects.** ACE inhibitors cause a dry cough in a substantial percent of the population (5–20%), especially in women, and swelling of facial and airway tissue (angioneurotic edema) to a lesser extent (0.1–0.2%), especially in African Americans. These effects may be mediated, in part, by bradykinin. These drugs increase the risk of excessive potassium levels in serum due to the reduction in aldosterone secretion. ACE inhibitors are contraindicated during the second and third trimester of pregnancy because of teratogenic effects on the kidney.

B. **Angiotensin Receptor Blockers**
1. **Agents. Losartan** (COZAAR) and many others.
2. **Site and Mechanism of Action.** Angiotensin receptor blockers have selective affinity for angiotensin II type 1 receptors (AT_1). They antagonize the interaction of angiotensin II with this receptor on smooth muscle of blood vessels and therefore cause vasodilation. Their effect on this receptor is generally insurmountable. Most of the other effects of angiotensin II are antagonized as well, including the stimulation of aldosterone release, the renal effects, and the vascular and cardiac structural changes. There is a prevailing view that these drugs may have a greater inhibitory effect than the ACE inhibitors, because angiotensin II can be synthesized through the action of enzymes other than ACE
3. **Side-effects.** These drugs do not affect the degradation of bradykinin, which may explain in part the lower risk of cough and angioedema. They cause an increase in the synthesis of angiotensin II and do not antagonize its effects mediated through the AT_2 receptor.

IV. **Vasodilators**
   A. **Calcium Channel Blockers**
1. **Agents.** Dihydropyridines such as **nifedipine** (PROCARDIA) and non-dihydropyridines such as **verapamil** (CALAN).
2. **Site and Mechanism of Action.** Calcium channel blockers act on a protein in the membrane of smooth and cardiac muscle cells that permits influx of calcium in response to a voltage change. The rise in intracellular calcium activates of the contractile machinery of the cell. These drugs differ in their selectivity for blood vessels and the heart. The dihydropyridines are more selective for calcium channels in blood vessels and primarily decrease total peripheral resistance. Others such as verapamil act on the heart as well and also decrease cardiac output. The cardioselective agents are indicated for their efficacy in treating abnormal rhythms of the heart and the pain associated with inadequate oxygen delivery to heart muscle (angina).
3. **Side-effects.** Calcium channel blockers can cause excessive depression of the heart and other adverse cardiac events such as infarctions and arrhythmias. These drugs can also cause constipation due to

inhibitory effects on smooth muscle of the gastrointestinal tract. Their hypotensive effect can cause reflex responses including increased output of aldosterone that leads to sodium and water retention and therefore, edema.

B. Other Vasodilators

1. **Hydralazine.** This older drug is a selective arteriolar vasodilator. Its mechanism of action is not known. Use of this drug is complicated by reflex tachycardia, which increases risk of angina and even heart attack. Other problematic side-effects include risk of immunologic reactions.

2. **Sodium nitroprusside.** Another drug among the older antihypertensives, this agent is now known to undergo biotransformation to release nitric oxide (NO). NO is a signaling molecule released in the vascular endothelium (and other tissues as well) in response to activation of endothelial receptors by agonists such as acetylcholine. The signaling cascade mediated by NO results in relaxation of vascular smooth muscle. This drug must be administered by intravenous infusion and so is only used for the short-term management of severe hypotension.

3. **Diazoxide.** This drug activates potassium channels in the smooth muscle membrane, which leads to cellular hyperpolarization and relaxation of the muscle. This drug, like sodium nitroprusside, is used intravenously for severe hypertensive crises.

V. Diuretics (see Appendix 2)

1. **Thiazides.** The thiazide diuretics reduce mean arterial blood pressure, primarily through a reduction in total peripheral resistance. The prototype in this large class is **chlorothiazide** (DIURIL). The mechanism of the effect on blood vessels is not entirely understood. The effect is dependent on thiazide-induced loss of sodium in response to the inhibitory action on the NaCl co-transporter in the renal distal convoluted tubule. Initially, the diuretic effect reduces extracellular fluid volume, but even when restored by compensatory mechanisms the blood pressure is lowered. The thiazides are currently recommended as drugs of first choice in hypertension, in part because of large clinical trials such as the Antihypertensive and Lipid Lowering Treatment to Prevent Heart Attack (ALLHAT, 2002), which demonstrated their efficacy in preventing the complications of hypertension. The risk of excessive potassium loss with thiazides can be reduced by use with angiotensin inhibitors or potassium-sparing diuretics.

2. **Loop diuretics.** These agents also reduce blood pressure but their use is complicated by relatively steep dose-response curves, resulting in excessive sodium and potassium loss, and short durations of action.

VI. Therapeutic Use of Antihypertensive Agents

Hypertension is generally a chronic condition that requires long-term drug therapy. The choice of a drug regimen involves consideration of factors such as the severity of the hypertension, the acceptability of expected side-effects, the presence of other diseases and the cost. Long-term compliance to a regimen of antihypertensive agents is one problem in the clinical use of these drugs. Survey estimates from 1999 to 2000 reveal that whereas 59% of hypertensive subjects are prescribed treatment only 34% experience blood pressure control. More than one class of antihypertensive agent may be required to achieve adequate blood pressure reduction and to minimize side-effects. Guidelines such as the Seventh Report of the Joint National Committee on Prevention, Detection, Evaluation, and Treatment of High Blood Pressure (JNC 7, 2003) recommend initiating a two-drug combination for patients who present with blood pressure of $\geq 160\,\mathrm{mm\,Hg}$ systolic or $\geq 100\,\mathrm{mm\,Hg}$ diastolic. The current recommendations favor thiazide diuretics with beta blockers, angiotensin inhibitors, or calcium channel blockers. Combinations of drugs that act on different targets generally increase the blood pressure-lowering effect. In addition, combinations of drugs can be chosen to reduce the risk of side-effects. For example, beta blockers inhibit the reflex tachycardia that occurs with vasodilators such as alpha blockers or vasoselective calcium channel blockers. Angiotensin inhibitors block the effects of increased angiotensin II that occur in response to the thiazide diuretics. Thiazide diuretics reduce the fluid retention that occurs in response to vasodilators. Epidemiologic data reveal a substantial reduction in morbidity and mortality rates from cardiovascular disease in the US over the last 30 years, and the greater use and efficacy of antihypertensive agents are two factors that have contributed to this positive outcome.

Appendix 5
Drugs for Reducing Pain and Consciousness

THE NATURE OF PAIN

> Remember that pain has this most excellent quality:
> if prolonged it cannot be severe, and if severe it cannot be prolonged.
> *Seneca* (4? BCE–CE 65), from
> *Moral Epistles to Lucilius, XCIV*

Pain, the symptom that most commonly brings a patient to consult a physician or dentist, is certainly the most intrusive of all symptoms. Although pain is one of our most useful sensations, indicating the presence and frequently the location of disease, and alerting us to threats of bodily injury, it often exceeds its protective function and becomes destructive. Relief of pain is, therefore, one of the great objectives in medicine.

Webster's dictionary defines pain as 'a basic bodily sensation induced by a noxious stimulus, received by naked nerve endings, characterized by physical discomfort (as pricking, throbbing, or aching) and typically leading to evasive action' (*Websters New Collegiate Dictionary*. Springfield, MA: Merriam, 1987). This definition recognizes several of the important phenomena that are associated with pain. It recognizes that the simple 'stimulus-response' concept – of stimuli activating receptors and giving rise to sensory impulses that are translated into a sensation or perception – is an integral part of the totality termed *pain*. The word *basic* incorporates the fact that, except for the very rare cases of individuals afflicted with congenital generalized analgesia, all humans are born with the gift of pain perception.

The dictionary definition also reflects the consensus of neurophysiologists that there are specific receptors for pain that are simple, unencapsulated nerve endings without specialized structure. Pain receptors are present in skin, mucous membranes, skeletal muscles, blood vessels, visceral organs and in most other areas of the body with the exception of the parenchyma of the lung and cerebral cortex. But these receptors are unlike the more specialized sensory receptors such as those for heat or cold, since pain receptors respond to a variety of stimuli, including mechanical (pressure or stretching), thermal, electric, and chemical. As the word *noxious* implies, however, painful sensations are elicited in healthy tissue by these various means only when the stimuli are relatively strong and potentially damaging. Pain receptors (nociceptors) in different areas, moreover, are frequently more sensitive to one type of stimulus than another; the viscera, for example, are fairly insensitive to cutting, whereas cutting the skin is usually painful.

A number of endogenous chemicals that are universally distributed and known to produce pain when applied exogenously have been implicated as the physiologic mediators of pain. The most important of these are serotonin (5-hydroxytryptamine, 5-HT), histamine, and bradykinin. These chemicals, known as algesic substances, are released soon after injury and activate rather specific chemically sensitive nociceptors. The prostaglandins, a complex group of fatty acids that do not themselves cause pain, play an important role in its modulation. The prostaglandins are generated from precursors in the cell membrane and these are released in response to noxious stimuli. The released prostaglandins, in turn, sensitize the nociceptors to the algesic substances.

The inclusion of the phrase 'leading to evasive action' in the Webster definition acknowledges that the total phenomenon of pain involves more than the physiology of the perception of pain – the awareness of a painful stimulus. It also involves the reaction to the stimulus. The physiology of pain perception is complex, since it involves discriminative capacity to identify the location, the onset, the intensity and the duration as well as the physical characteristics of the eliciting stimulus. Yet the physiology of the perception of pain may be almost the same in all mammals. But the reaction to pain is highly individualized in humans. It is determined by social mores, by the psychic state of the individual, by emotions, and by the individual's interpretation of the painful stimulus in terms of past and present events. The complete pattern of response to painful stimuli is, to some extent, also learned behavior, unlike pain perception, which is innate. Children, for example, react to pain much as their parents do. Animals kept isolated during the period of weaning to adulthood and deprived of normal sensory and social experiences learn very slowly, or not at all, to avoid painful stimuli after their release into a normal environment. Litter mates reared normally learn quickly to avoid the same painful stimuli. The reaction to pain is also influenced by the significance of the pain to the individuals. Athletes, for instance, who suffer injuries during a competition have shown a remarkable ability to postpone reaction to the painful stimulus until the excitement of the competition is over.

Since pain is such a complex phenomenon, it should be obvious that there are many ways to relieve pain and that the means to be used depend upon its cause – if it can be identified:

1. Removal of the cause: e.g. restoration or extraction of an aching tooth; neutralization of gastric acid in peptic ulcer.

2. Using physical measures: e.g. the application of heat, cold or pressure to a painful area. This type of procedure takes advantage of the fact that pain impulses can be modified and decreased through the generation of other concomitant stimuli, for example, the application of a liniment as a counterirritant.

3. By distraction of attention to the painful stimulus: e.g. the use of auditory stimuli – stereophonic music, sounds resembling a waterfall – in dental surgery. The converse is also true; i.e. the absence of distracting environmental stimuli enhances the perception of pain. This is apparent to anyone who has gone to bed unaware of an aching muscle or tooth and then gradually begins to perceive the painful condition.

4. By hypnotic suggestion or acupuncture.

5. By the use of drugs, including pharmacologically inactive substances, i.e. placebos (cf. pp. 282–284). Any drug that can alter the physiology or the subjective appreciation of pain can give relief from pain. Thus analgesia or the relief of pain can be effected anywhere along the pain pathways – in the pathways involved either in the perception of, or in the reaction to, pain.

    Perception – the awareness of a painful stimulus – is not dependent on consciousness but is dependent on intact afferent pathways: on receptors and sensory nerves conducting the impulses to the brain and the thalamus, where perception occurs. If a drug acts at any point along this pathway to interrupt the transfer of information to the brain, then pain cannot be perceived.

    The reaction to pain – the 'pain experience' – is a much more complex phenomenon requiring consciousness and occurring at the highest level of the brain – the cortex. Here, too, drugs can offer relief by altering the response to pain. Thus the use of agents that relieve anxiety – the anti-anxiety agents – can lower the subject's reaction to pain.

The following sections discuss the principal classes of drugs used to treat pain. We start with those agents that alter the perception of pain: (1) the local anesthetics that block nerve conduction and prevent afferent impulses from reaching the central nervous system (CNS); (2) the nonopioid, antipyretic-analgesics that inhibit perception by peripheral actions at receptors as well as by actions within the CNS. We then consider the opioid (previously termed 'narcotic') analgesics that interfere relatively selectively with the reaction to painful stimuli. Finally, we discuss ethanol and general anesthetic agents that nonselectively alter perception and reaction to painful stimuli by their general CNS depressant action.

LOCAL ANESTHETICS

I. Definition. Local anesthetics are drugs that produce a reversible loss of sensitivity to pain in the restricted area to which they are applied.

II. Chemistry. The clinically useful *injectable* local anesthetics are, almost without exception, *amines*. The structural configuration most consistently associated with effective agents is that of an *aliphatic* chain of two or more carbons, one end of which bears a hydrocarbon nucleus and the other an amino group. The link between the aliphatic chain and the hydrocarbon nucleus is either an ester or an amide group:

$$R_1 - (CH_2)_n - N \left\langle \begin{array}{l} R_2 \text{ (alkyl group)} \\ \\ R_3 \text{ (hydrogen or alkyl group)} \end{array} \right.$$

hydrocarbon   amine
nucleus

The hydrocarbon nucleus, usually a substituted benzene ring, provides the lipid solubility essential for penetration into nerves; the amino group provides the water solubility necessary for gaining access to the neuron.

III. Pharmacodynamics

A. Site and Mechanism of Action. The site of action is the nerve fiber. Local anesthetics act by reversibly blocking nerve conduction – by inhibiting impulse transmission along the nerve(s) from the point of drug application to the organs, tissues or other nerves that are usually stimulated by the blocked nerve(s). Local anesthetics produce this inhibition of impulse transmission by blocking the entry of sodium through sodium channels that is essential for impulse transmission.

B. Local Actions

1. **Local Anesthetic Activity.** The selectivity of action of the local anesthetics is the result of the differential sensitivity of nerve fibers of varying size; in general, nonmyelinated fibers of small diameter are more susceptible to blockade than larger or myelinated neurons. Consequently, after applying a local anesthetic to a mixed nerve, sensory fibers are usually blocked before motor fibers, and loss of sensory function generally occurs in the following order: pain, temperature, touch, and deep pressure.

2. **Effect on Local Blood Vessels**
   a. Arteriolar vasoconstriction with cocaine.
   b. Arteriolar vasodilatation with all other agents.

C. Systemic Actions

1. **On Cardiovascular System**
   a. Can produce a fall in blood pressure.
   b. Can slow impulse conduction in heart muscle. This property is of practical importance since some local anesthetics are used to suppress cardiac arrhythmias.

2. **On CNS.** Involves both stimulation and depression. Stimulation may be manifested by restlessness, apprehension, tremors, which may progress to convulsions. Central stimulation is followed by depression, and death is usually due to respiratory failure.

IV. Fate in the Body
  A. Absorption. Dependent on mode of administration, on physicochemical properties of individual agent and on presence of vasoconstricting agents.
  B. Distribution. No selective deposition in tissues; cross placenta.
  C. Biotransformation. See Chapter 8.
  D. Excretion. Metabolites and unchanged portion of drug are excreted in urine.
V. Modes of Administration
  A. Topical or Surface. Application of solutions, ointments, or sprays to skin or mucous membranes; blocks nerve fiber terminals.
  B. Infiltration. Injection into the intradermal layer or subcutaneous tissues; blocks small nerve fibers or their terminals.
  C. Nerve Block. Injection into immediate vicinity of the nerve supplying the area to be anesthetized.
  D. Spinal. Injection into the spinal fluid.
VI. Toxicity. Except for allergic or idiosyncratic reactions, is predictable and a result of overdosage. Thus, cardiovascular collapse and CNS stimulation and depression with respiratory failure may be expected as the toxic effects of overdosage.
VII. Commonly Used Agents
  A. Amides
    Lidocaine
    Dibucaine
    Prilocaine
    Bupivacaine
  B. Esters
    Procaine
    Tetracaine
    Benzocaine – lacks terminal amino group and used only topically.

ANALGESICS

I. Nonopioid Analgesics
  A. General Considerations. An analgesic drug is a substance that, through its action upon the nervous system, serves to reduce or abolish suffering from pain without producing unconsciousness. An antipyretic drug is a substance that reduces an elevated body temperature.

    All of the drugs listed below possess antipyretic and analgesic activity; they are frequently referred to as antipyretic-analgesics. With the exception of acetaminophen, they also belong to the class of agents known as nonsteroidal anti-inflammatory drugs (NSAIDs), which also includes drugs used to treat rheumatoid conditions and gout. They all share the ability to inhibit the conversions of unesterified fatty acids, such as arachidonic acid, to prostaglandins, thromboxanes, and prostacyclins.

The prostaglandins are naturally occurring acidic lipids that play an important role in mediating the inflammatory response.

1. **Derivatives of salicylic acid**
   a. Acetylsalicylic acid (aspirin).
   b. Methylsalicylate, used only topically.
2. **Acetaminophen** (paracetamol, TYLENOL, TEMPRA, APAP).
3. **Propionic acid derivatives**
   a. Ibuprofen (MOTRIN).
   b. Naproxen (NAPROSYN, ALEVE).
   c. Fenoprofen (NALFON).
4. **Cyclooxygenase-2 (COX-2) inhibitors**
   b. Celecoxib (CELEBREX).
   c. Rofecoxib (VIOXX)

B. **Mechanism of Analgesic Action.** The nonopioid analgesics alleviate pain by acting both in the CNS and at the periphery; the primary site of action is peripheral and at the nociceptor level to modify the cause of pain at the site where the pain originates. The sensation of pain is believed to be associated with the liberation or generation of endogenous substances, such as the prostaglandins, in response to other endogenous compounds like bradykinin. The salicylates inhibit the activity of cyclooxygenase (COX) and thereby suppress the synthesis of prostaglandins and, as a result, prevent the sensitization of pain receptors. The mechanism of action of other antipyretic analgesics is essentially the same as that of the salicylates.

However, the discovery of several subtypes of COX, particularly COX-1 and COX-2, has helped to explain the differences among the NSAIDs with regard to selectivity and the side-effects produced. The COX-1 subtype is expressed in many tissues, including the stomach, colon, kidneys and platelets, and may play a protective role in these tissues. The subtype COX-2 is the mediator of pain and inflammation.

The salicylates and the propionic acid derivatives, preferentially inhibit COX-1, but show variable selectivity for COX-1 over COX-2. Aspirin has a COX-1/COX-2 potency ratio of greater than 50, but for naproxen the ratio is about 1. The newer agents, such as celecoxib, are much more selective inhibitors of COX-2; they are equally as effective as the older agents, but have a greater margin of safety. Acetaminophen, which poorly inhibits COX-1 and COX-2, has been shown to inhibit a newly discovered cyclooxygenase, COX-3, found in the brain. This may explain its weak anti-inflammatory effects (see below).

The NSAIDs fulfill at least *one criterion of the ideal analgesic*: they have *selectivity* of action. In analgesic doses they cause no mental disturbance, anesthesia or changes in modalities of sensation other than pain. But, they are *not ideal* analgesics because they usually relieve pain of only low intensity, whether localized or widespread in origin, particularly pain of headache, muscles or joints, or other pains arising from external structures rather than from viscera.

C. **Mechanism of Antipyretic Effect.** Normal body heat is maintained within limits by a balance between the *heat-producing* and *heat-dissipating* mechanisms of the body. The peripheral mechanisms of production and loss of body heat are regulated by certain nuclei in the hypothalamus (cf. p. 31). The action of the antipyretics is mainly on the hypothalamus and not peripherally on blood vessels or sweat glands. Evidence for this is that high sectioning of the spinal cord prevents the antipyretic drugs from lowering the temperature of fevered animals. There is also evidence to indicate that certain fevers are caused by endogenous substances (pyrogens) released from white blood cells; these pyrogens act on the temperature-regulating center in the hypothalamus. The temperature-elevating effect of pyrogens is inhibited by the antipyretic analgesics, probably by inhibition of the synthesis of prostaglandins whose synthesis is stimulated by pyrogens.

The antipyretic action is usually rapid and effective in *febrile* patients but is demonstrated *rarely* when the body temperature is *normal.*

The antipyretics act to increase heat loss in febrile individuals by:
1. Increasing peripheral blood flow through peripheral vasodilatation;
2. Producing a shift in water to the bloodstream with a corresponding dilution of the blood;
3. Increasing perspiration.

The use of aspirin as an antipyretic is to be avoided in children with chickenpox or influenza because of the association with Reye's syndrome, a rare but often fatal consequence of infection with various strains of influenza virus or chickenpox virus *(varicella).*

D. **Mechanism of Anti-inflammatory Effect.** Certain of these drugs reduce the inflammatory response to a variety of stimuli, whether mechanical, chemical, or immunologic. Each of these stimuli induces the production of the enzyme COX-2, important in the synthesis of prostaglandins. All NSAIDs except acetaminophen inhibit COX-2, thereby reducing inflammation. These drugs are quite useful in treating diseases such as rheumatoid arthritis and the inflammation produced by injuries.

E. **The Salicylates (prototype, aspirin).** Aspirin has several pharmacologic actions in addition to its analgesic and antipyretic actions. Some of these provide the basis for additional therapeutic uses of aspirin, and others are largely responsible for the toxicities seen in some people.
1. **Anti-inflammatory Action.** The salicylates reduce the pain, immobility, swelling, and inflammation of the joints in rheumatoid arthritis. Due to gastrointestinal side-effects, their use has been replaced by more selective NSAIDs.
2. **Antiplatelet Aggregation Action.** Aspirin is a very selective inhibitor of COX-1 when used at low doses. This inhibits the production of thromboxane A_2, a potent stimulant of platelet aggregation. Because of its potent and long-lasting inhibition of platelet aggregation, aspirin in low doses is now used prophylactically as an

antithrombotic drug in the prevention of arterial and venous thrombosis (associated with surgery, cardiovascular disease, transplants, etc.). Aspirin has been shown to reduce the incidence in men of myocardial infarction or death in patients with unstable angina. It is also effective in reducing the incidence of stroke, especially after heart surgery, a heart attack, or a previous stroke.

3. **Side-effects.** The side effects of aspirin can be serious, especially when taken over long periods of time.

   a. **Gastrointestinal effects.** The commonest unwanted effects include gastric irritation, nausea and vomiting. Aspirin and other NSAIDs cause gastrointestinal blood loss, the severity of which depends on the dose and the formulation of the drug. Aspirin therapy of 1–3 g/day produces blood loss of 1–6 ml/day in 50% of the population, not a serious clinical problem. However, gastric ulceration and severe hemorrhage can occur, and it is estimated that patients who take NSAIDs have a four- to six-fold increased risk of developing peptic ulcers. The ulcerogenic effect of the salicylates and other NSAIDs is due mainly to inhibition of COX-1, which produces the prostaglandins that normally have a protective effect on the gastrointestinal wall. Proton-pump inhibitors and H_2 antagonists are effective in preventing NSAID-related ulcers. Misoprostol, a prostaglandin that maintains the integrity of the gastrointestinal lining, is effective as well, but causes diarrhea.

   b. **Prolonged bleeding time at ordinary analgesic doses.** Aspirin prolongs bleeding time by inhibiting the normal platelet-induced acceleration of plasma coagulation. This inhibition results, at least partly, from a block in the synthesis of thromboxane A_2. Other NSAIDs inhibit platelet aggregation but none do so as selectively as aspirin. Furthermore, the effect of aspirin, unlike the other NSAIDs, persists considerably beyond the time that the drug has been eliminated from the body. A single analgesic dose of aspirin (300 mg), for example, can double bleeding time for as long as 4–7 days (the lifespan of a platelet). The use of aspirin must, therefore, be avoided in patients with bleeding disorders and in patients prior to surgery.

   c. **Effects on respiration: disturbances in acid-base balance.** Salicylates stimulate respiration directly and indirectly. These effects are of paramount importance because they contribute to the serious acid-base balance disturbances that characterize poisoning by this class of compounds. The direct effect is produced by stimulation of the respiratory center in the medulla, and the indirect effect is a result of alterations in the metabolism of carbohydrates, proteins and fat.

   d. **Salicylism.** In addition to these effects of salicylate overdosage, there may be other effects which can jeopardize the patient. These take the form of a series of reactions called salicylism – resembling the side-effects seen with large doses of quinine. The symptoms are headache, dizziness, ringing in the ears (tinnitus), dimness of vision and mental confusion. As the dosage is increased, the symptoms become more severe – there is increased CNS stimulation, which may be followed by depression, stupor and coma. These symptoms occur along with the disturbances in acid-base balance and gastrointestinal symptoms.

    e. **Allergic-like reaction.** Skin rash – most frequent; edema; asthma – less frequent, but more than 16% of asthmatics show increased symptoms after aspirin. Cross-sensitivity occurs with all NSAID drugs.

  4. **Fate of Salicylates**

    a. **Absorption** (see pp. 85, 94). Rapidly and chiefly absorbed from the upper intestinal tract. Absorption of both Na-salicylate and aspirin occurs from the stomach itself, particularly if the pH is low. This is, again, an example of the fact that the nonionized form is more quickly absorbed. However, absorption is faster for both these agents in the upper part of the small intestine.

    b. **Biotransformation** (see pp. 159, 161, 166, 235–237).

F. Acetaminophen. Acetaminophen is an analgesic and antipyretic agent with little or no anti-inflammatory activity; it inhibits preferentially COX-3. It is similar to aspirin in analgesic potency and duration of action. Unlike aspirin this drug does not affect the gastric mucosa, platelets or uric acid excretion. It is unlikely to cause allergic symptoms in an aspirin-intolerant individual. The most serious consequence of acute overdosage is hepatic necrosis caused by minor metabolites of this drug. Acetaminophen is primarily biotransformed by sulfate and glucuronide conjugation. The minor pathway, mediated by microsomal enzymes, results in a quinone which reacts with hepatic glutathione to form mercapturates. If glutathione stores are depleted (a common occurrence in alcoholics), the quinone binds covalently to cellular macromolecules, which results in hepatic toxicity. Recommended treatment of acetaminophen poisoning includes administration of acetylcysteine (MUCOMYST). This compound prevents hepatotoxicity, possibly by repletion of hepatic glutathione content or by acting as conjugating substrate for the acetaminophen quinone. Chronic use of acetaminophen, as well as other nonopioid analgesics, can result in renal injury in the susceptible individual.

G. Propionic Acid Derivatives. The pharmacodynamic properties of the propionic acid derivatives do not differ significantly from each other or from those of aspirin; all have anti-inflammatory, antipyretic and analgesic activity. All these compounds alter platelet function, prolong bleeding time and produce gastrointestinal side-effects, although these effects are usually less severe with the propionic acid derivatives than with aspirin at effective anti-inflammatory doses. Naproxen is about 20 times more potent than aspirin, ibuprofen, or fenoprofen in inhibiting the biosynthesis of prostaglandins and it has a longer duration of action. It is the NSAID most preferred by patients with rheumatoid arthritis.

II. Opioid Analgesics
    A. Definition (see pp. 406–407).

    B. Agents (see p. 407).

    C. Pharmacodynamics. All of the opioids share the same pharmacologic properties and differ from each other only quantitatively with respect to analgesic potency, duration of action, etc. The opioids exert a number of extremely diverse effects on most of the systems and tissues in the body. Their major effects are on the CNS and gastrointestinal tract. Morphine is the prototype of the opioids.

        1. Analgesic Effect. Highly selective; little, if any, alteration of any other sensory phenomena, and analgesia occurs without loss of consciousness.

            a. Elevation in threshold for pain perception demonstrated experimentally in both humans and animals.

            b. Alteration in the reaction to pain; relief of anxiety, tension and fear associated with pain (see p. 408).

            c. Site of action – at a large number of widely but unevenly distributed sites within the brain and spinal cord, particularly in those areas or pathways associated with the phenomenon of pain and the regulation of mood and behavior. Actions on the reticular activating system are important since this system integrates the responses to pain through its projections to the cortex (see pp. 397–398). Sites of action outside the CNS are primarily in the small intestine.

            d. Mechanism of action – interaction with specific receptors in the CNS and other tissues (μ, δ, and κ, in the family of G-protein-coupled receptors). The binding of an opioid agonist to its receptor initiates the sequence of events that leads to the observed effect. The stereospecificity of the binding of opioid analgesics accounts for their selectivity of action. There is also very good correlation between the analgesic potency of the various opioids and their ability to bind to receptors. The sites to which the opioids bind are the receptors for endogenous ligands, the enkephalins, that produce effects similar to those of morphine (see also p. 410).

            e. The analgesic effect cannot be separated from the sedative effect because of the overall CNS depression produced by the opioids. Sedative effects are most profound in patients in bed at time of medication. The decrease in anxiety and relief of distress may produce euphoria in some patients.

2. **Respiratory Effects.** The respiratory center is very sensitive to morphine and its surrogates; severe respiratory depression is rarely seen with clinical doses; death from morphine overdosage is due to respiratory depression.

3. **Cardiovascular Effects.** Little effect on blood pressure or heart rate in the supine patient given low therapeutic doses. Most opioid analgesics decrease the capacity of the cardiovascular system to respond to stress of gravitational shifts. Thus, when the supine patient assumes head-up position, there may be a fall in blood pressure (orthostatic or postural hypotension), and fainting may occur. The release of histamine by morphine and other opioids may play a role in hypotension.

4. **Antitussive Effects.** All opioids can suppress the cough reflex by suppressing the cough center in the medulla. Codeine is the drug of choice in the United States. Dextromethorphan (ROMILAR) is a synthetic compound that is a good antitussive and exhibits no analgesic activity or other effects of the opioid analgesics since it does not act at opioid receptors.

5. **Stimulatory Effects**
   a. **Nausea and vomiting.** This is a major side-effect of opioid therapy that is caused by direct stimulation of the chemoreceptor trigger zone (CTZ) in medulla. After initial stimulation, morphine will depress CTZ.
   b. **Miosis** (pin-point pupils). Caused by stimulation of the pupillo-constrictor centers of the motor nerve controlling pupillary diameter. Miosis is characteristic of, and diagnostic for, intake of all opioid analgesics except meperidine (pethidine, DEMEROL). Little, if any tolerance develops to this effect.
   c. **Gastrointestinal tract.** Marked constipation due to contraction of sphincters, increased muscular tone and decreased propulsive movements; delays stomach emptying. Tolerance does not develop to these effects.
   d. **Effects on biliary tract.** Contraction of bile duct and increased pressure in biliary system; opioid analgesics, therefore, are contraindicated in gallbladder disease.

6. **Miscellaneous Effects**
   a. **Constriction of bronchi;** contraindicated in severe asthma.
   b. **Renal effects.** In therapeutic doses, no significant effect; with larger doses there is an antidiuretic effect mediated in part by the stimulation of pituitary secretion of the antidiuretic hormone (ADH) and in part by an increased tone of the bladder musculature which results in the retention of urine.

D. **Fate in the Body**
   1. **Absorption.** Morphine is well absorbed but rapidly conjugated in liver so oral bioavailability is low. Codeine is well absorbed and less

rapidly biotransformed in liver (to morphine); therefore a large proportion of oral dose of codeine reaches systemic circulation.

2. **Distribution.** Morphine is rapidly distributed. Although only a small percentage of the total dose reaches the brain, only a little is needed for CNS effects; heroin and codeine are more completely distributed to brain.

3. **Biotransformation.** (see Table 8-1). Conjugation with glucuronic acid is the main pathway for morphine.

4. **Excretion.** 7–10% of total morphine excreted in feces, remainder in urine.

E. **Toxicity**

1. **Acute.** Characterized by coma, pin-point pupils, severe respiratory depression. Treatment is usually with opioid antagonists, compounds that are specific competitive pharmacologic antagonists such as naloxone.

2. **Chronic** (see pp. 407–409).

ALCOHOL AND GENERAL ANESTHETIC AGENTS

I. General Considerations

Changes in the excitability of the central nervous system (CNS) occur in a gradual continuous fashion; decreases from normal progress from sedation to coma and increases in excitability range from mild hyperexcitability to severe convulsions. Drugs that have the ability to produce graded CNS depression with the administration of progressively larger doses are classified as *general depressants of the CNS.* (Analogously, drugs that increase excitability on this continuum as a function of dose are called *general CNS stimulants* [see Appendix 8]). The action of the general CNS depressants is relatively *nonselective* with respect to neuron type or brain region, affecting total brain function.

The ability to depress excitability at all levels of the CNS is a property shared by many compounds of diverse chemical structure including methanol and ethanol and other aliphatic alcohols; gaseous and volatile anesthetics; and intravenously administered anesthetics such as barbiturates and the nonbarbiturate sedative-hypnotic drugs. However, the mechanism by which the neuronal depression is brought about by the agents classified as general depressants of the CNS, the alcohols and the gaseous and volatile anesthetics, is not entirely clear. The most recent evidence indicates that each of these general CNS depressants enhances GABA neurotransmission (cf. Appendix 6). Thus, they can inhibit neuronal excitation via interactions with specific receptors as well as other components of neuronal membranes. In addition, various physical or metabolic effects, particularly inhibition of either energy consumption or production or both, have been implicated but not proved to be the basis of the neuronal depression. When an excitatory effect on some function is observed following low doses of a CNS depressant, in general it too is the result of neuronal depression – but of an inhibitory system. Depression of a system inhibitory to a particular function increases the level of excitability of other neurons involved in that function. The so-called stimulant effect of ethanol is an example of this release from inhibition (cf. p. 405).

The effects of the general CNS depressant drugs are additive not only with each other but also with the physiologic state at the time of drug administration. A given amount of ethanol, for example, will produce less sedation and drowsiness when consumed at a party than when imbibed in a quiet, nonsocial environment. The effects of the general CNS depressants can also be antagonized by other drugs, but this antagonism is physiologic rather than pharmacologic (cf. p. 307). Antagonism between the stimulants and depressants is brought about by opposite effects on the same physiologic function but not by opposition at the same site(s) of action. As a result, normal function cannot be entirely restored. The practice of using CNS stimulants to counteract the severe respiratory depression of intoxication by general depressants has been largely discontinued; measures that stress intensive supportive care have met with much greater success in such poisonings (cf. p. 355).

Individual general CNS depressant drugs differ from one another primarily with respect to potency. For instance, the concentration of anesthetic in the blood that is needed to produce surgical anesthesia is much less for isoflurane than for nitrous oxide. However, it is important to note that although the potency of a drug is a relatively unimportant characteristic (cf. pp. 194–196), the lack of potency may limit the maximum effect that can be achieved therapeutically. The low potency of nitrous oxide, for example, limits its usefulness as a safe, general anesthetic gas; the concentration that must be inhaled in order to produce anesthesia does not provide for adequate oxygenation. Consequently, nitrous oxide can be used for only very short procedures or in conjunction with other more potent agents.

The pattern of events that occurs as an individual is exposed to progressively increasing concentrations of a general CNS depressant is fairly predictable. The signs and symptoms that appear with increasing depth of depression permit the anesthesiologist to determine when conditions are favorable for surgical procedure and when a reaction constitutes a danger signal. The pattern of deepening CNS depression differs in specific ways for specific agents. But the 'stages' and 'signs' of anesthesia represent a framework upon which to build the exceptions for individual agents. The pattern of depression based on the signs produced by the action of anesthetics on different excitable tissues is arbitrarily divided into the following stages of anesthesia:

Stage I – Analgesia. The first stage is characterized by analgesia and amnesia and lasts until consciousness is lost. It is associated with depression of the ascending reticular activating system and of the relay systems in the thalamus. The areas of the brain concerned with message storage and retrieval are also susceptible to depression at this stage.

Stage II – Excitement. This stage, characterized by loss of consciousness and control, begins with unconsciousness and ends with the loss of the eyelid reflex.

The excitement of this stage involves the depression of additional areas in the brainstem and cerebellum. Purposeless movements and vomiting may occur; pupils are usually widely dilated, there is hyperreaction to stimuli and breathing is irregular. This stage is neither useful nor desirable clinically.

Stage III – Surgical Anesthesia. This stage, which involves progressive loss of reflexes and muscle tone, ends with cessation of spontaneous respiration. It is usually divided into four phases which are differentiated on the basis of the character of respiration, the presence or absence of certain reflexes, the eyeball movements and pupillary diameter.

Stage IV – Respiratory Paralysis. Complete respiratory paralysis occurs, which leads to and ends with complete circulatory failure.

II. Aliphatic Alcohols

A. **Definition.** The generic term *alcohol* designates an important class of organic compounds that are hydroxyl (–OH) derivatives of aliphatic (straight-chain) hydrocarbons. The compounds may have one or more hydroxyl groups. The important compounds in this class include methanol, ethanol, ethylene glycol (dihydroxy) and glycerol (the trihydroxy compound derived from the digestion of fats). When the simple term *alcohol* is used, it ordinarily refers to ethanol (ethyl alcohol).

B. **Physicochemical Properties.** The physicochemical properties of the aliphatic alcohols are extremely well correlated with their pharmacologic activity and their fate in the body (cf. pp. 62–63).

Ethanol is a universal solvent; it is able to dissolve substances that are soluble in water and in organic solvents. As a result, ethanol is widely used as a pharmaceutical agent in preparations of pure drugs from crude extracts and in compounding of solutions for medicinal use.

C. **Pharmacology**

1. **Actions on the CNS.** Although ethanol is not used as a general anesthetic agent, the events that occur as an individual is exposed to progressively increasing concentrations are similar to the pattern elicited by general anesthetics. The stages of neurological and behavioral changes exemplified by ethanol intoxication are presented in Table A-4-1 along with the blood alcohol content associated with each level of depression. The degree of CNS depression is directly related to the blood alcohol content because equilibrium between blood and brain tissue occurs very rapidly.

   The pharmacologic significance of ethanol lies not only in its direct action upon the individual who consumes it, but also in its indirect action in decreasing the ability of that individual to carry on societal responsibilities. Such considerations are of particular importance from the standpoint of operation of an automobile (cf. pp. 233–235). Impairment of visual acuity and reaction time occur in early stage I, at blood levels of ethanol much below 100 mg/100 ml, the level above which an individual is considered legally intoxicated in most states in the United States.

There is considerable evidence that the actions of alcohol to depress neuronal activity are based on its ability to enhance GABA neurotransmission by increasing the function of GABA receptors. In addition, alcohol blocks the function of the N-methyl-d-aspartate (NMDA) subtype of glutamate receptors, preventing excitatory neurotransmission. Its action at these two receptors forms the basis for many of the intoxicating effects of alcohol.

2. **Actions on Other Systems**

   a. The gastrointestinal tract. Hypertonic solutions stimulate acid production in the stomach, delay gastric emptying and promote injury to surface epithelium. Chronic alcoholics have malabsorption of many substances including fat, folic acid, thiamine and vitamin B_{12}.

   b. The liver. The chronic use of alcohol is associated with the accumulation of fat in the liver. There is considerable evidence to indicate that this deposition of fat is an indirect result of the biotransformation of ethanol itself. The oxidation of ethanol takes place by a series of steps (cf. pp. 232–234), and in each of these steps some energy is made available to the body – the oxidation of 1 g of ethanol yielding a total of 7 calories. The energy liberated by the metabolism of ethanol can be utilized by the body in the same way as energy from the oxidation of food substances. In the sense that ethanol is a source of energy it, too, is a food, but ethanol supplies only one compound that can enter into normal anabolic reactions – acetate. Some of the acetate required by the body is furnished by the oxidation of fatty acids. The oxidation of ethanol decreases the need for oxidation of fatty acids and promotes the preferential synthesis of the fatty acids to fats. Thus in addition to the nutritional deficiencies commonly associated with excessive or chronic use of alcohol, alcohol itself may be a factor in the etiology of alcoholic liver disease.

   The nonmicrosomal enzyme alcohol dehydrogenase is predominantly responsible for the oxidation of ethanol (cf. pp. 171, 232) and for the time course of ethanol elimination (cf. pp. 232–234). However, up to 20% of the ethanol in the body may be oxidized through an alternative pathway mediated by microsomal CYP450 (cf. pp. 167–171). Although this pathway plays only a minor role in the elimination of ethanol, it takes on considerable importance during chronic ethanol consumption or multiple drug use. The CYP450 activity is inducible and its activity can be increased by the chronic administration of ethanol itself or by other drugs. As a consequence, during chronic ethanol consumption there is an increase in the rate of metabolism of that fraction of ethanol oxidized by CYP450. This can

explain a part of the tolerance to ethanol that develops in alcoholics. Chronic consumption of ethanol can also induce other
microsomal enzymes and thereby accelerate the rate of biotransformation of other drugs such as diazepam and pentobarbital.
This can explain the well-known fact that alcoholics often have
an increased tolerance to a variety of drugs. This increased tolerance, however, is only seen in the *sober* alcoholic. In the presence of ethanol the activity of a variety of microsomal enzymes is
inhibited rather than accelerated. Thus the drinking alcoholic as
well as the inebriated individual is *more* susceptible to the effects
of other CNS depressants. The effects produced by the coadmin-
istration of ethanol and diazepam (VALIUM), for example, are
synergistic (cf. pp. 306–307); i.e. the degree of CNS depression
observed is greater than the algebraic sum of the individual
effects of ethanol and the benzodiazepine. This can be attributed
to the inhibition by ethanol of the biotransformation of
diazepam and their abilities to enhance GABA neurotransmission by different mechanisms.

    c.   The kidney. Ethanol produces diuresis by inhibiting the secre-
tion of antidiuretic hormone (cf. p. 142).

  3. **Fate in the Body**

    a.   Absorption (see pp. 61, 89).

    b.   Distribution. Ethanol distributes very rapidly to the total body
water and equilibrates very rapidly with its target organs. Therefore, ethanol blood concentration may be used to estimate the
level of ethanol in the brain. The equilibrium between the concentration of ethanol in the expired air and in blood is also
attained rapidly and, thus, ethanol blood levels can be estimated
by measuring its concentration in expired air.

    c.   Elimination (see pp. 232–233).

D. **Pharmacologic Actions of Other Aliphatic Alcohols.** The ability of the
aliphatic alcohols to produce CNS depression increases with increasing
molecular weight and is directly proportional to their lipid solubility (cf.
Table A-4-1) as well as their ability to enhance GABA receptor function.
Methanol, the first member of the homologous series, is a less potent
depressant than ethanol but is potentially more toxic because methanol
ingestion can lead to blindness (cf. p. 361).

Table A-4.1. Stages of behavioral neurological changes exemplified by alcohol intoxication

Whiskey dose (oz/hr)	Blood alcohol (mg/100 ml)	Function impaired	Physical state	Neurologic status			
				Conditioned reflexes	Superficial[1] reflexes	Deep[2] reflexes	Spontaneous function
1–4	0–100	Judgment; fine coordination	Happy; boastful; 'sociable'	+++→++	+++	+++	+++
4–12	100–300	Motor coordination; static reflexes; pain perception	Staggers; slurred speech; analgesia; amnesia	++→+	+++	+++	+++
12–16	300–400	Voluntary response to sensation	Emotional; restless; helpless	+→0	++++	++++	++++
16–24	400–600	Sensation voluntary movement; progressive loss of protective reflexes	Comatose	0	+−++	+++	+++
				0	0→+	+−++	+++
				0	0→+	0→+	++
				0	0	0	+
24–30	600–900	Spontaneous respiration; cardiovascular regulation	Dead	0	0	0	0

+ + + = essentially normal function.
+ + + + = hyperexcitability; increased response.
+ + or + = progressively decreasing functional response.
0 = total absence of function.
[1] e.g. eyelid reflex.
[2] e.g. pupillary response to light.

Appendix 6
Drugs for Producing Sedation and Sleep

I. **Definitions**
   A. A **sedative** is a drug that produces a mild degree of nonselective depression of the central nervous system (CNS) by decreasing the response of an individual to all sensory modalities.
   B. A **hypnotic** is a drug that produces more nonselective depression of the CNS than the sedative; it induces a state resembling natural sleep.

II. **General Considerations**
   The difference between sedatives and hypnotics is only quantitative. The different effects are a function of the dose of the drug administered. In theory, these agents have in common the ability to produce all degrees of depression of the CNS, starting with mild sedation and progressing through hypnosis, anesthesia, coma and death from respiratory paralysis. However, the sedative-hypnotic drugs used today (e.g. benzodiazepines, imidazopyridines) are quite safe, unlike their predecessors, the barbiturates. The designation of a particular agent for use as a sedative or a hypnotic is determined by its physicochemical and pharmacokinetic properties.

III. **The Benzodiazepines**
   A. **Physicochemical and Pharmacokinetic Properties**
      As a class, the benzodiazepines are highly lipophilic, with a few exceptions. The general structure includes a benzene ring fused to a seven-membered diazepine ring. An aryl ring in the number five position is required for activity. Several chemical substituents can be added to the aryl ring to provide differences in lipid solubility, half-life and the presence or absence of active metabolites. Benzodiazepines used as sedatives and hypnotics have short, intermediate and long durations of action:

Short:	Triazolam (HALCION)
	Midazolam (VERSED)
Intermediate:	Temazepam (RESTORIL)
	Flunitrazepam (ROHYPNOL)*
Long:	Diazepam (VALIUM)
	Chloridiazepoxide (LIBRIUM)

While the degree of lipid solubility determines how fast the drug enters and leaves the CNS, it is not the sole determinant of the duration of action of the drug. For example, diazepam is highly lipophilic and enters and leaves the brain rapidly, yet it has a relatively long duration of action. The longer duration of action usually reflects the metabolism of the benzodiazepine to an active metabolite (e.g. nordiazepam is an active metabolite of diazepam with a $t_{1/2}$ of up to 100 hours). Those benzodiazepines with shorter duration of action are generally more water-soluble, have no active metabolites and are metabolized by conjugation reactions directly. The benzodiazepines with a shorter half-life are more useful sedative/hypnotics, while those with a longer half-life are more useful as anxiolytics.

B. **Pharmacological Properties**

Benzodiazepines have several pharmacological properties including anxiolytic, sedative, hypnotic, anticonvulsant, muscle relaxant and amnesic actions. As discussed above, the physicochemical properties determine the most appropriate clinical use. As sedative and hypnotic drugs, the benzodiazepines replaced the barbiturates, which suffered from a low therapeutic index and a high abuse potential. Although all of the benzodiazepines are capable of progressively depressing the CNS as the dose is increased, they have an extremely wide margin of safety and a remarkably low capacity to produce profound respiratory depression (unless combined with alcohol); hypnotic doses are without effect on respiration.

The mechanism of action of benzodiazepines is clearly understood, although a specific site of action to cause sedation cannot be identified. Benzodiazepines bind to sites on γ-aminobutyric acid (GABA) receptors; activation of these sites potentiates the neuronal inhibition mediated by GABA to produce sedative, hypnotic, anti-anxiety, muscle relaxant, amnesic, and anticonvulsant activity. Clinical use of these agents depends not only on their pharmacokinetics but also on selectivity of action. For example, newer benzodiazepines have been developed to be more selective for anxiolytic and anticonvulsant activity at doses that do not produce sedation.

*This is marketed only outside the United States, but is used in combination with alcohol in the United States as the 'date-rape' drug, 'Roofies'.

C. Tolerance and Dependence

Tolerance develops to the sedating effects of benzodiazepines and dependence (physiologic) develops with long-term use. Withdrawal symptoms can be serious upon discontinuation of the drug, and the severity of the syndrome is related to the length of exposure and dosage used. Thus discontinuation of benzodiazepines must be controlled with a slow taper. Although the potential for abuse is considerably lower than that for barbiturates, their combination with alcohol produces synergistic actions and can result in coma.

The sedation produced by benzodiazepines can be reversed with a competitive antagonist, flumazenil. This is useful after surgery, when benzodiazepines may be used to produce sedation, and after a benzodiazepine overdose. Flumazenil is not effective at reversing sedation produced by other CNS depressants, including alcohol, barbiturates or antidepressants.

IV. Non-benzodiazepines

A. Agents. A new class of compounds with hypnotic properties has been developed with a structure distinct from benzodiazepines. These include zolpidem (AMBIEN, an imidazopyridine) and zaleplon (SONATA, a pyrazolopyrimidine). Although they are not benzodiazepines, they bind to benzodiazepine receptor sites on the GABA receptor, with selectivity for the subtype containing α_1 subunits (most benzodiazepines are non-selective for the various subtypes of benzodiazepine receptors). These drugs have become very popular for treating insomnia, and zolpidem is now the #1 selling hypnotic in the US and in Europe. They come close to being the ideal hypnotic drugs. They have a rapid onset and very short $t_{\frac{1}{2}}$, minimizing next day side-effects. They are tolerated very well by the elderly, who often suffer side-effects of benzodiazepines. The initial clinical trials indicated that little tolerance develops after 3 months of continuous use, but there are increasing reports indicating tolerance and the development of dependence and abuse.

V. The Barbiturates

A. General. Barbiturates have sedative/hypnotic actions but they are no longer used for treating insomnia because safer drugs have been developed, such as benzodiazepines. A few barbiturates are still used in anesthesia, such as thiopental (PENTOTHAL), and in the treatment of some forms of epilepsy, such as phenobarbital (LUMINAL). Barbiturates have a low therapeutic index; they readily depress respiration and cardiovascular function. Tolerance develops to their sedative/hypnotic effects, but not to their toxic effects. They used to be a major instrument of suicide and a leading cause of accidental poisoning. They also have a high abuse potential and cause physical dependence.

B. Mechanism of Action. Barbiturates also enhance GABA neurotransmission via an interaction with the $GABA_A$ receptor. They bind to a site on the receptor distinct from the benzodiazepine and GABA binding sites.

Barbiturates interact with all types of $GABA_A$ receptors to increase open time of GABA-gated chloride channels. This action, in turn, increases the duration of the GABA-induced inhibitory potentials. Because barbiturates act upon $GABA_A$ receptors throughout the brain, they are general CNS depressants. Their depressant actions range from mild sedation to general anesthesia, probably through depression of the reticular activating system.

Appendix 7
Drugs for Treating Mood Disorders

I. **General Considerations**

The use of drugs to treat psychiatric disorders became widespread following clinical studies in the mid-1950s with chlorpromazine which revealed its value in the treatment of psychotic states. It is estimated that about 20% of the prescriptions written in the United States today are for drugs in the treatment of *psychoses, disorders of mood,* and *anxiety*. The treatment of psychiatric disorders is complicated by uncertainties in the diagnosis and classification of the various mental illnesses. There is ample justification, however, to classify and discuss the various drugs used in these disorders under these three major categories.

II. **Antipsychotic Drugs**

These are agents used to improve mood and behavior of psychotic patients without excessive sedation. They are appropriately used in the therapy of schizophrenia and other acute psychotic illnesses. The classic 'target' symptoms that respond to antipsychotic drugs include: tension, hyperactivity, combativeness, hostility, hallucinations, delusions, insomnia, anorexia, self neglect, negativism, and seclusiveness. Clinical efficacy of the different drugs varies by individual, along with the spectrum of side-effects. The antipsychotic drugs comprise the following:

    Phenothiazine derivatives
        Chlorpromazine (THORAZINE)
        Thioridazine (MELLARIL)
    Haloperidol (HALDOL)
    Thiothixene (NAVANE)
    Atypical antipsychotics:
        Clozapine (CLOZARIL)
        Olanzapine (ZYPREXA)
        Risperidone (RISPERDAL)

A. **Phenothiazine Derivatives.** The phenothiazines not only act on the CNS but, in therapeutic doses, also exert significant effects upon other organ systems. The antipsychotic effects are attributed in part to their actions as antagonists of dopamine receptors in the brain. The phenothiazines also have important effects on the autonomic nervous system, including blockade of the actions of epinephrine and norepinephrine at sympathetic receptors and of acetylcholine at postganglionic parasympathetic receptors. This group also possesses antihistaminic and antiserotonin activity. Chlorpromazine (CPZ) is the prototype drug; it is one of the agents most widely used and differs from other phenothiazines only quantitatively with regard to primary action on the CNS and side-effects.

1. **CNS Effects**

   a. CPZ depresses the sensory input to the reticular formation and raises the threshold for stimuli impinging on the reticular formation. This sensory impairment produces a considerable degree of *sedation*. The sedative effect differs from that of the barbiturates since there is no ataxia or incoordination with CPZ and the subject can be easily aroused.

   b. Gross behavioral effects are the apparent indifference or slowing of responses to external stimuli and diminution of initiative and of anxiety without a change in the state of wakefulness or consciousness or of intellectual abilities. After single doses to normal subjects, there is impairment of performance of tasks that require attention but little effect on tests requiring intellectual function. Barbiturates affect preferentially those tasks that are dependent on intellectual functioning. On chronic administration of CPZ to patients, there is improvement in performance on tests, especially those tests requiring a great deal of attentive behavior.

   c. CPZ depresses the chemoreceptor trigger zone (CTZ) and is particularly effective against the nausea and vomiting induced by certain drugs and disease states. It is *not* effective in motion sickness.

   d. CPZ disrupts temperature-regulatory mechanisms in the hypothalamus; there is a resulting tendency for body temperature to fall if the subject is in a cool environment or rise due to high external temperature.

   e. CPZ can cause a variety of motor disorders ranging from involuntary muscle movements (tremors) to muscle weakness and fatigue. Some of these effects resemble the symptoms of Parkinson's disease. These effects result from the antagonism of dopamine, the neurotransmitter in the basal ganglia and forebrain. These symptoms are readily reversed when CPZ is discontinued.

2. **Effects on Autonomic Nervous System.** CPZ produces vasodilatation and a fall in blood pressure due to blockade of adrenergic receptors and to inhibition of hypothalamic regulatory centers. Blockade

of postganglionic parasympathetic (muscarinic) receptors results in dry mouth (inhibition of salivary secretion) and blurred vision.

3. **Other Effects**
   a. Mild antihistaminic activity.
   b. Endocrine system: CPZ reduces urinary levels of gonadotropins, estrogens and progestins. CPZ may block ovulation and induce lactation.

4. **Mechanism of Action.** The mechanism of action underlying the antipsychotic effects of CPZ and other antipsychotic drugs is not entirely clear. However, these drugs inhibit dopamine neurotransmission in several areas of the brain by blocking the D_2 subtype of dopamine receptors. Moreover, there is a strong correlation between the clinical potency of the antipyschotic drugs and their ability to bind to dopamine receptors. Their ability to block dopamine receptors may also underlie the extrapyramidal (Parkinson-like) motor side-effects that are produced by most antipsychotic agents (but see below).

5. **Side-Effects and Toxic Reactions**
   a. Many of the side-effects, such as dry mouth and muscular disorders, are due to actions described above. The most troublesome side-effect is postural hypotension; tolerance usually develops to this effect and it generally disappears after the first days of treatment.
   b. The occurrence of neurologic side-effects, particularly a Parkinsonian syndrome, is not unusual following the use of almost all antipsychotic drugs. Parkinsonian effects may be counteracted by the use of anti-Parkinsonian agents.
   c. The most dangerous effects of CPZ treatment are those resulting from allergic reactions. These include skin eruptions, disorders in blood cell formation, jaundice due to obstruction of the normal flow of bile and photosensitivity.

6. **Therapeutic Uses**
   a. For treatment of psychotic disorders such as schizophrenia.
   b. Formerly used as an anti-emetic to treat nausea and vomiting in radiation sickness and other diseases or emesis produced by drugs such as nitrogen mustards and tetracyclines.
   c. In the control of intractable hiccups (mechanism of action is unknown).

B. **Haloperidol and Thiothixene.** Similar to CPZ; no clinical advantages over phenothiazines but useful in those patients who tolerate phenothiazines poorly.

C. **Atypical Antipsychotic Drugs.** Newer antipsychotic drugs have been developed with markedly reduced extrapyramidal side-effects. These drugs include clozapine, olanzapine, risperidone, and aripiprazole. In some patients these drugs have provided superior efficacy over the traditional antipsychotic agents. Because these agents have significant interactions with receptors other than dopamine receptors, they have been termed 'atypical'.

1. **CNS Effects.** These agents produce actions in the CNS similar to other antipsychotic drugs. They improve many aspects of cognitive dysfunction in schizophrenics and improve attention and have significantly greater activity against the negative symptoms of schizophrenia than the older drugs. In addition, they have a fairly rapid onset of action (within 1–2 weeks) compared to typical antipsychotic drugs, which take at least 8 weeks to have efficacy.

2. **Mechanism of Action.** While the mechanism of action of the atypical antipsychotic drugs is not entirely clear, these compounds may produce their beneficial effects by interacting with more than one subtype of dopamine receptors and with other neurotransmitter systems. Each of these drugs interacts with enhanced antagonism at D_3, D_4, and serotonin (5-HT_2 subtype) receptors, compared to D_2 receptors. Both clozapine and olanzapine have antagonist activity at dopamine, serotonin, histamine, α-adrenergic and muscarinic receptors. The higher affinity for 5-HT_2 receptors compared to D_2 receptors might explain their increased efficacy against the negative symptoms of schizophrenia and the absence of extrapyramidal side-effects. Risperidone has high affinity for both serotonin (5-HT_2 subtype) and dopamine receptors (D_2 subtype), and it effectively treats both the positive and negative symptoms of schizophrenia. It does have some extrapyramidal side-effects at higher doses. The newest approved drug, aripiprazole, is a partial agonist at the $5HT_{1A}$ and D_2 receptor and an antagonist at the $5HT_2$ receptor. It reduces both the positive and negative symptoms of schizophrenia.

3. **Side-Effects and Toxic Reactions.** Because of the relative lack of selectivity of these compounds, they do produce side-effects. Clozapine can produce cardiovascular side-effects including orthostatic hypotension and tachycardia (increased heart rate). In addition, sedation may accompany its actions. These effects may be due to antagonist activity at adrenergic and muscarinic receptors. Clozapine has toxic side-effects as well, including the reduction of seizure threshold and the production of agranulocytosis (fall in white blood cell count). Since olanzapine does not produce agranulocytosis, this agent is now the drug of choice within the atypical class. Clozapine is only used for treatment-resistant schizophrenia.

III. Drugs Used in the Treatment of Mood Disorders

The drugs used to treat affective disorders include *antidepressants,* mood-elevating agents, and the *mood-stabilizing* drugs, principally lithium salts.

A. **Antidepressant Drugs.** Depressive disorders range from mild despondency and seasonal mood disorders to severe depression with suicidal risk. Treatment usually includes psychotherapy support, attempts to alter the stressful social situations, and pharmacology. The pharmacologic armamentarium for the treatment of depression has evolved over the last several decades to include three major classes of drugs: (1) the selective serotonin reuptake inhibitors (SSRIs), (2) the tricyclic antidepressants, and (3) the monoamine oxidase (MAO) inhibitors. Although these compounds have varying side-effect profiles, there is little difference in their clinical efficacies in the treatment of depression. Since their onset of action is usually delayed for several weeks, they may be unable to combat suicidal tendencies in the acute phase. In patients that are refractory to antidepressants, electroconvulsive therapy has often been remarkably effective. Another very effective treatment is the placebo. In clinical trials for many antidepressant drugs, as many as 40% of patients have responded positively to placebo in the treatment of depression!

1. **Selective Serotonin Reuptake Inhibitors (SSRIs)**

    Fluoxetine (PROZAC)

    Sertraline (ZOLOFT)

    Paroxetine (PAXIL)

    The SSRIs are the first-line therapy for treating unipolar depression. These drugs selectively inhibit the reuptake of serotonin by nerve terminals. There is no evidence that this selectivity provides better efficacy in the elevation of mood. However, the greater selectivity results in fewer side-effects, and they are safer if taken in an overdose. Thus the SSRIs have become a popular choice of physicians and patients alike.

    a. **Effects on the CNS.** Drugs such as fluoxetine elevate mood in depressed patients, but it takes several weeks for the antidepressant action to emerge. Their actions are predominantly at serotonin synapses (unlike the tricyclic antidepressants), which may limit the emergence of side-effects.

    b. **Other effects.** Fluoxetine and other SSRIs have considerably fewer anticholinergic side-effects compared to the tricyclics and MAO inhibitors. There are minimal cardiovascular effects and hypotension and a high margin of safety upon overdosage. The rate of convulsions is also lower with SSRIs compared to the tricyclics. Some patients do experience gastrointestinal distress and sexual difficulties in ejaculation. These side-effects are usually mild and short-lived.

2. **Tricyclic Antidepressants**

    Imipramine (TOFRANIL)

    Amitriptyline (ELAVIL; AMITRIL)

    Imipramine is the prototype drug for a group of antidepressant drugs with *no* MAO inhibitor activity. These compounds are closely related to the phenothiazines in structure and in pharmacologic activity. The tricyclics inhibit the reuptake of norepinephrine and serotonin, increasing adrenergic and serotonergic transmission. It is unclear whether these initial actions or the subsequent adaptive changes in neurotransmission underlie efficacy.

a.   **Effects on CNS.** The effects resembling those of the weaker phenothiazines include mild sedation and potentiation of CNS depressants.

   In contrast to the sedation produced in normal subjects, depressed patients respond with an elevation of mood, increased mental alertness and physical activity, improved sleep patterns and appetite and a reduction in morbid preoccupation with self-destruction.

   About 2–3 weeks of treatment must be given before the antidepressant action in patients is evident.

b.   **Other effects.** Imipramine possesses distinct parasympathetic postganglionic blocking activity which is manifested as dryness of the mouth, constipation, urinary retention and blurred vision. Postural hypotension and mild jaundice may also occur.

c.   **Therapeutic uses.** Imipramine and related compounds were once the drugs of choice in the treatment of depression and used in outpatient treatment, but have been largely replaced by the SSRIs .

3.   **Monoamine Oxidase (MAO) Inhibitors**
   Tranylcypromine (PARNATE)
   Phenelzine (NARDIL)

   The MAO inhibitors block the *intracellular* metabolism of naturally occurring amines such as epinephrine, norepinephrine, serotonin and tyramine. The chronic administration of MAO inhibitors results in the accumulation of these amines in various tissues including the brain, liver and sympathetic nerves. However, the MAO inhibitors inhibit not only the enzyme for which they are named but many other enzymes as well.

a.   **Pharmacologic effects**

   (1)   Behavioral effects are seen as an elevation of mood in certain depressed mental states; it takes several days or weeks for this effect to be discernible in depressed patients. They are just as effective as tricyclics, but because of the side-effect profile, they are used only when SSRIs and tricyclics produce an unsatisfactory response.

   (2)   Cardiovascular effects: either hypotension or hypertension may be produced depending on the dose, duration of use, co-medication or ingestion of tyramine-containing foods. The postural hypotension that occurs with the use of all MAO inhibitors cannot, at present, be attributed to enzyme inhibition.

      MAO inhibition is responsible, however, for the acute toxicity (hypertensive crisis) that develops when certain exogenous amines are ingested either as drugs (ephedrine) or as components in foods (tyramine in cheese) (see p. 316).

(3) Other effects: dry mouth, constipation, insomnia, nervousness. Because of their general enzyme-inhibiting properties, the MAO inhibitors also prolong and intensify the effects of CNS depressants such as barbiturates and alcohol, and opioid analgesics such as meperidine.

B. **Mood-Stabilizing Drugs.** Lithium salts are used in the treatment of bipolar or manic-depressive disorders. Despite decades of use, its mechanism of action is still unknown. Lithium differs from other psychotropic drugs in that it has no discernible effect in normal individuals and does not produce sedation, depression or euphoria. Although lithium has no primary sedative effects, it does correct the sleep disorder of manic patients. Lithium has a very low therapeutic index, and its concentration in plasma must be determined frequently to ensure safe use.

In therapeutic doses, patients may complain of fatigue and muscular weakness. Slurred speech, ataxia and tremor of hands are commonly noticed. Serious toxic effects are associated with high plasma levels; the CNS is primarily affected.

Other agents used as mood stabilizers include antiseizure drugs such as carbamazepine (TEGRETOL) and valproic acid (DEPAKOTE). These drugs inhibit glutamate neurotransmission, probably by keeping sodium channels in a closed state. They are often used when patients become resistant to lithium.

IV. Anti-anxiety Drugs

In addition to their sedative and hypnotic actions, benzodiazepines are also anxiolytics. Only a few, however, have been recommended for use in the treatment of anxiety: chlordiazepoxide (LIBRIUM) and diazepam (VALIUM) are prototypic agents (cf. p. 522). More selective benzodiazepines, such as alprazolam (XANAX) are anxiolytic at doses that do not produce sedation.

The pharmacology of all of these agents is much the same; they bind to GABA receptors to increase GABA neurotransmission. The continuous use of the anti-anxiety drugs often leads to physical dependence – intense anxiety can reemerge when a person stops taking the drug. Furthermore, seizures can occur following abrupt cessation of long-term benzodiazepine treatment. This is avoided by tapering off the drug slowly.

The anti-anxiety drugs produce muscular relaxation by an action in the CNS (not on the muscle). These agents also cause memory dysfunction, and should be avoided in the elderly.

Chlordiazepoxide and diazepam are also used in the treatment of alcohol withdrawal. Since both benzodiazepines and alcohol act at GABA receptors, the benzodiazepines can suppress alcohol withdrawal symptoms without causing intoxication.

Due to the dependence problems associated with the benzodiazepines, selective serotonin reuptake inhibitors (SSRIs) are now being used in a variety of anxiety disorders, including generalized anxiety, obsessive compulsive disorder, and panic disorder. The SSRIs do not produce dependence or have abuse potential, but they are probably not as effective as benzodiazepines in treating anxiety.

Appendix 8
Drugs for Stimulating the Central Nervous System

I. General Considerations
A great many agents can stimulate the central nervous system (CNS). Some of these produce central system stimulation as an adverse side-effect, but others produce this effect as their most prominent action. The latter group are classified as *general CNS stimulants* and are capable of increasing excitability on a continuum as a function of dose – from mild physiologic stimulation to severe convulsions. The general CNS stimulants can be divided into two major categories: the psychomotor stimulants and the methylxanthines.

II. Psychomotor Stimulants
A. **Amphetamines and Derivatives.** The amphetamines (amphetamine, dextroamphetamine and methamphetamine) produce their effects in part by increasing the release of norepinephrine and dopamine from stores in sympathetic and dopamine nerve terminals, respectively. Phenmetrazine (PRELUDIN) and methylphenidate (RITALIN) are also sympathomimetic amines that share the pharmacologic and toxic effects of the amphetamines.

1. **Peripheral Effects.** Vasoconstriction and increase in blood pressure. Except for a marked contraction of the urinary bladder sphincter making urination difficult, other smooth muscle effects are not notable; e.g. bronchial muscle is relaxed but not sufficiently to be of therapeutic value.

2. **CNS Effects**

   a. The effects of a single dose of amphetamine may be manifested as a general alerting action: increased alertness, attentiveness and wakefulness and a decreased sense of fatigue. Generally there is an elevation of mood, often elation and euphoria, although mentally retarded patients do not display euphoria and some patients may even feel dysphoric or be sedated. Amphetamine will improve performance of simple tasks when there is boredom, fatigue or lack of motivation; performance of complicated tasks is worsened by amphetamine.

The general alerting action is associated with stimulation of the reticular formation and lowering of the threshold to sensory stimuli. This effect on the CNS is presumably mediated by the release of catecholamines, i.e. norepinephrine and dopamine. Amphetamine also releases serotonin, but at higher doses than required to release catecholamines.

After chronic use, over 2–4 days, a model paranoid psychosis characteristic of amphetamine abuse is seen. There is some sleep deprivation but not enough to explain the psychosis. The paranoid psychosis is comparable to a true natural psychotic state (this is unlike the psychoses induced by LSD and mescaline). The amphetamine psychosis is normally self-limiting, reversing within 24–48 hours. Intervention, if necessary, is with a benzodiazepine. One cannot 'talk the patient down' as is possible with bad trips on LSD or mescaline. After chronic use, a state of depression occurs.

b.   The appetite depressant (anorexiant) effect of amphetamine which may result in weight loss is primarily due to appetite suppression rather than an increased rate of tissue metabolism or motor activity. Tolerance develops to this effect; if doses are raised to overcome tolerance, undesirable side-effects can occur.

c.   In normal subjects, usual doses of amphetamine do not appreciably increase respiration. When respiration is depressed by centrally acting drugs, amphetamine may stimulate respiration.

3.   **Fate of Amphetamine.** Well absorbed from gastrointestinal tract; distributed to brain rapidly. Amphetamines are not biotransformed by MAO, but are oxidized by microsomal enzyme systems. Urinary excretion is dependent on urine pH; increased rate of excretion with acid pH.

4.   **Therapeutic Uses.** While amphetamines were once used in the treatment of obesity and narcolepsy, their abuse potential is too high and they are no longer used for these conditions. Very low doses of amphetamine are used in the treatment of attention deficit hyperactivity disorder. The basis for improvement is not well-understood and the beneficial effects of the amphetamines are paradoxical. The mechanism of action may be due to stimulation in those parts of the brain involved in filtering information so that the patient can focus attention.

B.   **Other Agents.** Methylphenidate (RITALIN) has similar pharmacologic activity as the amphetamines, but produces fewer peripheral sympathomimetic effects due to lesser stimulation of norepinephrine release. Methylphenidate is used preferentially for treatment of attention deficit disorder in both children and adults, as it has better social acceptance than amphetamine.

III. The Methylxanthines
A. Agents
1. Caffeine
2. Theophylline
3. Theobromine

The three pharmacologically important xanthines listed above occur naturally in plants that have a wide geographic distribution. All three alkaloids are consumed worldwide in beverages derived from these plants. The principal xanthine in both coffee and tea is caffeine; coffee contains about 100–150 mg and tea about 30–40 mg of caffeine per average cup. Tea also contains small amounts of theophylline and theobromine, whereas cocoa and chocolate contain only theobromine and some caffeine. Cola drinks also contain significant amounts of caffeine (40 mg/12 oz) derived partly from extracts of nuts of *Cola acuminata* and partly from caffeine added during manufacturing.

Caffeine, theophylline, and theobromine have similar pharmacologic profiles, but differ in their potency to stimulate the CNS, produce diuresis and relax smooth muscle, their most prominent pharmacologic actions (Table A-7-1). These differences in potency also account for their therapeutic uses. The mechanism by which the xanthines produce these effects is related to their ability to block adenosine receptors.

B. Effects on CNS.
Caffeine in doses of 85–250 mg (equivalent to 1–3 cups of coffee) can improve performance in tasks requiring sustained intellectual effort but not in those involving fine muscular coordination.

Table A-7-1. *Comparative potency of the methylxanthines*

Xanthine	CNS stimulation	Bronchodilation	Diuresis
Caffeine	+ + + +	+ +	+ +
Theophylline	+ + +	+ + + +	+ + +
Theobromine	+	+	+

Although caffeine is traditionally considered to be more potent than theophylline as a CNS stimulant, theophylline stimulates the medullary respiratory center at lower doses and is more potent than caffeine in producing generalized convulsions.

Despite the ability to produce mild CNS stimulation, the xanthines, particularly caffeine, are not used in treating overdosage with barbiturates or other CNS depressants. There are, however, a number of over-the-counter caffeine-containing preparations which claim to improve or relieve, but actually do little to offset, physical fatigue.

C. Effects on Smooth Muscle.
The ability of the methylxanthines to relax smooth muscles is most important with regard to this action on the bronchi. Here theophylline is most potent and is of value in the treatment of bronchial asthma.

D. Effect on the Kidney. The methylxanthines, especially theophylline, increase urine flow. However, theophylline is no longer used as a primary diuretic. Some over-the-counter preparations claiming to be diuretics do contain caffeine but in doses that are well below potentially effective levels.

IV. Nicotine

Nicotine is the active alkaloid found in the tobacco plant. Although it is not classified as a psychomotor stimulant, nicotine does activate the CNS and it shares several actions of psychomotor stimulants. It has numerous pharmacologic actions within the CNS and the peripheral nervous system, yet it acts specifically at only one receptor, the nicotinic acetylcholine receptor. Its activation of nicotinic acetylcholine receptors within the CNS, at autonomic ganglia and at target tissues, explains its multitude of effects.

A. Actions in the CNS. Initially nicotine causes nausea and vomiting, due in part to its activation of the brainstem vomiting center. Tolerance develops rapidly to this effect. Nicotine also stimulates hypothalamic neurons to release antidiuretic hormone causing fluid retention, and it decreases appetite, probably via release of serotonin. Like other psychomotor stimulants, nicotine can increase attention, cognitive performance, and psychomotor activity. It has the ability to combat depression, alleviate anxiety, and produce euphoria. The positive reinforcing actions are mediated via activation of the reward pathway. Nicotine increases the release of dopamine within this pathway to produce its rewarding effects, similar to other psychomotor stimulants.

B. Actions on the Autonomic Nervous System. Nicotine increases heart rate and blood pressure due to the release of norepinephrine at sympathetic terminals and epinephrine from the adrenal glands. In addition, nicotine increases gastrointestinal muscle tone and activity.

C. Actions on the Somatic Nervous System. Nicotine increases muscle contraction by activation of nicotinic acetylcholine receptors at the neuromuscular junction. It can produce tremors and in cases of nicotine toxicity, paralysis of respiratory muscles can occur. Because of this action, nicotine has been included in some pesticides to produce death.

D. Tolerance and Dependence. Tolerance develops rapidly to the nausea initially produced by nicotine, but tolerance does not develop to other actions of nicotine. The smoker will smoke enough cigarettes per day to provide a blood (and brain) level that delivers the desired effect. With chronic use, nicotine produces dependence and the smoker continues to smoke to avoid withdrawal. This is especially evident in the morning, when smokers smoke their first cigarette upon awakening. Nicotine has been formulated in a patch as an aid to help smokers quit. The patch provides enough nicotine to avoid withdrawal, but does not lead to high enough blood levels to be pleasurable. The patch and other forms of nicotine replacement therapy increase abstinence 1.5–2-fold in certain populations over a 6-month period. However, abstinence rates decline when assessed 1 year after onset of nicotine replacement therapy.

Index

Note: Page references in *italics* indicate illustrations and tables